METHODS IN MOLECULAR BIOLOGY

Series Editor
John M. Walker
School of Life Sciences
University of Hertfordshire
Hatfield, Hertfordshire, AL10 9AB, UK

For further volumes:
http://www.springer.com/series/7651

Cancer Vaccines

Methods and Protocols

Edited by

Michael J.P. Lawman and Patricia D. Lawman

Morphogenesis, Inc., Tampa, FL, USA

Humana Press

Editors
Michael J.P. Lawman
Morphogenesis, Inc.
Tampa, FL, USA

Patricia D. Lawman
Morphogenesis, Inc.
Tampa, FL, USA

ISSN 1064-3745 ISSN 1940-6029 (electronic)
ISBN 978-1-4939-0344-3 ISBN 978-1-4939-0345-0 (eBook)
DOI 10.1007/978-1-4939-0345-0
Springer New York Heidelberg Dordrecht London

Library of Congress Control Number: 2014931086

Cover Illustration Caption: Taken from Figure 1 of Chapter 7.

Printed on acid-free paper

Humana Press is a brand of Springer
Springer is part of Springer Science+Business Media (www.springer.com)

Preface

Cancer immunotherapies, which include cancer vaccines, are novel therapeutic modalities being added to the armamentarium for cancer management/treatments that are finally becoming available to cancer patients around the world. In contrast to chemo- and radio-therapies, cancer vaccines are not normally associated with severe side effects, and unlike these therapies which directly kill the tumor cells and normal rapidly dividing cells in the body, cancer vaccines and other immunotherapies exert their effect by stimulating the body's immune system to focus on the cancer cells alone, remove them, and consequently reduce the severity of the disease, generally without toxicity. Given these characteristics, cancer vaccines offer cancer patients a more focused and gentler means of cancer treatment that is far less detrimental to their bodies and is cognizant of the patient's wish for a better quality of life.

The status of the patient's immune system is the vital biological element affecting the outcome of cancer immunotherapy. However, each individual's immune status is in turn affected by factors including age of the person, stage of the disease, prior treatment (chemotherapy or radiation therapy), tumor-induced immunosuppression, and the overall well-being of that person. As the term "immunotherapy" implies, the cells of the immune system perform the primary role in mediating the outcome of an immunotherapeutic regimen.

Most cancer vaccines to date have been designed to treat cancers that have already developed and therefore are termed "therapeutic." The purpose of these cancer vaccines is to stop cancer cell growth and eventually reduce the tumor burden. Some experts in the field believe that cancer vaccines may be best suited to prevent cancer from returning or to eliminate cancer cells that were not killed by other, more conventional treatments.

Whether used as adjunctive or stand-alone therapies, the development of effective cancer vaccines requires a thorough understanding of the innate and adaptive immune system, immune effector cells, and cancer cells. However, despite the plethora of clinical and basic knowledge of cancer and the immune system, the issue boils down to the simple fact that the immune system, in most cases, does not see cancer cells as being "nonself" and thus dangerous. Even when the immune system does recognize some element of danger, it does not usually mount a clinically significant response against well-established tumors. This is mainly due to the fact that cancer cells have developed mechanisms that make it challenging for the immune system to target them for removal. The most significant issue is that cancer cells express normal "self"-antigens on the cell surface in addition to specific cancer-associated antigens, giving the abnormal cells an advantage against immune surveillance. Furthermore, during their rapid proliferation, these cancer cells frequently undergo further genetic mutations that may consequently lead to the loss or down-regulation of the cancer-associated antigens. Finally, cancer cells generate soluble factors that function to suppress an anticancer immune response.

Producing an effective therapeutic cancer vaccine has proven to be challenging. To be effective, cancer vaccines must achieve two objectives. First, cancer vaccines must stimulate a robust tumor-specific immune responses against the correct target. Second, the immune responses must be potent enough to overcome the means by which cancer cells evade the adaptive immune response.

Therapeutic cancer vaccines can be divided into two broad categories, namely, (1) whole-cell vaccines, which encompass autologous, allogeneic, and dendritic cell vaccines, and (2) peptide or protein antigen vaccines. Dendritic cell vaccines fall into both "camps," since this category can include the use of peptide and/or protein antigens as well as whole-cell lysates in the production of these vaccines.

The whole-cell vaccine approach encompasses the use of inactivated whole-tumor cells and/or whole-cell lysate as the vaccine. As such, these whole-cell vaccines present an array of tumor cell-associated antigens to the patient's immune system. The approach of using whole-tumor cell as a vaccine eliminates the significant problem of having to identify the crucial antigen(s) for that cancer, most of which remain unknown, but almost always requires some type of immune adjuvant.

Peptide or protein antigen vaccines can be comprised of synthetic or purified native moieties that are representative of the tumor cell antigens displayed by the target tumors. These antigens can be used to immunize patients and have been shown to generate an immune response capable of destroying cells in the body that display these antigens. These types of cancer vaccines are dependent upon knowing the major tumor cell markers/antigens, their structure, and, if peptides are generated, the important epitope(s) required to generate a tumor-specific immune response. Dendritic cells, which orchestrate the function of immune cells, are often used as the "delivery vehicles" for these synthetic peptides and proteins to the immune system.

Researchers continue to acquire the elements and knowledge required in order to design cancer vaccines that can potentially accomplish both goals, i.e., to evoke a tumor-specific response and overcome the immuno-evasive mechanisms employed by the tumor cells. The purpose of this current volume is to gather many of the methods that have been developed to manufacture these cancer vaccines under one cover. The chapters are grouped according to the purpose or the aim of the cancer vaccine, namely, the manipulation and modification of immune cells; the manipulation and modification of tumor cells; and the manipulation of immune/tumor interactions and various delivery mechanisms. The volume also covers the subject of cancer vaccines in a more global sense with its section on the advances, challenges, and future of cancer vaccines.

In bringing this volume together, we have attempted to gather experts in the various subspecialty fields of cancer vaccines to share their expertise with current and future cancer vaccinologists, researchers, and clinicians. To this end, the authors have shared their experiences and given helpful "tips" through the Notes section in each chapter to aid in the development of future cancer vaccine design. It is hoped that the methods and protocols that have already been developed will lead to the further generation of cancer vaccines that are both safe and efficacious and that cancer vaccines will be the standard of care in the very near future.

The coeditors, Dr. Michael Lawman and Dr. Patricia Lawman, are grateful to the many authors who took time from their busy schedules to contribute to this volume. Without their efforts, this book would never have materialized. In addition, the coeditors offer special thanks to Dr. Venkata Narasimhulu Kuppala. Speaking for all the contributing authors, we also are very grateful for the advice, encouragement, and support given to us by Dr. John and Jan Walker, editors in chief for the series *Methods in Molecular Biology*, and to the publishers Humana Press and Springer Science + Business Media for the opportunity to attempt this project.

Tampa, FL, USA

Michael J.P. Lawman, Ph.D.
Patricia D. Lawman, Ph.D.

Contents

Part IV Manipulation of Immune/Tumor Interactions

Part V Delivery Mechanisms

Part VI The Advances, Challenges, and Future of Cancer Vaccines

Contributors

MOHAMED R. AKL • *College of Pharmacy, University of Louisiana at Monroe, Monroe, LA, USA*
LAURA ALANIZ • *Gene Therapy Laboratory, Facultad de Ciencias Biomédicas, Universidad Austral, Buenos Aires, Argentina*
RIYASAT ALI • *Department of Biochemistry, All India Institute of Medical Sciences, New Delhi, India*
NEHAD M. AYOUB • *College of Pharmacy, University of Louisiana at Monroe, Monroe, LA, USA*
CONSTANTIN N. BAXEVANIS • *Cancer Immunology and Immunotherapy Center, Saint Savas Cancer Hospital, Athens, Greece*
MAURIZIO BENDANDI • *Immunotherapy Program, University of Navarra Hospital, Pamplona, Spain*
FABIAN BENENCIA • *Biomedical Engineering Program, Russ College of Engineering and Technology, Ohio University, Athens, OH, USA; Molecular and Cell Biology Program, Department of Biomedical Sciences, College of Osteopathic Medicine, Ohio University, Athens, OH, USA*
DAPHNÉ BENTEYN • *Laboratory of Molecular and Cellular Therapy, Department of Immunology–Physiology and the Dendritic Cell Bank, Vrije Universiteit Brussel, Brussels, Belgium*
SANTWANA BHATNAGAR • *Department of Biochemistry, All India Institute of Medical Sciences, New Delhi, India*
AUDE BONEHILL • *Laboratory of Molecular and Cellular Therapy, Department of Immunology–Physiology and the Dendritic Cell Bank, Vrije Universiteit Brussel, Brussels, Belgium*
CHIARA CAMISASCHI • *Fondazione IRCCS Istituto Nazionale dei Tumori, Milan, Italy*
CHIARA CASTELLI • *Fondazione IRCCS Istituto Nazionale dei Tumori, Milan, Italy*
ASCENSIÓN LÓPEZ DÍAZ DE CERIO • *Immunotherapy Program, University of Navarra Hospital, Pamplona, Spain*
SOUNG-CHUL CHA • *Department of Lymphoma and Myeloma, The University of Texas MD Anderson Cancer Center, Houston, TX, USA*
TESS M. CHEE • *Cancer Immunology Program, Peter MacCallum Cancer Centre, East Melbourne, VIC, Australia; Sir Peter MacCallum Department of Oncology, University of Melbourne, Parkville, VIC, Australia*
NU-RI CHOI • *Research Center for Cancer Immunotherapy, Chonnam National University Hwasun Hospital, Hwasun, Jeollanamdo, Republic of Korea; Department of Hematology–Oncology, Chonnam National University Hwasun Hospital, Hwasun, Jeollanamdo, Republic of Korea; The Brain Korea 21 Project Center for Biomedical Human Resources, Chonnam National University, Gwangju, Republic of Korea*

PHILLIP K. DARCY • *Cancer Immunology Program, Peter MacCallum Cancer Centre, East Melbourne, VIC, Australia; Department of Pathology, University of Melbourne, Parkville, VIC, Australia; Sir Peter MacCallum Department of Oncology, University of Melbourne, Parkville, VIC, Australia; Department of Immunology, Monash University, Clayton, VIC, Australia*

KERRILYN R. DIENER • *Experimental Therapeutics Laboratory, Hanson Institute, Royal Adelaide Hospital, Adelaide, SA, Australia; Sansom Institute, School of Pharmacy and Medical Science, University of South Australia, Adelaide, SA, Australia; Discipline of Obstetrics and Gynaecology, School of Paediatrics and Reproductive Health, University of Adelaide, Adelaide, SA, Australia*

GIANPIETRO DOTTI • *Center for Cell and Gene Therapy, Department of Immunology and Department of Medicine, Baylor College of Medicine, Methodist Hospital and Texas Children's Hospital, Houston, TX, USA*

MAYER FISHMAN • *Experimental Therapeutics and Immunotherapy Programs, Department of Genitourinary Oncology, H. Lee Moffitt Cancer Center and Research Institute, Tampa, FL, USA*

AARON E. FOSTER • *Center for Cell and Gene Therapy, Baylor College of Medicine, Houston, TX, USA*

BERNARD A. FOX • *Laboratory of Molecular and Tumor Immunology, Robert W. Franz Cancer Research Center, Earle A. Chiles Research Institute, Providence Cancer Center, Portland, OR, USA; Department of Molecular Microbiology and Immunology, Oregon Health and Science University, Portland, OR, USA;Knight Cancer Institute, Oregon Health and Science University, Portland, OR, USA*

TOMONOBU FUJITA • *Division of Cellular Signaling, Institute for Advanced Medical Research, Keio University School of Medicine, Tokyo, Japan*

DMITRY GABRILOVICH • *H. Lee Moffitt Cancer Center, University of South Florida, Tampa, FL, USA*

SEAN M. GEARY • *College of Pharmacy, University of Iowa, Iowa City, IA, USA*

DAVID E. GILHAM • *Clinical and Experimental Immunotherapy, Department of Medical Oncology, Institute of Cancer Sciences, The University of Manchester, Manchester, UK*

AUDREY LE GOUËLLEC • *TIMC-TheREx Laboratory, La Tronche, France*

ORLANDO GRIMANY-NUNO • *Department of Microbiology and Immunology, Institute for Cellular Therapeutics, University of Louisville, Louisville, KY, USA; James Brown Cancer Center, University of Louisville, Louisville, KY, USA*

TANJA D. DE GRUIJL • *Department of Medical Oncology, VU University Medical Center, Amsterdam, The Netherlands*

RESHU GUPTA • *Department of Medical Genetics, Sir Ganga Ram Hospital, New Delhi, India*

JOHN D. HAYBALL • *Experimental Therapeutics Laboratory, Hanson Institute, Royal Adelaide Hospital, Adelaide, SA, Australia; Sansom Institute, School of Pharmacy and Medical Science, University of South Australia, Adelaide, SA, Australia; School of Medicine, University of Adelaide, Adelaide, SA, Australia*

SUMIT K. HIRA • *Immunobiology Laboratory, Department of Zoology, Banaras Hindu University, Varanasi, India*

YOSHIHIKO HIROHASHI • *Department of Pathology, Sapporo Medical University School of Medicine, Sapporo, Japan*

MY-DUNG HOANG • *Research Center for Cancer Immunotherapy, Hwasun Hospital, Chonnam National University, Hwasun, Jeollanamdo, Republic of Korea; Department of Hematology–Oncology, Hwasun Hospital, Chonnam National University, Hwasun, Jeollanamdo, Republic of Korea; The Brain Korea 21 Project Center for Biomedical Human Resources, Chonnam National University, Gwangju, Republic of Korea*

PAUL M. HOWLEY • *Sementis Ltd., Richmond, VIC, Australia; Experimental Therapeutics Laboratory, Hanson Institute, Royal Adelaide Hospital, Adelaide, SA, Australia; Sansom Institute, School of Pharmacy and Medical Science, University of South Australia, Adelaide, SA, Australia*

SUSANA INOGES • *Immunotherapy Program, University of Navarra Hospital, Pamplona, Spain*

MAYA M. JERALD • *Morphogenesis, Inc., Tampa, FL, USA*

ZHENGCAI JIA • *Institute of Immunology PLA, Third Military Medical University, Chongqing, China*

JANINA JIGA • *Department of Transplantation Immunology and Cell Therapies, Pius Branzeu Center, Victor Babes University of Medicine and Pharmacy, Timisoara, Romania*

LIZA B. JOHN • *Cancer Immunology Program, Peter MacCallum Cancer Centre, East Melbourne, VIC, Australia; Sir Peter MacCallum Department of Oncology, University of Melbourne, Parkville, VIC, Australia*

VIJAYA BHARTI JOSHI • *College of Pharmacy, University of Iowa, Iowa City, IA, USA*

TAKAYUKI KANASEKI • *Department of Pathology, Sapporo Medical University School of Medicine, Sapporo, Japan*

YUTAKA KAWAKAMI • *Division of Cellular Signaling, Institute for Advanced Medical Research, Keio University School of Medicine, Tokyo, Japan*

NAOSHI KAWAMURA • *Division of Cellular Signaling, Institute for Advanced Medical Research, Keio University School of Medicine, Tokyo, Japan*

CHRISTIAN KLEIST • *Department of Transplantation Immunology, Institute for Immunology, University of Heidelberg, Heidelberg, Germany*

DENNIS M. KLINMAN • *Cancer and Inflammation Program, Frederick National Laboratory for Cancer Research, NCI, Frederick, MD, USA*

RAMA P. KOTIPATRUNI • *Cancer Biology Division, Department of Radiation Oncology, Washington University School of Medicine, St. Louis, MO, USA*

K.K. KRISHNADATH • *Center of Experimental and Molecular Medicine, Academic Medical Center, Amsterdam, The Netherlands; Department of Gastroenterology and Hepatology, Academic Medical Center, Amsterdam, The Netherlands*

MING-LING KUO • *Department of Microbiology and Immunology, Graduate Institute of Biomedical Science, Chang Gung University, Kweishan, Taoyan, Taiwan*

LARRY KWAK • *Department of Lymphoma and Myeloma, The University of Texas MD Anderson Cancer Center, Houston, TX, USA*

ROELAND LAMERIS • *Department of Medical Oncology, VU University Medical Center, Amsterdam, The Netherlands*

ALVARO R. LARA • *Departamento de Procesos y Tecnología, Universidad Autónoma Metropolitana-Cuajimalpa, Del. Álvaro Obregón, Mexico*

MICHAEL J.P. LAWMAN • *Morphogenesis, Inc., Tampa, FL, USA*

PATRICIA D. LAWMAN • *Morphogenesis, Inc., Tampa, FL, USA*

HYUN-JU LEE • *Research Center for Cancer Immunotherapy, Hwasun Hospital, Chonnam National University, Hwasun, Jeollanamdo, Republic of Korea; Department of Hematology–Oncology, Hwasun Hospital, Chonnam National University, Hwasun, Jeollanamdo, Republic of Korea*
JE-JUNG LEE • *Research Center for Cancer Immunotherapy, Hwasun Hospital, Chonnam National University, Hwasun, Jeollanamdo, Republic of Korea; Department of Hematology–Oncology, Hwasun Hospital, Chonnam National University, Hwasun, Jeollanamdo, Republic of Korea; The Brain Korea 21 Project Center for Biomedical Human Resources, Chonnam National University, Gwangju, Republic of Korea; Vaxcell-Bio Therapeutics, Hwasun, Jeollanamdo, Republic of Korea*
PEI-TZU LEE • *Division of Asthma, Allergy, and Rheumatology, Department of Pediatrics, Chang Gung Memorial Hospital, Kweishan, Taoyuan, Taiwan*
YOUN-KYUNG LEE • *Research Center for Cancer Immunotherapy and Vaxcell-Bio Therapeutics, Hwasun, Jeollanamdo, Republic of Korea*
SYH-JAE LIN • *Division of Asthma, Allergy, and Rheumatology, Department of Pediatrics, Chang Gung Memorial Hospital, Kweishan, Taoyuan, Taiwan*
EVA LION • *Tumor Immunology Group, Laboratory of Experimental Hematology, Vaccine and Infectious Disease Institute, University of Antwerp, Antwerp, Belgium*
JUERGEN MAIRHOFER • *Department of Biotechnology, University of Natural Resources and Life Sciences, Vienna, Austria*
PARTHA P. MANNA • *Immunobiology Laboratory, Department of Zoology, Banaras Hindu University, Varanasi, India*
GUILLERMO MAZZOLINI • *Gene Therapy Laboratory, Facultad de Ciencias Biomédicas, Universidad Austral, Buenos Aires, Argentina*
FRANCESCA MILANO • *Section of Hematology and Clinical Immunology, Department of Internal and Experimental Medicine, University of Perugia, Perugia, Italy*
RENA MORITA • *Department of Pathology, Sapporo Medical University School of Medicine, Sapporo, Japan*
GANJI PURNACHANDRA NAGARAJU • *Department of Hematology and Medical Oncology, Winship Cancer Institute, Emory University, Atlanta, GA, USA*
MUNEHIDE NAKATSUGAWA • *Department of Pathology, Sapporo Medical University School of Medicine, Sapporo, Japan*
RAZA ALI NAQVI • *Department of Biochemistry, All India Institute of Medical Sciences, New Delhi, India*
BING NI • *Institute of Immunology PLA, Third Military Medical University, Chongqing, China*
AN M.T. VAN NUFFEL • *Laboratory of Molecular and Cellular Therapy, Department of Immunology–Physiology and the Dendritic Cell Bank, Vrije Universiteit Brussel, Brussels, Belgium*
CHIRANJIB PAL • *Cellular Immunology and Experimental Therapeutics Laboratory, Department of Zoology, West Bengal State University, Barasat, West Bengal, India*
MICHAEL PAPAMICHAIL • *Cancer Immunology and Immunotherapy Center, Saint Savas Cancer Hospital, Athens, Greece*
FERNANDO PASTOR • *Immunotherapy Program, University of Navarra Hospital, Pamplona, Spain*
GEORGE E. PEOPLES • *Department of Surgery, Brooke Army Medical Center, Houston, TX, USA*
SONIA A. PEREZ • *Cancer Immunology and Immunotherapy Center, Saint Savas Cancer Hospital, Athens, Greece*

SERENA K. PERNA • *Center for Cell and Gene Therapy, Baylor College of Medicine, Methodist Hospital and Texas Children's Hospital, Houston, TX, USA*
SAMUEL PIRRUCCELLO • *University of Nebraska Medical Center, Omaha, NE, USA*
HONG QIN • *Department of Lymphoma and Myeloma, The University of Texas MD Anderson Cancer Center, Houston, TX, USA*
GAMAL RAMADAN • *Zoology Department, Faculty of Science, Ain Shams University, Cairo, Egypt*
VIJAYAKUMAR K. RAMIYA • *Morphogenesis, Inc., Tampa, FL, USA*
MARCO RANDAZZO • *Department of Urology, Kantonsspital Aarau, Aarau, Switzerland*
D.N. RAO • *Department of Biochemistry, All India Institute of Medical Sciences, New Delhi, India*
LICIA RIVOLTINI • *Fondazione IRCCS Istituto Nazionale dei Tumori, Milan, Italy*
MANGLIO M. RIZZO • *Gene Therapy Laboratory, Facultad de Ciencias Biomédicas, Universidad Austral, Buenos Aires, Argentina*
DOMINIK RÜTTINGER • *Laboratory of Clinical and Experimental Tumor Immunology, Department of Surgery, Grosshadern Medical Center, Ludwig-Maximilians-University Munich, Munich, Germany*
PRADIP P. SACHDEVA • *Department of Medical Genetics, Sir Ganga Ram Hospital, New Delhi, India*
IPPEI SAKAMAKI • *Department of Lymphoma and Myeloma, The University of Texas MD Anderson Cancer Center, Houston, TX, USA*
TOSHIHARU SAKURAI • *Division of Cellular Signaling, Institute for Advanced Medical Research, Keio University School of Medicine, Tokyo, Japan*
MOHAMED L. SALEM • *Immunology and Biotechnology Unit, Zoology Department, Faculty of Science, Tanta University, Tanta, Egypt*
ALIASGER K. SALEM • *College of Pharmacy, University of Iowa, Iowa City, IA, USA*
NORIYUKI SATO • *Department of Pathology, Sapporo Medical University School of Medicine, Sapporo, Japan*
BARBARA SAVOLDO • *Center for Cell and Gene Therapy, Methodist Hospital and Texas Children's Hospital, Baylor College of Medicine, Houston, TX, USA; Department of Pediatrics, Baylor College of Medicine, Houston, TX, USA*
FAMKE L. SCHNEIDERS • *Department of Medical Oncology, VU University Medical Center, Amsterdam, The Netherlands*
JOSEPH SENESAC • *Bellicum Pharmaceuticals, Houston, TX, USA*
RAJESH K. SHARMA • *Department of Microbiology and Immunology, Institute for Cellular Therapeutics, University of Louisville, Louisville, KY, USA; James Brown Cancer Center, University of Louisville, Louisville, KY, USA*
HIDEKAZU SHIROTA • *Department of Clinical Oncology, Tohoku University, Sendai, Japan*
HAVAL SHIRWAN • *Department of Microbiology and Immunology, Institute for Cellular Therapeutics, University of Louisville, Louisville, KY, USA; James Brown Cancer Center, University of Louisville, Louisville, KY, USA*
EVELIEN L.J.M. SMITS • *Laboratory of Experimental Hematology, Tumor Immunology Group, Vaccine and Infectious Disease Institute, University of Antwerp, Antwerp, Belgium*
XIAO-TONG SONG • *Department of Immunology, Center for Cell and Gene Therapy, Baylor College of Medicine, Houston, TX, USA*
JAMES E. TALMADGE • *University of Nebraska Medical Center, Omaha, NE, USA*
MARCELLA TAZZARI • *Fondazione IRCCS Istituto Nazionale dei Tumori, Milan, Italy*

VIGGO F.I. VAN TENDELOO • *Laboratory of Experimental Hematology, Tumor Immunology Group, Vaccine and Infectious Disease Institute, University of Antwerp, Antwerp, Belgium*

PETER TERNESS • *Department of Transplantation Immunology, Institute for Immunology, University of Heidelberg, Heidelberg, Germany*

TOSHIHIKO TORIGOE • *Department of Pathology, Sapporo Medical University School of Medicine, Sapporo, Japan*

MASARU UDAGAWA • *Division of Cellular Signaling, Institute for Advanced Medical Research, Keio University School of Medicine, Tokyo, Japan; Department of Surgery, School of Medicine, Tokyo Medical and Dental University, Tokyo, Japan*

BERTRAND TOUSSAINT • *TIMC-TheREx Laboratory, La Tronche, France*

DEEPAK VERMA • *Immunobiology Laboratory, Department of Zoology, Banaras Hindu University, Varanasi, India*

HELENA VILLANUEVA • *Immunotherapy Program, University of Navarra Hospital, Pamplona, Spain*

HANS J. VAN DER VLIET • *Department of Medical Oncology, VU University Medical Center, Amsterdam, The Netherlands*

MANH-CUONG VO • *Research Center for Cancer Immunotherapy, Hwasun Hospital, Chonnam National University, Hwasun, Jeollanamdo, Republic of Korea; Department of Hematology–Oncology, Hwasun Hospital, Chonnam National University, Hwasun, Jeollanamdo, Republic of Korea; The Brain Korea 21 Project Center for Biomedical Human Resources, Chonnam National University, Gwangju, Republic of Korea*

LIYING WANG • *Norman Bethune College of Medicine, Jilin University, Changchun, China*

YAN WANG • *TIMC-TheREx Laboratory, La Tronche, France*

SOFIE WILGENHOF • *Laboratory of Molecular and Cellular Therapy, Department of Immunology–Physiology and the Dendritic Cell Bank, Vrije Universiteit Brussel, Brussels, Belgium; Department of Medical Oncology, Universitair Ziekenhuis Brussel, Brussels, Belgium*

CHARLOTTE M. DE WINDE • *Laboratory of Experimental Hematology, Tumor Immunology Group, Vaccine and Infectious Disease Institute, University of Antwerp, Antwerp, Belgium*

HAUKE WINTER • *Laboratory of Clinical and Experimental Tumor Immunology, Department of Surgery, Grosshadern Medical Center, Ludwig-Maximilians-University Munich, Munich, Germany*

YUZHANG WU • *Institute of Immunology PLA, Third Military Medical University, Chongqing, China*

TOMONORI YAGUCHI • *Division of Cellular Signaling, Institute for Advanced Medical Research, Keio University School of Medicine, Tokyo, Japan*

ESMA S. YOLCU • *Department of Microbiology and Immunology, Institute for Cellular Therapeutics, University of Louisville, Louisville, KY, USA; James Brown Cancer Center, University of Louisville, Louisville, KY, USA*

YONGLI YU • *Norman Bethune College of Medicine, Jilin University, Changchun, China*

HONG ZAHO • *Department of Microbiology and Immunology, Institute for Cellular Therapeutics, University of Louisville, Louisville, KY, USA; James Brown Cancer Center, University of Louisville, Louisville, KY, USA*

Part I

Manipulation and Modification of Immune Cells: Dendritic Cells

Chapter 1

Single-Step Antigen Loading and Maturation of Dendritic Cells Through mRNA Electroporation of a Tumor-Associated Antigen and a TriMix of Costimulatory Molecules

Daphné Benteyn, An M.T. Van Nuffel, Sofie Wilgenhof, and Aude Bonehill

Abstract

Dendritic cells (DC) are key players in several types of cancer vaccines. Large numbers of DC can easily be generated in closed systems from the monocyte fraction of the peripheral blood. They are the professional antigen-presenting cells, and electroporation of mRNA-encoding tumor antigens is a very efficient and a relatively simple way to load the DC with antigen. The co-electroporation of a tumor antigen of choice and the combination of 3 costimulatory molecules, including CD70, caTLR4, and CD40L (TriMix-DC), leads to fully potent antigen-presenting DC able to generate a broad immune response.

Here we describe the in vitro transcription of the mRNA and the subsequent generation and electroporation of autologous DC used for the treatment of melanoma patients.

Key words Leukapheresis, Dendritic cells, mRNA, Electroporation, Immunomonitoring, Tumor antigen, TriMix

1 Introduction

Dendritic cell (DC)-based cancer vaccines are hot topics in the antitumor immunology area. DC are the most professional antigen-presenting cells and are attractive candidates for therapeutic manipulation of the immune system to induce novel or enhance insufficient antitumor immune responses present in cancer patients. The types of tumor-associated antigens (TAA) for DC loading, DC culture, and maturation steps are key variables in the development of DC-based products. Different approaches have been used for antigen loading, and both defined (peptides, protein, mRNA) [1–7] and undefined (tumor mRNA, tumor lysates) antigens are used [8–10]. Also, for the maturation of immature DC, different clinical grade maturation protocols are used, among which are classical cytokine cocktails [11], Toll-like receptor ligands [12], and TriMix maturation [6, 13].

Michael J.P. Lawman and Patricia D. Lawman (eds.), *Cancer Vaccines: Methods and Protocols*, Methods in Molecular Biology, vol. 1139, DOI 10.1007/978-1-4939-0345-0_1, © Springer Science+Business Media New York 2014

Our expertise lies in the development of antigen-encoding mRNA-electroporated DC-based cancer vaccines. mRNA is a non-integrating molecule with a short half-life leading to a transient antigen expression mimicking an infection. When treating patients with mRNA-electroporated DC, there is no need for prior knowledge of the patient's HLA type as mRNA encoding the full-length TAA ensures presentation of the full antigenic spectrum of epitopes [5]. Both $CD8^+$ and $CD4^+$ T cells are necessary to coordinate an antitumor response leading to tumor regression [14–17]. mRNA coding for the TAA can be genetically modified to present peptides in both MHC class I and class II molecules by linking the TAA with a MHC class II targeting signal [18]. In addition, several parts of the mRNA can be optimized to enhance the transcription rate and stability. In general, mRNA is rapidly degraded because of its short half-life and several other characteristics that cause mRNA instability, including rare codon usage, low GC-content, or presence of negatively cis-acting motifs, hampering protein translation. Recently, it has been shown that a rational gene design, based on modern bioinformatics, followed by the de novo generation of a synthetic gene may help to circumvent this problem. Several studies have proven the positive impact of in silico cDNA optimization [19, 20].

To enable a DC-based vaccine to be fully potent, costimulatory signals are necessary. TriMix is the combination of three molecules, comprising CD40L, constitutive active TLR4 (caTLR4), and CD70-encoding mRNA, which in combination with the TAA are capable of generating functional mature antigen-presenting DC, further referred to as TriMix-DC, which are able to generate specific immune responses [21, 22]. All these molecules can be efficiently loaded into DC in a single step by co-electroporation. A major advantage of this approach is that there is no need to preincubate the DC for up to 48 h with soluble maturation signals like pro-inflammatory cytokines or TLR ligands to achieve maturation, which can render the cells "exhausted" and inferior for vaccination purposes. As a result, TriMix-DC can be injected into the patient within a few hours after electroporation and will mature and secrete most of their immunostimulatory cytokines and chemokines in situ.

Different routes of immunization can be combined to broaden the tissue distribution of antigen-specific T cells induced by the treatment. Investigators showed that immunization by different routes induces specific T cells situated at different tissue sites resulting in the eradication of tumors located at different body sites [23]. As reported by our group, the combination of intradermal (ID) and intravenous (IV) vaccination results in a broad T cell response induced by the DC treatment [13] and leads to enhanced clinical responses [24].

We here describe in detail the production and administration procedure of TriMix-DC.

2 Materials

2.1 Production of Capped mRNA

1. pST1/CD40L, pST1/CD70, pST1/sig-caTLR4, and pST1/sig-TAA-DC-Lamp plasmids (Fig. 1).
2. GenElute HP Endotoxin-Free Plasmid Maxiprep Kit (Sigma-Aldrich, Diegem, Belgium).
3. *Sap*I restriction enzyme (Fisher Scientific, Erembodegem, Belgium).
4. 3 M sodium acetate, pH 5.2 (nuclease-free).
5. 100 % and 70 % ethanol (EtOH).
6. Sterile RNase, DNase, and endotoxin-free water.
7. mMESSAGE mMACHINE® T7 Ultra Kit (Life Technologies, Merelbeke, Belgium).

2.2 Generation of Immature DC (iDC)

1. Peripheral blood mononuclear cells (PBMC) collected through leukapheresis (*see* **Note 1**).
2. 4-tray Cell Factories (*see* **Notes 2** and **3**) (VWR Nunc, Leuven, Belgium).

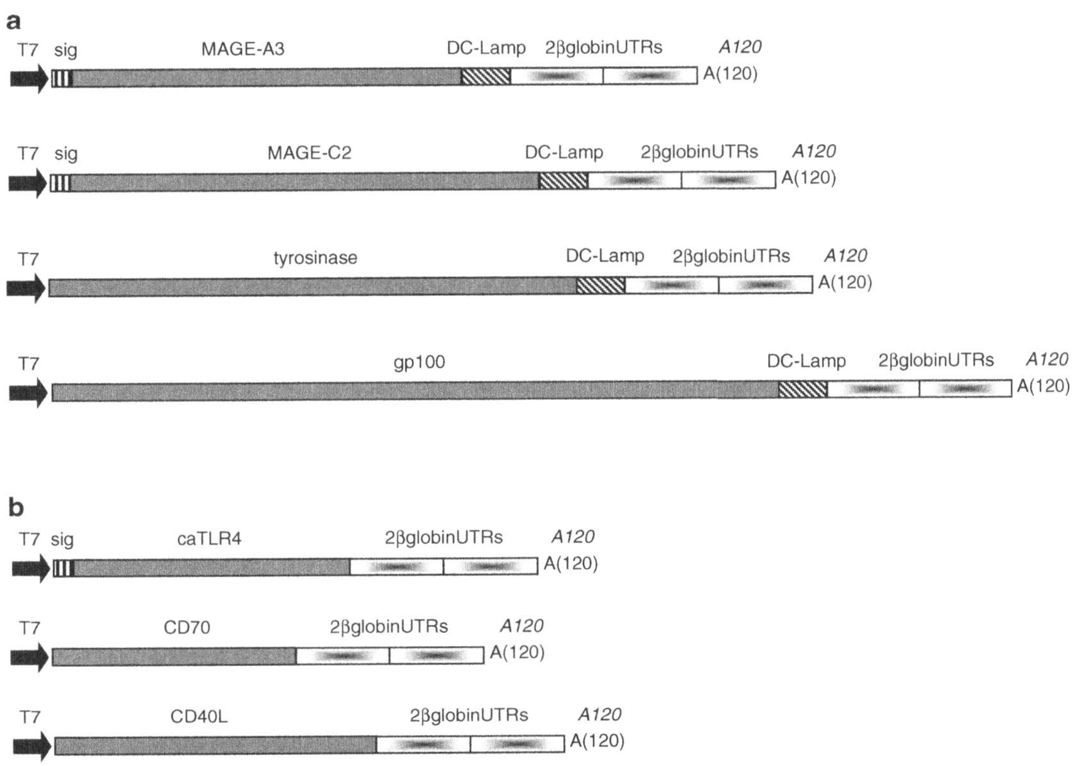

Fig. 1 Schematic representation of the different mRNAs. (**a**) Schematic representation of the mRNA encoding the 4 TAA comprising the vaccine. The T7 promoter, β-globin 3′ untranslated regions (UTRs), poly(A) tail (A120), signal sequence (sig) of Lamp-1, and the HLA class II targeting sequence (DC-Lamp) are shown. (**b**) Schematic representation of mRNAs coding for the TriMix molecules

3. X-VIVO™-15 medium.
4. Phosphate buffered saline (PBS).
5. Roswell Park Memorial Institute (RPMI)-1640 medium.
6. Granulocyte-macrophage colony-stimulating factor (GM-CSF) and interleukin-4 (IL-4) (*see* **Note 4**).
7. Heat-inactivated autologous plasma (AP) (*see* **Note 5**).
8. CELL-DYN Sapphire hematology analyzer (Abbott, Waver, Belgium).

2.3 Electroporation of DC for Vaccination

1. Serum-free RPMI-1640 medium.
2. Opti-MEM reduced serum medium without phenol red (Life Technologies).
3. 4-mm electroporation cuvettes (Immunosource Cell Projects, Schilde, Belgium).
4. Gene Pulser XCell electroporator (Bio-Rad, Nazareth, Belgium).
5. DC culture medium consisting of RPMI-1640 medium supplemented with 1 % AP, 1,000 U/mL of GM-CSF, and 500 U/mL of IL-4.
6. 15- and 50-mL tubes.
7. Ultra-Low Attachment T-75 flask (Elscolab Corning, Kruibeke, Belgium).
8. Cryopreservation medium consisting of AP+10 % DMSO (Acros Organics, Geel, Belgium) and 2 % glucose.
9. 1-mL cryopreservation tubes.
10. Cryofreezing container (Cryo 1 °C freezing container, rate of cooling −1 °C/min) (VWR Nalgene, Leuven, Belgium).
11. PBS.
12. Human serum albumin (HSA).
13. 1-mL and 20-mL syringes.

3 Methods

The methods below describe (1) the production of capped mRNA, (2) the generation of autologous immature DC, and (3) subsequent electroporation of the DC with TriMix and TAA for combined ID and IV administration to the patient.

3.1 Production of Capped mRNA

For the production of capped mRNA suitable for electroporation, the following procedures must be performed: (1) cloning of the gene(s) of interest into a suitable vector and production of plasmid DNA, (2) linearization of the plasmid DNA, and (3) in vitro transcription of capped mRNA.

For preparation of TriMix-mRNA, the DNA sequences encoding the CD40L, CD70, and caTLR4 proteins are cloned into the pST1 vector [25] (provided by Dr. U. Sahin, Johannes Gutenberg University, Mainz, Germany) by using standard molecular cloning techniques. The extracellular part of the TLR4 is deleted resulting in the caTLR4 with the intracellular and transmembrane fragments [26] flanked by a signal sequence. For preparation of TAA mRNA, the DNA sequence encoding full-length TAA, flanked by the signal sequence of the Lamp-1 and the HLA class II targeting sequence of DC-Lamp [18], is cloned into the pST1 vector by using standard molecular cloning techniques. The signal sequence will translocate newly synthesized proteins to the endoplasmic reticulum while the DC-Lamp targeting sequence will provide transport to the HLA class II compartments (*see* **Note 6**).

The pST1 vector contains a bacteriophage T7 promoter, which controls in vitro transcription. Downstream from the insert, a poly(A) tail of 120 adenines is present. Between the coding region and the poly(A) tail, 2 consecutive human β-globin 3′ untranslated regions (UTRs) are present. Before in vitro transcription of the mRNA, the plasmids are linearized (*see* **Note 7**) with the *Sap*I restriction enzyme, resulting in an unmasked poly(A) tail with a free 3′ end (Fig. 1). After cloning, sufficient amounts of plasmid DNA are prepared with the GenElute HP Endotoxin-free Plasmid Maxiprep Kit according to the manufacturer's instructions. Optionally, DNA sequences can be optimized in silico to maximize translational efficiency (*see* **Note 8**).

3.2 Production of In Vitro Transcribed Capped mRNA

Prior to the in vitro transcription, linearization of 100 μg plasmid with 100 U *Sap*I restriction enzyme in a total volume of 500 μL is performed, followed by ethanol precipitation. In vitro transcription of capped mRNA is performed with T7 RNA polymerase by using the mMESSAGE mMACHINE® T7 Ultra Kit according to the manufacturer's instructions. This kit is designed for the in vitro synthesis of large amounts of efficiently and correctly capped mRNA with a poly(A) tail suitable for cancer vaccines (*see* **Note 9**). After transcription, the remaining plasmid DNA is removed by DNase treatment to reduce the risk of introducing foreign DNA into the cells. Size and integrity of the mRNA are checked by gel electrophoresis and quantity and purity are determined by spectrophotometry. Good quality mRNA is then stored at −20 °C in small aliquots (*see* **Note 10**).

3.3 Generation of Immature DC

This method describes the generation of clinical grade DC in vitro from plastic adherent monocytes in GM-CSF and IL-4 containing medium.

1. Adjust the concentration of the washed peripheral blood mononuclear cells (PBMC) to 10×10^6 cells/mL X-VIVO™-15 medium supplemented with 2 % AP.

2. Bring 800 mL of the cell suspension into 1× 4-tray Cell Factory.
3. Allow plastic adherence of the DC precursors ($CD14^+$ monocytes) for 1.5–2 h at 37 °C (*see* **Note 11**).
4. Remove the nonadherent cells for cryopreservation and wash the Cell Factory once with 250 mL of X-VIVO™-15.
5. Bring 800 mL of RPMI-1640 medium supplemented with 1 % AP, 1,000 U/mL of GM-CSF, and 500 U/mL of IL-4 into the Cell Factory.
6. Incubate the cells at 37 °C and 5 % CO_2 in a humidified incubator.
7. On days 2 and 4 of DC culture, add the same amount of GM-CSF and IL-4 to the cells as on day 0 in 20 mL of RPMI-1640 medium supplemented with 1 % AP.
8. On day 6 of DC culture, the cells are harvested for subsequent vaccine preparation.
9. An in-process quality control is performed on day 6 including viability, sterility, and mycoplasma detection.

3.4 Electroporation of DC for Vaccination

1. Prepare a 50-mL tube with 30 mL of RPMI-1640 medium supplemented with 1 % AP, 1,000 U/mL of GM-CSF, and 500 U/mL of IL-4 (at 37 °C).
2. Adjust the physical parameters of the Gene Pulser XCell electroporator as follows: voltage 300 V, capacitance 450 μF, and resistance ∞Ω.
3. Wash 50×10^6 DC with 10 mL of Opti-MEM.
4. While performing the washing step, prepare the following mRNA electroporation mix in a final volume of 600 μL of Opti-MEM:

   20 μg of CD40L mRNA

   20 μg of CD70 mRNA

   20 μg of caTLR4 mRNA

   60 μg of sig-TAA-DC-Lamp mRNA
5. Resuspend the washed DC in the mRNA electroporation mix and transfer into a 4-mm electroporation cuvette.
6. Insert the cuvette into the electroporation chamber and trigger the pulse.
7. Immediately after the electroporation, transfer the DC to the 50-mL Falcon tube with 30 mL of RPMI-1640 medium supplemented with 1 % AP, 1,000 U/mL of GM-CSF, and 500 U/mL of IL-4 and rinse the electroporation cuvette twice with DC culture medium.

8. If you have performed different electroporations (with different TAA), pool the different DC into 1 Ultra-Low Attachment T-75 flask and incubate the electroporated DC for 3.5–4 h in a humidified incubator at 37 °C and 5 % CO_2 (*see* **Note 12**).
9. Harvest the electroporated DC and freeze them at $\pm 12.5 \times 10^6$ per cryotube (*see* **Note 13**).
10. Perform quality control (*see* **Note 14**).
11. For vaccination, thaw four cryotubes of electroporated DC (*see* **Note 13**) and let them rest for 1.2 h in X-VIVO™-15 supplemented with IL-4 and GM-CSF.
12. For intravenous administration, resuspend 20×10^6 electroporated DC in 15 mL of 0.9 % NaCl/1 % HSA and transfer the DC to a sterile 20-mL syringe.
13. For intradermal administration, resuspend 4×10^6 electroporated DC in 250 μL PBS supplemented with 1 % HSA and transfer the DC to a sterile 1-mL syringe.
14. The DC can now be used for vaccination.

3.5 Patients, Treatment Schedule, Clinical Evaluation, and Immunomonitoring

We treat patients with recurrent stage III or stage IV melanoma in academic, single-center clinical trials. These patients are incorporated in the study after written informed consent and with approval of the study protocol by the institutional ethical committee and national competent authorities.

DC therapy is administered by 4 biweekly intradermal (ID) and intravenous (IV) injections, and a 5th administration is scheduled 8 weeks after the 4th immunization in the absence of disease progression. TriMix-DC are administered IV during a 15-min infusion by constant flow rate in a peripheral vein. At the same time, TriMix-DC are injected ID at two different anatomical sites (axilla and inguinal region). Each patient is closely monitored for at least 1 h after the end of the IV administration (*see* **Note 15**).

Patients undergo two leukaphereses, one before treatment and one after the 4th administration (*see* **Note 16**). DC therapy is prepared from the first leukapheresis and the nonadherent fraction of both aphereses is frozen for immunomonitoring.

Tumor response assessments (by RECIST) are performed by [(18)F]-fluorodeoxyglucose positron emission tomography/computed tomography (FDG-PET/CT) at baseline and in weeks 8, 16, and 24.

Immunomonitoring is performed both on delayed type IV hypersensitivity (DTH) skin infiltrating lymphocytes (SKILs) [27] and on peripheral blood $CD8^+$ T cells [13]. One week after the fourth DC administration, a small amount of TriMix-DC (5×10^5) is injected ID to induce a DTH from which skin biopsies are taken 48 or 72 h later. After 2.5 weeks of in vitro culture in the presence of 100 U/mL IL-2, SKILs are harvested.

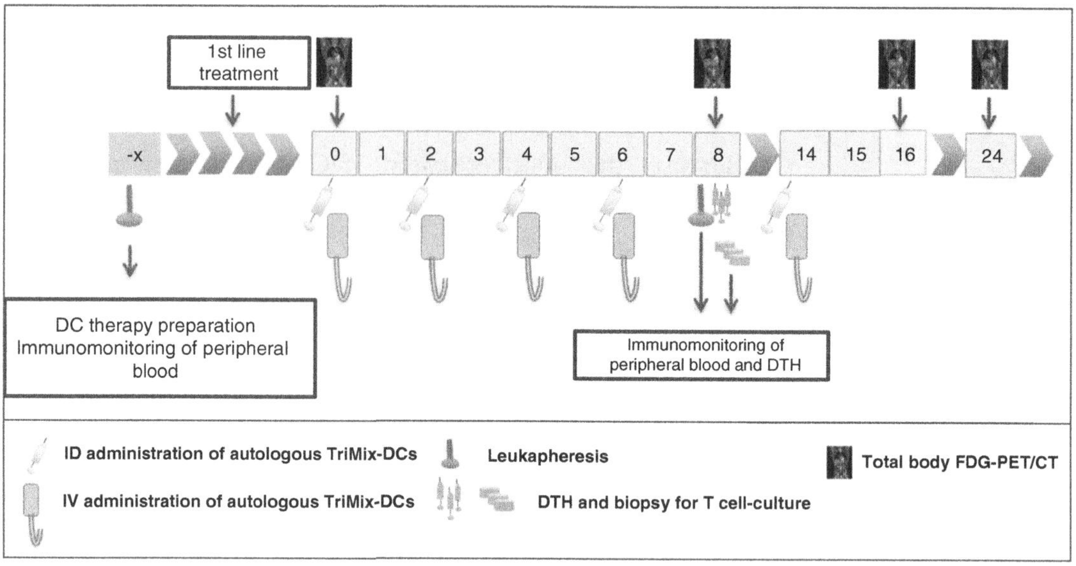

Fig. 2 Treatment schedule of melanoma patients receiving ID and IV administration of autologous TriMix-DC. Clinical evaluation and immunomonitoring time points are indicated

Their antigen-specific activation (CD137 upregulation [28]), cytolytic capacity (CD107a upregulation [29]), and cytokine release (IFN-γ and TNF-α) in response to autologous EBV-B cells expressing the antigens present in the TriMix-DC vaccine are assessed. For immunomonitoring of the peripheral blood of the patients, $CD8^+$ T cells are stimulated weekly with autologous TriMix-DC co-electroporated with one of four different tumor antigens at a 10:1 ratio for 2 or 3 weeks. Their antigen specificity is then determined as for the SKILs.

A schedule of the TriMix-DC administrations, leukaphereses, clinical evaluation, and immunomonitoring assays is given in Fig. 2.

4 Notes

1. Leukapheresis is performed with a COBE Spectra Apheresis System (CaridianBCT, Zaventem, Belgium) under continuous supervision of a trained physician, and approximately 12 L of blood is processed. The leukapheresed PBMC are then washed with a COBE 2991 Cell Processor (CaridianBCT) to remove contaminating platelets. Samples from the washed cell suspension are tested for hematocrit, total white blood cell count, and platelet count.
2. DC for vaccination must be produced in a clean room following the current guidelines of Good Manufacturing Practice. We have designed a system to produce large amounts of DC in

a closed system using Cell Factories suitable for clinical use [30]. Tubing sets with sterile connections and septa for injections to transfer the PBMC to the culture vessel and to perform the necessary washing steps, the addition of cytokines and AP, and the harvesting were designed. Typically, four to five Cell Factories can be filled with the PBMC of one single leukapheresis.

3. When granulocyte contamination of the leukapheresis product is less than 5 %, monocyte enrichment is performed by counterflow elutriation instead of by plastic adherence. Before elutriation, monocyte and granulocyte content of the PBMC are measured using the CELL-DYN Sapphire hematology analyzer. Continuous counterflow elutriation of leukapheresed PBMC is performed with the Elutra Cell Separation System (CaridianBCT) with single-use, functionally sealed disposable Elutra sets (CaridianBCT). After priming, the leukapheresis product is loaded via the inlet pump into the constantly rotating (2,400 rpm) elutriation chamber. The automation mode produces five elutriation fractions (F1–F5), each specified by a centrifuge speed, elutriation buffer flow rate, and a process volume. All fractions are collected in RPMI-1640 medium supplemented with 1 % AP. The final monocyte-enriched fraction (F5) is collected into the final collection bag when the centrifuge is stopped, i.e., the collection of the chamber content with the rotor off. All procedures are conducted according to the manufacturer's recommendations. After elutriation, DC culture is started by seeding $400–600 \times 10^6$ monocytes per 4-tray Cell Factory in 800 mL of RPMI-1640 medium supplemented with 1 % AP, 1,000 U/mL of GM-CSF, and 500 U/mL of IL-4.

4. GM-CSF and IL-4 are prepared in-house but are also commercially available. The cytokines prepared in-house are animal-protein- and endotoxin-free. Their biological activity is titrated against standards obtained from the National Institute for Biological Standards and Controls (NIBSC, South Hills, UK).

5. AP is collected from each patient and decomplemented at 56 °C for 50 min. Then, plasma is centrifuged at $23,000 \times g$ for 20 min at 4 °C. Human AB serum can be used as an alternative.

6. The primary aim of this approach is to obtain HLA class II-mediated presentation of antigen-derived $CD4^+$ helper T cells in addition to HLA class I-mediated $CD8^+$ cytotoxic T cells. Both are pivotal for the induction of an effective and long-lasting antitumor immunity [17]. Tumor-specific antigens MAGE-A3 and MAGE-C2 and differentiation antigens gp100 and tyrosinase were chosen. Almost every TAA-encoding sequence can be used for cloning.

7. Plasmid DNA must be linearized with a restriction enzyme downstream of the insert to be transcribed. Circular plasmid templates will generate extremely long, heterogenous RNA transcripts. It is important to examine the linearized template DNA on a gel to confirm that cleavage is complete.
8. Our observations report increased expression of CD40L and caTLR4 after in silico optimization (GENEART). Nevertheless, for some genes, no major impact on gene expression is observed, including CD70 expression.
9. A modified cap, Anti-Reverse Cap Analog (ARCA), is used which allows T7 RNA polymerase to synthesize RNAs capped exclusively in the correct orientation. Substitution of traditional cap analog with ARCA allows for synthesis of capped RNAs that are 100 % functional, in contrast to transcription reactions using traditional cap analog where only half of the cap analog is incorporated in the correct orientation. As a result, ARCA Cap mRNA molecules are more efficiently translated and much higher protein expression levels can be achieved than from mRNA made with the standard cap.
10. Gel electrophoresis of the transcribed mRNA should confer one single, sharp band. If not, mRNA might be degraded or improperly digested. mRNA quantity is measured at 260 nm and 280 nm. Pure RNA has an A260/A280 ratio of 1.9–2.1. If not, RNA might be contaminated with protein or DNA. After aliquoting and freezing, avoid freeze-thawing the mRNA.
11. Plastic adherence of the PBMC in Cell Factories is not feasible in RPMI-1640 medium. Therefore, we use X-VIVO™-15 medium.
12. We typically perform eight electroporations, 2× with 50×10^6 DC with TriMix-mRNA plus TAA (either gp100, MAGE-A3, MAGE-C2, or tyrosinase). This yields enough electroporated DC for one treatment cycle.
13. DC are frozen in cryotubes at $\pm 12.5 \times 10^6$ DC per tube in 1 mL of AP with 10 % DMSO and 2 % glucose. The DC are slowly frozen to −80 °C using a cryofreezing container and subsequently stored in liquid nitrogen until use. For thawing, DC are quickly thawed in a 37 °C water bath, transferred to DC culture medium, and pelleted at room temperature. The thawed DC are then resuspended in 5 mL of pre-warmed culture medium. Cell number and viability are determined with trypan blue. Typically, cells are >80 % viable and >90 % of the frozen cells are recuperated after thawing.
14. The final product must be monitored and reported prior to its release for clinical use. The endpoints for the quality control are the number of DC, purity (determined by flow cytometric light scatter properties) and viability (determined by trypan

blue exclusion), electroporation efficiency (measured by the % of cells expressing CD70), the immuno-phenotype (including CD40, CD80, CD83, CCR7, CD14 expression), and functional characterization by IL-12p70 secretion between 0–24 h and 24–48 h. DC-therapy samples are analyzed for sterility by long-term microbiological culture and tested for mycoplasma infection by PCR.

15. Post-infusion grade 2 chills are observed in some patients receiving IV infusion. Chills typically start about 15 min after the end of the IV infusion of TriMix-DC and resolve spontaneously within 30 min.

16. In an ongoing phase II clinical trial, patients are treated with a combined ID/IV [ID (4×10^6 DC) and IV (20×10^6 DC)] TriMix-DC therapy in combination with an antibody directed against the cytotoxic T-lymphocyte antigen 4 (anti-CTLA-4; ipilimumab). In this study, patients undergo a leukapheresis before the start of the treatment and a buffy coat at the end of the treatment.

Acknowledgements

TriMix-DC are the topic of a current patent application (WO2009/034172). A. B. and K. T. are mentioned as inventors of this application. None of the authors involved in this study receives any form of support or remuneration related to this platform.

This work was supported by grants from the Interuniversity Attraction Poles Program–Belgian State–Belgian Science Policy, the National Cancer Plan of the Federal Ministry of Health, the Stichting tegen Kanker, the Vlaamse Liga tegen Kanker, an Integrated Project and a Network of Excellence sponsored by the EU FP-6, an IWT-TBM program, the Fonds voor Wetenschappelijk Onderzoek Vlaanderen (FWO-Vlaanderen), and the Willy Gepts Wetenschappelijk Fonds of the UZ Brussel. S. W. is a Ph.D. fellow and A. B. is a postdoctoral fellow of the FWO-Vlaanderen.

References

1. Schnurr M et al (2005) Tumor antigen processing and presentation depend critically on dendritic cell type and the mode of antigen delivery. Blood 105:2465–2472
2. Hasegawa K et al (2006) In vitro stimulation of CD8 and CD4 T cells by dendritic cells loaded with a complex of cholesterol-bearing hydrophobized pullulan and NY-ESO-1 protein: identification of a new HLA-DR15-binding CD4 T-cell epitope. Clin Cancer Res 12:1921–1927
3. Keilholz U et al (2009) A clinical and immunologic phase 2 trial of Wilms tumor gene product 1 (WT1) peptide vaccination in patients with AML and MDS. Blood 113:6541–6548

4. Svane IM et al (2007) Vaccination with p53 peptide-pulsed dendritic cells is associated with disease stabilization in patients with p53 expressing advanced breast cancer; monitoring of serum YKL-40 and IL-6 as response biomarkers. Cancer Immunol Immunther 56:1485–1499
5. Van Nuffel AM et al (2012) Dendritic cells loaded with mRNA encoding full-length tumor antigens prime CD4(+) and CD8(+) T cells in melanoma patients. Mol Ther 20:1063–1074
6. Wilgenhof S et al (2011) Therapeutic vaccination with an autologous mRNA electroporated dendritic cell vaccine in patients with advanced melanoma. J Immunother 34:448–456
7. Henken FE et al (2012) Preclinical safety evaluation of DNA vaccines encoding modified HPV16 E6 and E7. Vaccine 30:4259–4266
8. Himoudi N et al (2012) Lack of T-cell responses following autologous tumour lysate pulsed dendritic cell vaccination, in patients with relapsed osteosarcoma. Clin Transl Oncol 14:271–279
9. Kalady MF et al (2004) Dendritic cells pulsed with pancreatic cancer total tumor RNA generate specific antipancreatic cancer T cells. J Gastrointest Surg 8:175–181
10. Win SJ et al (2012) Enhancing the immunogenicity of tumour lysate-loaded dendritic cell vaccines by conjugation to virus-like particles. Br J Cancer 106:92–98
11. Jonuleit H et al (1997) Pro-inflammatory cytokines and prostaglandins induce maturation of potent immunostimulatory dendritic cells under fetal calf serum-free conditions. Eur J Immunol 27:3135–3142
12. Medzhitov R (2001) Toll-like receptors and innate immunity. Nat Rev Immunol 1:135–145
13. Van Nuffel AM et al (2012) Intravenous and intradermal TriMix-dendritic cell therapy results in a broad T-cell response and durable tumor response in a chemorefractory stage IV-M1c melanoma patient. Cancer Immunol Immunother 61:1033–1043
14. Reiser M et al (2011) The immunodominant CD8 T cell response to the human cytomegalovirus tegument phosphoprotein pp 65 (495–503) epitope critically depends on CD4 T cell help in vaccinated HLA-A*0201 transgenic mice. J Immunol 187:2172–2180
15. De Veerman M et al (1999) Retrovirally transduced bone marrow-derived dendritic cells require $CD4^+$ T cell help to elicit protective and therapeutic antitumor immunity. J Immunol 162:144–151
16. Gao FG et al (2002) Antigen-specific $CD4^+$ T-cell help is required to activate a memory $CD8^+$ T cell to a fully functional tumor killer cell. Cancer Res 62:6438–6441
17. Bevan MJ (2004) Helping the CD8(+) T-cell response. Nat Rev Immunol 4:595–602
18. Bonehill A et al (2004) Messenger RNA-electroporated dendritic cells presenting MAGE-A3 simultaneously in HLA class I and class II molecules. J Immunol 172: 6649–6657
19. Fath S et al (2011) Multiparameter RNA and codon optimization: a standardized tool to assess and enhance autologous mammalian gene expression. PLoS One 6:e17596
20. Samorski R et al (2006) Codon optimized expression of HPV 16 E6 renders target cells susceptible to E6-specific CTL recognition. Immunol Lett 107:41–49
21. Bonehill A et al (2009) Single-step antigen loading and activation of dendritic cells by mRNA electroporation for the purpose of therapeutic vaccination in melanoma patients. Clin Cancer Res 15:3366–3375
22. Bonehill A et al (2008) Enhancing the T-cell stimulatory capacity of human dendritic cells by co-electroporation with CD40L, CD70 and constitutively active TLR4 encoding mRNA. Mol Ther 16:1170–1180
23. Mullins DW et al (2003) Route of immunization with peptide-pulsed dendritic cells controls the distribution of memory and effector T cells in lymphoid tissues and determines the pattern of regional tumor control. J Exp Med 198:1023–1034
24. Wilgenhof S et al (2013) Phase 1B study on intravenous synthetic mRNA electroporated dendritic cell immunotherapy in pretreated melanoma patients. Ann Oncol 24(10): 2686–2693
25. Holtkamp S et al (2006) Modification of antigen-encoding RNA increases stability, translational efficacy, and T-cell stimulatory capacity of dendritic cells. Blood 108: 4009–4017
26. Cisco RM et al (2004) Induction of human dendritic cell maturation using transfection with RNA encoding a dominant positive toll-like receptor 4. J Immunol 172: 7162–7168
27. Van Nuffel AM et al (2012) Epitope and HLA-type independent monitoring of antigen-specific T-cells after treatment with dendritic cells presenting full-length tumor antigens. J Immunol Methods 377:23–36
28. Wolfl M et al (2007) Activation-induced expression of CD137 permits detection, isolation,

and expansion of the full repertoire of CD8+ T cells responding to antigen without requiring knowledge of epitope specificities. Blood 110:201–210

29. Betts MR et al (2003) Sensitive and viable identification of antigen-specific CD8+ T cells by a flow cytometric assay for degranulation. J Immunol Methods 281:65–78

30. Tuyaerts S et al (2002) Generation of large numbers of dendritic cells in a closed system using Cell Factories. J Immunol Methods 264:135–151

Chapter 2

Generation of Multiple Peptide Cocktail-Pulsed Dendritic Cells as a Cancer Vaccine

Hyun-Ju Lee, Nu-Ri Choi, Manh-Cuong Vo, My-Dung Hoang, Youn-Kyung Lee, and Je-Jung Lee

Abstract

Cancer immunotherapy based on dendritic cell (DC) vaccination has promising alternatives for the treatment of cancer. A central tenet of DC-based cancer immunotherapy is the generation of antigen-specific cytotoxic T lymphocyte (CTL) response. Tumor-associated antigens (TAA) and DC play pivotal roles in this process. DCs are well known to be the most potent antigen-presenting cells and have the most powerful antigen-presenting capacity. DCs pulsed with various TAA have been shown to be effective in producing specific antitumor effects both in vitro and in vivo. Several types of tumor antigens have been applied in cancer treatment including tumor RNA, lysates, apoptotic bodies, heat shock protein, peptides from TAA, and allogeneic tumor cells. Among them, the use of immunogenic HLA-A*0201-specific epitopes from multiple TAA enhances induction of antigen-specific CTL and associated therapeutic efficacy in HLA-A*0201$^+$ cancer patients. The current chapter provides a detailed protocol of generating multiple peptide cocktail-pulsed DC to elicit CTL with a broad spectrum of immune responses against the related tumor antigens.

Key words Cancer immunotherapy, Dendritic cells, Multiple peptide, Tumor-associated antigens, Cytotoxic T lymphocytes

1 Introduction

Dendritic cells (DCs) are the most attractive and potent antigen-presenting cells for targeted immunotherapy in cancer. First, several physiological aspects of DC including DC type and maturation status can be easily manipulated during ex vivo generation. Second, tumor-associated antigens (TAA) can be loaded in a controlled and feasible manner using peptides, proteins, or RNA. Third, autologous tumor cells such as dying tumor cells or whole tumor RNA can be used as tumor antigens to target patient-specific DC vaccination for successful cancer immunotherapy [1–7]. Animal models demonstrated that TAA-loaded DCs are capable of eliciting protective and

Michael J.P. Lawman and Patricia D. Lawman (eds.), *Cancer Vaccines: Methods and Protocols*, Methods in Molecular Biology, vol. 1139, DOI 10.1007/978-1-4939-0345-0_2, © Springer Science+Business Media New York 2014

therapeutic antitumor responses [8, 9]. Clinical trials also showed immunologically and clinically promising effects of antigen-loaded DC administered as a cancer vaccine [10, 11].

Although DC-based immunotherapy is a promising approach to augment tumor antigen-specific cytotoxic T lymphocyte (CTL) responses in cancer patients, tumor immune escape mechanism via downregulation or complete loss of TAA and MHC class I molecules, escaping death receptor signaling, impaired antigen processing may limit the susceptibility of tumor cells to the immune attack [12]. Therefore, targeting of multiple TAA and concomitant generation of CTL responses may represent one strategy to circumvent this potential drawback. Recently, several studies demonstrated that cancer immunotherapy using DC pulsed with multiple peptide cocktail derived from multiple (4 or 5) TAA with repeated boosting generates feasible and efficient cellular antitumor responses in patients with hormone-refractory prostate cancer and multiple myeloma [13–15].

We describe here a universal protocol to generate DC pulsed with multiple peptide cocktail based on our and other groups. It is necessary that more suitable, immunogenic TAA and powerful DC should be chosen for a strong and efficient antitumor immune responses using multiple peptide cocktail-pulsed DC.

2 Materials

2.1 Isolation of CD14$^+$ Monocytes and CD3$^+$ Lymphocytes from Peripheral Blood

1. Vacutainer blood collection tubes with sodium heparin (Becton Dickinson, Franklin Lakes, NJ, USA).
2. 15-mL and 50-mL polypropylene tubes.
3. Lymphoprep $d = 1.077$ (Axis-Shield Po CAS, Oslo, Norway).
4. 1× phosphate-buffered saline (PBS).
5. Iscove's Modified Dulbecco's Medium (IMDM) (Invitrogen, Gibco® by Life Technologies™, Grand Island, NY, USA) with 10 % fetal bovine serum (FBS).
6. MACS buffer: 0.5 % bovine serum albumin (BSA) and 2 mM EDTA in PBS and pH 7.2 (Miltenyi Biotec, Auburn, CA, USA).
7. Medium for human CD14$^+$ monocytes: IMDM with 10 % FBS.
8. Medium for human CD3$^+$ T cells: Roswell Park Memorial Institute (RPMI)-1640 (Invitrogen) with 10 % FBS.
9. Isolation columns for human CD14$^+$ monocytes and CD3$^+$ T cells (Miltenyi Biotec).
10. MACS separation kit (Miltenyi Biotec).
11. CD14 microbeads, human (Miltenyi Biotec).

12. CD3 microbeads, human (Miltenyi Biotec).
13. MACS columns and MACS separators (MS, LS) (Miltenyi Biotec).
14. Allegra X-12 centrifuge (Beckman Coulter, Brea, CA, USA).

2.2 Generation of Immature and Mature DC

1. Medium for DC culture: IMDM with 10 % FBS.
2. Medium for washing the cells: 1× PBS.
3. 6-well or 24-well culture plates.
4. Cytokines for DC differentiation:
   (a) 50 ng/mL recombinant human granulocyte-macrophage colony-stimulating factor (GM-CSF) (Peprotech, Rocky Hill, NJ, USA) or 1,000 U/mL GM-CSF (Immunex, Seattle, WA, USA).
   (b) 20 ng/mL recombinant human interleukin-4 (IL-4) (Peprotech) or 1,000 U/mL IL-4 (R&D Systems, Minneapolis, MN, USA).
5. Cytokines for DC maturation 1 [13, 14]:
   (a) 20 ng/mL recombinant human tumor necrosis factor-α (TNF-α) and GMP grade (CellGenix, Freiburg, Germany).
   (b) 10 ng/mL recombinant human interleukin-1β (IL-1β) and GMP grade (CellGenix).
   (c) 1,000 U/mL recombinant human interleukin-6 (IL-6) and GMP grade (CellGenix).
   (d) 1 μg/mL prostaglandin 2 (PGE_2) (Pharmacia & Upjohn, Dubendorf, Switzerland).
6. Cytokines for DC maturation 2 [15]:
   (a) 1,000 U/mL recombinant human interferon-α (IFN-α) (R&D Systems, Minneapolis, MN, USA).
   (b) 10 ng/mL recombinant human TNF-α (TNF-α) (R&D Systems).
7. Cytokines for DC maturation 3 (with simple modification: αDC1-polarizing cocktails) [16]:
   (a) 50 ng/mL recombinant human TNF-α (Peprotech).
   (b) 25 ng/mL recombinant human IL-lβ (Peprotech).
   (c) 3×10^3 IU/mL recombinant human IFN-α; (Intron A-IFN-α-2b) (LG Life Science, Chonbuk, Korea).
   (d) 100 ng/mL recombinant human interferon-γ (IFN-γ) (Peprotech).
   (e) Poly-I:C 20 μg/mL (Sigma-Aldrich, St. Louis, MO, USA).

2.3 Synthesis of Multiple Peptide Cocktail Derived from Tumor Antigens

1. Two popular databases for MHC ligands and peptide motifs are available.
   (a) Peptide-binding database 1: Bioinformatics & Molecular Analysis Section (BIMAS), http://www-bimas.cit.nih.gov/molbio/hla_bind/
   (b) Peptide-binding database 2: SYFPEITHI, http://www.syfpeithi.de/.

2.4 Binding Affinity and Stability

1. T2 cell line (ATCC, Manassas, VA, USA).
2. Human β2-microglobulin (working concentration of 3 μg/mL) (Sigma-Aldrich).
3. PBS with BSA (PBA) [20]: 0.9 % sodium chloride (NaCl), 0.5 % BSA, 0.02 % sodium azide (NaN_3), or FACS buffer, 1× PBS and 1 % FBS.
4. The Brefeldin A (BFA) solution: 1,000×, working concentration of 3 μg/mL (eBiosciences Inc., San Diego, CA, USA).
5. Fluorescein isothiocyanate (FITC)-labeled anti-HLA-A*0201 monoclonal antibody (mAb) BB7.2 (Becton Dickinson Pharmingen).
6. FACS calibur cell sorter (Becton Dickinson Pharmingen).
7. Win MDI version 2.9 (Bio-Soft Net, developed by *John Trotter*, Salk Institute, San Diego, CA, USA).

2.5 DC Pulsing by Multiple Peptide Cocktail

1. Multiple peptides derived from tumor-associated antigen may be obtained from various sources.
2. 6-well culture plates (Becton Dickinson Pharmingen).
3. 15-mL polypropylene tubes.
4. IMDM medium with 10 % FBS.

2.6 DC Harvest and Storage

1. Cryotubes.
2. 2× freezing medium A: RPMI-1640 and 40 % FBS.
3. 2× freezing medium B: RPMI-1640 and 20 % dimethyl sulfoxide (DMSO).
4. Cryo 1 °C Nalgene™, freezing container (Thermo Fisher Scientific Inc, Rochester, NY, USA) with isopropanol.

2.7 Phenotypic Analysis of Multiple Peptide Cocktail-Pulsed DC

1. Mouse antihuman CD80 mAb conjugated with PE (Becton Dickinson Pharmingen).
2. Mouse antihuman CD83 mAb conjugated with FITC (Becton Dickinson Pharmingen).
3. Mouse antihuman CD86 mAb conjugated with PE (Becton Dickinson Pharmingen).
4. Mouse antihuman CCR7 mAb conjugated with FITC (R&D Systems).

5. Mouse IgG1, k, isotype control (Becton Dickinson Pharmingen).
6. Mouse IgG1, k, isotype control (Becton Dickinson Pharmingen).
7. Mouse IgG_{2A}, isotype control (R&D Systems).

2.8 In Vitro Induction of Multiple Peptide-Specific CTL

1. IL-2, 25 ng/mL (Peprotech).
2. Interleukin-7 (IL-7) 10 ng/mL (Peprotech).
3. 50 mL CTL medium: 22.5 mL RPMI-1640, 22.5 mL, AIM-V (Invitrogen), 5 mL FBS, and 0.5 mL penicillin-streptomycin. The AIM-V medium is a mixture of HEPES-buffered Dulbecco's Modified Eagle Medium and Ham's Nutrient Mixture F12 that had been supplemented with purified human albumin, transferrin, insulin, and a proprietary mixture of purified factors.

3 Methods

3.1 Isolation of Peripheral Blood Mononuclear Cells (PBMC)

1. Collect blood in heparinized tubes and dilute 1:2 with 1× PBS
2. Overlay 30 mL of diluted blood over 15 mL of Lymphoprep in each 50-mL tube.
3. Centrifuge at 1,000 × *g* for 25 min, at room temperature or 21 °C (acceleration, 5; deceleration, 0).
4. Harvest the buffy coat layer (PBMC fraction) after centrifugation.
5. Wash the cells twice with 1× PBS at room temperature.

3.2 Isolation of $CD14^+$ Monocytes and $CD3^+$ Lymphocytes from PBMC

1. Suspend PBMC in cold (4–8 °C) MACS buffer: PBS pH 7.2, 0.5 % BSA, and 2 mM EDTA.
2. Isolate $CD14^+$ monocytes and $CD3^+$ lymphocytes by the positive selection systems, respectively, according to the manufacturer's instructions (*see* **Note 1**).
3. Store the isolated $CD3^+$ lymphocytes in vapor phase of liquid nitrogen until needed.

3.3 DC Generation (See Note 2)

1. After the last wash of the monocytes, add fresh culture medium (IMDM with 10 % FBS), containing at least 50 ng/mL GM-CSF and 20 ng/mL IL-4 at a seeding density of 5×10^5 cells/mL/24-well plate or 2×10^6/2 mL/6-well plate.
2. On day 2 of the culture, discard half of the medium and add the same amount of fresh medium, pre-warmed to room temperature, with the 2× concentrated growth factors (100 ng/mL of GM-CSF and 40 ng/mL of IL-4).
3. On day 4 of the culture, repeat **step 2**.
4. On day 6, take out the half of the spent medium and add new medium containing GM-CSF (optional) and 2× concentrated

DC maturation cytokines, e.g., 1× αDC1-polarizing cocktail: 20 μg/mL of Poly-I:C, 50 ng/mL of TNF-α, 25 ng/mL of IL-1β, 3,000 IU/mL of IFN-α, and 100 ng/mL of IFN-γ.

5. Incubate for 42–48 h.

3.4 Analysis of Cytokine Production and Phenotypes in DC

1. On day 8, collect the supernatants from the cultures of mature DC. These supernatants represent "during maturation."
2. Harvest DC to 15-mL conical tubes and wash thoroughly to remove all the cytokines.
3. Plate the cells at 2×10^4 cells/100 μL/well in flat-bottomed 96-well plates.
4. Add the cytokine-inducing stimulus: 1 of 2 CD40 ligand (CD40L)-based stimuli, such as 5×10^4 cells/100 μL/well CD40L-transfected J558 cells [17] or 1 μg/mL of soluble CD40L [18, 19]. The induction of cytokine production is routinely performed in a final volume of 200 μL/flat-bottomed 96-well plates.
5. Following either of two methods of stimulation, the 24 h supernatants are harvested. These supernatants represent "after maturation and CD40L stimulation."
6. Perform the ELISA to measure human IL-12p70 and IL-10 secretion, for Th1 cytokine and Th2 cytokine, respectively, using the supernatants (during maturation and after maturation and CD40L stimulation) from cultures according to the manufacturer's instructions.

3.5 Synthesis of Multiple Peptide Cocktail

1. To predict T cell epitope candidates, select MHC type, e.g., HLA-A*0201. Choose a "mer," e.g., nonamers-9 amino acids; paste your amino acid sequence from source such as "MedLine"; and choose "run" to start analysis (*see* **Notes 3** and **4**).
2. Confirm the purity of commercially synthesized peptides (use >98 % purity by HPLC and Mass Spectrophotometry).
3. Dissolve the synthetic peptides in DMSO or distilled water according to the manufacturer's recommendations.
4. Store at –20 °C until needed.
5. Irrelevant peptides are used as controls.

3.6 Binding Affinity of Multiple Peptide Cocktail

1. Peptides binding to HLA-A*0201 molecules are measured using the T2 cell line according to a protocol described previously [20].
2. Wash T2 cells 2× in serum-free RPMI-1640 medium.
3. Place 8×10^4 cells T2 cells in serum-free RPMI medium into a V-bottom 96-well plate at total peptide concentrations ranging from 0 μg/mL to 50 μg/mL with 3 μg/mL of β2-microglobulin.

4. Incubate overnight at 37 °C in 5 % CO_2 in humidified air.
5. Wash T2 cells once with cold (4 °C) PBA: 0.9 % NaCl, 0.5 % BSA, 0.02 % NaN_3, or FACS buffer.
6. Stain T2 cells with the first antibody BB7.2 (HLA-A*0201-specific mAb).
7. Incubate for 30 min at 4 °C.
8. Wash 2× with cold PBA.
9. Stain T2 cells with FITC-labeled $F(ab')_2$ fragments of goat anti-mouse IgG as the second antibody.
10. Incubate for another 30 min at 4 °C.
11. Wash the cells 1×.
12. Measure the fluorescence at 488 nm on a FACScan flow cytometer.
13. Quantify the HLA-A*0201 expression according to the following formula:

$$\frac{\textit{Mean fluorescence with peptide} - \textit{Mean fluorescence without peptide}}{\textit{Mean fluorescence without peptide}} \times 100.$$

3.7 Stability of Multiple Peptide Cocktail

1. Wash the multiple peptide-pulsed T2 cells.
2. Incubate with BFA at 3 μg/mL to block the protein transport of newly synthesized HLA-A*0201 molecules.
3. Stain the cells with BB7.2 HLA-A*0201 mAb and FITC-labeled $F(ab')_2$ fragments of goat anti-mouse IgG sequentially at 0, 2, 4, 6, and 14 h post-BFA treatment.
4. Measure the peptide/HLA-A*0201 complex stability by flow cytometry.

3.8 DC Pulsing by Multiple Peptide Cocktail

1. Prepare 2×10^5 cells/mL in IMDM with 10 % FBS in each 15-mL tube.
2. Pulse the cells with multiple peptides at a concentration of 25–40 μg/mL (6.25–10 μg/peptide/mL) (*see* **Note 5**).
3. Incubate the cells for 2–4 h at 37 °C with multiple peptides and swing slightly every 30 min.
4. Harvest cells into a 15-mL conical tube and wash 2× using IMDM with 10 % FBS.
5. Count the cells.

3.9 DC Harvest and Storage

1. Spin the cells at $335\times g$ for 5 min at room temperature or 21 °C (acceleration, 5; deceleration, 0).
2. Prepare labeled cryotubes and store at 2–8 °C.
3. Resuspend the cells with 0.5 mL 2× cold freezing medium A.

4. Pipette 0.5 mL of DC in 2× cold freezing medium A into each cryotube and add 0.5 mL of 2× cold freezing medium B for a final concentration of 10^6 DC/mL.
5. Keep cryo 1 °C freezer container at −80 °C for at least 2 h or overnight.
6. Store DC in the vapor phase of liquid nitrogen.

3.10 Phenotypic Analysis of Multiple Peptide-Pulsed DC

Perform flow cytometric analysis of mDC. Stain the cells separately with mouse antihuman CD80 mAb conjugated with PE, mouse antihuman CD83 mAb conjugated with FITC, mouse antihuman CD86 mAb conjugated with PE, and mouse antihuman CCR7 mAb conjugated with FITC.

3.11 In Vitro Induction of Multiple Peptide-Specific CTL

1. Multiple peptide-specific CTL are generated ex vivo by repeated multiple peptide stimulation of $CD3^+$ T lymphocytes from HLA-A*0201 donors.
2. Harvest 2×10^5 cells/mL mDC to polypropylene tubes.
3. Wash thoroughly to remove all the cytokines.
4. Add multiple peptide at a concentration of 25–40 μg/mL (6.25–10 μg/peptide/mL) to mDC (*see* **Note 6**).
5. Incubate at 37 °C for 2–3 h.
6. Wash thoroughly to remove unbound peptides.
7. Resuspend the mDC in 1 mL of CTL medium.
8. Prepare 2×10^6 cells/mL $CD3^+$ T cells from the same (autologous) donor in 1 mL of CTL medium.
9. Plate mDC at 2×10^5 cells/mL/well in 24-well plates.
10. Add 2×10^6 cells/mL/well $CD3^+$ T cells in 24-well plates.
11. Co-culture mDC and $CD3^+$ T cells for 3 days.
12. After 3 days, add 25 ng/mL of rhIL-2 and 10 ng/mL of rhIL-7. The cells usually need to be fed with 50 % of fresh 25 ng/mL of rhIL-2-containing and 10 ng/mL of rhIL-7-containing medium every 2 days and transferred to new wells. The cultures reach quiescence about day 10–14 and need to be restimulated.
13. At 10–12 days after the first stimulation, restimulate the cells with irradiated (20 Gy), multiple peptide-pulsed autologous PBMC (at 1:1 ratio), with multiple peptide-pulsed T2 cells (at 2:1 ratio) or DC (at 10:1 ratio) (*see* **Note 7**).
14. The cells should be expanded for another 10–14 days in the presence of 25 ng/mL rhIL-2. This restimulation step allows the demonstration of the CTL activity induced by mDC and facilitates ELISPOT analysis of antigen-specific responses by reducing the nonspecific background. At days 20–24 (10–12 days after the second stimulation), the frequency of antigen-specific T cells is analyzed by IFN-γ ELISPOT according to the manufacturer's instructions (*see* **Note 8**).

4 Notes

1. Standard isotonic Percoll (SIP) solution and 10× concentrated "acidic" PBS can be used to isolate PBMC (the fraction of monocytes and lymphocytes) from the fresh blood [21].
2. It is important to select a batch of FBS and the source of medium. There can be significant differences between several different batches of FBS in their ability to support the DC1 maturation. DC1s are DC which can effectively elicit type 1 cytotoxic T lymphocytes (Tc1) production of high IFN-γ and low IL-4. The source of medium can make a difference as well.
3. Usually, naïve (unmodified) and/or heteroclitic (enhanced) nonapeptide can be used in multiple peptide cocktails. Heteroclitic peptides can be made by replacing one amino acid with the other different amino acid [22].
4. The sequence of multiple peptides from several tumor-associated antigens, which are associated with tumor pathogenesis and are highly expressed on the tumor cells, can be reviewed for peptides that could potentially bind to HLA-A*0201 using a peptide-binding database. After comparing the predictive binding scores, several peptide candidates are selected that could potentially bind with HLA-A*0201 molecules [5, 22].
5. If multiple peptides are applied, use one culture dish or one polypropylene tube for each peptide.
6. To avoid potential competition in HLA-A*0201 affinity among the specific peptides, do not avoid excess concentration of multiple peptide, e.g., 24–40 μg/mL total, 6.25–10 μg/peptide, to pulse the DC during CTL generation.
7. Cultures can be restimulated every 7–10 days with irradiated multiple peptide-loaded T2 cells, PBMC, or DC for a total of 2–4 cycles to generate multiple peptide-specific CTL.
8. In order to further characterize the function of antigen-specific CTL, MHC class I peptide multimer (tetramer) staining and cytolytic assays are available.

Acknowledgments

This study was financially supported by grant no. 2011-0005285 from General Researcher Program Type II of the National Research Foundation of Korea; grant no. RTI05-01-01 from the Regional Technology Innovation Program of the Ministry of Commerce, Industry and Energy; grant no. A000200058 from the Regional Industrial Technology Development program of the Ministry of Knowledge and Economy; grant no. 1120390 from the National

R&D Program for Cancer Control, Ministry for Health and Welfare; and grant no. 2011-0030034 from Leading Foreign Research Institute Recruitment Program through the National Research Foundation of Korea (NRF) funded by the Ministry of Education, Science and Technology (MEST), Republic of Korea.

References

1. Steinman RM (1991) The dendritic cell system and its role in immunogenicity. Annu Rev Immunol 9:271–296
2. Fong L, Engleman EG (2000) Dendritic cells in cancer immunotherapy. Annu Rev Immunol 18:245–273
3. Nestle FO, Farkas A, Conrad C (2005) Dendritic-cell-based therapeutic vaccination against cancer. Curr Opin Immunol 17: 163–169
4. Yang DH et al (2010) Alpha-type 1-polarized dendritic cells loaded with apoptotic allogeneic myeloma cell line induce strong CTL responses against autologous myeloma cells. Ann Hematol 89:795–801
5. Lee HJ et al (2012) Identification of novel HLA-A*0201-restricted epitopes from anterior gradient-2 as a tumor-associated antigen against colorectal cancer. Cell Mol Immunol 9: 175–183
6. Lee HJ et al (2012) In vitro induction of anterior gradient-2-specific cytotoxic T lymphocytes by dendritic cells transduced with recombinant adenoviruses as a potential therapy for colorectal cancer. Exp Mol Med 44:60–67
7. Nguyen-Pham TN et al (2012) Cellular immunotherapy using dendritic cells against multiple myeloma. Korean J Hematol 47:17–27
8. Mayordomo J et al (1995) Bone marrow-derived dendritic cells pulsed with synthetic tumour peptides elicit protective and therapeutic antitumour immunity. Nat Med 1:1297–1302
9. Nair SK et al (2000) Induction of cytotoxic T cell responses and tumor immunity against unrelated tumors using telomerase reverse transcriptase RNA transfected dendritic cells. Nat Med 6:1011–1017
10. Hsu FJ et al (1996) Vaccination of patients with B-cell lymphoma using autologous antigen-pulsed dendritic cells. Nat Med 2:52–58
11. Nestle FO et al (1998) Vaccination of melanoma patients with peptide- or tumor lysate-pulsed dendritic cells. Nat Med 4:328–332
12. Ahmad M et al (2004) Escape from immunotherapy: possible mechanisms that influence tumor regression/progression. Cancer Immunol Immunother 53:844–854
13. Waeckerle-Men Y et al (2006) Dendritic cell-based multi-epitope immunotherapy of hormone-refractory prostate carcinoma. Cancer Immunol Immunother 55:1524–1533
14. Bae J et al (2012) Myeloma-specific multiple peptides able to generate cytotoxic T lymphocytes: a potential therapeutic application in multiple myeloma and other plasma cell disorders. Clin Cancer Res 18:4850–4860
15. Fuessel S et al (2006) Vaccination of hormone-refractory prostate cancer patients with peptide cocktail-loaded dendritic cells: results of a phase I clinical trial. Prostate 66:811–821
16. Mailliard RB et al (2004) alpha-type-1 polarized dendritic cells: a novel immunization tool with optimized CTL-inducing activity. Cancer Res 64:5934–5937
17. Cella M et al (1996) Ligation of CD40 on dendritic cells triggers production of high levels of interleukin-12 and enhances T cell stimulatory capacity: T-T help via APC activation. J Exp Med 184:747–752
18. Fanslow WC et al (1994) Structural characteristics of CD40 ligand that determine biological function. Semin Immunol 6:267–278
19. Kalinski P et al (1999) Final maturation of dendritic cells is associated with impaired responsiveness to IFN-gamma and to bacterial IL-12 inducers: decreased ability of mature dendritic cells to produce IL-12 during the interaction with Th cells. J Immunol 162:3231–3236
20. Nijman HW et al (1993) Identification of peptide sequences that potentially trigger HLA-A2.1-restricted cytotoxic T lymphocytes. Eur J Immunol 23:1215–1219
21. Kalinski P et al (2010) Generation of stable Th1/CTL-, Th2-, and Th17-inducing human dendritic cells. Methods Mol Biol 595: 117–133
22. Qian J et al (2007) Dickkopf-1 (DKK1) is a widely expressed and potent tumor-associated antigen in multiple myeloma. Blood 110: 1587–1594

Chapter 3

Pulsing Dendritic Cells with Whole Tumor Cell Lysates

Laura Alaniz, Manglio M. Rizzo, and Guillermo Mazzolini

Abstract

One of the strategies employed in immunotherapy for cancer is to use of ex vivo-generated dendritic cells (DC) pulsed with tumor antigens. Several approaches have been used to obtain and load tumor antigens in DC. One such technique is to use whole tumor cell lysate from one or more tumor cell lines of the tumor type to be treated. The advantage of applying this method is that it provides a large spectrum of tumor antigens. However, some considerations must be taken into account to obtain a lysate with appropriate biological activity, such as cell line harvest and the method to lyse the cells. In this chapter, we describe the steps to obtain whole tumor cell lysates from human tumor cell lines by repetitive freeze–thaw cycles in sufficient amount and quality to pulse DC.

Key words Tumor antigens, Hepatocellular carcinoma cell lines, Whole tumor cell lysate, Necrotic cells, Antigen pulsing, Immunotherapy

1 Introduction

The efficiency of using DC as a tool to treat cancer depends on their capability to activate the specific host's T cells against tumor antigens [1]. Despite the fact that tumor-associated antigens (TAA) or tumor-specific antigens (TSA) have been identified for several tumors [2], it is still necessary to perform a full characterization of their capability to induce an active immune response. The use of only 1 TAA or TSA is frequently unable to generate a potent immune response; therefore, using poly-antigenic sources is a good approach for loading DC. A method to cover a wide range of antigens is through the use of allogeneic tumor cell lines. The mix obtained contains not only proteins but also other molecules which are able to induce a potent immune response, such as RNA, DNA, and cellular components [3]. Established tumor cell lines that share one or even several tumor antigens provide a simple source of delivering antigens in tumor immunotherapy. Another advantage that this method offers is the possibility to obtain standardized and controlled preparations to be used clinically under good

Michael J.P. Lawman and Patricia D. Lawman (eds.), *Cancer Vaccines: Methods and Protocols*, Methods in Molecular Biology, vol. 1139, DOI 10.1007/978-1-4939-0345-0_3, © Springer Science+Business Media New York 2014

manufacturing practice (GMP) [4, 5]. However, the method to yield the lysates may affect the efficacy of tumor vaccines, and data about preparation methods are controversial [6, 7]. The quality of tumor cell lysates is dependent on how the cells are harvested, the concentration of cells, and the method used to lyse the cells. For example, it is well known that trypsinization as a method to harvest adherent tumor cells could affect immunogenicity and biologic activity of tumor lysates by degradation of important protein antigens [6]. Here, we describe the principal steps in harvesting cells cycles from human adherent tumor cell lines grown as monolayer and obtaining whole tumor lysates by repetitive freeze–thaw in adequate concentration and sterility to pulse ex vivo-generated peripheral blood monocyte-derived DC. Finally, these DC present an adequate maturation status to induce a potent immune response. Thus, we use the direct coculture of lysates with DC for loading tumor antigens into the cells in order to develop an anticancer immunotherapy.

2 Materials

Use all reagents and culture medium at room temperature and under sterile conditions.

2.1 Tumor Cell Extract

1. Hep3B and Huh7 hepatocellular carcinoma (HCC) tumor cell lines passaged to 80–90 % confluency and a viability of greater than 90 % (*see* **Note 1**).
2. 0.9 % sterile saline solution (NaCl).
3. Sterile 2 mM ethylenediaminetetraacetic acid (EDTA) in saline solution.
4. Cell scrapers.
5. Liquid nitrogen container.
6. Thermostat-controlled water bath.
7. 50-mL conical centrifuge tubes.
8. 0.22-μm (Millipore Express®) filters low-binding protein membrane.
9. Temperature-controlled centrifuge (ThermoElectron Centra CL3R with 243 horizontal rotor or equivalent).
10. Coomassie blue protein assay kit.

2.2 Pulsing DC with Tumor Lysate

1. Dendritic cell suspension (monocyte-derived DC) [7, 8].
2. Complete culture medium: serum-free AIMV medium, 100 U/mL of penicillin, 100 μg/mL of streptomycin, 350 ng/mL of macrophage colony-stimulating factor (GM-CSF), and 500 IU/mL of human recombinant interleukin-4 (IL-4).

3. 0.05 M β_2 mercaptoethanol.
4. Humidified 37 °C and 5 % CO_2 incubator.

2.3 Counting Viable Cells

1. Neubauer cell counting chamber.
2. Trypan blue solution.

3 Methods

Work at all times under sterile conditions using a level II biosafety laminar flow cabinet.

3.1 Necrotic Tumor Cell Lysates from Tumor Cell Lines

1. Remove medium from culture dish by aspiration; wash the monolayer cells 2× with saline. Place the culture dishes on ice (*see* **Note 2**).
2. Using the plastic cell scraper, scrape the confluent monolayer of adherent cells and harvest. Collect the cell suspension in a 50-mL conical centrifuge tube (*see* **Note 3**). Centrifuge at 530×*g* at 4 °C for 5 min. Wash cells 2× and resuspend in 2.5 mL of saline per 5×10^7 cells.
3. Cells can be detached and harvested using sterile 10 mL/148 cm^2 of 2 mM EDTA solution in a Petri dish accompanied by gentle rocking to remove the cells from the dish (*see* **Note 4**). Collect the cell suspension in a 50-mL conical centrifuge tube (*see* **Note 3**). Centrifuge at 530×*g* at 4 °C for 5 min. Wash cells 2× and resuspend in 2.5 mL of saline per 5×10^7 cells.
4. Disrupt the cell suspension by freezing at −196 °C (in a liquid nitrogen container) followed by thawing at 37 °C in a prewarmed water bath for 5 min. Repeat this freeze/thaw procedure 5× in rapid succession.
5. Centrifuge at 97×*g* at 18–20 °C for 10 min to remove large particles of cellular debris. Filter the supernatant with a 0.22-μm sterile low protein-binding filter unit (*see* **Note 5**).
6. Measure protein concentration using the Bradford method (*see* **Note 6**).
7. Aliquot the cell lysate and store at −80 °C until needed.

3.2 Pulsing DC

1. Incubate $1–5 \times 10^6$ dendritic cells in 1 mL of complete culture medium directly with 500 μg of tumor cell extract for 12 h in a humidified incubator at 37 °C and 5 % CO_2 before checking viability using the Trypan blue dye exclusion test (*see* **Note 7**).
2. Following the pulsing with antigen, the DC are centrifuged at 530×*g* for 10 min at 18–20 °C. The cells are resuspended in 0.9 % saline solution and centrifuged again under the same centrifugation parameters. This washing step is repeated 2×.

3. Following the washing step, the cells are finally resuspended in 0.9 % sterile saline solution and checked for viability using the Trypan blue exclusion test (*see* **Note 8**). These antigen-pulsed DC are ready to use for subsequent immune assays.

4 Notes

1. For cells growing in suspension culture, take into account the cell density and viability.
2. Ice helps to easily harvest the cells using scrapers or EDTA, avoiding the use of trypsin which could degrade some cell surface proteins or peptides.
3. Although the final volume is 5 mL, we use a 50-mL conical centrifuge tube given that it facilitates sample handling in the following steps.
4. 2 mM EDTA solution is an alternative method to harvest cells. Keep the solution on ice in order to provide satisfactory cell detachment.
5. Carry out the filtration gently to prevent the filter from clogging, since the final suspension has a concentration of proteins and other cellular components. We use a polyethersulfone filter which has a low protein-binding capability to prevent protein loss.
6. The Bradford assay measures only protein concentration, but the lysates contain other components which cannot be measured by this method. The yield of proteins depends on the tumor cell quantity and type. We obtain approximately 5 mg of total protein from 5×10^7 tumor cells.
7. The DC were generated following the protocol described by Mazzolini et al. [8]. Six-day post-cultured DC are used in the pulsing with tumor cell lysates. Once the lysate is added, the DC cultures are further incubated for 24 h with the differentiation factors, GM-CSF, and IL-4. To avoid large dilution of the culture, the final volume should not exceed 1.5 mL.
8. In order to obtain a potent response, viability of the DC must be greater than 90 %. Furthermore, the phenotype and the maturation stage of the DC should be tested by flow cytometry using antibodies directed against cell surface and co-stimulator markers, e.g., CD11c, HLA-DR, CD80, and CD86.

Acknowledgement

This work was supported by grants from Austral University, Agencia Nacional de Promoción Científica y Tecnológica, Argentina.

References

1. Palucka K, Banchereau J (2012) Cancer immunotherapy via dendritic cells. Nat Rev Cancer 12:265–277
2. Novellino L et al (2005) A listing of human tumor antigens recognized by T cells: March 2004 update. Cancer Immunol Immunother 54:187–207
3. Chiang CL et al (2010) Whole tumor antigen vaccines. Semin Immunol 22:132–143
4. Ribas A et al (2010) Multicenter phase II study of matured dendritic cells pulsed with melanoma cell line lysates in patients with advanced melanoma. J Transl Med 8:89
5. Prins RM et al (2011) Gene expression profile correlates with t-cell infiltration and relative survival in glioblastoma patients vaccinated with dendritic cell immunotherapy. Clin Cancer Res 17:1603–1615
6. Herzog GI et al (2011) Quality of tumor lysates used for pulsing dendritic cells is influenced by the method used to harvest adherent tumor cells. BMC Res Notes 4:153
7. Schuler G et al (1995) Production and properties of large numbers of dendritic cells from human blood. In: Banchereau J, Schmitt D (eds) Dendritic cells in fundamental and clinical immunology. Springer, New York, pp 43–52
8. Mazzolini G et al (2005) Intratumoral injection of dendritic cells engineered to secrete interleukin-12 by recombinant adenovirus in patients with metastatic gastrointestinal carcinomas. J Clin Oncol 23:999–1010

Chapter 4

Antigen Trapping by Dendritic Cells for Antitumor Therapy

Chiranjib Pal

Abstract

Dendritic cells (DC) are potent antigen-presenting cells (APC) that are capable of stimulating both naive CD4+ T helper cells and CD8+ cytotoxic T cells. Therefore, DC are being extensively evaluated as vehicles for antigen delivery in immunotherapies for the treatment of patients with cancer. Many techniques have been used to load DC with tumor-associated antigens (TAA), including pulsing with synthetic peptides that represent T cell epitopes. This strategy has been used in several human clinical vaccination trials; however, it is limited to patients who express the particular peptide MHC-restricting molecule. Alternatively, DC have been pulsed with recombinant proteins or transduced with recombinant viruses. These approaches circumvent the MHC restrictions associated with peptides but are generally limited to individual proteins. Because many tumors display heterogenous expression of target antigens, strategies that induce T cell responses against multiple proteins may be more efficacious. Another concern is that some of these antigen-loading techniques facilitate the presentation of immunogenic viral or bacterial epitopes in addition to those from the tumor-associated protein.

Key words Dendritic cells, Immunotherapy, Cancer, Tumor antigens, Antigen pulsing

1 Introduction

Developing more effective anticancer vaccines has been one of the major goals of cancer immunotherapy. Recent advances in generation and manipulation of DC provide opportunities to design powerful tumor vaccines. DC are ideal vehicles for polyvalent tumor vaccination as they readily process and present tumor antigen taken up from dying tumor cells. DC pulsed with apoptotic tumor cells have been used successfully to induce tumor vaccination [1–4], although controversy surrounds the ability of necrotic versus apoptotic tumor cells to serve as a source of multivalent antigen to pulse DC [5, 6].

Several reports have described the use of tumor-extracted RNA as source of tumor antigen for the preparation of DC and have indicated its potential use for antigen-specific or polyvalent tumor vaccination in the absence of identified tumor antigens [7, 8]. Such an approach may address important limitations in the

Michael J.P. Lawman and Patricia D. Lawman (eds.), *Cancer Vaccines: Methods and Protocols*, Methods in Molecular Biology, vol. 1139, DOI 10.1007/978-1-4939-0345-0_4, © Springer Science+Business Media New York 2014

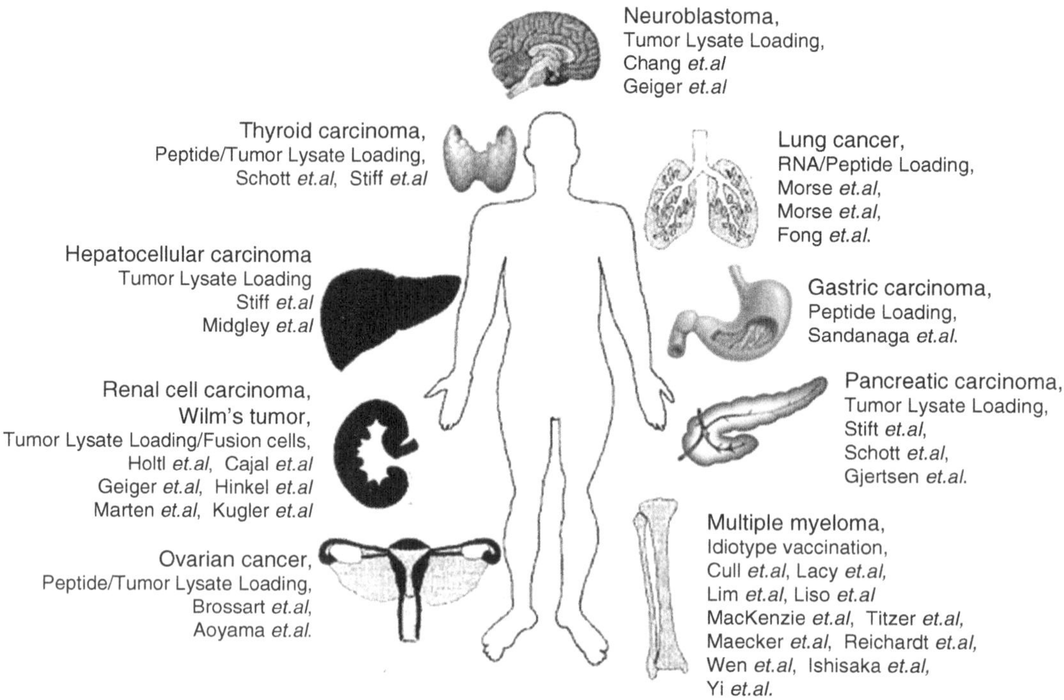

Fig. 1 Cancer indications tested in human immunotherapeutic trials using ex vivo-generated dendritic cells

procurement of tumor antigen since primary tumor cell cultures may not be feasible for a large number of patients.

Numerous DC-based immunotherapeutic trials with ex vivo-generated DC (Fig. 1) aiming for the initiation or amelioration of antitumor T cell immunity have been performed for a wide range of tumors and recently reviewed [9–12]. In some of these trials, clinical responses were reported, and in a few selected ones, the induction or enhancement of tumor-specific T cells has been demonstrated. The antigen-loading methods applied in most trials to achieve the major histocompatibility complex (MHC)-restricted presentation of tumor antigen were either peptide pulsing, involving immune-dominant sequences of defined TAAs, or different whole tumor cell preparations. The synthesis of large quantities of clinical grade eight- to ten-amino-acid-long peptides that fit into the MHC class I groove is technically rather easy, and peptide pulsing of DC populations is thus a method to achieve the desired TAA presentation. It has been shown that peptide-pulsed DC expand peptide-specific cytotoxic T lymphocytes (CTL) in healthy subjects [13] and melanoma patients [14]. However, there are certain caveats with this approach. The longevity of MHC-peptide complexes in vivo is unknown; the affinity of peptides for their various

HLA molecules varies; competition between peptides may affect immunogenicity; MHC class II-restricted epitopes for activation of $CD4^+$ T cells are still scarce, and the approach is inherently tailored for individuals as it is dependent upon the HLA type.

In contrast to peptide pulsing, using whole tumor cell preparations for DC loading avoids the need for detailed tumor analysis and individual HLA typing as it is assumed that tumor antigens, including as yet undefined TAA and rare mutations, will be presented on MHC class I and II molecules by autologous DC. The latter argument is of special importance as in principle, it is desirable to aim for the parallel presentation of HLA class I- and II-restricted antigens since the absence of $CD4^+$ helper cells affects the generation of long-term $CD8^+$ T cell memory [15], and $CD4^+$ helper T cells are considered important for effective antitumor immune responses [16].

Interest in DC maturation stems from the rationale that mature DC should function as more potent antigen-presenting cells and stimulators of tumor-specific immunity than immature DC. However, the definition of a "mature" DC remains the subject of ongoing debate and further investigation [17]. While the maturation state of DC may be defined phenotypically, based on markers expressed on the cell surface, maturation may also be defined functionally, e.g., based on the ability to secrete cytokines or induce antigen-specific T cell responses. DC may be matured phenotypically using a variety of stimuli such as TNF-α, CD40 ligand (CD40L), bacillus Calmette-Guerin (BCG), lipopolysaccharide, calcium ionophores, or other agents. Interestingly, while single agents have the capacity to induce the upregulation of cell surface maturation markers such as CD83, combinations of signals appear to be necessary to induce fully functional maturation as defined by IL-12 production and the ability to induce antigen-specific T cell responses [18–20]. Consequently, there has been growing interest in identifying optimal combinations of factors to induce functional DC maturation [17].

2 Materials

2.1 Buffer

1. For 1 L of phosphate-buffered saline (PBS), mix 8 g of NaCl, 0.2 g of KCl, 1.44 g of Na_2HPO_4, and 0.24 g of KH_2PO_4.
2. Dissolve salts in 800 mL of distilled water.
3. Adjust to pH 7.4 with HCl.
4. Add water to 1 L. Dispense into aliquots.
5. Sterilize by autoclaving.
6. For PBS/FBS: sterile PBS, fetal bovine serum (FBS) to a final concentration of 2 %.

2.2 Media for Cell Culture

1. Add 700 mL of distilled water to 15.8 g of Roswell Park Memorial Institute (RPMI)-1640 powder medium (or as specified by the manufacturer for 1 L final volume).
2. Add 2 0 mL of 10 % sodium bicarbonate ($NaHCO_3$): 10 g of $NaHCO_3$, 90 mL of double-distilled water for 100 mL of 10 % $NaHCO_3$.
3. Filter $NaHCO_3$ with 0.45-μm-pore-size membrane.
4. Add 200 mM of l-glutamine to a final concentration of 1 %.
5. Add 10 mL of PenStrep stock: 10,000 IU of penicillin and 10,000 mg/mL of streptomycin.
6. Add 160 mL of distilled water.
7. Adjust the pH 7.2–7.4. If pH is high, adjust it with 1 N HCl; if pH is low, adjust it with 1 N NaOH.
8. Sterilize by filtering through a filter with 0.22-μm pore size using vacuum air pump.
9. Add 100 mL of FBS.

2.3 Cytokines

1. Granulocyte-macrophage colony-stimulating factor (GM-CSF).
2. Interleukin-4 (IL-4).
3. Tumor necrosis factor-alpha (TNF-α).

2.4 Miscellaneous

1. Histopaque-1077.
2. 15-mL and 50-mL conical tubes.

3 Methods

3.1 Sourcing DC

DC comprises less than 1 % of mononuclear cells in the peripheral blood [21]. Leukapheresis can be used to isolate approximately 10^6–10^7 DC and may be adapted with positive or negative selection techniques. While the direct isolation of DC from peripheral blood allows rapid preparation of DC, it may require repeated leukapheresis if multiple immunizations are required in a protocol. This can present a significant problem, particularly for those cancer patients with functionally defective or decreased numbers of DC [22, 23]. An alternative method of preparing DC is to generate them ex vivo. Most commonly, DC are cultivated from peripheral blood monocytes or $CD34^+$ hematopoietic precursors. DC precursors may be enriched from peripheral blood mononuclear cells by techniques such as plastic adherence, density gradient centrifugation, positive selection of $CD14^+$ cells, negative selection of B and T cells, and/or elutriation.

1. Pipet 5 mL of Histopaque-1077 into a 15-mL conical tube.
2. Overlay Histopaque-1077 with 10 mL of blood and centrifuge at 750×*g* for 20 min at 20 °C in a swinging-bucket rotor without brake [interphase must not be disturbed].
3. Remove the upper layer leaving the mononuclear cell layer undisturbed at the interphase. Carefully transfer the interphase cells (lymphocytes and monocytes) to a new 50-mL conical tube in chilled PBS.
4. Add PBS/BSA to 50-mL mark, mix, and centrifuge at 350×*g* for 10 min at 4 °C. Remove the supernatant carefully.
5. Resuspend the cell pellet in 25 mL of PBS/BSA and centrifuge at 160×*g* for 15 min at 4 °C. Remove the supernatant carefully.
6. Resuspend the cell pellet in 25 mL of PBS/BSA and centrifuge at 300×*g* for 10 min at 4 °C. Remove the supernatant carefully.
7. Resuspend cell pellet in 5 mL of PBS/BSA and count the cells.
8. Plate 1–1.5 × 10^6 PBMC in a T162 flask with 25 mL of complete RPMI-1640 medium.
9. Incubate for 2–3 h in a humidified 37 °C incubator with 5 % CO_2.
10. Discard medium containing nonadherent cells.
11. Add 25 mL of RPMI-1640 supplemented with 50 ng/mL of GM-CSF and 100–200 ng/mL of IL-4. Cell density should be adjusted between 1 and 3 × 10^5/mL.
12. Culture cells in a humidified incubator at 37 °C with 5 % CO_2 for 6 days. Replacing medium once after 3 days with fresh RPMI-1640 supplemented with 50 ng/mL of GM-CSF and 100–200 ng/mL of IL-4 is recommended. Save all nonadherent or loosely adherent cells by centrifuging the removed culture medium for 10 min at 200×*g* and adding the pellet to the fresh culture medium.
13. After 6 days, the loosely adherent or nonadherent cells, approximately 3–6 × 10^6 per T162, should display typical dendritic cell morphology and surface markers (CD1a, CD80, CD86, HLA-DR). If possible, check an aliquot of cells for expression of these markers.

3.2 Preparation of Whole Tumor Lysates

1. Take tumor materials at a concentration of 10^7 cells per mL in PBS. In case of tumor masses from patients or animals, tease the tumor materials in PBS to get single cell suspension (10^7 cells per mL) and pass it through cheesecloth to avoid the large masses.
2. Treat the cells with five cycles of heating and freezing in a 15-mL centrifuge tube. One cycle consists of 10 min at room temperature and successional 1 min in liquid nitrogen.

3. Use an ultrasonic homogenizer to dissolve the clots of cell components.
4. Irradiate the lysates with 12,000 rad (120 Gy) to avoid the live cells, if any.
5. Pass through a syringe-driven 0.2-μm filter to obtain the sterile whole tumor lysate.

3.3 Pulsing DC with Tumor Lysates

1. Take DC cultures containing 10^7–10^8 cells and wash in complete RPMI-1640.
2. Pulse the cells with 50 μg/mL tumor lysate overnight for 18 h at 37 °C and 5 % CO_2.
3. Mature the dendritic cells by adding 10–50 ng/mL of TNF-α to the culture and incubating for 1 or 2 more days. Mature dendritic cells should display CD83 as an additional surface marker and upregulation of HLA-DR, CD80, and CD86.
4. Maturation of DC after tumor lysate pulsing is recommended as immature DC are inefficient in providing signals to T cells compared to mature DC (*see* **Note 1**).

4 Notes

1. Because a large number of tumor antigens and antigenic epitopes have been defined, loading DC with specific tumor antigen proteins or immunodominant peptides is feasible and represents a widely utilized approach. Advantages of loading DC with a specific peptide include the following: (1) because peptide epitopes are precisely defined, specific immune responses may be monitored easily; (2) the immunodominant epitope(s) can be targeted specifically in an effort to enhance vaccine potency; (3) most peptides can be produced in large quantities adequate for performance of clinical trials; (4) peptide sequences can be modified easily to enhance binding to MHC molecules and/or immunogenicity. The use of whole proteins also offers a number of advantages: (1) proteins may contain multiple immunogenic epitopes; (2) whole proteins should incorporate both class I- and class II-restricted epitopes; and (3) proteins, in contrast to peptides, are not restricted to specific HLA types. Unfortunately, whole protein tumor antigens may be difficult to produce in large quantities. Several ongoing challenges remain before truly efficacious dendritic cell vaccines will be available for the treatment of cancer. The first is to understand the key immunoregulatory processes at the molecular level so that they can be modulated in a predictable manner. The second is to identify, optimize, and determine the appropriate combination of molecular signals that results in

the induction of potent and clinically significant antitumor immunity. The third is to develop standard cellular processing and immune monitoring methodologies that will make pivotal multicenter cancer vaccine trials feasible. Finally, the best vaccine candidates and most appropriate subset(s) of patients in whom to test each vaccine must be identified for testing in large-scale trials.

Acknowledgement

This work was supported by DBT grant BT/PR8217/MED/14/1239/2006 and ICMR grant 5/8-7(94)/2011-ECD-II.

References

1. Chen W et al (2006) Efficient induction of antitumor T cell immunity by exosomes derived from heat-shocked lymphoma cells. Eur J Immunol 36(6):1598–1607
2. Chen Z et al (2001) Efficient antitumor immunity derived from maturation of dendritic cells that had phagocytosed apoptotic/necrotic tumor cells. Int J Cancer 93(4):539–548
3. Henry F et al (1999) Antigen-presenting cells that phagocytose apoptotic tumor-derived cells are potent tumor vaccines. Cancer Res 59(14):3329–3332
4. Hoffmann TK et al (2000) Generation of tumor-specific T-lymphocytes by cross-priming with human dendritic cells ingesting apoptotic tumor cells. Cancer Res 60(13):3542–3549
5. Scheffer SR et al (2003) Apoptotic, but not necrotic, tumor cell vaccines induce a potent immune response in vivo. Int J Cancer 103(2):205–211
6. Basu S et al (2000) Necrotic but not apoptotic cell death releases heat shock proteins, which deliver a partial maturation signal to dendritic cells and activate the NF-kappa B pathway. Int Immunol 12(11):1539–1546
7. Boczkowski D et al (1996) Dendritic cells pulsed with RNA are potent antigen-presenting cells in vitro and in vivo. J Exp Med 184(2):465–472
8. Geiger C et al (2005) A generic RNA-pulsed dendritic cell vaccine strategy for renal cell carcinoma. J Transl Med 3(29):18–23
9. Fong L, Engleman EG (2000) Dendritic cells in cancer immunotherapy. Annu Rev Immunol 18:245–273
10. Banchereau J et al (2001) Dendritic cells as vectors for therapy. Cell 106:271–274
11. Jenne L, Bhardwaj N (2001) Perspectives of DC based immunotherapies. In: DeVita VT, Hellman S, Rosenberg SA (eds) Principles and practice of oncology. Lippincott Williams & Wilkins, New York, USA, pp 1–15
12. Pal C et al (2007) Dendritic cells and antigen trapping technology—a revolution in vaccine/immunotherapy strategy. Indian J Exp Biol 45(6):491–504
13. Dhodapkar MV et al (1999) Rapid generation of broad T cell immunity in humans after a single injection of mature dendritic cells. J Clin Invest 104:173–180
14. Schuler-Thurner B et al (2000) Mage-3 and influenza-matrix peptide-specific cytotoxic T cells are inducible in terminal stage HLA-A2.1+ melanoma patients by mature monocyte-derived dendritic cells. J Immunol 165:349–3496
15. Zajac AJ et al (1998) Viral immune evasion due to persistence of activated T cells without effector function. J Exp Med 188:2205–2215
16. Toes RE et al (1999) CD4 T cells and their role in antitumor immune responses. J Exp Med 189:753–756
17. Morse MA et al (2002) Dendritic cell maturation in active immunotherapy strategies. Expert Opin Biol Ther 2:35–43
18. Snijders A et al (1998) High-level IL-12 production by human dendritic cells requires two signals. Int Immunol 10:1593–1598
19. Mosca PJ et al (2002) A subset of human monocyte-derived dendritic cells expresses high levels of interleukin-12 in response to combined CD40 ligand and interferon-gamma treatment. Blood 96:3499–3504
20. Mosca PJ et al (2002) Multiple signals are required for maturation human dendritic cells

mobilized in vivo with Flt3-ligand. J Leukoc Biol 72:546–553
21. Fearnley DB et al (1999) Monitoring human blood dendritic cell numbers in normal individuals and in stem cell transplantation. Blood 93:728–736
22. Ratta M et al (2002) Dendritic cells are functionally defective in multiple myeloma: the role of interleukin-6. Blood 100:230–237
23. Gabrilovich DI et al (1997) Decreased antigen presentation by dendritic cells in patients with breast cancer. Clin Cancer Res 3:483–490

Chapter 5

Ex Vivo Loading of Autologous Dendritic Cells with Tumor Antigens

Manglio M. Rizzo, Laura Alaniz, and Guillermo Mazzolini

Abstract

Ex vivo-generated antigen-loaded dendritic cells (DC) have been shown to be immunogenic in patients with cancer. Loading DC with autologous whole tumor antigens is a strategy to arm DC against tumor without human leukocyte antigen (HLA) restriction. Furthermore, this approach allows the presentation of a full antigen range to the immune system. We describe the methods to obtain whole antigens from autologous tumor tissues in order to load DC generated ex vivo from patients with gastrointestinal cancer.

Key words Tumor specimen, Autologous tumor tissue, Immunotherapy, Tumor-associated antigens, Colon carcinoma

1 Introduction

The use of DC for cancer could require the ex vivo loading with tumor in order to induce a specific immune response against tumors [1, 2]. Antigens obtained from autologous tumor tissues could induce a broad response and cover a large variety of peptide–MHC complexes, providing sufficient amounts of a number of tumor antigens [3–5]. The type of tumor antigens delivered into DC is crucial to achieve a clinical response [6, 7]. Tumor-associated antigen (TAA) HLA-restricted immunodominant peptides are identified as the most widely used for tumor vaccination. However, this approach has several disadvantages: (1) only expressing specific HLA haplotypes are eligible, (2) immune responses are limited to the epitopes used for immunization and may be insufficient, and (3) longevity of MHC–peptide complexes in vivo is unknown [3, 8]. A hopeful alternative is loading ex vivo DC for vaccination using whole tumor lysates without defined antigens. Tumor tissues express a whole array of TAA and tumor-specific antigens that are

Michael J.P. Lawman and Patricia D. Lawman (eds.), *Cancer Vaccines: Methods and Protocols*, Methods in Molecular Biology, vol. 1139, DOI 10.1007/978-1-4939-0345-0_5, © Springer Science+Business Media New York 2014

both characterized and uncharacterized. These antigens are processed by immune cells expressing MHC II and I and promote the activation of both $CD8^+$ cytotoxic T and $CD4^+$ helper T cells against tumor cells [9]. Although whole tumor lysate may increase the risk of autoimmunity by shared epitopes, clinical studies have shown its safety [4, 10]. In our laboratory, we have applied a method to prepare autologous antigens from tumor tissue by mechanical disruption, freeze, and thawing to finally obtain an antigen suspension to load human DC by direct coculture.

2 Materials

Use all reagents and culture media at room temperature and in sterile conditions.

2.1 Tumor Extract

1. Fresh tumor specimen obtained under sterile conditions (*see* **Note 1**).
2. 100-mm Petri dishes.
3. Surgical scalpel blade #20.
4. 0.9 % NaCl saline solution.
5. Liquid nitrogen container.
6. Water bath with thermostat.
7. 50-mL sterile conical centrifuge tubes.
8. Thermo Electron Centra CL3R with 243 horizontal rotor (or equivalent temperature-controlled centrifuge).
9. 0.22-μm sterile, low-binding proteins filter unit.
10. Quick Start™ Bradford Coomassie protein assay kit (BioRad, Hercules, CA, USA).

2.2 Pulsing Dendritic Cells

1. Complete culture medium: liquid RPMI-1640, 100 U/mL of penicillin, 100 U/mL of streptomycin, 350 ng/mL of human recombinant GM-CSF, and 500 IU/mL of human recombinant IL-4.
2. 0.05-M 2β mercaptoethanol.
3. Humidified 37 °C, 5 % CO_2 incubator.

2.3 Counting Viable Cells

1. Neubauer chamber.
2. Trypan blue solution.

3 Methods

Work at all times in sterile conditions under biosafety level II.

3.1 Tumor Lysate from Fresh Tumor Tissue

1. Take approximately 5-mm^3 fresh tumor specimen in sterile conditions and place it in a sterile tube with 15-mL saline solution.
2. Place tumor tissue in a Petri dish and disperse it with needle and scalpels, adding a volume of saline solution until a suspension is obtained (*see* **Note 2**).
3. Collect the final suspension in a 50-mL conical centrifuge tube (*see* **Note 3**).
4. Disrupt suspension by freezing (−196 °C, in a liquid nitrogen container) and thawing (37 °C in a water bath) for 5 min each. Repeat this procedure 5× in rapid succession.
5. To remove large debris, centrifuge at 70×*g*, 18–20 °C for 10 min.
6. Filter the sample with a 0.22-μm sterile, low-binding proteins filter unit (*see* **Note 4**).
7. Quantify protein by Bradford or other method (*see* **Note 5**).
8. The resulting tumor lysate can be aliquoted and stored at −80 °C until needed.

3.2 Pulsing Dendritic Cells

1. Check viability by Trypan blue dye exclusion (*see* **Note 6**).
2. Incubate 1–5×10^6 DC in 1-mL complete culture medium with 200 μg of tumor extract for 12 h in a humidified 37 °C, 5 % CO_2 incubator.
3. Centrifuge for 10 min at 18–20 °C, at 390×*g*.
4. Resuspend the cells, count viable cells by Trypan blue, and use (*see* **Note 7**).

4 Notes

1. Patients who agree to participate in our study read and sign the corresponding informed consent prior to tissue sampling.
2. Carefully add 2–5-mL saline solution in small amounts in order to allow the total extract dispersion. The optimal final volume of the mix depends on the tumor size and quality. In general, with a tumor of 5 mm^3 in size, one can obtain 5 mL of a solution at final concentration around to 2 mg/mL.
3. Although the final volume is small, we use 50-mL conical centrifuge tubes given that their use facilitates handling of the sample in the following steps.

4. Given that final suspension has a high density of proteins and other cellular components, carry out the filtration gently to prevent filter getting clogged. We use polyethersulfone filters which have a low-protein-binding capability to prevent protein loss.
5. The Bradford assay measures only protein concentration. However, the tumor tissue lysate contains other components which cannot be measured by this method.
6. The DC were generated following protocol describe by Mazzolini [11]. DC are cocultured with tumor cells lysate at 6 day of DC culture, completing a culture of 7 day with differentiation factors GM-CSF and IL-4. Note that the final volume should not exceed 1.5 mL to avoid large dilution of the culture.
7. We observe that some tumor extract can modify DC viability after the coculture. Thus, we check DC viability which must be around 90 % in order to obtain a functional response. Further, DC markers and costimulator molecules are tested by flow cytometry for CD11c, HLA-DR, CD80, and CD86 in order to confirm maturation state.

Acknowledgement

This work was supported by grants from Austral University, Agencia Nacional de Promoción Científica y Tecnológica, Argentina.

References

1. Palucka K, Banchereau J (2012) Cancer immunotherapy via dendritic cells. Nat Rev Cancer 12:265–277
2. Schuler G et al (1995) Production and properties of large numbers of dendritic cells from human blood. In: Banchereau J, Schmitt D (eds) Dendritic cells in fundamental and clinical immunology. Springer, New York, USA, pp 43–52
3. Chiang CL et al (2010) Whole tumor antigen vaccines. Semin Immunol 22:132–143
4. Geiger JD (2001) Vaccination of pediatric solid tumor patients with tumor lysate-pulsed dendritic cells can expand specific T cells and mediate tumor regression. Cancer Res 61:8513–8519
5. Nestle FO (1998) Vaccination of melanoma patients with peptide- or tumor lysate-pulsed dendritic cells. Nat Med 4:328–332
6. Andersen BM, Ohlfest JR (2012) Increasing the efficacy of tumor cell vaccines by enhancing cross priming. Cancer Lett 325:155–164
7. Heath WR, Carbone FR (2001) Cross-presentation, dendritic cells, tolerance and immunity. Annu Rev Immunol 19:47–64
8. Novellino L et al (2005) A listing of human tumor antigens recognized by T cells: March 2004 update. Cancer Immunol Immunother 54:187–207
9. Bhardwaj N (2001) Processing and presentation of antigens by dendritic cells: implications for vaccines. Trends Mol Med 7:388–394
10. Iwashita Y et al (2003) A phase I study of autologous dendritic cell-based immunotherapy for patients with unresectable primary liver cancer. Cancer Immunol Immunother 52:155–161
11. Mazzolini G et al (2005) Intratumoral injection of dendritic cells engineered to secrete interleukin-12 by recombinant adenovirus in patients with metastatic gastrointestinal carcinomas. J Clin Oncol 23:999–1010

Chapter 6

Tumor Antigen-/Cytokine-Pulsed Dendritic Cells in Therapy Against Lymphoma

Sumit K. Hira, Deepak Verma, and Partha P. Manna

Abstract

Adoptive cell therapy using dendritic cells (DCs) is a strategy to deliver tumor antigens in cancer immunotherapy. Co-delivery of antigens to DC with essential components like genes encoding cytokines, chemokines, and other molecules or stimulation with recombinant cytokines is a potential method for designing an effective tumor vaccine protocol. Here, we describe the stimulation of purified splenic- or bone marrow-derived DC with recombinant interleukin-15 (IL-15) in the presence of intact soluble antigen from metastatic lymphoma tumor cells in an experimental animal model.

Key words Dendritic cells, Cytokines, Antigens, IL-15, Adoptive cell transfer, Kaplan–Meier survival curve, Tumor metastasis

1 Introduction

The key role of DC in the generation and regulation of T-cell immunity has led to attempts to target tumor antigens to DC. This includes both the generation and antigen loading of DC ex vivo prior to adoptive transfer and targeting DC directly in situ and is being increasingly appreciated to improve the efficacy of existing vaccine strategies [1]. Active immunization of DC via adoptive transfer has been facilitated by the development of newer methods of generating DC from blood monocytes or $CD34^+$ hematopoietic progenitors [2]. Advantages of ex vivo manipulation of DC include the control of DC quality, e.g., maturation status, DC subset, and expression of desired antigens. These studies have recognized the competence of these DC to stimulate both $CD4^+$ and $CD8^+$ T-cell responses in vivo, both in healthy volunteers and cancer patients [3, 4]. One of the concerns, however, is the use of peptide-pulsed DC against tumor. The duration and efficacy of the MHC-peptide complexes in vivo is unknown with

Michael J.P. Lawman and Patricia D. Lawman (eds.), *Cancer Vaccines: Methods and Protocols*, Methods in Molecular Biology, vol. 1139, DOI 10.1007/978-1-4939-0345-0_6, © Springer Science+Business Media New York 2014

variable affinities of peptides for diverse HLA molecules besides peptide competition which affects immunogenicity in several possible ways. This may demand detailed knowledge of HLA-restricted epitopes from tumor antigens, which could limit its application in many patients. Other approaches like loading tumor antigens to DC, use of viral vectors, tumor-derived RNA, DNA, immune complexes, apoptotic tumor cells, tumor cell lysates, or heat shock proteins may have significance considering the versatility of malignancy in different cancers [2, 5]. DC pulsed with killed autologous primary ovarian tumor cells induced antigen-specific T cells that secreted interferon-gamma (IFN-γ) upon stimulation with autologous tumor cells suggesting that antigen-pulsed DC may be a viable option for therapeutic vaccination against cancer [6, 7]. Because of their critical role in orchestrating the immune response, DCs are now widely applied in vaccines for the treatment of various cancers [8]. The vast majority of DC vaccination clinical trials have utilized autologous monocyte-derived DC with only few trials utilizing DC derived from $CD34^+$ precursors [8]. Nevertheless, this approach has been ineffective with respect to clinical efficacy [9]. Multiple hurdles like effective standardization of clinical trials, insufficient T-cell stimulatory phenotypes from advanced stage cancer patients, etc., have made it difficult for cancer patient to benefit from autologous DC precursor-based immunotherapies [10, 11].

One effective alternative is the use of allogeneic DC as vaccine vehicles. This approach has a higher degree of feasibility for preparing large clinical-grade batches that may be useful for all patients. This could provide a more standardized DC vaccine in terms of phenotype and maturation status, inducing stronger vaccine-specific immune responses [12]. Vaccination with allogeneic DC has reported to provide superior antitumor protection compared to syngeneic DC [13, 14]. Recently, we showed that adoptive cell therapy with allogeneic natural killer (NK) cells cured established infection with *Leishmania donovani* in susceptible mice [15].

Here, we will describe and demonstrate the approaches to load IL-15-stimulated DC from the bone marrow and spleen with tumor antigens that take advantage of the ability of DC to present tumor-derived antigens in an experimental lymphoma model. The Kaplan–Meier estimate of the survival probabilities suggests a very high survival in groups treated with antigen-pulsed IL-15-stimulated DC compared to others. Although several major gaps remain in our understanding of the mechanism of cross presentation by DC in vivo in humans, improved understanding of the process suggests several steps that might regulate the efficiency of DC as a cellular adjuvant.

2 Materials

Prepare all reagents and buffers in deionized double-distilled water and bring them at room temperature before use. Waste disposal should be conducted carefully as per institutional regulations.

2.1 Culture Medium, Antibodies, and Cytokines

1. Roswell Park Memorial Institute (RPMI)-1640 supplemented with 10 % fetal bovine serum (FBS), 100 U/mL of penicillin, and 100 μg/mL of streptomycin, henceforth referred to as complete medium.
2. 1× phosphate buffered saline (PBS) prepared in deionized double-distilled water.
3. GM-CSF diluted in PBS containing 2 % FBS and further diluted with complete medium.
4. IL-15 diluted in PBS containing 2 % FBS and further diluted with complete medium.
5. Anti-mouse MHC class I, MHC class II, CD11c, CD40, CD86, CD69, CD3, CD14, CD19, and CD56 monoclonal antibodies.
6. Dynal beads (Dynal M-450).
7. Trypan blue dye.
8. 6-well tissue culture plates.
9. Red blood cell (RBC) lysis buffer.
10. Collagenase D.

2.2 Tumor Antigens

1. Tumor cells should be cultured in complete medium, maintained at stationary phase at the time of antigen preparation, and kept mycoplasma-free.
2. Tumor cells should be passaged in normal mice in order to maintain the tumorigenic potential.
3. Labsonic 2000 sonifier (Bender & Hobein, Zurich, Switzerland).
4. Sodium dodecyl sulfate polyacrylamide gel electrophoresis (SDS-PAGE): 4.5 %, acrylamide/bis-acrylamide stacking gel and 12.5 % resolving gel with 0.5 M Tris–HCl, pH 6.8 and 1.5 M Tris–HCl, pH 8.8, respectively, 10 % ammonium persulfate, 0.1 % sodium dodecyl sulfate, 5 μL *N*,*N*,*N*′,*N*′-tetramethylethylenediamine (TEMED).
5. SDS-PAGE running buffer: 25 mM Tris–HCl, pH 8.3, 192 mM glycine, 0.1 % SDS.
6. Coomassie Brilliant Blue stain solution: 40 % methanol, 10 % acetic acid, 0.025 % Coomassie Brilliant Blue R-250.

2.3 Experimental Animals

1. Six–eight-week-old AKR, $H2^k$ female mice, kept at clean and in a pathogen-free condition.
2. Provide mice with a diet of standard mouse pellets and sterile water.
3. Statistical analysis software OriginPro 8 SR0 v8.0724 (B724) (Origin Lab Corporation, Northampton, MA, USA).

3 Methods

Carry out all procedures at room temperature unless otherwise specified. Animal experiments are to be carried out following the institutional regulations.

3.1 Preparation of DC from the Bone Marrow

1. Prepare single cell suspensions from the bone marrow in PBS. Lyse the RBC using 2 mL lysis buffer. Wash the cells 2× in complete medium, and count and set the concentration at 3×10^6 cells/mL (*see* **Note 1**).
2. Adhere the bone marrow cells in a 6-well plate for 4–6 h at 37 °C with 5 % CO_2. Remove the nonadherent cells by washing in 1× PBS and add fresh culture medium to the plate-bound adherent cells (*see* **Note 2**).
3. Culture the adherent cells in the presence of 1,000 U/mL GM-CSF. Replace the culture medium every other day with fresh supplements of GM-CSF (*see* **Note 3**).
4. The DC should grow the characteristic processes, visible from day 4, and become more conspicuous as the culture progresses (Fig. 1).
5. After 7 days, harvest the nonadherent cells and treat with saturating concentrations of anti-mouse CD3, CD14, CD19, and CD56, plus immunomagnetic Dynal beads to remove T cells, monocytes, B cells and NK cells, respectively [16, 17]. Use azide-free antibodies and recommended concentrations of the antibodies (*see* **Note 4**).
6. The bead-adhered cells are removed with a magnet, and the process is repeated 3×. The supernatant should contain more than 97 % DCs as judged by flow cytometry (*see* **Note 5**).
7. Assess the cell viability by Trypan blue dye exclusion. Cell viability should be always >98 % (*see* **Note 6**).
8. Characterize DC by fluorescence-activated cell sorting (FACS) using monoclonal antibodies against MHC class I, MHC class II, CD40, and CD86.
9. Incubate DC with 500 pg/mL recombinant IL-15 for 12 h for further maturation and differentiation (Fig. 1).
10. Pulse the DC with 10 μg/mL soluble tumor antigen for 12 h before injecting into tumor-bearing mice.

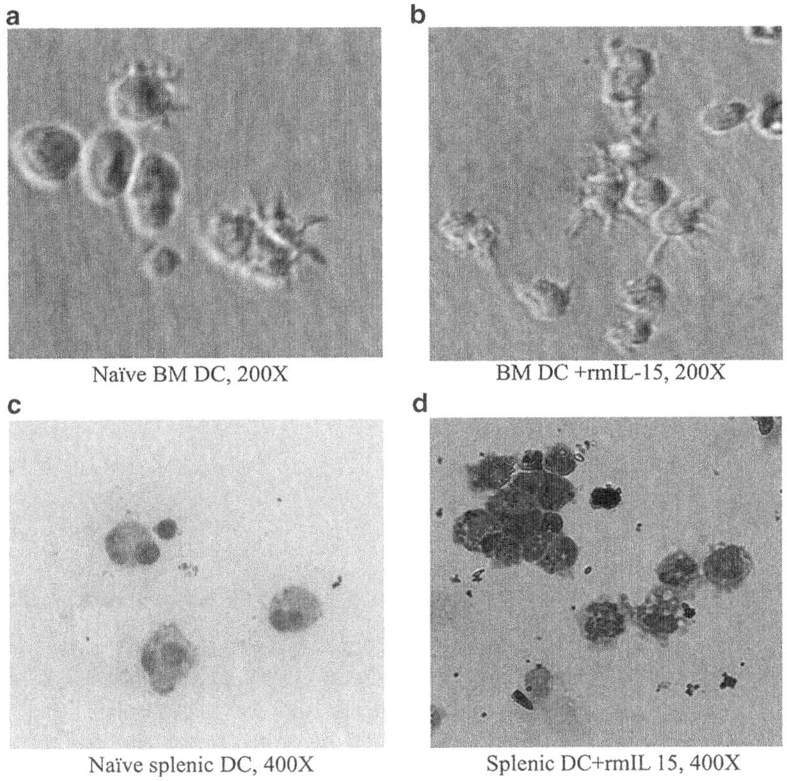

Fig. 1 DC preparation from the bone marrow (BM) (**a**, **b**) and spleen (**c**, **d**). Recombinant mouse IL-15 (rmIL-15)

Prior to administration, the DCs are washed in complete medium for the removal of excess tumor antigens (*see* **Notes 6** and 7).

3.2 Preparation of DC from Spleen

1. Following mechanical disruption, treat the spleen cells and tissues from normal 6–8-week-old mice with 0.1 mg/mL collagenase D for 1–2 h at 37 °C (*see* **Note 8**).
2. Remove the cellular debris by strainer. Wash the single cell suspension in 1× PBS.
3. Lyse the RBC using lysis buffer, wash in 1× PBS, and resuspend in PBS containing 2 % FBS.
4. Treat the single cell splenic suspension with anti-mouse CD3, CD14, CD19, and CD56 monoclonal antibodies plus immunomagnetic Dynal beads to remove T cells, monocytes, B cells, and NK cells, respectively (*see* **Note 4**).
5. Stain the naïve DC with CD11c to confirm its DC phenotype. Treat the DC with indicated cytokine(s) (GM-CSF or IL-15) in the presence or absence of tumor antigen as mentioned for bone marrow-derived DC.

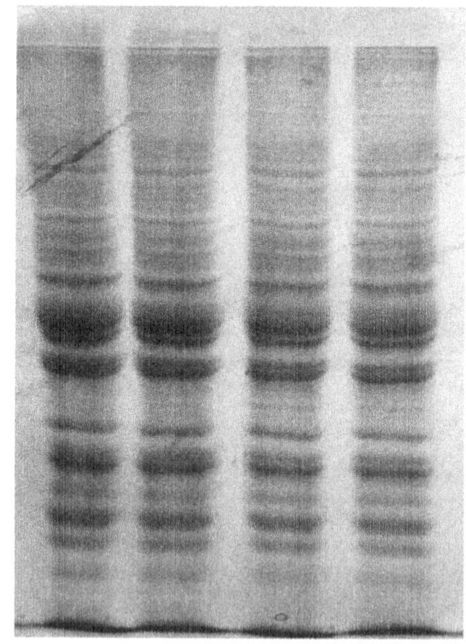

Fig. 2 Protein profile of whole DL tumor antigens. In each lane, 30 μg protein was electrophoresed on 4.5 % stacking and 10 % resolving denaturing PAGE followed by staining with Coomassie Brilliant Blue. *DLA* represents protein from ascites, and *DLC* represents the protein derived from cultured tumor cell in duplicate determination

3.3 Preparation of Tumor Antigens

1. Prepare crude soluble tumor antigens (DLC) from stationary stage tumor cells by repeated freeze thawing of cell suspension.
2. Sonicate 2×10^7 tumor cells in 1× PBS for 45 s 5× at 20 kilocycles per minute on ice using a Labsonic sonifier.
3. Centrifuge the contents at 5,000 × *g* for 20 min at 4 °C. Collect the supernatant; measure the protein concentration spectrophotometrically and store in aliquots at −80 °C until use.
4. To make the DLA, collect the ascitic fluid from the peritoneum of the mouse, measure the protein content, and analyze using a 4.0 % stacking and 12.5 % resolving SDS-PAGE mini gel at a constant voltage of 75 V for 3 h (*see* **Note 9**).
5. A representative protein profile of the tumor antigens is presented in (Fig. 2).

3.4 Stimulation of DC with Antigens and Cytokines

1. Harvest 3×10^6 splenic- or bone marrow-derived DC in complete medium. Incubate with whole cell tumor lysates in a 6-well plate in a total volume of 2 mL for 12 h at 37 °C with 5 % CO_2. Cell viability should be assessed by Trypan blue dye exclusion following the antigen stimulation (*see* **Note 7**).
2. Simultaneously, stimulate other sets of the 3×10^6 DC with recombinant mouse 10 μg/mL of GM-CSF or IL-15 in the

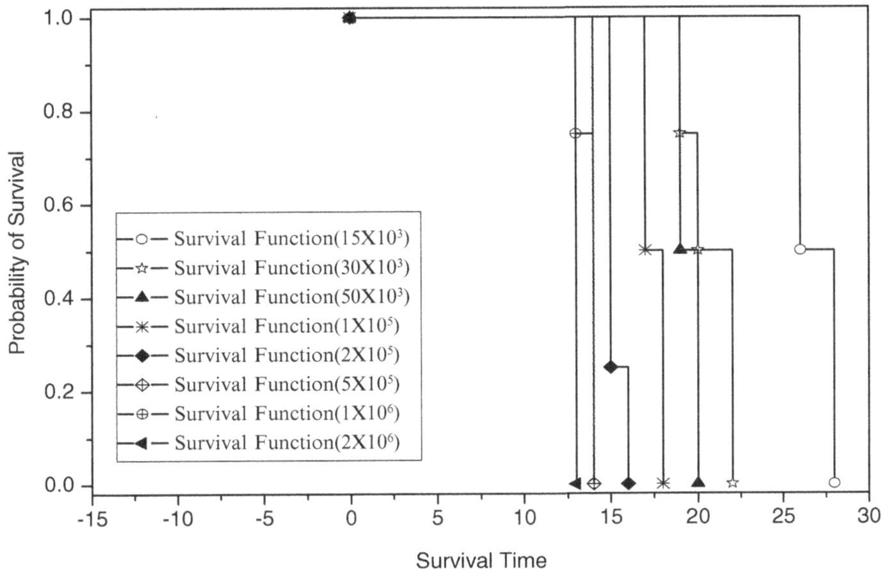

Fig. 3 Survival (in days) of different groups of AKR mice from the day of intraperitoneal tumor cell transplantation. The number of transplanted tumor cells is given in *brackets*

presence or absence of tumor antigens for 12 h. Wash the cells in 1× PBS before injecting inside the mouse peritoneum.

3. DC from the bone marrow or spleen stimulated with antigens or IL-15 can be stained with FITC-conjugated anti-mouse CD69 to show activation.

3.5 Tumor Transplantation in Mice

1. The tumor model used in our previous study is a lymphoma which develops in mouse peritoneum and rapidly metastasizes in organs like the liver, spleen, and lung causing death in 20–22 days. The lymphoma (also called Dalton's lymphoma, DL) should be maintained in RPMI-1640 supplemented with 10 % FBS and antibiotics.
2. The tumor cells form ascites within 15–18 days in AKR/J mice when challenged intraperitoneally. Mice are injected intraperitoneally with 1×10^5 tumor cells for routine maintenance of the tumor (*see* **Note 10**).
3. A Kaplan–Meier survival curve was generated with variable number of tumor cells (1.5×10^4–2×10^6 cells per mouse) which gives the optimum cell number for the tumor development to be used for subsequent studies (Fig. 3).
4. Monitor the mouse colony routinely for tumor growth. Tumor size will be measured by observing the increase in circumference of the abdomen measured using a Vernier caliper (*see* **Note 11**).

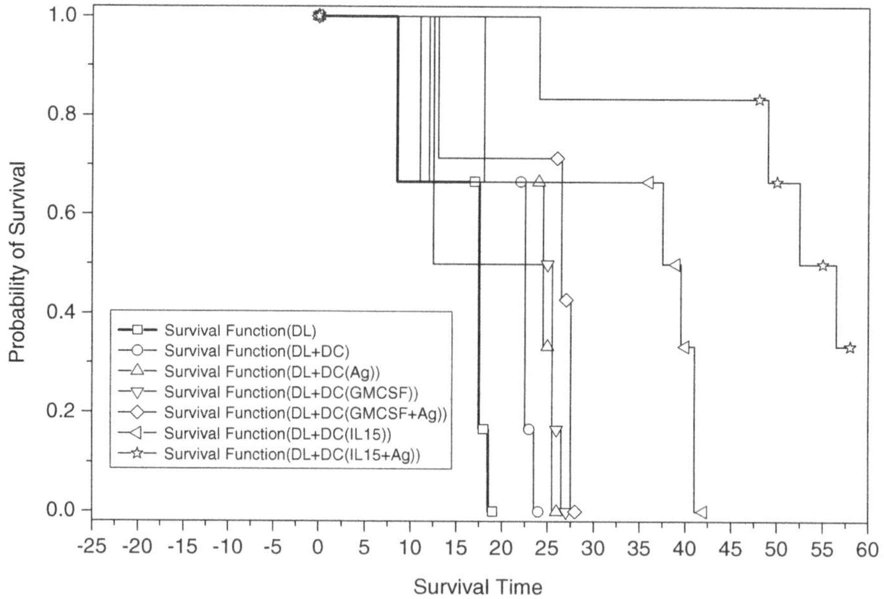

Fig. 4 Survival (in days) of different groups of mice from the day of tumor cell transplantation followed by therapy with cytokine (GM-CSF or IL-15)-activated DC pulsed with or without whole tumor cell antigen (Ag)

5. Maintain the cage and the animal room pathogen-free. Give sterile food and water to avoid infection (*see* **Note 12**).

3.6 Adoptive Therapy with Antigen-/Cytokine-Activated DC

1. Use 3×10^4 DL cells for tumor development in six to eight female mice and allow the tumor to form for 5 days.
2. Immunize tumor-bearing animals with 1×10^6 tumor antigen-pulsed DC with or without activation with GM-CSF or IL-15 and injected intraperitoneally. Give a total of five injections in a span of 2 weeks.
3. Take a minimum of seven to nine mice per group in order to get complete statistical data which could also avoid any loss of data on account of animal death during the experimentation (*see* **Note 10**).
4. Deliver DC vaccination after 5 days following tumor transplant.
5. Generate survival curves using the Kaplan–Meier method and make the comparisons by logrank tests. Statistical analysis software OriginPro 8 SR0 v8.0724 (B724) can be used for all statistical analysis in the study [18, 19] (Fig. 4) (*see* **Notes 13** and **14**). Results from our study show that spleen sizes from different groups and near normal abdominal circumference after 40 days following tumor challenge and subsequent therapy suggest the effectiveness of the therapy to reverse the metastasis

a

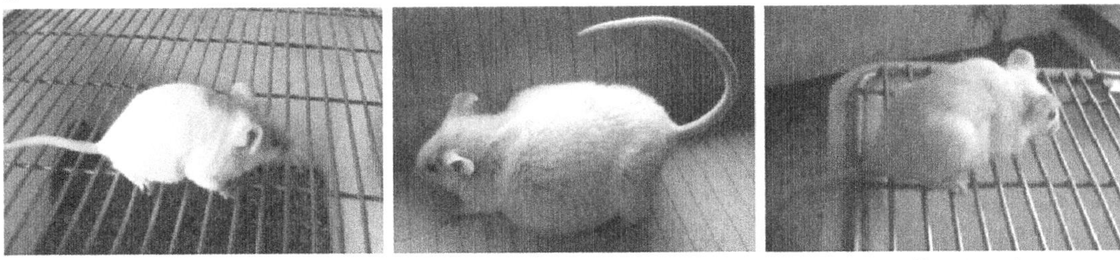

b

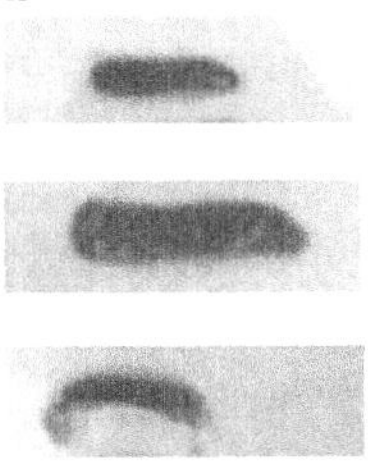

Abdominal circumference

	Day 0	Day 18
Normal Mouse	7.15±0.55	7.23±0.34
DL Mouse	7.29±0.09	12.68±0.55
Treated Mouse	7.01±0.51	7.22±0.49

Fig. 5 (**a**) Tumor development following transplant of tumor cells and IL-15-activated DC therapy in AKR mice. (**b**) Representative spleen size in normal, tumor cell transplanted and mice with transplanted tumor cells followed by therapy with IL-15-activated DC pulsed with whole tumor antigen

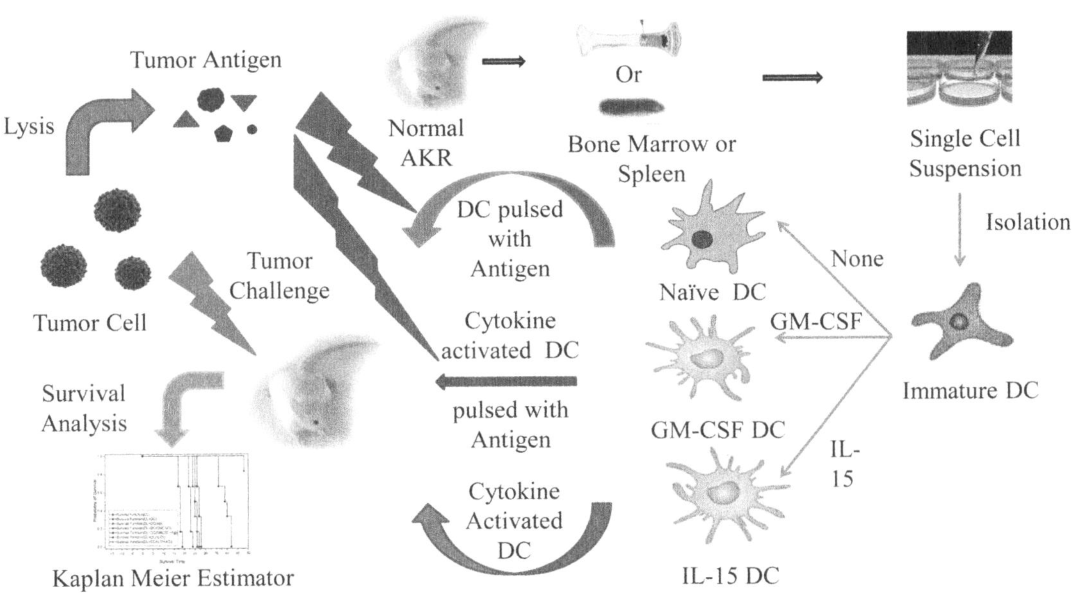

Fig. 6 Graphic representation of experimental design

and reduce disease progression (Fig. 5). The spleen size estimation was made in a mouse which survived 60 days and beyond following therapy.

6. Measure the abdominal circumference with a Vernier caliper which measures the peritoneal size (*see* **Note 15**).
7. A graphic presentation of the scheme is illustrated in Fig. 6 and reflects the entire protocol from tumor development.

4 Notes

1. Bone marrow preparation from mouse femur requires care to avoid contamination. Take care to avoid contact with fur. The femurs with muscle can be kept in 1× PBS for 30 min which loosens the muscle from the bone and makes it easy to detach with forceps and scissors. The use of medium could make it difficult to tease the muscles from the femur and should be avoided at this step.
2. Isolation and enrichment of DC from mouse spleen is a critical step. DC and macrophages tend to adhere simultaneously to glass Petri dishes. The washing of nonadherent cells following incubation of total splenocytes is crucial to minimize contamination with nonadherent cells in the final preparation of the DC. Care should be taken in order to prevent loss of adherent cells during washing. Do not use jet force on the adhered cells.
3. Add GM-CSF to culture in optimal concentration. Addition of GM-CSF should be made following the completion of adherence of the cells. Absence of GM-CSF for 12 or more hours could damage the cells and may have a drastic effect on the DC generation.
4. Use the antibodies and the Dynal beads under optimum conditions in order to obtain the best results. Repeat the Dynal beads step at least 2× to get the maximum removal of the undesired cell populations. The magnet and the cell-containing tube should have a tight grip. Use BD FACS tubes containing 5×10^6 cells for individual preparations.
5. A negative selection process is suitable for DC isolation for the current purposes since magnetic beads do not pose any problem for the harvested DC. This also facilitates further phenotypic characterization. Also, negative selection does not affect the DC viability.
6. Viability of cells is the most important factor for this study. Always use the Trypan blue dye exclusion method to assess the cell viability before use.

7. The antigen-pulsed or cytokine-stimulated DC must be assessed for any unwanted cell death before the use for the adoptive cell therapy. Annexin FITC staining can be used for activation-induced cellular apoptosis. Trypan blue staining can be carried out to assess the viability of the cells. Use 3×10^6/mL DC for stimulation with IL-15 and tumor antigen. Stimulation with cytokine and antigen can be performed together.
8. Collagenase D treatment is required for releasing the DC from the cellular matrix. Without collagenase D treatment, the DC recovery will be low.
9. Care should be taken in making the components for preparing the gel. Specific care should be taken in handling acrylamide since it is neurotoxic in the unpolymerized state. Skin contact should be avoided.
10. The number of animals used in each set should not be less than seven, preferably nine which gives more flexibility to assess the overall survival kinetics. This is critically important for therapy groups with antigen-pulsed DC stimulated with IL-15.
11. The tumor model used in our study is highly vigorous and invasive, causing metastasis in organs like the spleen, liver, and lung leading to the rapid death of the animal.
12. The animals should be maintained in clean and pathogen-free condition without any secondary infection during the course of the experimentation. The metastasis of the spleen and liver makes the organs much larger compared to normal which could be similar to the enlargement of those organs due to unwanted secondary infection.
13. Survival analysis is the study of the time until a certain event, such as a death due to treatment. The time until the event is known as the survival time. If the event occurs during the study period, the survival time represents complete data. Otherwise, if the event does not happen to a particular study participant, the survival time is called censored time.
14. The survival rate can be described as a survival function, $S(t)$, from the sample survival time. A survival function, $S(t)$, is the probability of surviving until at least time t with $S(t) = 1 - F(t)$, where $F(t)$ is the cumulative distribution function of the failure times. Since there are censored values, which mean an incomplete observation, special methods should be introduced to estimate $S(t)$.
15. The measurements of the spleen and the animal weight are clear indicators of the extent of the metastasis following tumor transplantation. The therapy regimen with IL-15 plus antigen drastically reduces the extent of metastasis and prevents the accumulation of tumor cells in the form of ascites and thus increases the chances of survival of the animal.

Acknowledgements

This work was supported by a grant from the Department of Science and Technology, New Delhi, India, No. SR/SO/AS-55/2009 (G) and a grant from the Department of Biotechnology, New Delhi, India, No. BT/PR11490/BRB/10/675/2008.

References

1. Steinman RM, Pope M (2002) Exploiting dendritic cells to improve vaccine efficacy. J Clin Invest 109:1519–1526
2. Banchereau J et al (2001) Dendritic cells as vectors for therapy. Cell 106:271–274
3. Nestle FO et al (1998) Vaccination of melanoma patients with peptide- or tumor lysate-pulsed DCs. Nat Med 4:328–332
4. Dhodapkar MV et al (1999) Rapid generation of broad T-cell immunity in humans after a single injection of mature dendritic cells. J Clin Invest 104:173–180
5. Zhou Y et al (2002) Current methods for loading dendritic cells with tumor antigen for the induction of antitumor immunity. J Immunother 25:289–303
6. Schlienger K et al (2003) TRANCE- and CD40 ligand-matured dendritic cells reveal MHC class I-restricted T cells specific for autologous tumor in late-stage ovarian cancer patients. Clin Cancer Res 9(4):1517–1527
7. Martin JC, O'Brien TJ (2009) Cellular immunotherapy for ovarian cancer. Expert Opin Biol Ther 9(6):677–688
8. Davis ID et al (2003) Rational approaches to human cancer immunotherapy. J Leukoc Biol 73:3–29
9. Small EJ et al (2006) Placebo-controlled phase III trial of immunologic therapy with sipuleucel-T (APC8015) in patients with metastatic, asymptomatic hormone refractory prostate cancer. J Clin Oncol 24:3089–3094
10. Lesterhuis WJ et al (2008) Dendritic cell vaccines in melanoma: from promise to proof? Crit Rev Oncol Hematol 66(2):118–134
11. Neves AR et al (2005) Dendritic cells derived from metastatic cancer patients vaccinated with allogeneic dendritic cell-autologous tumor cell hybrids express more CD86 and induce higher levels of interferon-gamma in mixed lymphocyte reactions. Cancer Immunol Immunother 54:61–66
12. Fabre JW (2001) The allogeneic response and tumor immunity. Nat Med 7:649–652
13. Suzuki T et al (2005) Vaccination of dendritic cells loaded with interleukin-12-secreting cancer cells augments in vivo antitumor immunity: characteristics of syngeneic and allogeneic antigen-presenting cell cancer hybrid cells. Clin Cancer Res 11:58–66
14. Yasuda T et al (2007) Superior anti-tumor protection and therapeutic efficacy of vaccination with allogeneic and semiallogeneic dendritic cell/tumor cell fusion hybrids for murine colon adenocarcinoma. Cancer Immunol Immunother 56:1025–1036
15. Manna PP et al (2010) Innate immune defense in visceral leishmaniasis: cytokine mediated protective role by allogeneic effector cell. Vaccine 28:803–810
16. Manna PP, Mohanakumar T (2002) Human dendritic cell mediated cytotoxicity against breast carcinoma cells in vitro. J Leukoc Biol 72(2):312–320
17. Manna PP, Frazier WA (2003) The mechanism of CD47-dependent killing of T cells: heterotrimeric G_i-dependent inhibition of protein kinase A. J Immunol 170:3544–3553
18. Lee ET, Wang JW (2003) Statistical methods for survival data analysis, 3rd edn. Wiley, Berlin
19. Kaplan EL, Meier P (1958) Non-parametric estimation from incomplete observations. J Am Stat Assoc 53:457–481

Chapter 7

Dendritic Cells Primed with Protein–Protein Fusion Adjuvant

Liying Wang and Yongli Yu

Abstract

To develop efficient T cell priming cancer vaccines, various recombinant fusion proteins have been developed by fusing a tumor antigen with a protein capable of stimulating or targeting dendritic cells (DC), the most important antigen-presenting cells for inducing $CD8^+$ cytotoxic T lymphocytes (CTL) which can efficiently kill tumor cells expressing the tumor antigen. The DC-stimulating or DC-targeting proteins, including granulocyte/macrophage colony-stimulating factor (GM-CSF), anti-DEC-205 monoclonal antibodies, flagellin, and heat shock proteins (HSP), function as promising intermolecular adjuvants. Herein, we describe in vitro assays on human DC pulsed with HSP fusion proteins, which might be useful in preclinical studies for the screening and assessment of candidate cancer vaccines.

Key words Dendritic cells, Fusion protein, GM-CSF, Antibody, Flagellin, Heat shock protein, Cancer vaccine, Adjuvant

1 Introduction

Current vaccines work primarily by inducing protective antibodies. However, medicine does need to develop T cell-based vaccines that induce resistance to cancers. Efforts have been made to fuse tumor antigens with various proteins with the capacity of stimulating or targeting dendritic cells (DC), the most efficient antigen-presenting cells for T cells, especially $CD8^+$ T cells which can differentiate into cytotoxic T lymphocytes (CTL) to efficiently kill tumor cells expressing the tumor antigen [1, 2].

In April 2010, the Food and Drug Administration approved Provenge™ (sipuleucel-T) as a viable approach to cancer treatment for advanced prostate cancer [3]. Provenge™ is an autologous DC-based vaccine [4], comprising autologous peripheral blood mononuclear cells (PBMC) pulsed with a fusion protein (PAP-GM-CSF) composed of prostatic acid phosphatase (PAP), a tumor-associated differentiation antigen, and granulocyte/macrophage colony-stimulating factor (GM-CSF). Provenge™ is manufactured

Michael J.P. Lawman and Patricia D. Lawman (eds.), *Cancer Vaccines: Methods and Protocols*, Methods in Molecular Biology, vol. 1139, DOI 10.1007/978-1-4939-0345-0_7, © Springer Science+Business Media New York 2014

by culturing PBMC collected from patients by leukopheresis with medium containing PAP-GM-CSF for 36–44 h at 37 °C. Provenge™ refusion achieved a 4.1-month improvement (25.8 months vs. 21.7 months) in median survival in patients [3]. It has been established that GM-CSF is a critical factor for the differentiation of DC [5]. In response to GM-CSF and other environmental changes, DC respond quickly to differentiate into matured DC which are capable of presenting tumor antigens to T cells [6, 7]. The DC in Provenge™ could be matured by the fused GM-CSF in PAP-GM-CSF in vitro. In the patients, the matured PAP loading DC would present PAP to $CD8^+$ T cells to generate PAP-specific CTL with the capacity of finding and killing PAP-expressing prostate cancer cells.

Discovery of antigen uptake receptors on DC has enabled the development of engineered monoclonal antireceptor antibodies with tumor antigen as a vaccine to specifically target DC [8]. One such receptor is DEC-205 [9] which is expressed mainly on DC in T cell areas of human and mouse lymphoid tissues [10]. Anti-DEC-205 monoclonal antibodies fused with foreign antigens have been tested in extensive preclinical studies in mice and in proof of concept studies in human [11–13]. Foreign antigens, once fused into the constant region of the heavy chain in an anti-DEC-205 monoclonal antibody, become highly immunogenic in low doses which can lead to a significant $CD4^+$ T cell response and cross-priming of $CD8^+$ T cells in mice. More importantly, the anti-DEC-205 monoclonal antibodies can achieve cross-priming of $CD8^+$ T cells in many different MHC haplotypes [14], thus providing an excellent approach to developing cancer vaccines. A DEC–HER2 fusion monoclonal antibody was reported capable of delivering HER2 protein to DC in vivo. The DC in turn processed the HER2 protein to liberate peptides for presentation on MHC class I and II complexes to $CD8^+$ and $CD4^+$ T cells, respectively, finding in vivo rare clones of HER2-specific T cells, expanding them, and inducing critical helper and killer anticancer T cell functions. In a mouse transplantable tumor model, vaccination with DEC-205-HER2 induced significant long-term survival benefits to mice challenged with HER2-expressing tumors [15].

Over the past several years, an interest has emerged in developing flagellin, a major protein constituent of bacterial flagella involved in motility and a ligand for Toll-like receptor 5 (TLR5) [16], as an adjuvant for vaccines [17]. TLR5, a transmembrane protein, is expressed on antigen-presenting cells including monocytes and DC [18]. In response to flagellin, DC produces interleukin-12 (IL-12) and present antigen to $CD4^+$ T cells that produce interferon-γ (IFN-γ) to polarize a Th1 response [19]. Direct stimulation of TLR5 expressing DC is necessary for the adjuvant activity of flagellin [20]. In mice, $CD8\alpha^+$ DC are particularly efficient at sensing bacterial flagellin through NOD-like receptor (NLR)-4

NLRC4 inflammasomes, releasing interleukin-18 (IL-18) and interleukin-1 β (IL-1β) [21]. Neuronal apoptosis inhibitory protein (NAIP), a BIR domain NOD-like receptor (NLR) protein required for *Legionella pneumophila* replication in mouse macrophages, has been identified as a receptor for flagellin in the NLRC4 inflammasomes, mediating a flagellin–NLRC4 pathway for activating innate immune responses [22]. Indicatively, the TLR5 and inflammasome-activating property allows flagellin to enhance changes in antigen presentation and cellular activation, and the incorporation of flagellin could result in more efficacious vaccines. Based on these findings, various recombinant flagellin–antigen fusion proteins have been constructed and tested in animal models to induce potent T and B cell responses [23] to a number of microbial antigens, including influenza M2e Ag [24], *Plasmodium vivax* merozoite surface protein-1 [25], and *Mycobacterium tuberculosis* Ag p27 [26]. In addition, flagellin has also been fused with tumor antigens such as MUC1, a tumor-associated antigen overexpressed in many carcinomas. A recombinant flagellin fused with a 25-residue fragment of MUC1 was tested in human MUC1 transgenic mice in which spontaneous breast cancer and metastases occur. The fusion protein induced a significant reduction of both the size and growth rate of the tumor, a lower number of metastases, and increased life span [27]. The feasibility of using flagellin as a cancer vaccine adjuvant could be substantiated by vaccination with irradiated flagellin-expressing tumor cells which prevented tumor development and, by disrupting flagellin recognition by TLR5 or NLRC4/NAIP5, impaired protective immunization against existing or subsequent tumors [28].

There is growing evidence that heat shock proteins (HSPs), derived from mammalian cells or microbes, function as modulators for innate and adaptive immune responses and can be used as an adjuvant. Extracellular HSPs generated by passive release from necrotic cells or by active release in exosomes activate innate immune responses through TLRs and augment their associated TLR ligands such as lipopolysaccharide (LPS) to stimulate cytokine production and maturation of DC [29, 30]. More interestingly, HSPs have been found to facilitate the cross-priming of exogenously applied antigens in DC [31, 32]. HSP–peptide complexes isolated from tumor cell could be taken up by DC and be presented to MHC class I-restricted T cells. Interestingly, mycobacterial HSP65 (mHSP65) can be fused with peptides of various lengths, and DC can take up these fusion proteins for cross-priming to $CD8^+$ T cells specific for the fused peptides [33]. This unique property allows HSP65 to be used to generate recombinant fusion proteins with tumor antigens for developing tumor vaccines. HSPE7, a recombinant fusion protein composed of mHSP65 linked to E7, an oncogenic protein of human papilloma virus (HPV), was found capable of inducing E7-specific CTL in experimental animal models.

E7-expressing tumors in C57BL/6 mice can be eradicated by treatment with the HspE7. In phase II clinical trials, HSPE7 displayed significant clinical benefit for the immunotherapy of HPV-related diseases. HSPE7 primes potent E7-specific CTL that can differentiate into memory T cells with effector functions in the absence of CD4^{+} T cell help. The memory cells persist for at least 17 weeks and can confer protection against E7-positive murine tumor cell challenge [34]. To explore the possibility of utilizing the specific antitumor immunity induced by variable numbers of tandem repeat (VNTR) peptide of MUC1 and the nonspecific immunity induced by HSP, we constructed a recombinant protein (HSP65–MUC1) by fusing mHSP65 with the MUC1 VNTR peptide and tested its ability to induce antitumor activities in a tumor challenge model. The growth of MUC1-expressing tumors was significantly inhibited in mice immunized with HSP65–MUC1 both before and after tumor challenge. A much larger percentage of immunized mice survived the tumor challenge than nonimmunized mice. Correlating with the antitumor activity, HSP65–MUC1 was shown to induce MUC1-specific CTL as well as nonspecific antitumor immunity. In the human system, HSP65–MUC1-loaded human DC induced the generation of autologous MUC1-specific CTL in vitro [35]. The HSP65–MUC1 was evaluated for single-dose toxicity and repeat-dose toxicity both in mice and rhesus monkeys and the evaluation contributed to the approval of initiating a phase I clinical trial with HSP65–MUC1 for the treatment of patients with MUC1-positive breast cancer in China [36].

Considering that the development of HSP fusion proteins as cancer vaccines will depend on reliable assays to assess their efficacy on the activation of DC, in this chapter, we will describe in vitro systems for the analysis of adjuvant effects of the fusion proteins on human DC and the subsequent generation of tumor antigen-specific CTL. These systems are based on the use of human monocyte-derived DC generated in vitro and three recombinant HSP fusion proteins, including HSP65–MUC1 [35] between mHSP65 and the VNTR peptide of MUC1, HSP65–HBV of hepatitis B virus (HBV) [37] between mHSP65 and HBV multiple epitopes, and HSP65–HER2 [38] between mHSP6- and HER2-derived peptides.

2 Materials

Prepare all solutions and medium at room temperature. Store all Fluorochrome-conjugated monoclonal antibodies at 4 °C unless indicated otherwise. Human PBMC (buffy coat) cells are better used at the time of isolation, otherwise should be kept at 4 °C for next day use. HSP fusion proteins are stored at −20 °C in aliquots.

2.1 Induction of Monocyte-Derived Dendritic Cells

1. Human buffy coat.
2. Ficoll–Paque Plus (Ficoll) (GE Healthcare, Life Sciences, Piscataway, NJ, USA), stored at room temperature.
3. Percoll (GE Healthcare): 100 % Percoll: 90 mL of Percoll, 10 mL of 10× phosphate-buffered saline (PBS), stored at room temperature and 52 % Percoll: 100 mL of 100 % Percoll, 92.3 mL of 1× PBS, stored at room temperature.
4. Complete culture medium (CM): Roswell Park Memorial Institute (RPMI)-1640 medium, 2 mM L-glutamine, 20 μg/mL of gentamicin, 50 μM of β-mercaptoethanol, 1 % nonessential amino acids, 10 % fetal bovine serum (FBS), stored at 4 °C.
5. Recombinant GM-CSF (R&D Systems, Minneapolis, MN, USA): 1 μg/mL of GM-CSF in CM as stock solution, filtered and stored at −20 °C (use a 10× dilution as a working solution).
6. Recombinant interleukin-4 (IL-4) (R&D Systems): 2,000 U/mL of IL-4 in CM as stock solution, filtered and stored at −20 °C (use a 10× dilution as a working solution).
7. Cytokine cocktail: CM, 10 ng/mL of tumor necrosis factor-α (TNF-α), 10 ng/mL of interleukin-6 (IL-6), 10 ng/mL of interleukin-1β (IL-1β), 1 μg/mL of prostaglandin E2 (PGE2).
8. Recombinant HSP fusion protein (*see* **Note 1**): HSP65–MUC1 [35], HSP65–HBV [37], and HSP65–HER2 [38].
9. PBS/Ethylenediaminetetraacetic acid (EDTA) buffer: PBS, pH 7.2, 2 mM EDTA, stored at room temperature.
10. PBS/EDTA/human serum: PBS, pH 7.2, 2 mM EDTA, 2 % human serum (AB type, heat inactivated at 56 °C for 30 min, aliquoted and stored at −20 °C).

2.2 Analysis of Fusion Protein-Induced DC Activation

1. Fluorochrome-conjugated monoclonal antibodies (mAbs) to CD80, CD83, CD86, CD40, human leukocyte antigen (HLA)-A2 (BD Biosciences, San Jose, CA, USA).
2. Staining buffer (FACS buffer): PBS, pH 7.2, 2 % human serum (heat inactivated at 56 °C for 30 min), 0.5 mM EDTA, stored at 4 °C.
3. Giemsa staining buffer: 20× dilution of Giemsa stain with deionized water.
4. IL-12p70 ELISA kit (U-CyTech Biosciences, Utrecht, Netherlands).

2.3 Analysis of HSP Fusion Protein-Pulsed DC

1. mAbs to human CD14, CD19, CD56, HLA-DR, CD4, γδTCR, CD45RO (BD Biosciences).
2. Anti-mouse IgG magnetic beads (Miltenyi Biotec, Teterow, Cologne, Germany).

3. Fluorochrome-conjugated antibodies for surface staining: FITC-conjugated mouse antihuman CD4, CD14, CD16, and CD20, PE-conjugated mouse antihuman CD27, Tc-conjugated mouse antihuman CD45-RA (BD Biosciences).
4. PBS, pH 4.0: PBS, pH 7.2, 4.2 mM magnesium chloride ($MgCl_2$), 0.01 % sodium azide (NaN_3). Adjust pH to 4.0 with hydrochloric acid (HCl).
5. Bead-preserving solution: PBS, pH 4.0, 50 μL of 5 μg/mL DNase I.
6. ^{3}H-thymidine (NEN Life Science, Boston, MA, USA).
7. Recombinant human interleukin-7 (IL-7) (R&D Systems): 100 U/mL of IL-7 in CM as stock solution, filtered and stored at −20 °C (use a 10× dilution as a working solution).
8. Recombinant human interleukin-2 (IL-2) (R&D Systems): 100 U/mL of IL-2 in CM as stock solution, filtered and stored at −20 °C (use a 10× dilution as a working solution).
9. ^{51}Cr sodium chromate: 1 mCi/mL in sterile saline as stock solution (use a 10× dilution as a working solution).
10. 10 % Triton X-100: 10 mL of Triton X-100 in 90 mL of distilled water, stored at room temperature.
11. Fluorescein isothiocyanate (FITC)-conjugated mAbs to CD45RA and CD8 (BD Biosciences).
12. Brefeldin A: Brefeldin A in dimethyl sulfoxide (DMSO) or ethanol stored at −20 °C.
13. Saponin buffer: PBS, pH 7.2, 1 % FBS, 1 % sodium azide, 0.1 % saponin (Sigma-Aldrich, St. Louis, MO, USA). Adjust pH to 7.4–7.6. Filter, aliquot, and freeze at −20 °C.
14. 4 % Paraformaldehyde: 5 mL of PBS, pH 7.2, 0.2 g of paraformaldehyde dissolved at 60 °C in a water bath or boiled. The solution should be freshly prepared from paraformaldehyde powder before use.
15. ^{3}H-thymidine.
16. Enzyme-linked immunosorbent spot (ELISPOT) human IFN-γ Set (BD Biosciences).
17. For the ELISPOT assay, the following buffers are used:
    (a) Coating buffer: PBS, pH 7.2.
    (b) Blocking solution: RPMI 1640, 10 % FBS, 1 % L-glutamine, and antibiotics.
    (c) Wash buffer I: PBS/0.05 % Tween-20, pH 7.2.
    (d) Wash buffer II: PBS, pH 7.2.
    (e) Dilution buffer: PBS/10 % FBS, pH 7.2.
    (f) Substrate solution: 10 mL of 0.1 M acetate solution and 333.3 μL of 3-amino-9ethylcarbazole (AEC) stock solution.

Filter through a 0.45-μm filter, and then add 5 μL of hydrogen peroxide for immediate use. The AEC stock solution is made by mixing 100 mg AEC in 10 mL N, N-dimethylformamide.

(g) Streptavidin-HRP.

18. BD™ Dimer X kit (BD Biosciences).
19. PKH-26 (Sigma-Aldrich).
20. 5-, 6-carboxyfluorescein diacetate succinimidyl ester (CFSE) (Molecular Probes, Eugene, OR, USA).
21. Dulbecco's phosphate-buffered saline (DPBS): PBS, pH 7.2, 1 % FBS, 0.09 % NaN_3.

3 Methods

Human buffy coat cells or PBMC are a source of monocytes which are used for inducing monocyte-derived DC. Maturation or activation of DC can be analyzed based on cell morphology, cell surface molecule, or ability for priming T cells. Many immune stimulators are able to activate DC. Here, we focus on the activation of DC primed by HSP65–MUC1, HSP65–HBV, and HSP65–HER2, respectively.

3.1 Induction of Monocyte-Derived DC

There are two steps for inducing monocyte-derived DC. One is monocyte purification from human buffy coat. The other is to culture monocytes in CM containing GM-CSF and IL-4 for inducing DC (*see* **Note 2**).

3.1.1 Purification of Monocytes

1. In order to purify monocytes, aliquot 12.5 mL of Ficoll into a 50-mL tube. For one buffy coat, four tubes are usually needed.
2. Wash the external surface of the blood bag with 70 % ethanol, and then put the blood into the flask containing PBS/EDTA. The total volume in the flask should be 100 mL.
3. Transfer 25 mL of the blood/PBS mixture from the flask into one tube containing 12.5 mL of Ficoll. When adding the PBMC to the Ficoll, great care needs to be taken to avoid disturbing the Ficoll.
4. Centrifuge the tubes at 1,200 × *g* for 20–25 min at room temperature without the centrifuge brake. Discard the upper supernatant by aspiration and finally, using a pipette, aspirate the PBMC at the interface and transfer them into a new tube.
5. Wash the PBMC with large volume of PBS/EDTA. After the first wash, the cells are spun at 450 × *g* for 10 min at 4 °C and after the second washing, at 180 × *g* for 7 min at 4 °C. Following the second wash, place the cell pellets on ice.

6. Suspend the cell pellets with PBS/EDTA/human serum buffer and adjust the cell density to 50×10^6/mL.
7. Transfer 3 mL of the cell suspension onto 6 mL of a 52 % Percoll gradient. When adding the PBMC to the Percoll, great care needs to be taken to avoid disturbing the gradient, and then centrifuge the tubes at $500 \times g$ for 20 min at 4 °C without engaging the centrifuge brake.
8. Using a sterile pipette, aspirate the interface cells into a new tube and then transfer the remaining cells into another tube for HLA typing.
9. Wash the interface cells 2× with cold PBS/EDTA/human serum buffer at $200 \times g$ for 10 min at 4 °C, again without engaging the centrifuge brake.
10. Filter the cells with a nylon mesh to remove dead cells, which should be clumped together, then finally, count the remaining cells (monocytes) using Trypan blue dye exclusion.

3.1.2 Induction of Immature DC Derived from Monocytes

1. Dilute the purified monocytes from Subheading 3.1 with CM to a cell concentration of 2×10^6 cells/mL (50 % of cells purified by Percoll should be monocytes).
2. Add 1 mL of the cell suspension into one well of a 12-well plate containing 1 mL of CM.
3. Culture the cells in 2 mL (total volume/well) for 2 h in an incubator set at 37 °C in an atmosphere of 5 % CO_2 in air.
4. Remove the nonadherent cells from the wells after 2 h and then, using CM, wash once gently by sucking the medium "in and out" with a pipette remembering to keep the pipette tip facing the wall of the well to avoid disturbing the adherent cells.
5. Add 2 mL of CM containing 100 ng/mL of 200 U GM-CSF and 200 U/mL of IL-4 to one well of 12-well plate.
6. Culture the cells for 5 days with the incubator set at 37 °C in an atmosphere of 5 % CO_2 in air. Change medium every 2–3 days by replacing half the medium with fresh CM containing GM-CSF and IL-4 at the above stated concentrations.

3.2 Analysis of Fusion Protein-Induced DC Activation

Cell morphology and phenotype analysis can be primarily used for evaluating the activation of DC stimulated with HSP fusion protein. DC morphology is gradually changing during their maturation and can be checked dynamically using light microscopy. Herein, we describe a method of making a slide preparation using a cytocentrifuge to analyze DC morphology. DC phenotype analysis can be done by surface staining for CD80, CD83, CD86, CD40, and HLA molecules expressed on the surface of DC.

1. To culture DC with fusions proteins (*see* **Note 3**), remove half of the medium from the immature DC culture plate on day 5 of DC induction and add fresh CM containing GM-CSF and IL-4.
2. Directly add HSP65 fusion protein to the medium of immature DC to make final concentration of the fusion protein of 10 μg/mL.
3. Mix the medium by gently shaking the plate by fingers.
4. Culture the plate for 48 h in an incubator set at 37 °C in an atmosphere of 5 % CO_2 in air.
5. Harvest the DC after 48 h (*see* **Note 4**) and count using Trypan blue dye exclusion.

3.3 Analysis of DC Morphology by Making Slides Using Cytocentrifugation

1. Using a pipette remove an aliquot of DC and spot onto a slide.
2. Spin the slide at 10 × *g* for less than 3 min (several seconds should be enough).
3. Place the slide at room temperature overnight.
4. Fix the DC slide using methanol for 20 min and air dry at room temperature.
5. Stain the slide with a 20× diluted Giemsa staining buffer and incubate the slice for 15–20 min at room temperature.
6. Gently wash the slide with deionized water and dry at room temperature.
7. Check the staining DC morphology under the microscope. As an example, Fig. 1 shows the morphology of monocyte-derived DC matured by a cytokine cocktail including 10 ng/mL of TNF-α, 10 ng/mL of IL-6, 10 ng/mL of IL-1β, and 1 μg/mL of PGE2.

3.4 Surface Staining of DC

1. Aliquot $1–2 \times 10^4$ DC or less per 100 μL into one well of a round-bottom 96-well plate for each surface staining reaction.
2. Centrifuge the plate at 180 × *g* for 5 min at 4 °C.
3. Wash the DC 2× with staining buffer by centrifuging at 180 × *g* for 5 min at 4 °C and discard the supernatant.
4. Vortex the plate to suspend DC in remaining buffer.
5. Add the desired antibodies to the well at suitable dilution, e.g., 1:50, and mix well by vortexing. For analyzing DC activation, FITC-conjugated anti-CD11c mAb and phycoerythrin (PE)-conjugated mAbs against CD80, CD83, CD86, CD40, HLA-A2, and HLA-DR may be used.
6. Incubate the plate for 30 min on ice in the dark and then wash the plate 2× with staining buffer.

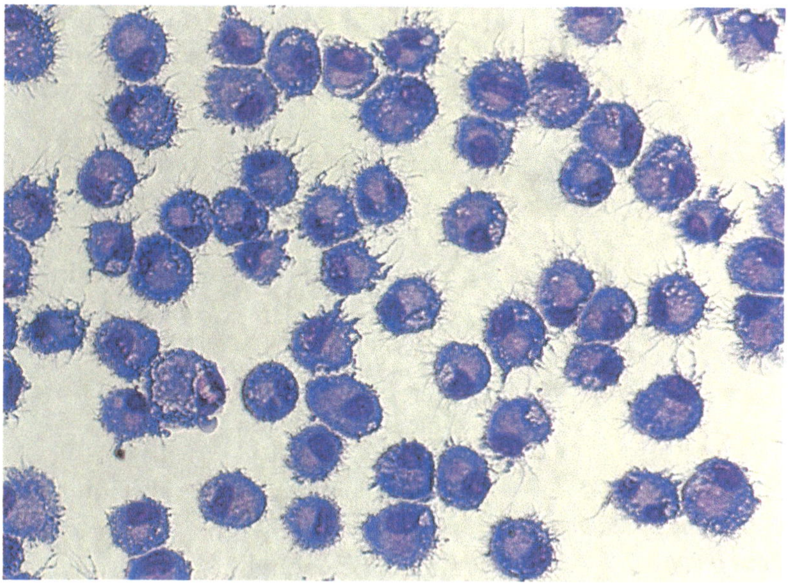

Fig. 1 Morphology of matured monocyte-derived DC. On day 5 of DC induction, add cytokine cocktail to cultured immature DC and continue to culture the DC for 48 h. Harvest DC and make a slide of the cells using a cytocentrifuge. Stain with Giemsa. Observe and photograph the DC under light microscopy (×400 magnification shown)

7. Resuspend the DC with 200 μL of staining buffer and transfer into tubes for the fluorescent-activated cell sorter (FACS) assay.

Note: (1) Use isotype-labeled mAb as a negative control. (2) 2×10^4 DC/mL is an adequate cell concentration for single color staining. (3) For 3-color or 4-color staining, set up 4 controls [isotype, FITC, PE, tri/color (Tc), or allophycocyanin (APC)] and increase the cell number to 0.5×10^6 DC/mL.

3.5 Detection of Cytokines Released by DC Primed with Fusion Protein

Activation of DC stimulated by HSP fusion protein is accompanied by cytokine release in the culture supernatants. Here, IL-12p70 released from DC pulsed by HSP–HBV fusion protein is detected by ELISA [37].

1. Directly add HSP65–HBV into the supernatant of immature DC on day 5 of the induction and continually culture for 48 h.
2. Harvest the supernatants of the cultured DC.
3. Detect IL-12p70 level in the supernatants with an ELISA kit according to the manufacturer's instructions.

3.6 Analysis of HSP Fusion Protein-Pulsed DC

HSP fusion protein-loaded DC can stimulate proliferation of autologous $CD8^+$ T cells and generation of antigen-specific CTL. The CTL can be evaluated by cytotoxic assay for tumor cell killing capacity, dimer assay for frequency of specific CTL, and ELISPOT assay for IFN-γ production.

3.7 Isolation of Human Autologous CD8+ Naïve T Cells by Negative Selection (See Note 5)

1. Isolate purified human PBMC from buffy coat and check the cell concentration and viability using Trypan blue dye exclusion.
2. Make a cell suspension containing 20×10^6 cells/mL in PBS/EDTA/human serum buffer.
3. Freshly prepare 5 mL of an antibody cocktail by adding 1:1,000 dilutions in PBS/EDTA/human serum buffer of the following antibodies: antihuman CD4, CD14, CD19, CD56, CD45-RO, and HLA-DR. The antibody cocktail is finally filtered using a 0.2-μm filter.
4. Combine together the cell suspension and antibody cocktail.
5. Incubate the mixture for 30 min on ice with agitation. Centrifuge the cells at $200 \times g$ and then resuspend the cell pellet in 25 mL of PBS/EDTA/human serum buffer.
6. Prepare anti-mouse IgG magnetic beads by washing 3× with PBS, pH 7.4. Using a magnet to hold the beads in place, remove the wash supernatant. Following the wash steps, transfer the cell suspension into tube containing the beads at a ratio of 1:4 cells/bead.
7. Incubate the cell/bead mixture for 20 min on ice. To keep the cell/bead mixture in suspension, use a bidirectional rotation.
8. Harvest the supernatant by placing the tube in a magnet for 2 min. Resuspend the cell/beads in the same volume of PBS/EDTA/human serum buffer and very gently agitate using your fingers, and then repeat the harvest of the supernatant as before. Mix the two supernatants together.
9. Count the cells in the combined supernatant. Centrifuge at $180 \times g$ and resuspend the cell pellet at a cell concentration of 40×10^6/mL with PBS/EDTA/human serum buffer.
10. Using flow cytometry, identify, sort, and collect $CD45RA^+CD27^+$ T cells (naive $CD8^+$ T cells) from the negatively selected $CD8^+$ T cells obtained above:
    (a) Surface staining with FITC-conjugated anti-CD4, CD14, CD16, and CD20, PE-conjugated anti-CD27, Tc-conjugated CD45RA, and FITC-conjugated anti-CD1a (isotype antibody control).
    (b) Set up 4 controls for surface staining: isotype control (isotype antibodies), FITC control (FITC cocktail including anti-CD4, CD14, CD16, and CD20), PE control (PE-anti-CD27), and Tc control (Tc-anti-CD45RA). For the controls, 5×10^5 cells/mL is sufficient for each staining. For sorting, 40×10^6 cells/mL is required. The staining volume is 100 μL and the antibody dilution is 1:10.
    (c) Incubate the reactions for 30 min on ice with shaking in the dark.

(d) Wash 1× for controls and 2× for sorted cells.

(e) Filter cells with a nylon mash to remove dead cells.

(f) Resuspend cells at concentration of $\leq 5 \times 10^6$ cell/mL with PBS/EDTA/human serum buffer into a tube previously blocked by CM containing 20 % FBS for at least 20 min at 37 °C.

(g) Using FACS sort and collect the $CD45RA^+CD27^+$ $FITC^-$ cells.

3.8 Proliferation of Autologous $CD8^+$ T Cells Primed by Fusion Protein-Loaded DC

1. Plate HSP fusion protein-loaded DC at 2×10^4/well of a 96-well plate.
2. Add purified autologous naïve $CD8^+$ T cells at 20×10^4/well into the well containing 2×10^4 DC. The ratio of DC to $CD8^+$ T cells is 1:10.
3. Coculture the mixture of DC and $CD8^+$ T cells in CM containing 10-U/mL IL-7 (*see* **Note 6**) for 6 days at 37 °C in an atmosphere of 5 % CO_2 in air.
4. On day 7, add 0.5 μCi of ^3H-thymidine/well into the culture and incubate for 16 h at 37 °C in an atmosphere of 5 % CO_2 in air.
5. Harvest the cells and using a scintillation counter, count the counts per minute (cpm) incorporated into each sample.

3.9 Generation of Fused Peptide-Specific CTL

1. Culture HSP fusion protein-loaded DC (*see* **Note 7**) with autologous PBMC or purified $CD8^+$ T cells at $0.5–1 \times 10^5$ DC/mL and 2×10^6 T cells/mL in CM containing 10 U/mL of IL-7 at a final volume of 3 mL/well on a 24-well plate for 7 days (first cycle).
2. On day 7, harvest cells and wash 2× with CM. Replate the cells and culture them with HSP fusion protein-loaded DC in CM containing 2.5 U/mL of IL-2 for another 7 days (second cycle).
3. Harvest the cells and wash 2× with CM. Replate the cells and culture them with HSP fusion protein-loaded DC in CM containing 2.5 U/mL of IL-2 for 7 days (third cycle).
4. Harvest the cells and wash 2×. The cells are the generated fused peptide-specific CTL.

3.10 ^{51}Cr-Release CTL Assay

1. Using 100 μCi ^{51}Cr in a volume of 100 μL, label $1–2 \times 10^6$ cells T2 cells (*see* **Note 8**), which were previously pulsed with 50 μg/mL of MUC1 peptide for 2 h at 37 °C with occasionally mixing. Wash the cells 3× with CM and then adjust the cell concentration to 1×10^5/mL in assay medium: RPMI-1640, 10 % FBS, 1 mM glutamine, antibiotics.

2. Harvest the generated CTL to be used as effector cells in the ^{51}Cr-release CTL assay on day 5 after the last stimulation.
3. Seed varying number of CTL per well in a 96-well round-bottom plate based on an effector/target (E:T) ratios 100:1, 50:1, 25:1, and 12.5:1.
4. Add 50 μL of ^{51}Cr-labeled target 5×10^3 T2 cells into the wells containing effector cells in a final volume of 200 μL/well. Set up two controls: spontaneous release control, 50 μL target cells plus 150 μL of assay medium, and maximum release control, 50 μL target cells plus 150 μL of 1 % Triton X-100.
5. Centrifuge the plate for 5 min at $10 \times g$ and then incubate the plate for 4 h at 37 °C in an atmosphere of 5 % CO_2 in air.
6. At the end of the incubation period, harvest 50 μL of supernatant from each well and count on a γ-counter for ^{51}Cr release.
7. Calculate of specific lysis (%):

$$\text{Specific lysis}(\%) = \left[\frac{(\textit{Mean cpm} - \textit{Mean spont release cpm})}{(\textit{Mean maximum release cpm} - \textit{Mean spont release cpm})}\right] \times 100\%$$

3.11 PKH-26/CFSE Assay

1. Label HBcAg$_{18\text{-}27}$ peptide-loaded T2 cells with 2.5×10^{-6} mol/L PKH-26 and 1.7×10^{-6} mol/L CFSE for 40 min [37, 39] and then wash 3× with assay medium.
2. Harvest the generated CTL to be used as effector cells in a PKH-26/CFSE assay on day 5 following the last stimulation.
3. Incubate CTL with 1×10^4 labeled T2 cells per well into 96-well round-bottom plate at an E:T ratio of 30:1 [37], for 4 h at 37 °C in an atmosphere of 5 % CO_2 in air.
4. Collect the cells and analyze their CFSE mean fluorescence intensities (MFI) in PKH-26$^+$ cells by flow cytometry. The decrease of CFSE fluorescence from target cells (PKH-26$^+$) denotes the release of cytoplasm from the target cells.
5. Calculate the specific lysis according to the following formula:

$$\text{Specific lysis}(\%) = \left[1 - \frac{(\textit{MFI of CFSE in target cells incubated with effector cells})}{(\textit{MFI of CFSE in intact labeled target cells})} \times 100\%\right]$$

3.12 Dimer Assay for Detecting the Frequency of Peptide-Specific CTL

The dimer assay is developed for determining the frequency of peptide-specific T cells using an HLA-A2:Ig fusion protein comprising three extracellular domains of major histocompatibility complex (MHC) class I HLA-A2 and VH regions of mouse IgG1. In order for the MHC class I to be functional, i.e., capable of binding HLA-A2 associated peptides, β2 microglobulin (β2M) must be present. BD™ DimerX consists of recombinant HLA-A2:Ig fusion protein supplemented with recombinant β2M. The BD™ DimerX is used for studying T cell function by immunofluorescent staining and flow cytometry analysis of peptide-specific T cells which can bind the peptide-HLA-A2:Ig fusion protein through the T cell receptors (TCR) on their surface [40].

1. Dilute the peptide solution to 2 mg/mL in sterile DPBS, pH 7.2, for use in the HLA-A2:Ig loading.
2. Mix HLA-A2:Ig protein with specific or control peptide at 40, 160, or 640 molar excess together in PBS, pH 7.2, and then incubate at 37 °C overnight. The peptide-loaded HLA-A2:Ig can be stored at 4 °C for up to 1 week.
3. Incubate 2 μg peptide, e.g., $HBcAg_{18\text{-}27}$-loaded HLA-A2:Ig, with 1×10^6 generated CTL for 1 h at 4 °C. Prior to the incubation, resuspend the generated CTL with 50 μL of purified polyclonal human IgG at 1 mg/mL in FACS buffer for 10 min to block nonspecific binding of DimerX to Fc receptors on the cell surface.
4. Wash the cells, then incubate with 100 μL of purified polyclonal human IgG in FACS buffer for 10 min.
5. Stain the cells with 0.5 μL of PE-conjugated A85-1 mAb (anti-mouse IgG1) for 30 min on ice in the dark.
6. Wash the cells with FACS buffer and then stain with FITC-conjugated mouse antihuman CD8 mAb for 30 min on ice in the dark.
7. Wash the cells with FACS buffer and then analyze the cells by flow cytometry.

3.13 IFN-γ ELISPOT Assay

The ELISPOT assay is the current method of choice for monitoring immune responses. It can be used to identify and enumerate cytokine-producing cells at the single-cell level. Each spot represents a single reactive cell. Here, we describe an IFN-γ ELISPOT assay using ELISPOT human IFN-γ Set [41, 42] to enumerate IFN-γ-producing $CD8^+$ T cells induced by DC loaded with HSP fusion proteins.

1. Dilute capture antibody (anti-IFN-γ mAb) in coating buffer. Add 100 μL of diluted antibody solution to each well of an ELISPOT plate and store the plate at 4 °C overnight.
2. Discard the coating antibody and wash wells 1× with 200 μL blocking solution/well. Add 200 μL blocking solution/well and incubate for 2 h at room temperature.
3. Discard the blocking solution. Add 100 μL of generated CTL primed by antigen-loaded DC/well at density of 2×10^4 cells/well and 100 μL/well of peptide-loaded T2 cells at a ratio of 15:1 to an ELISPOT plate.

4. Incubate the plate for 36 h at 37 °C in an atmosphere of 5 % CO_2 in air.
5. Aspirate the cell suspension. Wash wells 2× by soaking 3–5 min at each wash step with deionized water and 3× with 200 μL/well of wash buffer.
6. Add 100 μL of diluted detection antibody (biotinylated anti-IFN-γ mAb)/well to the ELISPOT plate and incubate for 2 h at room temperature.
7. Discard detection antibody solution. Wash wells 3× with 200 μL/well of wash buffer.
8. Add 100 μL/well of diluted streptavidin–HRP to the ELISPOT plate and incubate for 1 h at room temperature.
9. Discard the streptavidin–HRP solution. Wash wells 4× with 200 μL/well of wash buffer I and 2× with wash buffer II.
10. Add 100 μL of final substrate solution (AEC) to each well.
11. Monitor spot development 5–60 min.
12. Stop substrate reaction by washing the wells with deionized water.
13. Air-dry plate for 2 h or overnight at room temperature in the dark until the plate is completely dry. Store the plate in the dark prior to analysis.
14. Enumerate the spots. Each spot represents an IFN-γ-producing cell. Set up controls: no stimulation and unrelated peptide-loaded DC control.

3.14 IFN-γ Intracellular Staining

Cytokine intracellular staining is a method to detect cytokines at the single-cell level to study the contribution of different cells to cytokine production in heterogeneous cell populations. IFN-γ intracellular staining enables the detection of IFN-γ-producing peptide-specific $CD8^+$ T cells restimulated with peptide-loaded DC by flow cytometry.

1. Restimulate the generated CTL with peptide-loaded DC at ratio of 10:1 in 1 mL of complete medium supplemented with 10 U/mL of IL-2, and incubate for 8 h at 37 °C in an atmosphere of 5 % CO_2 in air.
2. Add 10 μg/mL of Brefeldin A for 5 h into the culture before the end of restimulation.
3. Wash the cells with staining buffer and then stain the cells with anti-cell surface molecules, e.g., FITC-conjugated anti-CD8 mAb, for 30 min on ice in the dark.
4. Wash the cells 1× with staining buffer and then resuspend the cells in 75 μL of 4 % paraformaldehyde and 25 μL of PBS and incubate for 20 min at room temperature.

5. Wash the cells with 2 mL of PBS and then resuspend the cells in 50 μL of saponin buffer containing anti-IFN-γ mAb and incubate for 30 min at room temperature.
6. Wash the cells 2× with 2 mL of PBS and then resuspend the cells in 0.3 mL of PBS and analyze by flow cytometry. For later analysis, resuspend the cells in 0.3 mL of 1–2 % paraformaldehyde. Set up controls: no stimulation control, isotype surface staining control, and isotype intracellular staining control.

4 Notes

1. Endotoxin or LPS may exist in the recombinant HSP fusion proteins expressed in *E. coli* and purified from whole lysate of *E. coli* despite performing endotoxin removal during protein purification. LPS can nonspecifically activate DC via CD14 and TLR4 on the cell membrane, causing the deviation of the results. To avoid this, we use polymyxin B to inhibit the activity of trace endotoxin in HSP fusion protein, setting up a control of HSP fusion protein plus polymyxin B. Also, HSP fusion proteins need to be checked for endotoxin levels before use.
2. For inducing human monocyte-derived DC, GM-CSF and IL-4 are added into complete medium. The optimal concentrations of the cytokines need to be determined before use since the activity of different sources of the cytokines is varied. Monocyte-derived DC can be induced in monocyte-conditioned medium which can be prepared as follows: (1) Add 4 mL of 10 mg/mL human γ-globulin to a 100 mm bacteriologic plate for 1 min immediately before use, (2) remove the residual γ-globulin and wash the plate for 3× with PBS prior to use, (3) layer 35×10^6 PBMC onto the Ig-coated plate for 1 h in 6–8 mL of complete medium with 5 % human serum or 1 % autologous plasma at 37 °C in an atmosphere of 5 % CO_2 in air, (4) wash off the nonadherent cells and incubate adherent cells in fresh complete medium with 5 % human serum or 1 % autologous plasma at 37 °C for no more than 24 h, and (5) collect the medium and freeze at −20 °C before use [43, 44].
3. It is recommended to determine the optimal dose of the HSP fusion proteins for activating DC by stimulating DC with various concentrations of the fusion proteins and checking the morphology of DC using light microscopy. The more sensitive method would be to check expression levels of CD80, CD83, CD86, CD40, or HLA-A2 molecules on DC by flow cytometry. Results may vary because of donor to donor variation. We strongly recommend the use of DC from at least three donors.

4. HSP fusion protein-pulsed mature DC can be preserved by freezing in a freezing solution: autologous serum, 10 % DMSO, 5 % glucose, at a cell density of 10×10^6/mL [45]. The following procedure is for preserving the mature DC: (1) Harvest mature DC on day 7 following culturing with HSP fusion protein, (2) make a cell suspension of 10×10^6/mL in complete medium, (3) mix the cell suspension with freezing solution at a 1:1 ratio and then immediately transfer the mixture to 1-mL or 1.8-mL cryo tubes, (4) slowly freeze the tubes to −80 °C using a cryofreezing container and finally transfer the tubes into liquid nitrogen. If a cryofreezing container isn't available, the tubes can be wrapped up with about 2–3 cm thick of cold cotton, put into −80 °C freezer overnight, and then transferred into liquid nitrogen.
5. To collect peptide-specific $CD8^+$ T cells, a negative selection method is used to avoid nonspecific activation of $CD8^+$ T cells by antibodies during T cell sorting.
6. To generate specific CTL with DC pulsed with HSP fusion protein in vitro, IL-7, not IL-2, is added into the culture in the first 7 days since IL-7 can support T cell survival to respond to MHC class I peptide complex on the surface of DC.
7. To generate peptide-specific CTL, peptide-pulsed DC rather than peptide alone are incubated with the $CD8^+$ T cells since the TCR on the surface of T cells can only bind and recognize peptide associated with MHC class I complex on DC.
8. T2 cells (HLA-$A2^+$), from American Type Culture Collection, are defective in transporting MHC class I-presented antigenic peptides across mitochondrial membrane, expressing "empty" HLA-A2 molecules on their surface. The T2 cells are cultured in Iscove's modified Dulbecco's medium supplemented with 10 % FBS. Peptides can be loaded onto "empty" HLA-A2 molecules on T2 cells to make peptide–HLA-A2 complexes which can be recognized and bound by TCR on the surface of T cells. For this reason, T2 cells are usually used as target cells for seeking peptide-specific T cells.

Acknowledgement

This work was partly supported by the National Nature Scientific Foundation of China (31270982).

References

1. Steinman RM, Banchereau J (2007) Taking dendritic cells into medicine. Nature 449:419–426
2. Steinman RM (2012) Decisions about dendritic cells: past, present and future. Annu Rev Immunol 30:1–22
3. Kantoff PW et al (2010) Sipuleucel-T immunotherapy for castration-resistant prostate cancer. N Engl J Med 363:411–422
4. Small EJ et al (2000) Immunotherapy of hormone-refractory prostate cancer with antigen-loaded dendritic cells. J Clin Oncol 18:3894–3903
5. Witmer-Pack MD et al (1987) Granulocyte/macrophage colony-stimulating factor is essential for the viability and function of cultured murine epidermal Langerhans cells. J Exp Med 166:1484–1498
6. Romani N et al (1989) Presentation of exogenous protein antigens by dendritic cells to T cell clones: intact protein is presented best by immature, epidermal Langerhans cells. J Exp Med 169:1169–1178
7. Sallusto F, Lanzavecchia A (1994) Efficient presentation of soluble antigen by cultured human dendritic cells is maintained by granulocyte/macrophage colony-stimulating factor plus interleukin 4 and down-regulated by tumor necrosis factor α. J Exp Med 971:81–9011
8. Tacken PJ et al (2007) Dendritic-cell immunotherapy: from ex vivo loading to in vivo targeting. Nat Rev Immunol 7(10):790–802
9. Jiang W et al (1995) The receptor DEC-205 expressed by dendritic cells and thymic epithelial cells is involved in antigen processing. Nature 375(6527):151–155
10. Granelli-Piperno A et al (2005) Dendritic cell-specific intercellular adhesion molecule 3-grabbing nonintegrin/CD209 is abundant on macrophages in the normal human lymph node and is not required for dendritic cell stimulation of the mixed leukocyte reaction. J Immunol 175(7):4265–4273
11. Cheong C et al (2010) Improved cellular and humoral immune responses in vivo following targeting of HIV Gag to dendritic cells within human anti-human DEC205 monoclonal antibody. Blood 116(19):3828–3838
12. Idoyaga J et al (2011) Comparable T helper 1 (Th1) and CD8 T-cell immunity by targeting HIV gag p24 to CD8 dendritic cells within antibodies to Langerin, DEC205, and Clec9A. Proc Natl Acad Sci U S A 108(6):2384–2389
13. Trumpfheller C et al (2012) Dendritic cell-targeted protein vaccines: a novel approach to induce T-cell immunity. J Intern Med 271(2):183–192
14. Bozzacco L et al (2007) DEC-205 receptor on dendritic cells mediates presentation of HIV gag protein to $CD8^+$ T cells in a spectrum of human MHC I haplotypes. Proc Natl Acad Sci U S A 104(4):1289–1294
15. Wang B et al (2012) Targeting of the non-mutated tumor antigen HER2/neu to mature dendritic cells induces an integrated immune response that protects against breast cancer in mice. Breast Cancer Res 14(2):R39
16. Hayashi F et al (2001) The innate immune response to bacterial flagellin is mediated by Toll-like receptor 5. Nature 410(6832):1099–1103
17. Mizel SB, Bates JT (2010) Flagellin as an adjuvant: cellular mechanisms and potential. J Immunol 185:5677–5682
18. Edwards AD et al (2003) Toll-like receptor expression in murine DC subsets: lack of TLR7 expression by CD8 $alpha^+$ DC correlates with unresponsiveness to imidazoquinolines. Eur J Immunol 33(4):827–833
19. Vicente-Suarez I et al (2009) TLR5 ligation by flagellin converts tolerogenic dendritic cells into activating antigen-presenting cells that preferentially induce T-Helper 1 responses. Immunol Lett 125(2):114–118
20. Bates JT et al (2009) Direct stimulation of tlr5+/+ $CD11c^+$ cells is necessary for the adjuvant activity of flagellin. J Immunol 182(12):7539–7547
21. Kupz A et al (2012) NLRC4 inflammasomes in dendritic cells regulate noncognate effector function by memory $CD8^+$ T cells. Nat Immunol 13(2):162–169
22. Zhao Y et al (2011) The NLRC4 inflammasome receptors for bacterial flagellin and type III secretion apparatus. Nature 477(7366):596–600
23. Mizel SB et al (2009) Flagellin-F1-V fusion protein is an effective plague vaccine in mice and two species of nonhuman primates. Clin Vaccine Immunol 16(1):21–28
24. Huleatt JW et al (2008) Potent immunogenicity and efficacy of a universal influenza vaccine candidate comprising a recombinant fusion protein linking influenza M2e to the TLR5 ligand flagellin. Vaccine 26(2):201–214
25. Bargieri DY et al (2008) New malaria vaccine candidates based on the Plasmodium vivax

Merozoite surface Protein-1 and the TLR-5 agonist Salmonella Typhimurium FliC flagellin. Vaccine 26(48):6132–6142
26. Le Moigne V et al (2008) Flagellin as a good carrier and potent adjuvant for Th1 response: study of mice immune response to the p27 (Rv2108) Mycobacterium tuberculosis antigen. Mol Immunol 45:2499–2507
27. Machluf N, Arnon R (2012) Therapeutic MUC1-based cancer vaccine expressed in flagella-efficacy in an aggressive model of breast cancer. World J Vaccines 2(3):109–120
28. Garaude J et al (2012) Simultaneous targeting of toll- and nod-like receptors induces effective tumor-specific immune responses. Sci Transl Med 4(120):120
29. Tamura Y et al (2012) New paradigm for intrinsic function of heat shock proteins as endogenous ligands in inflammation and innate immunity. Curr Mol Med 12(9):1198–1206
30. Tamura Y et al (2012) Heat-shock proteins as endogenous ligands building a bridge between innate and adaptive immunity. Immunotherapy 4(8):841–852
31. Srivastava PK, Heike M (1991) Tumor-specific immunogenicity of stress-induced proteins: convergence of two evolutionary pathways of antigen presentation? Semin Immunol 3:57–64
32. Srivastava PK, Maki RG (1991) Stress-induced proteins in immune response to cancer. Curr Top Microbiol Immunol 167:109–123
33. Cho BK et al (2000) A proposed mechanism for the induction of cytotoxic T lymphocyte production by heat shock protein fusion proteins. Immunity 12(3):263–272
34. Liu H et al (2007) Induction of CD4-independent E7-specific CD8+ memory response by heat shock fusion protein. Clin Vaccine Immunol 14(8):1013–1023
35. Li D et al (2006) Heat shock fusion protein induces both specific and nonspecific anti-tumor immunity. Eur J Immunol 36(5):1324–1336
36. Huo Y et al (2007) Pre-clinical safety evaluation of heat shock protein 65-MUC1 peptide fusion protein. Regul Toxicol Pharmacol 49(1):63–74
37. Hua W et al (2011) Recombinant heat shock protein 65 carrying PADRE and HBV epitopes activates dendritic cells and elicits HBV-specific CTL responses. Vaccine 29(12):2328–2335
38. Yu F et al (2007) Purification of a non-tagged recombinant BCG heat shock protein 65-Her2 peptide fusion protein from Escherichia coli. Protein Expr Purif 53(2):390–395
39. Sheehy ME et al (2001) A novel technique for the fluorometric assessment of T lymphocyte antigen specific lysis. J Immunol Methods 249(1–2):99–110
40. BD™ DimerX, Technical Data Sheet, DimerX I: recombinant soluble dimeric human HLA-A2:Ig fusion protein
41. BD™ ELISPOT, Technical Data Sheet: human IFN-γ ELISPOT pair
42. Czerkinsky C et al (1983) A solid-phase enzyme-linked immunospot (ELISPOT) assay for enumeration of specific antibody-secreting cells. J Immunol Methods 65(1–2):109–121
43. Bender A et al (1996) Improved methods for the generation of dendritic cells from nonproliferating progenitors in human blood. J Immunol Methods 196(2):121–135
44. Anita R et al (1997) A monocyte conditioned medium is more effective than defined cytokines in mediating the terminal maturation of human dendritic cells. Blood 90(9): 3640–3646
45. Feuerstein B et al (2000) A method for the production of cryopreserved aliquots of antigen-preloaded, mature dendritic cells ready for clinical use. J Immunol Methods 245:15–29

Chapter 8

Antigen-Specific mRNA Transfection of Autologous Dendritic Cells

Fabian Benencia

Abstract

Several reports have described the use of tumor-extracted RNA as source of tumor antigen for the preparation of vaccines based on dendritic cells (DC) and its potential use for antigen-specific or polyvalent tumor vaccination. Upon transfection, RNA is transcribed into proteins that enter the cytoplasmic degradation pathway and can be presented by DC through class I major histocompatibility complex (MHC)-I, thus inducing specific T cell cytotoxic responses. In this chapter, we present a protocol to transfect murine dendritic cells with tumor mRNA by means of electroporation.

Key words Dendritic cells, mRNA, Electroporation, Vaccine, Transfection

1 Introduction

The capacity of the immune system to fight cancer relies on the presence of tumor-specific antigens and tumor-associated antigens (TAA). While tumor-specific antigens are expressed only by tumor cells due to mutations or expression of viral antigens or normally suppressed oncogenes in cancer, TAA are expressed both in cancer and noncancerous cells, but at higher levels in the former cells. TAA can also be expressed by normal cells during the embryonic state of differentiation [1]. For the purposes of this chapter, tumor antigens are generically referred as TAA. TAA can be used for vaccination purposes as genetic material, e.g., as RNA. The advantage of using RNA instead of DNA as a means of delivering TAA is that with the former, the possibility of genomic integration is avoided. Both types of genetic material also have the potential to further stimulate the immune response upon recognition of CPG sequences by toll-like receptor (TLR)-9 (DNA) or by activation of TLR-3 (RNA). RNA vaccination strategies include delivery of naked RNA to either tissue or pulsing DC with RNA molecules.

Michael J.P. Lawman and Patricia D. Lawman (eds.), *Cancer Vaccines: Methods and Protocols*, Methods in Molecular Biology, vol. 1139, DOI 10.1007/978-1-4939-0345-0_8, © Springer Science+Business Media New York 2014

DC are powerful antigen-presenting cells with the capability to stimulate specific T cell responses [2–4]. As such, they have been used as a platform for cell-based vaccines against tumors as previously reviewed [5]. The efficacy of DC vaccines pulsed with TAA in an RNA format has been widely investigated. In the mouse model, DC have been pulsed with whole tumor RNA or mRNA harboring specific antigens [6–11]. Likewise, whole tumor RNA or mRNA has been be used to transfect human DC by electroporation or lipofection [12, 13]. In addition, RNA recovered from tumor cell lines, e.g., leukemia KL562 cell line, has also been used to pulse human DC [14]. It has been shown that the best TAA expression upon RNA transfection of DC is achieved in the absence of antisense RNA, which indicates that better results can be achieved by using mRNA and also emphasizes the need to prepare high-quality RNA for these kinds of studies [15]. In contrast to the delivery of TAA as protein/peptide formulations, TAA synthesized in the cytosol of the cells using an RNA template can enter the degradation pathway of intracellular molecules, yielding peptides that can be directly presented by MHC-I molecules and hence inducing a robust CD8 (cytotoxic) T cell immune response. In addition, some reports indicate that pulsing DC with RNA encoding TAA fused with molecules that augment the delivery of the synthesized proteins to the endoplasmic reticulum could be a valuable strategy to increase the efficiency of the presentation. To this end, TAA RNA have been linked with ubiquitin RNA to target the ubiquitin-proteasome, MHC-I and II pathways by fusion with LAMP1 or DC.LAMP sequences or with immunogenic helper proteins such as EGFP [16–19].

In order to prepare DC vaccines pulsed with TAA as RNA, these cells have been generated from bone marrow precursors in the mouse and mostly from monocytes in humans as previously reviewed [20]. Different steps in the antigen presentation process have been evaluated, such as antigen loading, DC maturation, and delivery route and dose scheme as we have recently reviewed [20]. The majority of RNA-DC vaccination protocols, both in mouse and human settings, induce activation of these cells after transfection. To this end, different maturation cocktails or immunostimulatory factors have been assayed in order to activate these RNA-pulsed cells [21]. Alternatively, mRNA encoding for cytokines that promote DC maturation or function such as interleukin-12 (IL-12) or granulocyte monocyte-colony-stimulating factor (GM-CSF) can be simultaneously transfected into the same cells [22–25]. In this chapter, we describe a protocol for preparing murine DC vaccines by means of transfection with mRNA molecules encoding tumor antigens.

2 Materials

2.1 General Reagents

1. Phosphate buffered saline (PBS).
2. Bovine serum albumin (BSA).
3. Roswell Park Memorial Institute (RPMI)-1640 medium.
4. Minimum essential medium (MEM).
5. Fetal bovine serum (FBS).
6. 5,000 U/mL penicillin-streptomycin.
7. Trypsin.
8. Sodium azide.
9. FACS buffer: PBS, 2 % BSA, 0.05 % sodium azide.
10. Flow cytometry (FACSAria, BD Biosciences, San Jose, CA, USA).

2.2 Dissection of Mouse Femurs and Tibiae and Differentiation of Bone Marrow Cells

1. C57BL/6 mice, 8–12 weeks of age (The Jackson Laboratory, Bar Harbor, Maine, USA) (*see* **Note 1**).
2. Sterilized surgical tools: forceps, scissors.
3. Tissue paper.
4. 70 % Ethanol.
5. 25-mm Petri dishes.
6. 100-mm microbiological grade Petri dishes.
7. Hemocytometer chamber.
8. Cytokines: mouse recombinant (rm) GM-CSF and tumor necrosis factor alpha (TNFα) (Peprotech, Rocky Hill, NJ, USA).
9. Lipopolysaccharide (LPS).
10. Monoclonal antibodies: CD11b (M1/70), CD11c (clone N418), CD45 (30-F11), CD80 (16-10A1), and CD86 (GL1) (eBioscience, San Diego, CA, USA).
11. Anti-mouse CD16/CD32 purified antibody (eBioscience).
12. ACK lysing buffer (Lonza, Allendale, NJ, USA).
13. 0.4 % Trypan Blue solution.
14. BD Via-Probe Viability Solution (BD Biosciences).

2.3 Materials for mRNA In Vitro Transcription, Purification, and Electroporation

1. Murine ovarian cancer cell line (ID8).
2. mMESSAGE mMACHINE® Kit High Yield Capped RNA Transcription Kit (Life Technologies, Grand Island, NY, USA).
3. MEGAclear™ Kit for RNA purification from in vitro transcription experiments (Life Technologies).
4. Dynabeads® mRNA DIRECT™ Kit (Life Technologies).
5. DynaMag™-2 magnet (Life Technologies).
6. Opti-MEM® Reduced Serum Medium (Life Technologies).

7. Electroporator: Gene Pulser II (BIO-RAD Laboratories, Hercules, CA, USA).
8. Electroporation cuvettes Gene Pulser/MicroPulser Cuvettes 0.2 cm gap sterile (BIO-RAD).

3 Methods

3.1 Dissection of Mouse Femurs and Tibiae and Culture of Bone Marrow Cells

1. Sacrifice the mice following the institution/AVMA approved method and carefully dissect tibias and femurs without cutting the bone ends. Two mice will be appropriate for the following procedure.
2. Eliminate all tissue attached to the bone, first using scissors and finally by using tissue paper. Be careful not to break the bones.
3. Inside a biosafety cabinet, immerse the bones in 70 % ethanol for 10 min to sterilize their external surface.
4. Then, using previously sterilized forceps and scissors, cut the femurs in half and the tibia at its thinnest tip. To recover the bone marrow cells, use a sterile syringe to infuse 1 mL of RPMI-1640 medium (with antibiotics but without serum) inside the marrow, collecting the cell suspension on a sterile Petri dish.
5. Wash the cell suspension two times by centrifugation for 10 min at $300 \times g$ in a swinging bucket rotor at 4 °C in 10 mL of the same medium in a 15-mL Falcon centrifuge tube.
6. After the last wash, eliminate the supernatant completely. Resuspend the cells in 2 mL of ACK lysing buffer and incubate for 5 min at room temperature to eliminate contaminating erythrocytes.
7. Then, flood the tubes with RPMI-1640 with 10 % FBS and wash 2× in the same medium by centrifugation as above.
8. After the last washing, resuspend the cell suspension in 10 mL of RPMI-1640 with 10 % FBS. Collect 10 μL of the cell suspension and dilute 1:10 in a solution containing Trypan Blue in order to identify dead cells. Count the cells in a hemocytometer chamber, adjust the original cell suspension to 2×10^5 cells/mL in RPMI-1640 with 10 % FBS, and add 20 ng/mL of rmGM-CSF [26] (*see* **Note 2**).
9. Add 10 mL of the cell suspension to a sterile, microbiological quality, 10-cm Petri dish and culture at 37 °C, 5 % CO_2.
10. After 3 days, add to each of the culture plates 10 mL of RPMI-1640 with 10 % FBS and 20 ng/mL of freshly added rmGM-CSF.
11. On day 6 of culture, collect 10 mL of supernatant from each Petri dish, centrifuge as above, and resuspend the pellet in 10 mL of RPMI-1640 with 10 % FBS and 20 ng/mL of freshly

added rmGM-CSF. Return this suspension to the Petri dish and incubate for two additional days at 37 °C in a CO_2 incubator.

12. On day 8 of culture, recover the floating cells together with the loosely adherent cells by gently washing the Petri dishes with PBS. This protocol renders around $2–4 \times 10^8$ DC in our hands when using two mice. Cells are then analyzed for DC phenotype by flow cytometry in order to use them for RNA transfection procedures.

3.2 Analysis of Bone Marrow-Derived DC by Flow Cytometry

1. Collect an aliquot of freshly prepared DC and resuspend in 500 μL of FACS buffer in order to obtain a concentration of 10^6 cells/mL.
2. Block nonspecific binding by adding 1:100 dilution of anti-mouse CD16/CD32 antibody. Incubate on ice for 15 min.
3. Add a 1:100 dilution of anti-murine CD11c, CD11b, CD45, and MHC-II antibodies or respective isotype controls in a similarly prepared tube and incubate for 45 min on ice.
4. Wash 2× in FACS buffer by centrifugation at $300 \times g$ in a swinging bucket centrifuge.
5. Resuspend in 500 μL of FACS buffer and read in a multicolor flow cytometry such as the FACSAria. The DC population should be 100 % $CD45^+$ and $CD11b^+$, and more than 80 % of the population should express high levels of CD11c [26]. In addition, the obtained population should be positive for MHC-II expression.
6. Simultaneously, viability is measured by adding 20 μL of Via-Probe solution to the cell suspension 15 min before reading in the flow cytometry. Dead cells, into which the dye has diffused, will appear as bright PerCP positive cells.

3.3 Isolation of Whole mRNA from Tumor Cells

Whole cellular mRNA can be recovered from tumor tissues or tumor cell lines using commercially available reagents. Here, we describe a protocol to extract whole mRNA from a murine ovarian cancer cell line using the Dynabeads® mRNA DIRECT™ Kit. Other tumor cell lines can be used as a source of RNA for electroporation as we have previously demonstrated [27].

1. Grow the murine ID8 cell line in T75-culture flasks in MEM with 10 % FBS up to 75 % confluence. Detach the cells by trypsin treatment and wash the cell pellet 2× in PBS by centrifugation at $300 \times g$ for 10 min in a 15-mL Falcon tube at 4 °C in order to eliminate all protein residues from the cell culture medium.
2. Resuspend the pellet in 1,250 μL of the Lysis/Binding Buffer provided by the kit for each flask (approximately 4×10^6 cells). Homogenize by repeated passage through a micropipette tip. Collect in a 2 mL microcentrifuge tube.

3. In order to shear the co-extracted DNA, the lysate must then be passed through a 21 gauge needle 5× using a 2-mL syringe.
4. After washing, add the provided oligo dT Dynabeads to the lysate and incubate with rotation for 5 min at room temperature.
5. Place the centrifuge tube on a DynaMag magnet for 2 min and then remove the supernatant.
6. Wash the beads/mRNA complex 2× with 1,250 μL of the provided Washing Buffer A. Use the magnet to separate the beads from the solution between each washing step.
7. Wash the beads/mRNA complex 1× with 1.5 mL of the provided Washing Buffer B.
8. To elute the mRNA from the beads, add 25 μL of the provided Elution Buffer (10 mM Tris–HCl, pH 7.5) to the pellet outside the magnet and incubate at 65 °C for 2 min. Then, place the microcentrifuge tube on the magnet and transfer the supernatant containing the mRNA to a new tube.
9. The quality of the RNA can be checked by agarose-formaldehyde gel electrophoresis.

3.4 Preparation of Antigen-Specific mRNA

mRNA encoding specific molecules can be prepared by using in vitro transcription protocols (*see* **Note 3**). To this end, researchers must clone their gene of interest in a plasmid that allows for in vitro transcription studies. If using the mMESSAGE mMACHINE kit as described here, the plasmid should have either T7, T3, or SP6S RNA polymerase promoter sites. In addition, the plasmid should be able to be linearized without affecting the integrity of the sequence being transcribed.

1. Prepare 0.5 μg/μL of a linearized plasmid containing the gene of interest with T7, T3, or SP6S RNA polymerase promoter sites in RNAse-free water.
2. By following the manufacturer's instruction, the reaction will take place in a 20 μL volume and the mRNA will be obtained in approximately 2 h. In these conditions, the in vitro transcription process might yield up to 30 μg of mRNA. This will be enough to transfect $1–2 \times 10^6$ DC as discussed below.
3. Purification of the in vitro-transcribed mRNA can be performed by using the MEGAclear Kit following the manufacturer's instructions. The purity of the recovered RNA will allow for transfection studies.

3.5 Electroporation of DC with mRNA

1. DC are resuspended in OptiMEM at a concentration of 10^7 cells/mL. Two million DC are then mixed with 1–25 μg mRNA per 10^6 DC and added to a 0.2-cm cuvette and electroporated using Gene Pulser II under 300 V and 150 μF of

capacitance [27] (*see* **Note 4**). DC electroporated in the presence of nonspecific mRNA can be used as controls. The reaction is performed in a total volume of 200 μL (*see* **Note 5**).

2. Immediately after electroporation, place the cuvette containing the cells on ice for 5 min to increase the efficacy of the transfection process. Then, resuspend the cells in RPMI-1640 medium containing 10 % FBS with antibiotics and 3 ng/mL of GM-CSF and incubate for 24 h at 37 °C, 5 % CO_2 at a concentration of 10^6 cells/mL.
3. After 6 h of incubation, DC maturation can be induced by adding 20 ng/mL of TNF-α and 100 ng/mL of LPS (*see* **Note 6**).
4. Cells are harvested for phenotypic analysis 24 h later. To this end, maturation can be determined by flow cytometric analysis of activation markers such as CD80 and CD86. Cells are stained as above using CD86, CD80, MHC-II, CD45, and CD11c. When compared with nonactivated cells, the levels of expression of all costimulatory molecules should be increased. Viability can be determined by flow cytometry by addition of Via-Probe as above. In this example, taking into account that ID8 cells express GFP, the efficacy of the transfection process can also be determined by flow cytometry, since GFP gives a signal in the FITC channel. In case of a particular protein, intracellular flow cytometry staining will allow to determine the levels of expression and percentage of cells harboring the protein of interest as we have previously shown [27].

4 Notes

1. Older animals tend to have fewer precursors and render lower number of dendritic cells.
2. Some protocols use IL-4 in addition of GM-CSF to differentiate murine DC from bone marrow precursors, but as previously described, at a concentration of 20 ng/mL of GM-CSF as the one used here, no differences are obtained [28]. In order to generate other DC populations, such as CD8 positive cells which are not present when GM-CSF is used as the solely growth factor for differentiation, treatment with different cytokines such as FLT3 ligand has also been proposed [29].
3. In vitro-transcribed mRNA has been successfully used for DC transfection by means of electroporation as described in various manuscripts [19, 22, 30–32]. It is important to design the plasmid construct in a manner that allows the in vitro transcription event to generate sense RNA. It is important to highlight that the length of the gene to be transcribed will affect the efficacy of the whole transfection process and requires a great deal of

attention from the researchers. Longer RNA molecules will have a higher possibility of suffering degradation compared to smaller ones, affecting the efficiency of the process in respect to the amount of RNA used for a successful transfection. Also, in order to obtain better results during the in vitro transcription process, the linearized plasmid should be as free from contaminating proteins and RNA as possible.

4. To optimize DC pulsing, different concentrations of RNA should be assayed. In our hands, a range between 5 and 50 μg/10^6 DC was appropriate. We were not able to obtain a significant increase in protein expression when using more than 50 μg/10^6 DC.
5. If there is a need to scale up the process, larger electroporation cuvettes, i.e., 0.4 cm, can be used. The researchers must assay the appropriate voltage and capacitance conditions in order to obtain the maximum transfection efficacy with the lowest possible cell death.
6. A study suggests that RNA transfection of DC can also be performed after maturation of these cells [33]. Some reports also indicate that mature DC can be cryopreserved without loss of function, thus indicating that DC vaccines can be prepared and stored for further use [34].

Acknowledgement

This work was supported in part by the NIH under Grant R15 CA137499-01, the NSF grant CBET-1039869, and the RSAC grant (RP1206) from the Heritage College of Osteopathic Medicine, OU.

References

1. Aly HA (2012) Cancer therapy and vaccination. J Immunol Methods 382(1–2):1–23
2. Bonasio R, von Andrian UH (2006) Generation, migration and function of circulating dendritic cells. Curr Opin Immunol 18(4): 503–511
3. Lanzavecchia A, Sallusto F (2001) The instructive role of dendritic cells on T cell responses: lineages, plasticity and kinetics. Curr Opin Immunol 13(3):291–298
4. Banchereau J et al (2000) Immunobiology of dendritic cells. Annu Rev Immunol 18:767–811
5. Ridgway D (2003) The first 1000 dendritic cell vaccines. Cancer Invest 21(6):873–886
6. Pan K et al (2010) Comparative analysis of cytotoxic T lymphocyte response induced by dendritic cells loaded with hepatocellular carcinoma-derived RNA or cell lysate. Int J Biol Sci 6(7):639–648
7. Jarnjak-Jankovic S et al (2007) mRNA transfection of DC in the immature or mature state: comparable *in vitro* priming of Th and cytotoxic T lymphocytes against DC electroporated with tumor cell line-derived mRNA. Cytotherapy 9(6):587–592
8. Ashley DM et al (1997) Bone marrow-generated dendritic cells pulsed with tumor extracts or tumor RNA induce antitumor

immunity against central nervous system tumors. J Exp Med 186(7):1177–1182
9. Liao X et al (2004) Transfection of RNA encoding tumor antigens following maturation of dendritic cells leads to prolonged presentation of antigen and the generation of high-affinity tumor-reactive cytotoxic T lymphocytes. Mol Ther 9(5):757–764
10. Nair SK et al (2000) Induction of cytotoxic T cell responses and tumor immunity against unrelated tumors using telomerase reverse transcriptase RNA transfected dendritic cells. Nat Med 6(9):1011–1017
11. Edlich B et al (2010) Dendritic cells transfected with Her2 antigen-encoding RNA replicons cross-prime CD8 T cells and protect mice against tumor challenge. Vaccine 28(49): 7764–7773
12. Ponsaerts P et al (2002) Messenger RNA electroporation of human monocytes, followed by rapid *in vitro* differentiation, leads to highly stimulatory antigen-loaded mature dendritic cells. J Immunol 169(4):1669–1675
13. Van Tendeloo VF et al (2001) Highly efficient gene delivery by mRNA electroporation in human hematopoietic cells: superiority to lipofection and passive pulsing of mRNA and to electroporation of plasmid cDNA for tumor antigen loading of dendritic cells. Blood 98(1): 49–56
14. Gao L et al (2007) Impact of transfection with total RNA of K562 cells upon antigen presenting, maturation, and function of human dendritic cells from peripheral blood mononuclear cells. Transfusion 47(2):256–265
15. Harris J et al (2005) An improved RNA amplification procedure results in increased yield of autologous RNA transfected dendritic cell-based vaccine. Biochim Biophys Acta 1724(1–2): 127–136
16. Kim SG et al (2008) Modification of CEA with both CRT and TAT PTD induces potent anti-tumor immune responses in RNA-pulsed DC vaccination. Vaccine 26(50):6433–6440
17. Hosoi A et al (2008) Dendritic cell vaccine with mRNA targeted to the proteasome by polyubiquitination. Biochem Biophys Res Commun 371(2):242–246
18. Steitz J et al (2006) Effective induction of anti-melanoma immunity following genetic vaccination with synthetic mRNA coding for the fusion protein EGFP.TRP2. Cancer Immunol Immunother 55(3):246–253
19. Bonehill A et al (2004) Messenger RNA-electroporated dendritic cells presenting MAGE-A3 simultaneously in HLA class I and class II molecules. J Immunol 172(11): 6649–6657
20. Benencia F et al (2012) Dendritic cells the tumor microenvironment and the challenges for an effective antitumor vaccination. J Biomed Biotechnol 2012:425–476
21. Onaitis MW et al (2003) CD40 ligand is essential for generation of specific cytotoxic T cell responses in RNA-pulsed dendritic cell immunotherapy. Surgery 134(2):300–305
22. Bontkes HJ et al (2008) Tumor associated antigen and interleukin-12 mRNA transfected dendritic cells enhance effector function of natural killer cells and antigen specific T-cells. Clin Immunol 127(3):375–384
23. Naka T et al (2008) Tumor vaccine therapy against recrudescent tumor using dendritic cells simultaneously transfected with tumor RNA and granulocyte macrophage colony-stimulating factor RNA. Cancer Sci 99(2): 407–413
24. Bontkes HJ et al (2007) Dendritic cells transfected with interleukin-12 and tumor-associated antigen messenger RNA induce high avidity cytotoxic T cells. Gene Ther 14(4): 366–375
25. Koido S et al (2000) Induction of antitumor immunity by vaccination of dendritic cells transfected with MUC1 RNA. J Immunol 165(10):5713–5719
26. Lutz MB et al (1999) An advanced culture method for generating large quantities of highly pure dendritic cells from mouse bone marrow. J Immunol Methods 223(1):77–92
27. Benencia F et al (2008) Whole tumor antigen vaccination using dendritic cells: comparison of RNA electroporation and pulsing with UV-irradiated tumor cells. J Transl Med 6:21
28. Lutz MB et al (2000) Immature dendritic cells generated with low doses of GM-CSF in the absence of IL-4 are maturation resistant and prolong allograft survival *in vivo*. Eur J Immunol 30(7):1813–1822
29. Brasel K et al (2000) Generation of murine dendritic cells from flt3-ligand-supplemented bone marrow cultures. Blood 96(9): 3029–3039
30. Grunebach F et al (2005) Cotransfection of dendritic cells with RNA coding for HER-2/neu and 4-1BBL increases the induction of tumor antigen specific cytotoxic T lymphocytes. Cancer Gene Ther 12(9):749–756
31. Dorfel D et al (2005) Processing and presentation of HLA class I and II epitopes by dendritic cells after transfection with *in vitro*-transcribed MUC1 RNA. Blood 105(8):3199–3205

32. Bonehill A et al (2003) Efficient presentation of known HLA class II-restricted MAGE-A3 epitopes by dendritic cells electroporated with messenger RNA encoding an invariant chain with genetic exchange of class II-associated invariant chain peptide. Cancer Res 63(17):5587–5594
33. Schaft N et al (2005) Generation of an optimized polyvalent monocyte-derived dendritic cell vaccine by transfecting defined RNAs after rather than before maturation. J Immunol 174(5):3087–3097
34. Feuerstein B et al (2000) A method for the production of cryopreserved aliquots of antigen-preloaded, mature dendritic cells ready for clinical use. J Immunol Methods 245(1–2): 5–29

Chapter 9

Electroporation of Dendritic Cells with Autologous Total RNA from Tumor Material

Francesca Milano and K.K. Krishnadath

Abstract

Dendritic cells (DC) are unique antigen-presenting cells that initiate and orchestrate adaptive immunity. Theoretically, cancer cells that express tumor-specific antigens can be destroyed by cytotoxic T cells. However, inherent antitumor responses are often not efficient, since tumor cells can mask their antigens and do not activate DC, an event required for the development of tumor antigen-specific cytotoxic T cell responses. Over a decade ago, the ex vivo preparation of autologous tumor antigen-loaded monocyte-derived DC vaccines as a novel potent anticancer strategy was launched. Phase I and II trials have been performed employing this strategy to treat several malignancies, such as B cell lymphoma, myeloma, melanoma, prostate, colon, ovarian, pancreatic, breast cancer, and renal cell carcinoma. So far, DC immunotherapy is well tolerated with little side or toxic effects. An issue of concern is the way DC are loaded with tumor antigens. An effective strategy is the loading of DC with tumor antigen through electroporation with tumor RNA. In this chapter, a comprehensive description of a protocol for loading of ex vivo-derived DC with total tumor RNA through electroporation is provided.

Key words Electroporation, RNA, Tumor, Dendritic cells, Cytotoxic T cells

1 Introduction

Dendritic cell (DC)-based cancer vaccination is a strategy that utilizes the patient's immune system to reject cancer by using DC. DC are professional antigen-presenting cells able to prime naïve T cells to induce a specific immune response against cancer. For DC-based cancer immunotherapy, DC are loaded ex vivo with tumor antigens and then given back to patients. After activation of the DC, T cells become effector cytotoxic T lymphocytes (CTL). A very important part of the ex vivo generation of potent antitumor DC is the loading of DC with tumor-associated antigens (TAA), which can be performed in various ways. DC can either be loaded with defined antigens or with whole tumor preparations. Loading DC with short peptides derived from defined antigens such as carcinoembryonic antigen (CEA), MelanA, gp100, and HER-2 is currently the most applied method [1–4]. These pep-

Michael J.P. Lawman and Patricia D. Lawman (eds.), *Cancer Vaccines: Methods and Protocols*, Methods in Molecular Biology, vol. 1139, DOI 10.1007/978-1-4939-0345-0_9, © Springer Science+Business Media New York 2014

tides are able to directly bind to either class 1 or class 2 major histocompatibility (MHC) molecules and can easily be produced on large scale according to good manufacturing practice (GMP) regulations, while immunomonitoring can be easily performed for instance by using human leukocyte antigen (HLA)-specific tetramers/pentamers. On the other hand, there are substantial limitations to this method: these peptides are HLA specific, thus making them only suitable for a restricted group of patients. Moreover, for several cancers the number of defined antigen peptides that can be used to load DC is limited. Loading DC with whole TAA preparations such as modified whole proteins, viral vectors, antigen-coding DNA, or messenger RNA (mRNA) allows DC to naturally process the antigen and to select multiple antigens for presentation on both MHC class 1 and 2, including antigenic peptides that have not been previously defined. Moreover, these methods do not require HLA restrictions and can thus be used for a larger group of patients. A variety of whole tumor preparations such as exosomes, tumor lysates, apoptotic cells, and total tumor mRNA have been used. The first report on the use of mRNA to load DC has come from E. Gilboa et al. [5–7]. Gilboa and his group applied passive RNA pulsing or RNA lipofection to introduce the coding RNA into DC. Later, several other groups reported to have successfully loaded DC with antigens using different methodology such as lipofection, passive pulse, or transfection through electroporation, with DNA, total RNA, or mRNA of defined tumor antigens [8–10]. In general, most assays employ blood or bone marrow monocytes that are first stimulated to become immature or mature DC before cells are loaded with the antigens [11]. Electroporation proves to be a more efficient and frequently applied method for antigen loading of DC compared to other methods [9]. When DC reach the immature stage, DC are specifically able to capture and process antigens and therefore can be employed at this stage of maturation for electroporation [12]. Yet, electroporation of monocytes directly isolated from blood has been described [13]. In a previous study published by our group, we demonstrated that electroporation of monocytes directly isolated from blood is an efficient procedure that results in a three times higher yield of immunopotent DC when compared to the more conventional electroporation of immature DC [14]. The protocol described herein is a detailed description of the monocyte electroporation procedure.

2 Materials

2.1 Isolation and Culture of DC from Peripheral Blood

1. Heparinized vials for collection of peripheral blood mononuclear cells (PBMC) (*see* **Note 1**).
2. Ficoll-Hypaque solution (*see* **Note 2**).

3. 10× Phosphate-buffered saline (PBS), pH 10 (*see* **Note 3**).
4. Standard isotone Percoll (SIP): 19.8 mL Percoll, 2.2 mL 10× PBS, pH 10.
   (a) 47.5 % SIP: 11.45 mL IMDM (no FBS, no Pen/Strep), 10.55 mL SIP.
   (b) 34 % SIP: 6.6 mL of IMDM, 3.4 mL of SIP.
5. Roswell Park Memorial Institute (RPMI)-1640 medium with 10 % fetal bovine serum (FBS) and 1 % penicillin/streptomycin, no glutamine.
6. Iscove's Modified Dulbecco's Medium (IMDM), no FBS/penicillin/streptomycin.
7. Cytokines: interleukin-4 (IL-4), granulocyte-macrophage colony-stimulating factor (GM-CSF), transforming growth factor-β (TGF-β), tumor necrosis factor-α (TNF-α), lipopolysaccharide (LPS). Store at −20 °C (*see* **Note 4**).

2.2 Electroporation of DC

1. Amaxa Nucleofector device (Amaxa GmbH, Cologne, Germany).
2. Amaxa Cell Line Nucleofector Kit V (Amaxa GmbH, Cologne, Germany). Store at 4 °C (*see* **Note 5**).

2.3 Isolation of RNA from Human Cancer Biopsy Specimens (Without a Kit)

1. Trizol Reagent (Life Technologies Inc., Invitrogen, Breda, The Netherlands).
2. Phenol/chloroform.
3. Isopropanol.
4. 70 % ethanol.
5. RNase-free H_2O.
6. Nano-Drop device and software.
7. Bioanalyzer device and software.

2.3.1 Isolation of RNA from Human Cancer Biopsy Specimens (with a Kit)

1. RNeasy Midi Kit (Qiagen, Breda, The Netherlands).
2. TissueRuptor (230 V, 50/60 Hz, EU/CH).
3. TissueRuptor disposable probes.
4. RNase-free H_2O.
5. Nano-Drop device and software.
6. Bioanalyzer device and software.

3 Methods

3.1 RNA Isolation

3.1.1 RNA Isolation Without a Kit

1. Collect biopsies from cancer tissues in Trizol Reagent adding 300 μL of Trizol. Set centrifuge to 4 °C.
2. Add 60 μL of chloroform to the material collected in Trizol.

3. Shake the Eppendorf tube vigorously and incubate for 3 min at room temperature. Centrifuge at 12,000 × *g* for 15 min at 4 °C.
4. Collect aqueous phase (upper layer) in a new Eppendorf tube. Add 500 μL isopropanol.
5. Incubate for 10 min at room temperature.
6. Centrifuge at 12,000 × *g* for 10 min at 4 °C.
7. Pour off isopropanol.
8. Add 1 mL 75 % ethanol and vortex.
9. Centrifuge at 7,500 × *g* for 5 min at 4 °C.
10. Pour off ethanol and remove remaining fluid with pipette (*see* **Note 6**).
11. Air-dry for 5 min.
12. Add 30 μL RNAse-free H_2O.
13. Measure RNA concentration with Nanodrop.

3.1.2 RNA Isolation with RNA Midi Kit from Qiagen

Prior to starting: (*see* **Note 7**)

1. Place the weighed tissue (previously collected in RNAlater and left overnight at 4 °C) in a suitably sized vessel for the homogenizer (15-mL tube). Add the appropriate volume of buffer RLT (follow instructions from the Qiagen kit handbook). Homogenize immediately using a TissueRuptor homogenizer for 45 s until the sample is uniformly homogeneous.
2. Centrifuge the tissue lysate for 10 min at 3,000–5,000 × *g*. Carefully transfer the supernatant to a new 15-mL tube by pipetting. Use only this supernatant (lysate) in subsequent steps.
3. Add 1 volume of 70 % ethanol to the homogenized lysate and mix immediately by shaking vigorously. Ensure that any precipitates are resuspended. *Do not centrifuge.*
4. Apply the sample to an RNeasy Midi column placed in a 15-mL centrifuge tube and close the tube gently. Maximum loading volume is 4 mL. Centrifuge for 5 min at 3,000–5,000 × *g*. Discard the flow-through.
5. Add 4 mL buffer RW1 to the RNeasy column. Close the centrifuge tube gently and centrifuge for 5 min at 3,000–5,000 × *g* to wash the column. Discard the flow-through.
6. Add 2.5 mL buffer RPE to the RNeasy column. Close the centrifuge tube gently and centrifuge for 2 min at 3,000–5,000 × *g* to wash the column. Discard the flow-through.
7. Add another 2.5 mL buffer RPE to the RNeasy column. Close the centrifuge tube gently and centrifuge for 5 min at 3,000–5,000 × *g* to dry the RNeasy silica-gel membrane.

8. To elute, transfer the RNeasy column to a new 15-mL collection tube. Pipet 150 μL RNase-free water directly onto the RNeasy silica-gel membrane. Close the tube gently. Let it stand for 1 min and then centrifuge for 3 min at 3,000–5,000 × *g*.
9. Repeat the elution step as described with a second volume of RNase-free water.

3.2 Isolation of Monocytes and Lymphocytes from Peripheral Blood

1. Add 30 mL RPMI-1640 to a T75 flask and then add the 64 mL of collected human peripheral blood.
2. QS to 150 mL with RPMI-1640 with no additives.
3. Take 6 × 50 mL Falcon tubes and add 14 mL of Ficoll per tube.
4. Very carefully add 25 mL of blood onto every tube (*see* **Note 8**).
5. Centrifuge at 1,710 × *g* for 30 min; brake speeds must be set at 0 and 1, at 22 °C (*see* **Note 9**).
6. Collect the white ring of cells which will be visible on top of the bottom layer (erythrocytes) and the Ficoll layer.
7. Put the entire amount in 4 × 50-mL tubes.
8. Fill up the tubes to 45 mL with RPMI-1640.
9. Centrifuge at 490 × *g* for 10 min at 10 °C.
10. Remove the supernatant, resuspend the pellet in 10 mL of RPMI-1640, and pool them in two tubes.
11. Centrifuge at 490 × *g* for10 min at 10 °C.
12. Remove the supernatant, add 4 mL of IMDM (with FBS/Pen/Strep) per tube, and resuspend the cells.
13. Add 6 mL of SIP to the cell suspension so that the cells are in 60 % SIP.
14. Add 2.5 mL of the cell suspension per tube (4 × 15-mL tubes), then pipette very carefully 5 mL of 47.5 % SIP (gravity mode for the PIPETBOY and keep pipette on same spot on the wall of the tube).
15. Very carefully add 2 mL of 34 % SIP on top of this (on the same spot on the wall of the tube).
16. Centrifuge at 2,105 × *g* for 45 min; brake speeds must be set at 0 and 1.
17. At the end of the centrifugation, there are two interfaces and two rings: the upper one contains monocytes and the lower one contains lymphocytes.
18. Collect each of the two rings in two different 50-mL tubes and QS to 45 mL with IMDM.
19. Centrifuge at 490 × *g* for 10 min.
20. Resuspend the cell pellet in 10 mL of IMDM.
21. Count cells or freeze them: cells are ready to use.

3.3 Nucleic Acid Measurement

1. On the Nanodrop software, select "Nucleic acid measurement."
2. Add 1-μL H_2O and click "Blank." "Sample type = RNA-40."
3. Clean device between sample measurements with a tissue.
4. "Start report" to record all concentrations and other parameters such as 260/280 ratio and 260/230 ratio.
5. Add 1 μL of sample. Fill in "Sample ID."
6. Click "Measure."
7. Change "Sample ID."
8. When finished, click on "Show report," "Print," and "Exit."
9. Clean device with H_2O. Click "Exit" and then "Ok."
10. Store RNA at −80 °C until further use.

3.4 Electroporation of Monocytes with Autologous Tumor Total RNA

1. Wash monocytes characterized as $CD14^+$, $CD45^+$, $CD80^-$, $CD86^-$, $CD83^-$, and $CD209^-$ freshly isolated from blood 2× in IMDM by centrifuging at 342 × *g* for 10 min at 10 °C.
2. Remove *all* the supernatant (*see* **Note 10**).
3. Electroporate the monocytes using the Amaxa Cell Line Nucleofector Kit V. The desired number of cells is usually from 0.5 to 10×10^6 cells.
4. Add 100 μL of the solution to the cell pellet and resuspend.
5. Take a cuvette from the kit, add 2 μL of isolated RNA (concentration range: 500 ng/mL–20 μg/mL RNA) (*see* **Note 11**).
6. Add 100 μL of the solution on top of the RNA previously dropped on the wall of the cuvette so that it mixes properly to the cell suspension.
7. Use the U16 program of the Amaxa transfection device: insert the cuvette, select the program, press the proper button (X) on the Amaxa device, and wait until "ok" appears on the screen.
8. Add quickly culture medium with FBS (*see* **Note 12**) and resuspend the cells.
9. Culture 1×10^6/mL of monocytes in 24-well plates using IMDM with 10 % FBS and 2 % Pen/Strep.
10. Place cells at 37 °C and 5 % CO_2 for 1 h (*see* **Note 13**).
11. Wash 2× with IMDM (*see* **Note 14**).
12. Add 1 mL of fresh IMDM supplemented with 10 % FBS, 1 % Pen/Strep, 1 % L-glutamine, and 1,000 U/mL of IL-4 and 800 U/mL of GM-CSF to initiate the maturation process.
13. After 3 days, remove half of the medium (0.5 mL), and add fresh medium and fresh IL-4 and GM-CSF.
14. After 3 days at the stage of immature DC: remove half of the medium of the wells (0.5 mL) and add the maturation cytokines (depending on the protocol used by each laboratory, the

protocol used in our laboratory is the following: 10 ng/mL of IL-1β, 25 ng/mL of TNF-α, and 0.02 ng/mL of LPS).

15. Analyze cells by flow cytometry for the expression of maturation markers at day 6 and at day 8 of culturing.
16. Use the cells for further functional analysis of antigen expression (such as T cell proliferation, IFN-γ production, and cytotoxicity assay).

4 Notes

1. When collecting the blood, always flick the tubes up and down to avoid blood clotting. Process the blood rapidly after collection to keep the quality of the isolated cells elevated.
2. Ficoll solutions must be stored at room temperature, in the dark, to avoid degradation and keep the quality of the solution. When the blood is diluted, carefully pipette small volumes at a time in order to avoid disruption of the cells from the Ficoll solution. Pipetting cautiously will create a layer between the blood and the Ficoll, and cells will not be damaged.
3. When preparing standard isotonic Percoll (SIP), carefully pipette up and down in order for the components to mix properly. This will ensure that the gradient separation will be carried out properly and monocytes and lymphocytes will be efficiently separated.
4. Preferably, make aliquots of the stock solutions of cytokines since this will avoid degradation due to thawing and freezing cycles.
5. Once the transfection solution is prepared, it is stable for up to 3 months. When the cells are in solution and centrifuged for transfection, carefully remove all the supernatant since traces of FBS will inhibit the transfection procedure. When the cell pellet is resuspended in the transfection solution (provided by the kit), the transfection must be carried out rapidly since the transfection solution can harm the cells and induce cells death. After transfection, centrifuge the cells at 342 × *g* for 5 min and resuspend them in culture medium with the addition of the maturation cytokine cocktail.
6. At this point, there will be a pellet of RNA which will not be visible; therefore, pour off the ethanol and then with a small 10-μL pipette, carefully remove the residual ethanol since the pellet is invisible (it is usually better to do it at the other side wall of the tube). This will prevent contamination of ethanol in the final sample and will also permit a quicker evaporation of residual ethanol. If left too long, the RNA will be difficult to dissolve in water.

7. Add 10 μL β-mercaptoethanol per 1 mL buffer RLT (see instruction from kit). Add 4 volumes of ethanol (96–100 %), as indicated on the bottle, to obtain a working solution (see instruction from kit). The collection of the material in RNAlater must be performed as follows: immediately after collection, the material must be placed in RNAlater and left overnight in the refrigerator in order for the RNAlater to soak into the tissue, then either used for isolation or stored at −80 °C.
8. Since the smaller pipettes are easier to control for pipetting speed, use a 10-mL pipette to first pipette 13 mL of blood at the "gravity" mode and subsequently the other 12 mL to fill up one Falcon tube. This step is crucial for the isolation of the PBMCs in case the cells are damaged from the Ficoll. Otherwise, this process would not result in a high yield of viable cells. Do not wait too long for centrifuging (following step) as the cells will begin to sink to the bottom and prevent a proper gradient separation. Do not wait as well after the centrifuge is complete as the ring of PBMCs will also start to sink to the bottom layer.
9. If the brake speeds of the centrifuge are not set at 0 and 1, the separated layers will mix and the gradient separation of the layers will be lost. Therefore, the centrifuge settings are crucial for the successful separation of the cells.
10. This step is as well very crucial, since if the pipetting is not done carefully, the layers will not separate properly. Use gravity mode on the pipette and proceed with extreme care.
11. Add the RNA drop on the side wall of the cuvette. In this way, the cells can be added on top of the drop of RNA and will automatically mix with it.
12. This step is crucial for the survival of the cells since the transfection solution is very toxic for the cells. Quickly add medium containing FBS and plate the cells in culture plates.
13. This step will be needed for the monocytes to attach to the plate. It is as well possible to wait for 2 h for the attachment step.
14. This step will serve to remove unwanted dead cells and unattached cells from the plate. When washing, carefully pipette the medium to avoid detaching of the cells.

References

1. Erdmann M et al (2007) Effective clinical-scale production of dendritic cell vaccines by monocyte elutriation directly in medium, subsequent culture in bags and final antigen loading using peptides or RNA transfection. J Immunother 30:663–674
2. Lesterhuis WJ et al (2010) Immunogenicity of dendritic cells pulsed with CEA peptide or transfected with CEA mRNA for vaccination of colorectal cancer patients. Anticancer Res 30:5091–5097
3. Morse MA, Clay TM et al (2003) HER2 dendritic cell vaccines. Clin Breast Cancer 3(Suppl 4):S164–S172
4. Pezeshki AM et al (2011) Forced expression of HLA-DM at the surface of dendritic cells

increases loading of synthetic peptides on MHC class II molecules and modulates T cell responses. J Immunol 187:74–81

5. Ashley DM et al (1997) Bone marrow-generated dendritic cells pulsed with tumor extracts or tumor RNA induce antitumor immunity against central nervous system tumors. J Exp Med 186:1177–1182
6. Boczkowski D et al (1996) Dendritic cells pulsed with RNA are potent antigen-presenting cells *in vitro* and *in vivo*. J Exp Med 184: 465–472
7. Nair SK et al (1998) Induction of primary carcinoembryonic antigen (CEA)-specific cytotoxic T lymphocytes in vitro using human dendritic cells transfected with RNA. Nat Biotechnol 16:364–369
8. Brossart P et al (2001) The epithelial tumor antigen MUC1 is expressed in hematological malignancies and is recognized by MUC1-specific cytotoxic T-lymphocytes. Cancer Res 61:6846–6850
9. Van Tendeloo VF et al (2001) Highly efficient gene delivery by mRNA electroporation in human hematopoietic cells: superiority to lipofection and passive pulsing of mRNA and to electroporation of plasmid cDNA for tumor antigen loading of dendritic cells. Blood 98: 49–56
10. O'Neill DW et al (2004) Manipulating dendritic cell biology for the active immunotherapy of cancer. Blood 104:2235–2246
11. Porgador A et al (1996) Induction of antitumor immunity using bone marrow-generated dendritic cells. J Immunol 156:2918–2926
12. Sallusto F et al (1995) Dendritic cells use macropinocytosis and the mannose receptor to concentrate macromolecules in the major histocompatibility complex class II compartment: downregulation by cytokines and bacterial products. J Exp Med 182:389–400
13. Ponsaerts P et al (2002) Messenger RNA electroporation of human monocytes, followed by rapid *in vitro* differentiation, leads to highly stimulatory antigen-loaded mature dendritic cells. J Immunol 169:1669–1675
14. Milano F et al (2007) An improved protocol for generation of immuno-potent dendritic cells through direct electroporation of $CD14^+$ monocytes. J Immunol Methods 321:94–106

Chapter 10

Dendritic Cells Transfected with Adenoviral Vectors as Vaccines

Joseph Senesac, Dmitry Gabrilovich, Samuel Pirruccello, and James E. Talmadge

Abstract

Dendritic cells (DCs) are critical to the initiation of a T-cell response. They constitute the most potent antigen-presenting cell (APC) endowed with the unique capacity to stimulate an antigen-specific T-cell responses by naïve T cells. Adenoviruses (Ad) have high transduction efficiency for many cell types including cells of hematopoietic origin independent of their mitotic status, and replication-defective Ad have demonstrated a safety profile clinically. Further, Ad vectors provide a high level of transgene expression, and Ad-transduced DCs can effectively present antigenic proteins. In this chapter, we outline a functionally closed, good manufacturing protocol for the differentiation of monocytes into DCs and transduction by Ad vectors. Basic functional and phenotypic release assays are provided, as well as contrasting research approaches for Ad-transduced DC-based vaccines.

Key words Monocytes, Dendritic cells, Adenovirus, Vaccine, Release assays

1 Introduction

Immunotherapy has entered a new era in which therapeutic concept has been clinically proven using autologous products [1]. However, because of the low frequency of DCs within the vaccine and minimal therapeutic efficacy, improvements to this approach may be achievable. The general strategy to produce Ad-transduced DCs utilizes autologous monocytes obtained by apheresis, enriched by one of several methods and differentiated into DCs by 5–7 days of culture. The resultant immature DCs are transduced by vectors with transgenes for tumor-associated antigen(s), or cytokines, and delivered by a variety of injection routes, subcutaneous, intramuscular, or intratumoral, to the patient.

This approach is not without logistical and technical challenges including, from a clinical perspective, manufacturing within a closed system to limit contamination, as well as provide cost containment. An ideal vector to transduce DCs is simple to produce

Michael J.P. Lawman and Patricia D. Lawman (eds.), *Cancer Vaccines: Methods and Protocols*, Methods in Molecular Biology, vol. 1139, DOI 10.1007/978-1-4939-0345-0_10, © Springer Science+Business Media New York 2014

and capable of high levels of transduction and antigenic transgene expression. The vector choice is challenging as not all vectors easily infect DCs and/or do so without cellular toxicity. Thus, a compromise between transduction efficiency and toxicity is critical to process scaling. In some instances, antigen-loaded DCs are differentiated *ex vivo* to facilitate clinical induction and to boost antigen-specific T-cell mediated immunity. Ad-transduced DC vaccination has been shown to induce tumor-specific cytotoxic T-lymphocyte responses capable of limiting tumor growth and, in a few reports, introducing tumor regression [2, 3]. However, there are numerous variables associated with using Ad vectors including, but not limited to, the transgene utilized and the associated toxicities, and the viral serotype with the associated differences in transduction efficiencies.

The generation-recombinant serotype 5 Ad vectors deficient in E1 and/or E2 and partial E3 expression that can be manufactured to high titer and number have been the primary vector used in vaccination trials [4]. However, there are multiple challenges to their use, including inefficient DC transduction, and, as they are human pathogens, preexisting immunity, which can potentially limit the induction of T-cell responses. The challenge of limited transduction has been overcome, in part, by the use of Ad35 vectors [5] or hybrids, although these vectors may have increased DC toxicity perhaps due to the improved transduction efficiency. Similarly, recombinant technologies to modify the viral capsid components, which are key targets of the immunity to Ad vectors, have been undertaken. However, apparently, this approach has not meaningfully affected immunogenicity in clinical trials [6]. An additional challenge to transduction and potential immunogenicity is an assessment of antigen expression and transduction efficacy. Further, challenges to developing and accessing Ad-transduced DC vaccines include defining a DC phenotype in addition to its innate and antigen-specific presenting function. Immunization using immature DCs would use cells with improved antigen-processing capabilities, as compared to mature or activated DCs with superior antigen-presenting capabilities. Further, the definition of immature vs. mature/activated DCs and their assessment has yet to achieve a consensus. It should be stressed that adenovirus transduction of growth factor-differentiated monocytes into DCs can induce DC maturation and activation resulting in differentiation of $CD83^{-}CD11c^{+/-}CD14^{+}$ DCs into $CD11c^{+}CD14^{-}CD83^{+}$ DC [7, 8].

Initially, monocytes were enriched and cultured in media containing fetal bovine serum (FBS); however, from a regulatory perspective, defined, serum-free media are superior, and most media currently use autologous or AB plasma, although human serum albumin (HSA) can also be used for serum-free culture of monocytes/DCs. The timing of monocyte culture for differentiation into harvest of immature DCs is frequently controversial and ranges from 2 to 7 days, although 5 to 7 days seems optimal. Monocytes represent the primary source of progenitors for DC differentiation. However, $CD34^+$ cells can also be differentiated, and a few trials have directly isolated circulating DCs for use as vaccines. Numerous techniques can be utilized to isolate monocytes including elutriation [9–11]; tangential flow filtration [12]; adherence [13], including the closed system developed by Aastrom [14]; and positive [15, 16] or negative [17, 18] selection. At present, the primary strategies used to isolate monocytes include adherence and elutriation, although adherence cannot be currently performed in a closed fashion. Elutriation and positive or negative selection can both be undertaken in a functionally closed manner; however, on a cost basis, elutriation is more attractive. Further, obtaining sufficient DCs for multiple cycles of immunization requires a large number of monocytes, which can only be obtained by a 10–15 L apheresis.

In this chapter, we discuss what we believe are the most effective, commonly used approaches, methods, and strategies to manufacture Ad-transduced DCs as vaccines. However, the primary emphasis is on an approach that we believe represents the best compromise between transduction efficiency and toxicity within a closed system. Further, we provide parameters and insight into optimization strategies to facilitate the clinical development of new vectors, antigens, and/or cytokines as part of a therapeutic vaccine. The constraints this format affords limit the detail that can be provided, and so, a basic understanding of good manufacturing practices (GMP) and aseptic processing is assumed.

2 Materials

2.1 Blood Products

1. Apheresis products: These leukocyte populations can be collected using a variety of leukapheresis devices. However, the characteristics of the population obtained are critical. Notably, the product should be high in monocytes and low in granulocytes, red blood cells (RBCs), and platelets. Thus, a mononuclear cell (MNC) apheresis protocol, rather than a stem cell apheresis protocol, should be used. These criteria are essential for subsequent monocyte isolation (*see* **Note 1**).
2. Whole blood: As an alternative to apheresis, especially when fewer DCs are needed, whole blood can be collected and MNCs isolated by Ficoll-Hypaque density gradient centrifugation.

2.2 Monocyte Isolation

1. Monocyte enrichment by plastic adherence: MNCs can be isolated from leukapheresis products by density gradient centrifugation, washing, and incubation for 2 h in plastic flasks containing DC media supplemented with 1 % human pooled AB plasma or HSA. Nonadherent cells are removed by repeated rinsing of the plate.

2. Monocyte enrichment by positive selection: The CliniMACS® cell selection system (Miltenyi, Bergisch Gladbach, Germany) is used for positive selection of monocytes. Briefly, leukapheresis products are washed to remove platelets, the remaining leukocytes are incubated with CD14 monoclonal antibody (mAb) (Miltenyi), and the mAb-coated cells are isolated with magnetic beads (alternatively, beads conjugated with anti-CD14 mAb can be used). Removal of the beads following isolation is required [19]. These cells are processed using the CliniMACS® system in which an automated procedure guides all subsequent steps including retention of the magnetic bead-coated cells on a magnetic column, removal of unbound cells by washing, and the release of enriched monocytes from the magnetic column.
3. Monocyte enrichment by depletion of T and B lymphocytes: The leukapheresis products are processed as above except T and B cells are depleted with anti-CD2 and anti-CD19 mAbs using the Isolex 300i Magnetic Cell Selector (Nexell, Irvine, CA) according to the manufacturer's instructions. These cells are retained on the magnetic column, and the monocytes are in the elutriate.
4. Elutriation: The Elutra® Cell Separation System is a closed system to isolate monocytes based on the Spectra apheresis unit that can enrich monocytes from an apheresis product within 1 h (Caridian BCT Inc., Lakewood, CO, USA). The monocytes are separated based on size and, to a lesser extent, density by elutriation in a 40-mL conical chamber. The total monocyte recovery following elutriation has been reported to be as high as 98 % and a mean purity of >80 % [20]. This system (Elutra®) allows for fast and easy enrichment of monocytes within a closed system and does not require a density gradient step to enrich peripheral blood mononuclear cells (PBMCs) from leukapheresis products, nor does it require xenogeneic antibodies to isolate monocytes.

2.3 Materials Considerations

1. Ad vector: Recombinant adenoviruses (rAd) are widely used in gene therapy and immunization. These replication-incompetent vectors have an established safety record and a number of advantages including production to high viral titers, relatively large transgene coding capacity (up to 8 kb), and immunogenicity resulting in vaccine adjuvant activity. Several different human rAd serotypes are being studied clinically as vectors to assess the induction of T-cell responses by Ad-transduced DC vaccines. The majority of studies performed to date have utilized human Ad5-based constructs, which limits ease of use as monocytes, and DCs have a relatively low incidence of the coxsackievirus and adenovirus receptor (CAR), the primary membrane receptor utilized by subgroup C adenovirus [21].

This necessitates the use of high viral particle/DC ratios to achieve effective transduction levels. Alternative serotypes, such as Ad35 (subgroup B), or the hybrid Ad5f35 (Ad5 with the Ad35 fiber), are more efficient at transducing cells of hematopoietic origin, as the CD46 receptor is used for infection [22].

2. Media: Several different media formulated for DC differentiation and maturation are available. These include CellGenix DC medium (CellGenix, Portsmouth, NH, USA), Aim V® medium (Life Technologies, Grand Island, NY, USA), and X-VIVO™-15 (Lonza, Walkersville, MD, USA). Considerations in media choice include availability to obtain media manufactured under GMP, volume per bottle or bag, and the availability of pigtails on the bag to facilitate sterile docking. Some media also incorporate non-animal-derived protein that facilitates compounding the media. Indeed, some media are available with GM-CSF and IL-4, although this limits the stability (shelf life). In addition, glutamine supplementation may be needed due to its poor stability. Another consideration is the inclusion of phenol red; while useful for a visual indication of pH control, it can also be a residual impurity that carries over into the final product.

3. HSA or autologous serum: Serum can improve DC differentiation and function, although FBS has potential to transmit bovine-related infectious agents and potential serum contaminants that affect differentiation as well as induce anti-bovine immune reactivity limiting multiple vaccinations. Autologous serum can also be used, although there is potential for contamination by chemotherapeutic drugs or high levels of inflammatory cytokines that can affect DC differentiation. Pooled human AB serum is one alternative, but, optimally, would incorporate the use of a single lot to avoid variation. Thus, arguably, the best approach is the use of protein supplementation with HSA resulting in serum-free DC media, such as provided by CellGenix DC media in a preconfigured formulation. Alternatively, X-VIVO™-15 and Aim V® can also be formulated with HSA.

4. COBE 2991® Cell Processor (Terumo Group, Lakewood, CO, USA): The COBE 2991® cell processor has been used in cell processing applications for over 30 years. A number of alternatives have become available including the Baxter/Nexell CytoMate™ (note, the CytoMate™ has gone off market) and most recently the Biosafe Sepax® (Biosafe America Inc., Houston, TX, USA). The COBE 2991® can wash cells with high yield as well as allow Ficoll-Hypaque density gradient separation of blood in a functionally closed manner.

5. Peristaltic pumps: Peristaltic pumps combined with sterile docking allow the transfer of media and cells in a closed fashion. The choice of pump depends upon frequency of use and volume to be transferred.

6. Bag centrifuges: Bag centrifuges, either tabletop or freestanding, can be modified with block inserts or used as designed to pellet cells within bags and, when used in combination with the plasma press, allow closed washing and concentration of cells.
7. Plasma press: The use of a conventional V-shaped plasma press allows separation of centrifuged cells from the supernatant or plasma. Together with sterile docking, bag centrifuges, and/or a syringe transfer system using a two- or three-way valve, one can wash, transfer, and/or concentrate cells using a plasma press.
8. Sterile docking device: Sterile connections between tubes, bags, and media bags, outside of a biosafety cabinet (BSC), can be accomplished using a sterile docking device. This approach maintains a functionally closed system (*see* **Note 2**).
9. Granulocyte macrophage colony-stimulating factor (GM-CSF): GM-CSF is the primary growth factor used to differentiate monocytes into DCs in vitro. It is a 20–30-kDa glycoprotein, synthesized by lymphocytes, monocytes, fibroblasts, and endothelial cells, and it is available as a GMP protein either from *Escherichia coli* (non-glycosylated) or yeast (glycosylated). Its major function is to prolong cellular survival and promote monocyte differentiation into large macrophage-like cells, increasing their metabolism and function as APCs by enhancing major histocompatibility complex II expression. Early studies with human peripheral blood suggested that other factors were required to differentiate monocytes into DC. Studies have shown that culturing monocytes with either interleukin-4 (IL-4) or interleukin-13 (IL-13) results in their differentiation into DC. The concentration of GM-CSF used to culture monocytes for differentiation into DC is normally close to 1,000 IU/mL. Note, once incorporated into media, it has a relatively short shelf life, especially at 37 °C.
10. IL-4 and IL-13: IL-4 is critical to the differentiation of monocytes into DCs as it suppresses overgrowth of DCs by macrophages. Thus, monocytes have the ability to develop into macrophages unless suppressed by the addition of IL-4 or IL-13. While a combination of GM-CSF and IL-4 is commonly used to differentiate immature DC from monocytes, other cytokines, such as IL-13, can be used in combination with GM-CSF for this purpose.
11. Gas-permeable bags: Afc Fluoroethylene Propylene (AFP)® bags (American Fluoroseal Corporation, Gaithersburg, MD, USA) are impermeable to liquid, while remaining permeable to gas exchange. This allows adequate gas exchange while all ports remain fully sealed, so vapor cannot escape the bag. Thus, no medium loss occurs, and it is unnecessary to keep water in the incubator for humidification, reducing contamination risk.

12. Racks for culturing using Gas-permeable bags: The racks in most incubators limit gas exchange at the bag surface that rests on the incubator rack. Thus, we place the bags onto wire racks allowing gas exchange on all sides of the bags.
13. Clinical blood analyzer (*see* **Note 3**): An automated hematology blood analyzer rapidly provides cell numbers and differentials using blood/sample volumes of 20–40 μL.
14. Controlled rate freezer: A controlled rate freezer is recommended to prevent the significant decrease in viability that occurs following thawing of dendritic cells frozen using a dump protocol.

2.4 Freezing Materials

1. CryoStor™ 5 (CS5) (Sigma-Aldrich Corporation, St. Louis, MO, USA).
2. 6-mL KryoSure™ 6-F bags (Afc, Gaithersburg, MD).

2.5 Cell Phenotyping

1. Anti-CD45 mAb.
2. Anti-HLA-DR mAb.
3. Anti-CD11c mAb.
4. Anti-CD14 mAb.

2.6 Cell Fixation and Manipulation

1. Fix/Perm intracellular IL-12 kit (Becton Dickinson, Franklin Lakes, NY, USA) (BD).
2. HSA/HBSS: Add 1 % human serum albumin (HSA) to a 4-L bag of GMP-grade Hanks balanced salt solution (HBSS).

3 Methods

A standardized method to isolate, culture, and differentiate monocytes into DCs has not been developed, although it should include a simple, economical, functionally closed, and reproducible GMP-compatible system. Multiple strategies are used, and we discuss the approach we have developed to produce human DCs from leukapheresis products [11]. Critically, the quality attributes of the final product must be assessed and reported on a certificate of analysis prior to release. These quality attributes include safety, quality, identity, potency, and purity, where a complete product characterization contains one or more methods from each category.

3.1 GMP vs. Research Manufacturing of DC (See Note 4)

1. Research: A variety of production methods can be used to manufacture DC vaccines ranging from manual approaches to semiautomated, functionally closed systems for monocyte isolation, culture, Ad transduction, and final product formulation. Normally, for research, whole blood is density gradient centrifuged and the MNCs subjected to adherence isolation of

monocytes. The resultant product frequently has a high lymphocyte contamination due to the "poor" monocyte separation by adherence and a low yield due to the inefficiencies of Ficoll-Hypaque and adherence purification.

2. GMP manufacture: The manufacturing of Ad-infected DCs for clinical use has as its goal a closed processing system and a high DC yield. Thus, an apheresis is the most common starting cell product. Typically, scaling studies are undertaken prior to validation, and, frequently, research approaches may be initially used to assess specific parameters to optimize steps in the process.

3.2 Apheresis

1. Target apheresis characteristics: Our preferred monocyte isolation procedure is elutriation using the Terumo Elutra®, allowing the process to occur in a functionally closed manner. Specific characteristics, including cellularity, monocyte number, and RBC and granulocyte contamination, are all critical (*see* **Note 5**). An increased RBC contamination can be addressed by debulking, requiring a longer processing time and resulting in a lower monocyte yield. It is important to note that an apheresis designed to obtain a monocyte product utilizes parameters that differ from a stem cell apheresis, and close attention should be paid to this.
2. Fresh vs. frozen apheresis product: A fresh apheresis for processing will result in improved cellular viability and DC yield despite a 24-h delay associated with transport. However, pragmatically, if there is a delay of more than 24 h between shipment and the initiation of processing, the apheresis product should be frozen (*see* **Note 6**). Elutra® isolation of frozen cells can be problematic as contaminating granulocytes lyse, and the released DNA can aggregate the monocytes (*see* **Note 7**).
3. Mobilized mononuclear cell product: Growth factor-mobilized MNC products, which have a higher frequency of monocytes, can also be used to manufacture DC; however, they have increased numbers of degranulated and immature neutrophils, which reduce monocyte purity following elutriation.

3.3 Monocyte Isolation: Elutra® (See Note 8)

1. Take samples of the apheresis product for sterility testing, cellularity (CBC), viability, and flow analysis (*see* **Note 9**).
2. Undertake all processes within a class 10,000 facility and within a BSC (class 100). Utilize sterile technique at all times.
3. Add 1 % HSA to a 4-L bag of GMP-grade HBSS.
4. Dilute the apheresis 1:1 with the 1 % HSA-HBSS.
5. Place a disposable Elutra® tubing set into the BSC after spraying with 70 % alcohol.
6. Clamp the tube with the blue breather cap and then all other clamps on the tubing set.

7. Attach the 4-L HBSS and 1 % HSA bag to the white spike on the primary media line.
8. Attach the 1-L bag of DC media bag to the second spike on the primary media line.
9. Attach a 1-L saline bag to the white spike on the secondary media line.
10. Attach the diluted apheresis bag to the orange spike on the cell inlet line.
11. Attach the disposable Elutra® tubing set and attached bags to the Elutra® outside of the BSC, but within the class 10,000 suite.
12. Label all bags from the tubing set and hang on the IV pole.
13. Follow instructions for mounting the tubing set to the Elutra®.
14. Turn power switch to on and allow self-check to complete.
15. Place separation chamber into bracket in Elutra®.
16. Execute the start-up routine and enter the requested characteristics as per menu instructions.
17. Utilize profile 2, which will allow monocyte collection in supplemented DC media eliminating need to pellet cells and replace saline with culture media.
18. If the RBC volume is ≥10 mL, the product will need to be debulked, which can occur in automated fashion on the Elutra®.
19. Assure product is at room temperature prior to execution of Elutra® enrichment.
20. Follow instructions from menu on Elutra®.
21. Heat-seal and remove bags as completed for cell count, viability, and flow analysis (*see* **Note 9**).
22. The characteristics of the cells in each bag are shown in Fig. 1.

3.4 Adherence Isolation of Monocytes

1. The vessel used for monocyte enrichment depends upon the number of monocytes to be cultured. Thus, T-75s, T-125s, T-225s, or cell factories can be used (*see* **Note 10**).
2. PBMCs are seeded onto the plastic at 1–1.5 × 10^6 cells/cm^2 surface area in medium with 1–2 % heat-inactivated autologous or AB plasma.
3. The monocytes are allowed to adhere for 2 h at 37 °C.
4. Nonadherent cells are removed by gently shaking the flask by hand for approximately 10 s and decanting the medium.
5. The flasks are washed to remove nonadherent cells by the addition of medium, gentle shaking, and decanting. This may be repeated as optimized by the individual manufacturing facility.
6. Cultured medium is then added for DC differentiation.

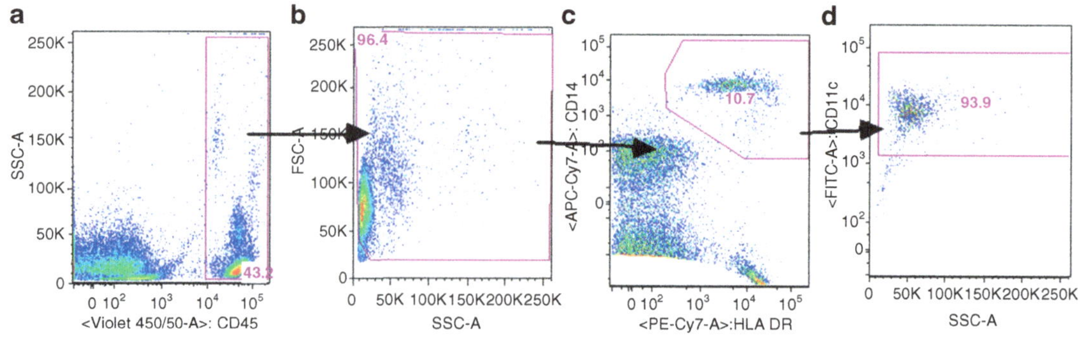

Fig. 1 Gating strategy to assess monocyte/DC cell frequency in monocyte preparations. The viable leukocytes are gated as CD45 intermediate to bright cell events (**a**) and are then gated via forward angle light scatter to remove any remaining cellular debris (**b**). The monocytes are identified as CD14 and HLA-DR bright cell events (**c**). The monocytes will also be brightly positive for CD11c expression (**d**)

3.5 Monocyte Culture and DC Transduction

1. Obtain a sample from bag 6 following Elutra® isolation of monocytes for flow cytometry, viability, and cell differential and count.
2. Weigh bag 6 and calculate volume.
3. Calculate the total number of monocytes.
4. Determine number and size of semipermeable culture bags required for culture at 2×10^6/mL monocytes.
5. Cells are cultured in bags at 80 % of the volume to fill to a 1 cm thickness. The 1 cm thickness should not be exceeded allowing gas exchange (*see* **Note 11**).
6. Bag clips (*see* **Note 12**) can also be used to retain a 1 cm thickness at all times during the culture such that the bag is extended following refeed.
7. The use of media at 80 % of the maximum allows refeeding on day 3 or 4 of the 6 days of culture with additional media and growth factors.
8. Using a peristaltic pump or a 60-mL syringe, a three-way value, injection ports, and sterile tubing transfer sets, together with a sterile docking machine, transfer cells and media into the culture bags.
9. Place the labeled, semipermeable culture bags on top of a VueLife bag cassette (stainless steel mesh, to allow for greater gas exchange) inside a validated, constantly monitored, and alarmed incubator at 37 °C, 5 % CO_2, ambient humidity, for 3–4 days.
10. On day 3 or 4, add additional media with growth factors to the culture bags as above.
11. On day 6 of culture, remove bags from the incubator and attach a bag to a COBE 2991® blood cell processing set.

12. Load the blood cell processing set on the COBE 2991®.
13. Sequentially process all culture bags via sterile docking.
14. When all media and cells have been transferred to the processing donut and the supernatant expressed, heat-seal the donut, cut between heat seals, and place donut in a BSC.
15. Resuspend cells in donut.
16. Spike the donut with a COBE 2991® coupler.
17. Using a peristaltic pump or syringe transfer set, remove the cells to a culture bag, rinse donut twice with additional media, and transfer to the culture bag.
18. Obtain sample for flow, cell count, viability, differential, and mycoplasma testing (*see* **Note 13**).
19. Weigh the bag and calculate the total volume.
20. Determine the cell number in the bag.
21. Pellet the cells using a bag centrifuge.
22. Transfer the bag to the BSC and sterile dock an extension set to the bag. Drain the media into a waste container using a plasma press.
23. Resuspend cells in remaining media inside the bag and calculate volume. Dilute cells to 2×10^6 viable cells/mL and aliquot to the needed number of 72-mL bags.
24. Add Ad vector to the DCs to achieve a predetermined virus particle (VP): viable DC ratio.
25. Achieve infection of DCs in a gas-permeable bag on a wire cassette to increase gas exchange at 37 °C for a predetermined time. Typically, this is 1–3 h.
26. The cell concentration during infection will be determined based on the vector used and culture conditions established. We found that $1–5 \times 10^6$ viable cells/mL provides the best infection efficiency and cellular viability.
27. Concentrate and wash cells 3× using a bag centrifuge and a plasma press with sterile docking.
28. Obtain a sample for flow, cell count, viability, and differential.

3.6 Transduction Parameters

There are multiple parameters involved in optimizing Ad infection of DCs. This includes the serotype of the vector, the DC concentration, the duration of co-incubation, and the virus particle to DC ratio. Confounding these parameters is their interrelationship, and extensive studies may be required to optimize parameters for transduction frequency and minimal toxicity.

1. Vector serotypes: Ad gene therapy typically uses either serotype Ad5 or Ad35 vectors. When targeting hematopoietic cells, such as DCs, serotype 35 Ad has the advantage that hematopoietic

cells have a large number of receptors (CD46) such that a lower VP to DC ratio can be used [23].

2. Duration of incubation: Transgene expression following Ad transduction of DCs is incubation time dependent [24]. However, as transgene expression is detected beginning at ~8 h post-initiation of transduction and peaks around 24 h. The duration of infection required is a challenging parameter to assess. We have found that optimal co-incubation of Ad and DCs is 2–3 h, and a more prolonged incubation can result in virus-associated toxicity.
3. DC concentration: The concentration of DCs during co-incubation with Ad vectors also contributes to the frequency of transduction.
4. VP to DC ratio: The multiplicity of infection or VP to DC ratio is a critical parameter for the frequency of DC transduction [25]. Our studies, in an Ad-serotype-dependent manner, have shown that the optimal VP to DC ratio ranges from 3,000:1 to 20,000:1, with a defined cell concentration of 2×10^6 viable DC/mL.

3.7 Ad Vectors

1. Ad vector serotype: The majority of Ad vectors utilized for gene therapy are based on serotype 5 viruses due to our extensive understanding of their characteristics. However, Ad5 infection requires coxsackievirus Ad receptor (CAR) expression for infection [26], and the transduction efficiency of the Ad5-based vectors is associated with CAR membrane density [27]. Thus, Ad5 vector-mediated gene transfer to cells lacking sufficient CAR expression is inefficient, which includes DCs [28] despite their expression the secondary Ad5 receptor, alpha-v integrins [29]. In contrast to Ad5, Ad35 uses CD46 as the primary attachment receptor. CD46 is a histiocyte marker and is expressed on most subtypes of DC [23].
2. Replicative defective Ad: Replication incompetent rAd vectors are generated in mammalian packing cells lines, such as HEK293 or PER.C6, and are in common use. These vectors are rendered replication incompetent by genetic deletion of early genes that are required for viral replication. Numerous packaging cell lines have been developed that provide deleted early genes in trans. These rAd vectors have the capacity for transgenes of up to 7.5 kb under control of various promoters, although the promoter type can affect transgene expression, and promoter activity is dependent on cell type [30]. Multiple transgene insertions in different adenovirus regions can be used to advantage to result in combined functions from the same genetic construct.

3.8 Freeze (See Note 14)

1. Calculate total viable cell number and cell number/mL.
2. Pellet cells using a bag centrifuge.
3. Remove all supernatant using a plasma press.
4. Sterile dock a bag with CryoStor™ 5 (CS5) using an extension set, three-way valve, and syringe to the bag with a cell pellet.
5. Using a syringe, transfer ice cold CS5 to the cell pellet to achieve the target cell number/mL for the vaccine.
6. Mix the cells by manual manipulation.
7. Remove sample for release testing (*see* **Note 15**), including gram stain, endotoxin testing, and sterility testing.
8. Using a syringe transfer approach with a three-way value (*see* **Note 2**), 6-mL KryoSure™ 6-F bags, and a sterile welding device, transfer desired cell volume to the freezing bag. Attention to hub/tubing volume is critical.
9. Perform three seals across the fluorinated ethylene propylene material at the tubing end of the bag.
10. In addition to vaccine aliquots, reserve at least two samples using the same freezing bags (although a lower volume can be used). Be prepared for additional release testing or stability testing as required (*see* **Note 16**).
11. Cut through the middle seal and transport for control rate freezing.
12. Affix labels via string, pouches, etc., using labeling approaches that are resistant to cold, aqueous solutions, and solvents.
13. Within 45 min of CS5 addition, freezing using a controlled rate freezer should be initiated (*see* **Note 17**).
14. Prepare the controlled rate freezing device so that it is ready to perform a run, following the manufacturer's instructions. This usually involves attaching the liquid nitrogen dewar using a hose connection or opening the hose connection from a central liquid nitrogen line and initializing the machine's freezing program. It should take 2–3 min for the machine to stabilize at its start temperature (4 °C).
15. Load the filled cryobags into the freezer chamber of the mechanical freezing device and initiate the freezing run.
16. At the end of the run, remove the frozen bags and place in a transfer container with crushed dry ice. Transfer the cryobags immediately into a liquid nitrogen freezer for long-term storage in the vapor phase of the freezer, not submerged in liquid nitrogen.
17. Log the patient name and freezer location.
18. Inspect the temperature chart from the freezing run as part of quality control (QC). Verify that the expected results were obtained for the shape of the freezing curve, including the crystallization point.

3.9 Quality Control (Release) Testing and Batch File Records and Review

1. Batch release testing per the FDA 21 CFR 211 and 610 (see also USP29) requires that the vaccine meets predetermined criteria for dose; safety (mycoplasma, sterility, endotoxin tests); identity (membrane markers); purity (percent of cells that are viable, transduced and with specific membrane markers); and potency (viability and bioassays).
2. The manufacturing batch files must be reviewed and occurrences analyzed and reported for product release.

3.10 Injection Preparation

1. Rapidly thaw the cryobag containing the vaccine designated "for injection" in a 37 °C water bath filled with sterile water. This is performed ideally with removal of the cryobag from the water bath just prior to complete thaw to ensure no unnecessary warming of the dose occurs.
2. Some studies use a wrapper bag prior to insertion into the water bath in case of bag rupture. However, this also delays thawing, which can impact viability.
3. Check for leaks in the bag.
4. Rinse the bag with 70 % alcohol.
5. Using scissors, open the end of the bag with the rubber septum.
6. Using a sterile alcohol wipe, wash the septum and withdraw the volume needed for vaccination into the desired syringe and needle.
7. If being prepped in a pharmacy, place the syringes on ice and transport to the clinic for injection.
8. Regardless of preparation site (pharmacy vs. bedside), the vaccine should be stored on ice and administered within 30 min.

3.11 Monocyte Phenotype Analysis

1. Ficolled, plastic-adhered, or antibody/magnetic bead-based monocyte preparations require RBC lysis prior to flow cytometric analysis. Elutriated monocyte samples generally do not.
2. The primary antibodies used to evaluate the monocyte products include CD45, HLA-DR, CD11c, and CD14 (Figs. 1 and 2).
3. Most conventional flow cytometry software packages can be utilized for analysis. We demonstrate analysis using FlowJo (Figs. 1, 2, 3, and 4).
4. Acquired cells are initially gated using an SSxCD45 histogram to eliminate any remaining RBCs, platelets, and cell debris (Fig. 2).
5. Remaining apoptotic cells are eliminated using a forward light scatter discriminator window or by an FSxSS gate.
6. Monocytes are identified based on bright CD14 and HLA-DR expression (Figs. 1 and 2). Granulocytes are excluded as CD14 dim or negative and HLA-DR negative cell events.
7. The monocyte population can be confirmed based on light scatter characteristics and bright CD11 expression.

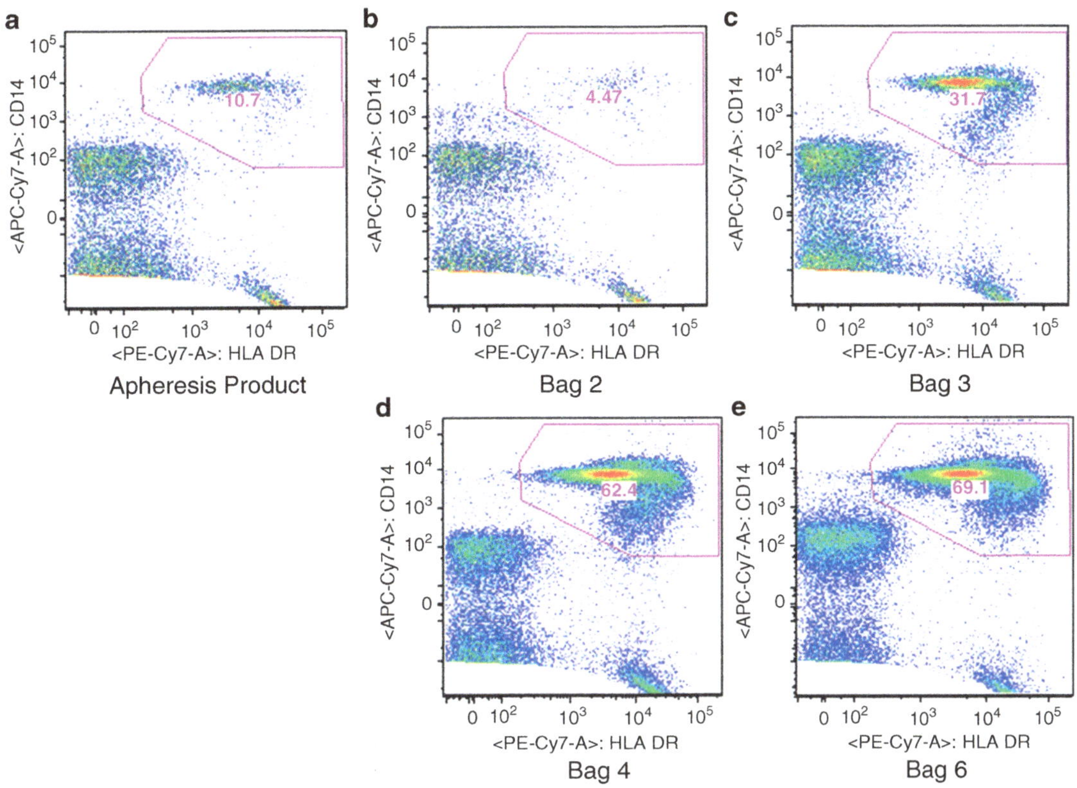

Fig. 2 Monocyte frequency in apheresis and Elutra® monocyte preparations. Cells were initially gated as shown in Fig. 1. The monocytes are identified as CD14 and HLA-DR bright events within the CD45+ leukocyte population. Monocyte frequency is highest in Elutra bags 4–6. The histograms are labeled as apheresis product (**a**) and bags 2 (**b**), 3 (**c**), 4 (**d**), and 6 (**e**) from the elutration using the Terumo Elutra®

3.12 DC Phenotype (See Note 18) Analysis (Fig. 3)

1. RBC lysis is not required prior to staining.
2. An aliquot of cultured cells is incubated with anti-CD45, HLA-DR, CD11c, and CD14 mAbs to assess DC precursor frequency/purity. CD14 expression provides a baseline assessment of DC maturation.
3. One can assess the expression of the transgene (membrane or intracellular, for instance interleukin-12 (IL-12) expression) to determine transduction efficiency.
4. We routinely evaluate expression of CD80, CD86, CD83, CD40, and CCR7 to determine DC maturation and activation, but, to date, we have not required specific expression levels for product release.
5. The acquired cells are gated as above using an SSxCD45 histogram to select CD45+ events and a forward light scatter discriminator window or gate to further eliminate cell debris.
6. The DC population is identified based on bright HLA-DR and CD11c expression (Figs. 3a and 4a).

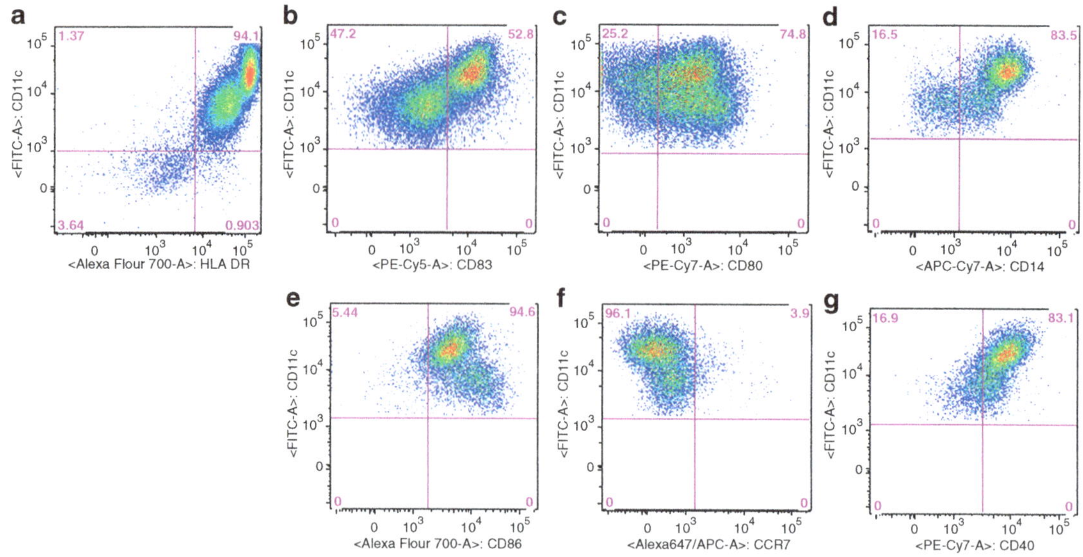

Fig. 3 DC maturation assessment of cultured cell preparations at day 6. Using the same cell-gating approach as shown in figs. 1 and 2, the monocyte/DC population is identified as CD11c and HLA-DR$^+$ (**a**). These HLA-DR and CD11c$^+$ cells were then evaluated for expression of CD83 (**b**), CD80 (**c**), CD14 (**d**), CD86 (**e**), CCR7 (**f**), and CD40 (**g**). In the cultured cell preparation shown, the resultant mature DCs had approximately 52.8 % expression of CD83, 74.3 % expression of CD80, 94.6 % expression of CD86, 83.5 % expression of CD14, 83.1 % expression of CD40, and very low level expression of the chemokine receptor CCR7 (3.9 %)

7. A decrease in CD14 expression density on the HLA-DR and CD11c positive cells accompanies DC cell maturation (Fig. 4b).
8. Acquisition of CD80, CD86, CD40, CD83, and CCR7 provides additional evidence of DC maturation and activation.
9. Note, DCs prepared using monocytes isolated by Elutra® are typically less mature compared to plastic adhesion or magnetically selected monocyte-prepared DCs at similar culture time points (Fig. 4b, e).

3.13 DC Function

1. IL-12 secretion: The secretion of IL-12 is an important characteristic of mature DCs and can be triggered by exposure to lipopolysaccharide, PGE-2, interferon-γ (IFN-γ), Ad infection, etc. We determined IL-12 levels in the culture supernatants of DCs 18–24 h following transduction (*see* **Note 19**). The immature DCs are cultured at 2×10^4 DC/mL in a 24-well dish containing 2 mL of DC culture media. A direct comparison to noninfected DCs provides a negative control; alternatively, a comparison of DCs cultured with or without activating agents is undertaken. The supernatants are separated from the DCs by centrifugation and multiple aliquots frozen for analysis. IL-12 levels are determined by enzyme-linked immunosorbent assay (ELISA) using serial dilutions to assure the analysis of IL-12 levels within protocol parameters (*see* **Note 20**).

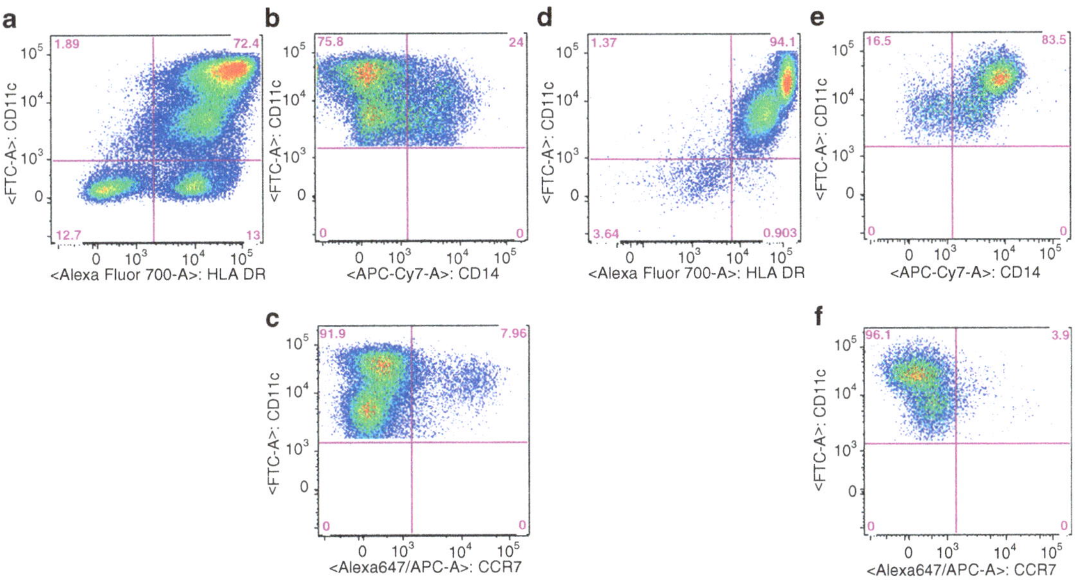

Fig. 4 Comparison of DC maturation in monocytes isolated by plastic adherence vs. elutriation. Histograms of culture day 6 DCs isolated by adherence and cultured in flasks (histograms **a**–**c**) compared to DCs isolated by elutriation and cultured in nonadherent gas-permeable bags (histograms **d**–**f**). The CD11c and HLA-DR, double-positive DCs are selected and evaluated for CD14 and CCR7 expression. The DC isolated by adherence are more mature with few cells expressing CD14 (**b**) and a higher percentage of cells expressing CCR7 (**c**). This contrasts with the DCs isolated by elutriation and cultured in gas-permeable bags where the majority of the cells express CD14 (**e**) and few expressed CCR7 (**f**)

2. Intracellular IL-12 levels: The cells separated from the supernatants are stained using the BD intracellular IL-12 kit, the BD Fix/Perm. We do this in combination with membrane staining for CD11c and HLA-DR. This provides insight into the frequency of infected cells as opposed to a population response.
3. Transgene expression ELISA and membrane or intracellular expression of transgene (antigen) expression: The approach and logic is similar to that of Subheading 3.11, **steps 1** and **2**. The use of membrane vs. intracellular transgene expression depends on the promoter utilized (*see* **Note 21**).
4. Mixed lymphocyte reaction (MLR): To measure the DC capacity to present antigens and mediate T-lymphocyte activation, an allogeneic MLR can be utilized. This also measures the maturation/activation of DCs as activated DCs will stimulate a higher T-lymphocyte proliferation when assessed in a serial dilution of activator (DC) and responder (T cells) cells. Typically, ratios ranging from 1:2 to 1:128 are used. Cells are pulsed during the last 16 h of a 5-day culture period, harvested on glass fiber filters, and analyzed in a liquid scintillation counter. Results are expressed based on the mean counts per minute (cpm) of the experimental group. Alternatively, results can be

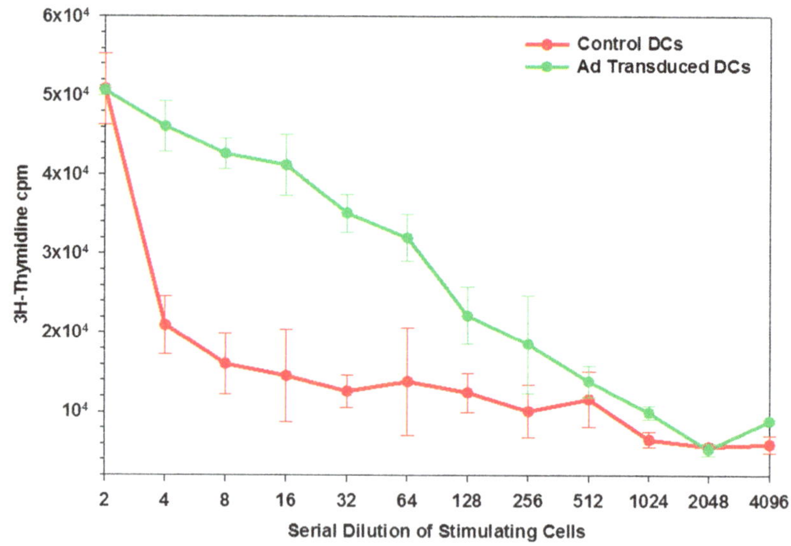

Fig. 5 One-way MLR comparing the allogeneic T-cell response to cultured immature DC (control) versus Ad-transduced DC as stimulator cells. A serial dilution of irradiated DC was used as stimulators beginning at 100,000 cells/well (96-well plates) with 200,000 Ficoll-Hypaque isolated mononuclear cells

reported as the stimulation index of the experimental group (responder cells cultured with stimulators) cpm divided by the cpm of responders cultured without stimulators. One expects to observe a difference in the stimulation of T-cell proliferation between transduced and control DCs (Fig. 5).

4 Notes

1. Leukapheresis products must be obtained by a qualified cell collection facility or contractor. To obtain PBMCs, we request that the facility process 12 L of blood (approximately 2 blood volumes) with the blood cell separator set to obtain MNCs. The cells and plasma should be processed as soon as possible following collection, although we have obtained good results with products that have been shipped overnight on blue ice.
2. http://www.toafc.com/document-library/instructions-for-use/6-f/.
3. The differentials obtained from clinical blood analyzers can be suspect due to the high concentration of monocytes and/or the abnormal phenotype of DCs. Given the need to obtain this information frequently in real time, we normally confirm differentials using flow analysis and/or a manual diff.
4. In the United States, clinical protocols using DCs for immunotherapy in human subjects must first be approved by the

Food and Drug Administration (FDA) as an Investigational New Drug and an Institutional Review Board. All cell processing steps should be carried out in an appropriate controlled environment, i.e., a clean room with HEPA-filtered air, following current good tissue practices as per 21-CFR-1271. Further, work should be performed in a class II BSC using aseptic technique. Workers should be fully gowned and gloved, including shoe covers, a head cover, and a face mask. Regular environmental monitoring during operations should be conducted to ensure an appropriate working environment.

5. Specific apheresis product characteristics required for the Elutra include $0.5–3 \times 10^{10}$ nucleated cells, <10 mL RBC contamination, and $>1 \times 10^9$ monocytes as well as a neutrophil frequency of ≤20 %. We have also found that patients with degranulated granulocytes, and/or increased numbers of immature granulocytes, can be challenging as the low density of the granulocytes results in their collection at the interface with monocytes during Ficoll-Hypaque separation or elutriation.

6. It is our experience that mononuclear cells are more fragile following freezing and thawing and prefer to use fresh transported apheresis products.

7. Optimally, the cryopreservation media used to freeze the apheresis products is supplemented with 25 U/mL of DNAse (either dornase alpha or Benzonase®) to prevent cellular aggregation associated with the DNA from lysed cells following freezing and thawing. In addition, 3 U/mL of DNAse should be added to the HBSS used for Elutra® processing to further limit cellular aggregation.

8. In this section of the methods, we discuss the major steps in Elutra® isolation, but due to the complexity of this process and the constrained word limit, the full process needs to be based on the documentation from Terumo BCT and appropriate training.

9. To evaluate DC precursor frequency, cell aliquots from the apheresis and from each bag of the Elutra® are analyzed using antibodies to CD45, HLA-DR, and CD14 (Fig. 1). Lymphocyte and granulocyte contamination can be assessed based on light scatter properties. Granulocytes are also bright CD11c positive but are HLA-DR negative.

10. The open culture system of DC generation using flasks is useful for laboratory studies; however, it has an increased risk of contamination. A similar approach for manufacturing clinical-grade DCs in a closed system using Cell Factories and sterile connections has been developed, employing standard operating procedures. Cell Factories are more labor intensive and have the potential for operator skill-based variation, as washing non-attached cells can be challenging.

11. Bags are cultured at no more than a 1 cm thickness to allow gas exchange. To allow for media refeed on days 3 or 4, use <80 % of the culture bag's volume to achieve a 1 cm thickness.
12. The use of bag clips allows for volumes less than that needed to achieve a 1 cm thickness. The clips are applied to allow a 1 cm thickness and then removed as the culture is refed. American Fluoroseal supplies appropriate clips, but any plastic clip that would not damage the bags work.
13. Mycoplasma testing requires a larger culture volume including a meaningful number of cells, and, thus, we sample at this stage of processing as there is significant loss of yield during Ad infection. As mycoplasma contamination would be expected to occur from the original monocytes, we feel this time for testing is justified. This is in agreement with the recommendation in 21CFR610.30, which suggests that a culture harvest is the most appropriate processing point to detect mycoplasma contamination in biologic products.
14. In most cell processing facilities, freezing of cells is an established procedure, and, as such, we have dealt with this in a relatively superficial manner herein. The critical aspects include the use of a specific cryoprotectant, which in our case is CryoStor™ 5, which provides a pre-manufactured, GMP-compliant cryoprotectant.
15. In the United States, the FDA requires that therapeutic cells, like any other biologic product, be tested for identity, purity, potency, and stability before they can be used in human subjects. We test a QC aliquot of each manufactured DC batch for viability (Trypan blue staining), sterility (BACTEC™-validated to the USP sterility test), mycoplasma PCR (validated to give comparable results to the USP culture analysis), and absence of bacterial endotoxin (Limulus amoebocyte lysate assay) using a sensitive kinetic chromogenic assay. Because in some protocols, the first vaccine dose is given prior to completion of the BACTEC™ analysis (8 days), we also perform a gram stain with BACTEC™ confirmation. Our current QC (release) criteria include >80 % viable cells, negative results for all sterility tests, endotoxin levels as identified in USP 85 as ≤5 EU/kg/h, although specifications may also be based on process capability, and >75 % of the cells having the characteristics of mature DC by flow cytometry (large, $CD45^{+}HLA^{-}DR^{+}CD11c^{+}$ cells). We routinely obtain close to 90 % mature DCs, with cell viability usually >80 % post-thaw. The goal is to have a cellular product >70 % viable post-thaw. Most of the remaining cells are lymphocytes.
16. The QC aliquot for each batch is kept frozen in case future testing is needed.
17. We have found that manufacturing a 10–15 L apheresis in this manner allows freezing of up to eight vaccines at $2–5 \times 10^{7}$

cells/bag, allowing a single processing event as opposed to undertaking multiple processing events on frozen cells or multiple aphereses. Further, we have confirmed that the expression of transgene, phenotype, and cytokine secretion remains stable as compared to pre-freeze [25] and that the viability of the cells remains >70 %.

18. We have validated our processing approach to ensure the identity, potency, and stability of the cells by testing frozen/thawed DCs for cell-surface phenotype (high level expression of HLA-DR and CD11c) and assessed for maturation/activation markers including CD86, CD80, CD83, CCR7, CD40, IL-12 secretion, and transgene expression.
19. The use of an Ad vector requires culture for >8–12 h to obtain upregulated transgenes and activate the required DCs.
20. For the assessment of potency of the transduced DC vaccine, we assess the production of IL-12 following activation as compared to inactivated DCs (non-transduced). It is important to note that in non-transduced DCs (immature DCs), the production of IL-12p70 is very low, although 8–24 h following transduction, IL-12 levels are increased. If the DCs are being activated via various stimulation methods, very high levels of IL-12 (>100 ng/20,000 DC/mL over 24 h) can be secreted.
21. We typically observe a median transduction frequency of 15–40 % based on the analysis of transgene expression.

Acknowledgement

The authors would like to thank Richard E. Neubiser, Afc, for his contributions to this chapter and Alice S. Cole for her assistance in with manuscript preparation.

References

1. Kantoff PW et al (2010) Sipuleucel-T immunotherapy for castration-resistant prostate cancer. N Engl J Med 363:411–422
2. Morse MA et al (1999) Migration of human dendritic cells after injection in patients with metastatic malignancies. Cancer Res 59:56–58
3. Reichardt VL et al (1999) Idiotype vaccination using dendritic cells after autologous peripheral blood stem cell transplantation for multiple myeloma—a feasibility study. Blood 93:2411–2419
4. Gallo P et al (2005) Adenovirus as vehicle for anticancer genetic immunotherapy. Gene Ther 12(Suppl 1):S84–S91
5. Sakurai F (2003) Characterization of *in vitro* and *in vivo* gene transfer properties of adenovirus serotype 35 vector. Mol Ther 8:813–821
6. Schoggins JW, Falck-Pedersen E (2006) Fiber and penton base capsid modifications yield diminished adenovirus type 5 transduction and proinflammatory gene expression with retention of antigen-specific humoral immunity. J Virol 80:10634–10644
7. Rouard H et al (2000) Adenoviral transduction of human 'clinical grade' immature dendritic cells enhances costimulatory molecule expression and T-cell stimulatory capacity. J Immunol Methods 241:69–81

8. Lyakh LA et al (2002) Adenovirus type 5 vectors induce dendritic cell differentiation in human CD14(+) monocytes cultured under serum-free conditions. Blood 99: 600–608
9. Cao H et al (2000) *In vitro* generation of dendritic cells from human blood monocytes in experimental conditions compatible for *in vivo* cell therapy. J Hematother Stem Cell Res 9:183–194
10. Lemarie C et al (2007) Purification of monocytes from cryopreserved mobilized apheresis products by elutriation with the Elutra device. J Immunol Methods 318:30–36
11. Gulen D et al (2008) Closing the manufacturing process of dendritic cell vaccines transduced with adenovirus vectors. Int Immunopharmacol 8:1728–1736
12. Zhou Y et al (2003) Commercial scale production of dendritic cells for cancer immunotherapy. Proc Am Assoc Cancer Res 44:2876A
13. Thurner B et al (1999) Generation of large numbers of fully mature and stable dendritic cells from leukapheresis products for clinical application. J Immunol Methods 223:1–15
14. Whiteside TL et al (2009) Production of a dendritic cell-based vaccine containing inactivated autologous virus for therapy of patients with chronic human immunodeficiency virus type 1 infection. Clin Vaccine Immunol 16: 233–240
15. Padley DJ et al (2001) Mature myeloid dendritic cells for clinical use prepared from cd14+ cells isolated by immunomagnetic adsorption. J Hematother Stem Cell Res 10:427–429
16. Wong EC et al (2002) Development of a closed-system process for clinical-scale generation of DCs: evaluation of two monocyte-enrichment methods and two culture containers. Cytotherapy 4:65–76
17. Bender J (2000) Next generation clinical systems for the production of dendritic cells. Clin Appl Immunol Rev 1:37–44
18. Suen Y et al (2001) Comparison of monocyte enrichment by immuno-magnetic depletion or adherence for the clinical-scale generation of DC. Cytotherapy 3:365–375
19. Gajdosikova A et al (2006) Acute toxicity of magnetic nanoparticles in mice. Neuro Endocrinol Lett 27(Suppl 2):96–99
20. Berger T et al (2005) Efficient elutriation of monocytes within a closed system (Elutra™) for clinical-scale generation of dendritic cells. J Immunol Methods 298:61–72
21. Stockwin LH et al (2002) Engineered expression of the Coxsackie B and adenovirus receptor (CAR) in human dendritic cells enhances recombinant adenovirus-mediated gene transfer. J Immunol Methods 259:205–215
22. Verhaagh S et al (2006) Human CD46-transgenic mice in studies involving replication-incompetent adenoviral type 35 vectors. J Gen Virol 87:255–265
23. Lore K et al (2007) Myeloid and plasmacytoid dendritic cells are susceptible to recombinant adenovirus vectors and stimulate polyfunctional memory T cell responses. J Immunol 179:1721–1729
24. Dietz AB et al (2001) Maturation of dendritic cells infected by recombinant adenovirus can be delayed without impact on transgene expression. Gene Ther 8:419–423
25. Adams WC, Loré K (2011) Recombinant adenovirus vector infection of human dendritic cells. DOI:10.5772/20255
26. Bergelson JM et al (1997) Isolation of a common receptor for coxsackie B viruses and adenoviruses 2 and 5. Science 275:1320–1323
27. Hemmi S et al (1998) The presence of human coxsackievirus and adenovirus receptor is associated with efficient adenovirus-mediated transgene expression in human melanoma cell cultures. Hum Gene Ther 9:2363–2373
28. Tillman BW et al (1999) Maturation of dendritic cells accompanies high-efficiency gene transfer by a CD40-targeted adenoviral vector. J Immunol 162:6378–6383
29. Einfeld DA et al (2001) Reducing the native tropism of adenovirus vectors requires removal of both CAR and integrin interactions. J Virol 75:11284–11291
30. Papagatsias T et al (2008) Activity of different vaccine-associated promoter elements in human dendritic cells. Immunol Lett 115:117–125

Chapter 11

Genetic Modification of Dendritic Cells with RNAi

Xiao-Tong Song

Abstract

Gene silencing with RNAi is an invaluable technique in cell biology to knock down the target gene expression. Dendritic cells (DC) are the most effective antigen-presenting cells (APC), and the efficacy of antigen presentation is tightly controlled by the stimulatory as well as inhibitory mechanisms. In recent studies, RNAi technology has been employed to silence the expression of the intrinsic inhibitors of antigen presentation in DC, improving the efficacy of DC vaccines against tumor antigens in pre-clinical studies. Here, we describe the technique of using siRNA oligonucleotides, adenovirus expressing shRNA (Ad-shRNA), or lentivirus expressing shRNA (Lv-shRNA) to knock down inhibitors of antigen presentation in both mouse and human DC.

Key words RNAi, siRNA, shRNA, Dendritic cells, Knock down, Antigen presentation

1 Introduction

Dendritic cells (DC) are the most effective antigen-presenting cells (APC) with key regulatory roles in the initiation and maintenance of immune response [1]. Toll-like receptor (TLR) signaling promotes DC maturation by activating nuclear factor-κB (NF-κB), which then mediates the expression of various cytokines and chemokines. The magnitude and duration of adaptive immunity are tightly controlled by the strength and duration of NF-κB signaling and their regulatory mechanisms, including stimulatory and inhibitory mechanisms [2–6]. A20 is a unique negative regulator that suppresses the tumor necrosis factor receptor (TNFR) signaling pathway and both MyD88-dependent and MyD88-independent TLR signaling pathways in DC. A20-deficient mice are hypersensitive to TLR ligands and tumor necrosis factor (TNF) and neonatally lethal with severe inflammation in multiple organs. A20-deficient macrophages displayed prolonged NF-κB activity and failed to properly terminate TNF- and TLR-induced NF-κB responses [7–12]. In our and other recent studies, siRNA for mouse or human A20 has been designed and utilized to silence the

Michael J.P. Lawman and Patricia D. Lawman (eds.), *Cancer Vaccines: Methods and Protocols*, Methods in Molecular Biology, vol. 1139, DOI 10.1007/978-1-4939-0345-0_11, © Springer Science+Business Media New York 2014

expression of A20 in DC. A20 siRNA effectively silenced the expression of A20 in DC, endowing the DC with enhanced T cell stimulatory capacity [13–16]. Therefore, DC-based cancer vaccines could be enhanced by genetic modification with RNAi.

Here, we describe the protocols for genetically modifying both mouse bone marrow-derived DC (BM-DC) and human monocyte-derived DC using RNAi technology. In the protocol for mouse DC, mouse DC were first generated from mouse bone marrow cells in the presence of mouse granulocyte-monocyte colony-stimulating factor (GM-CSF) and interleukin-4 (IL-4) followed by transduction with lentivirus or adenovirus expressing A20 shRNA. We demonstrated that A20 expression in mouse BM-DC was knocked down by 90 %. In addition, human DC were generated from human peripheral monocytes in the presence of human GM-CSF and IL-4 followed by transduction with adenovirus expressing A20 shRNA or A20 siRNA oligos. Thus, expression of a target gene in both mouse BM-DC and human DC can be successfully knocked down by RNAi using this protocol [13–16].

2 Materials

Diligently follow all biohazard or waste disposal regulations when disposing biohazard and waste materials.

2.1 Mouse DC Culture and shRNA Transduction

1. Peripheral blood should be obtained with informed consent from healthy donors on a protocol approved by an institutional review board or similar oversight. Alternatively, peripheral blood of buffy coat can be purchased from institutions such as the Gulf Coast Regional Blood Center, Houston, TX, USA.
2. Roswell Park Memorial Institute (RPMI)-1640 medium.
3. GlutaMax-1 (Invitrogen, Carlsbad, CA, USA).
4. Fetal bovine serum (FBS) (Hyclone, Logan, UT, USA).
5. 1× sterile cell culture grade phosphate buffered saline (PBS).
6. Red blood cell lysis buffer (Sigma-Aldrich, St. Louis, MO, USA).
7. Mouse GM-CSF (Proleukin) (Chiron, Emeryville, CA, USA).
8. Mouse IL-4 (Chiron).
9. Lipopolysaccharide (LPS).
10. Polybrene.
11. Ethylenediamine acetic acid (EDTA).
12. 10-cm tissue culture-treated dishes.
13. 6-well tissue culture-treated plates.
14. 50- and 15-mL conical centrifuge tubes.
15. Lymphoprep (LP).

2.2 Human DC Culture and shRNA Transduction

1. Peripheral blood (Gulf Coast Regional Blood Center, Houston, TX, USA).
2. CellGenix DC medium (CellGenix, Freiburg, Germany).
3. GlutaMax-1.
4. 1× sterile cell culture grade PBS.
5. Lymphoprep (LP, Nycomed, Oslo, Norway).
6. Human GM-CSF.
7. Human IL-4.
8. Human IL-1β.
9. Human IL-6.
10. Human TNF-α.
11. PGE-2.
12. Gentamicin.
13. Polybrene.
14. EDTA.
15. 24-well tissue culture-treated plates.
16. 50- and 15-mL conical centrifuge tubes.
17. Sterile pipettes.

3 Methods

Unless otherwise noted, the procedure is carried out in the cell culture hood at room temperature (15–30 °C).

3.1 Lv-shRNA Transduction of Mouse DC

3.1.1 Generation of Mouse Bone Marrow-Derived DC (BM-DC)

1. On day 0, sacrifice a C57bL/6 mouse (*see* **Note 1**) and carefully remove all muscle tissues with gauze from the femurs and tibias (*see* **Note 2**). Dissect the femurs and tibias and place in a 10-cm dish. Wash 1× with 10 mL of 70 % alcohol and then 2× with 10 mL PBS (*see* **Note 3**). Spray scissors with 70 % alcohol and cut both ends of the bones with the scissors in the dish. Flush out the marrow using 2 mL of RPMI-1640 with a 5-mL syringe and 21-gauge needle. To completely flush out all the marrow, flush the bone 2× using additional fresh 2 mL of RPMI-1640. Then suspend the marrow with a 5-mL syringe and 16-gauge needle gently. Using a sterile pipette, flush the marrow cell suspension through a 70-μm wide cutoff cell strainer to remove small pieces of bone and debris.
2. Centrifuge at 400 × *g* for 5 min at room temperature.
3. Gently remove the centrifuge tube from the centrifuge and check the cell pellet. Aspirate supernatant without disturbing the cell pellet. To lyse the red cells, resuspend the pellet in

5 mL red cell buffer, and mix gently and thoroughly into a homogenous cell suspension. Let the cells sit in the cell culture hood at room temperature for 4 min (*see* **Note 4**).

4. Using a sterile pipette, add 10 mL of RPMI medium.
5. Centrifuge at 400 × *g* for 5 min at room temperature.
6. Gently remove the centrifuge tube from the centrifuge and check the cell pellet. Aspirate the supernatant without disturbing the cell pellet.
7. Resuspend pelleted cells in RPMI medium supplemented with 10 % FBS, 20 μg/mL of GM-CSF, and 20 μg/mL of IL-4. Seed the bone marrow cells from one mouse in a 10-cm cell culture dish in 20 mL of conditioned medium (*see* **Note 5**).
8. Incubate overnight at 37 °C in a humidified atmosphere of 5 % CO_2 in air.
9. On day 1, to enrich for proliferating DC, using a sterile pipette, gently remove the medium containing the nonadherent cells (*see* **Note 6**). Do not wash the cells. Using a sterile pipette, add 20 mL of fresh RPMI medium supplemented with 10 % FBS, 20 μg/mL of GM-CSF, and 20 μg/mL of IL-4.
10. Incubate overnight at 37 °C in a humidified atmosphere of 5 % CO_2 in air.
11. On day 3, feed the culture. Using a sterile pipette, gently harvest the 20 mL of medium.
12. Centrifuge at 400 × *g* for 5 min at room temperature.
13. Gently remove the centrifuge tube from the centrifuge and check the cell pellet. Aspirate the supernatant without disturbing the cell pellet. Using a sterile pipette, add 20 mL of fresh RPMI medium supplemented with 10 % FBS, 20 μg/mL of GM-CSF, and 20 μg/mL of IL-4. Transfer the cell suspension back to the 10-cm cell culture dish with the adherent cells (*see* **Note 7**).
14. On day 5, harvest the cells for shRNA transduction. Using a sterile pipette, harvest the supernatant and gently wash the plate 1× with 5 mL of pre-warmed PBS. Add 5 mL of 2 mM EDTA and incubate for 2 min at 37 °C in a humidified atmosphere of 5 % CO_2 in air. Using a sterile pipette, collect the cells, and wash the dish 1× with PBS.
15. Centrifuge at 400 × *g* for 5 min at room temperature.
16. Gently remove the centrifuge tube from the centrifuge and check the cell pellet. Aspirate the supernatant without disturbing the cell pellet. Using a sterile pipette, add 5 mL of fresh RPMI medium supplemented with 10 % FBS, 5 % antibiotics, 20 μg/mL of GM-CSF, and 20 μg/mL of IL-4.

17. Count the viable cells using Trypan blue and a hemocytometer. Mix cells gently but thoroughly prior to sampling for the count. Determine the cell concentration. Adjust the medium volume to reach 1×10^6 cells/mL.
18. Seed 2 mL of cells into one well of a 6-well cell culture plate. The cells are ready for virus transduction. Usually, BM-DC are ready for experimental use between days 7 and 9. Since it takes 2 days for virus-delivered shRNA to knock down the target gene expression, transduce BM-DC with virus at day 5 and then harvest the BM-DC at day 7 for experimental use (*see* **Note 8**).

3.1.2 Lv-shRNA Transfection of Mouse BM-DC

1. On day 5 of BM-DC culture, thaw Lv-shA20 and GFP shRNA (Lv-shGFP) at room temperature and mix gently. Keep thawed shRNA lentiviral stock on ice (*see* **Note 9**). Add the lentiviral stock into the wells containing the BM-DC. The proper multiplicity of infection (MOI) for mouse BM-DC transduction is an MOI of 5. For example, 1×10^7 virus particles are required for 2×10^6 cells in one well from Subheading 3.1.1, **step 18,** to reach an MOI 5 (*see* **Note 10**). Mix by pipetting gently.
2. Add polybrene at final concentration of 5 μg/mL (*see* **Note 11**). Gently swirl the cell culture plate to mix.
3. Incubate overnight at 37 °C in a humidified atmosphere of 5 % CO_2 in air.
4. On day 6 of BM-DC culture, centrifuge at $400 \times g$ for 5 min at room temperature.
5. Gently remove the 6-well cell culture plate from the centrifuge. Remove the medium containing virus and polybrene. Replace with 2 mL of fresh complete RPMI 1640 culture medium supplemented with 10 % FBS, 5 % antibiotics, 20 μg/mL of GM-CSF, and 20 μg/mL of IL-4.
6. To mature the mouse BM-DC, add LPS at the final concentration of 100 ng/mL.
7. Incubate overnight at 37 °C in a humidified atmosphere of 5 % CO_2 in air.
8. On day 7 of BM-DC culture (48 h after shRNA lentivirus transduction), harvest the BM-DC for experimental use. Using a sterile pipette, harvest the supernatant and gently wash the plate 1× with 5 mL of pre-warmed PBS. Add 5 mL of 2 mM EDTA and incubate for 2 min at 37 °C in a humidified atmosphere of 5 % CO_2 in air. Using a sterile pipette, collect the cells and wash the dish 1× with PBS. To detect the knock down of the target gene expression, use Q-PCR or Western blot analyses. The BM-DC are also ready for phenotype analysis and antigen presentation assays (Fig. 1).

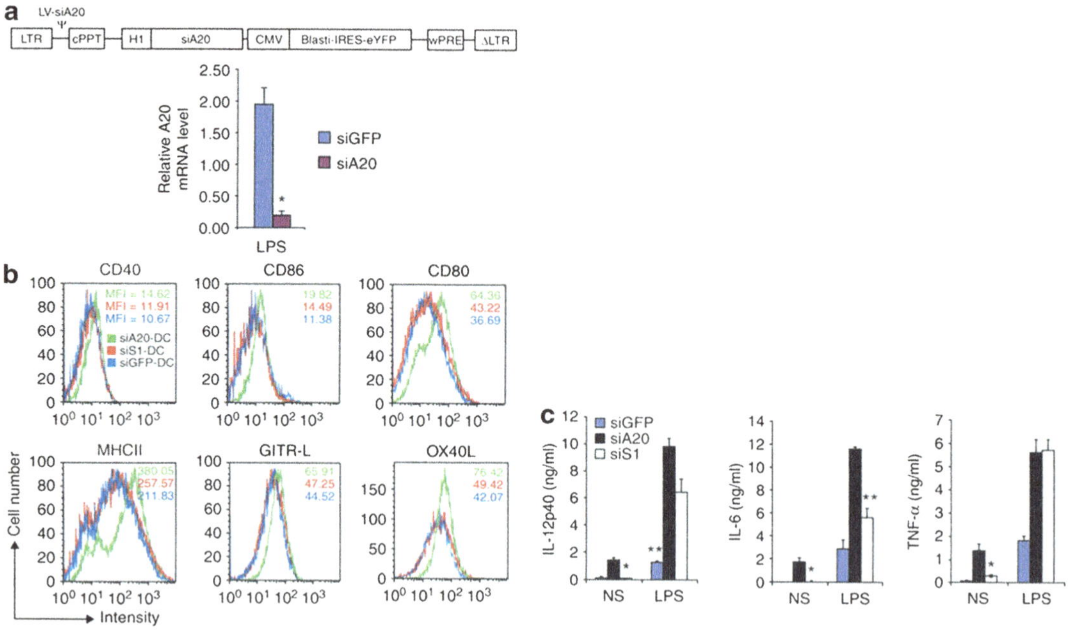

Fig. 1 Silencing A20 in mouse BM-DC. (**a**) qRT-PCR analysis of A20 mRNA levels in YFP+ siA20-DC (siA20) and siGFP-DC (siGFP) after stimulation with LPS for 12 h. Experiments were repeated 2× with similar results. *$P<0.01$ versus siGFP-DC. Schematic diagram of the recombinant lentiviral vector LV-siA20 (*top*) is presented. *LTR* long terminal repeat, *H1* H1 RNA promoter, *cPPT* central polypurine tract sequence, *IRES* internal ribosome entry site, *wPRE* Woodchuck posttranscriptional regulatory element sequence. (**b**) Surface expression of costimulatory and MHC class II molecules on CD11c+YFP+-gated DC 48 h after viral transfection, as determined by FACS analysis. Experiments were repeated 3× with similar results. *MFI* mean fluorescence intensity. (**c**) ELISA measurement of the amounts of cytokines secreted by transfected DC (5×10^5 cells/mL) in response to stimulation with LPS (100 ng/mL) for 16 h from one representative experiment of three. *NS* no stimulation. *$P<0.01$ versus siA20-DC (Reproduced from [12] with permission from Elsevier)

3.2 Ad-shRNA Transduction of Mouse DC

3.2.1 Ad-shRNA Transduction of Mouse BM-DC

1. On day 5 of BM-DC culture, thaw adenovirus particles at room temperature and keep thawed adenovirus particles on ice (*see* **Note 12**). Gently mix the adenovirus stock and add the shRNA adenovirus stock into the wells containing the BM-DC at MOI 500. For example, 1×10^9 virus particles are required for 2×10^6 cells in one well to reach MOI 500 (*see* **Note 10**). Mix by pipetting gently.
2. Incubate overnight at 37 °C in a humidified atmosphere of 5 % CO_2 in air.
3. On day 6 of BM-DC culture, to mature the mouse BM-DC, add LPS at the final concentration of 100 ng/mL. Return the plates to incubator.
4. On day 7 of BM-DC culture (48 h after shRNA adenovirus transduction), harvest the BM-DC for experimental use. Using a sterile pipette, harvest the supernatant and gently wash the plate 1× with 5 mL of pre-warmed PBS. Add 5 mL of 2 mM

EDTA and incubate for 2 min at 37 °C in a humidified atmosphere of 5 % CO_2 in air. Using a sterile pipette, collect the cells and wash the dish 1× with PBS. To detect the knock down of the target gene expression, use Q-PCR or Western blot analyses. The BM-DC are ready for antigen presentation analysis.

3.2.2 Generation of Human Monocyte-Derived DC

1. On day 0, dilute fresh peripheral blood 1:1 in PBS in 50-mL conical centrifuge tubes and mix gently and thoroughly by pipetting.
2. Using a sterile pipette, add 20 mL of LP into a new 50-mL conical centrifuge tube. Carefully overlay 25 mL of diluted blood over 20 mL of LP (ratio of lymphoprep to diluted blood is 5:4).
3. Centrifuge at 400 × *g* for 40 min at room temperature with the brake off (*see* **Note 4**).
4. After pelleting, carefully remove the 50-mL conical centrifuge tube from the centrifuge so as not to disturb the layers. Using a new sterile pipette, carefully harvest the cloudy interface band between the plasma-PBS fraction and the clear separation medium solution into 20 mL of PBS in a 50-mL conical centrifuge tube.
5. Centrifuge at 400 × *g* for 10 min at room temperature.
6. Gently remove the 50-mL conical centrifuge tube from the centrifuge and check the cell pellet. Aspirate supernatant without disturbing the cell pellet. Resuspend the pellet in 20 mL of PBS. Mix gently and thoroughly into a homogenous cell suspension.
7. Centrifuge at 400 × *g* for 5 min at room temperature.
8. Gently remove the 50-mL conical centrifuge tube from the centrifuge and check the cell pellet. Aspirate the supernatant without disturbing the cell pellet. Resuspend the pellet in PBS. Mix gently and thoroughly into a homogenous cell suspension. If more than one tube was used for one blood sample, the cells should be combined into one tube in about 1/3 the starting blood volume of PBS.
9. Count cells using Trypan blue and a hemocytometer. Mix cells gently but thoroughly prior to sampling for the count. Determine the cell concentration.
10. Resuspend the PBMC at 5×10^6 cells/mL in complete RPMI medium containing 10 % FBS.
11. Using a sterile pipette, seed 2 mL of PBMC into one well of a 6-well culture plate. The final cell number is 1×10^7 cells/well.
12. Incubate at 37 °C in a humidified atmosphere of 5 % CO_2 in air for 2 h.
13. Using a sterile pipette, collect the supernatant containing nonadherent cells and gently wash the plate 1× with 2 mL of pre-warmed PBS. Use the adherent cells to generate monocyte-derived DC.

Freeze the nonadherent cells for further experiments as autologous T cells.

14. To collect the adherent cells, add 5 mL of 2 mM EDTA and incubate for 2 min at 37 °C in a humidified atmosphere of 5 % CO_2 in air. Using a sterile pipette, collect the cells, and wash the dish 1× with PBS.
15. Centrifuge at 400 × *g* for 5 min at room temperature.
16. Gently remove the 50-mL conical centrifuge tube from the centrifuge and check the cell pellet. Aspirate the supernatant without disturbing the cell pellet. Resuspend the pellet in CellGenix DC media with L-glutamine. Mix gently and thoroughly into a homogenous cell suspension.
17. Count the cells using Trypan blue and a hemocytometer. Mix cells gently but thoroughly prior to sampling for the count. Determine the cell concentration.
18. Adjust the DC culture medium volume at 2×10^6 cells/mL CellGenix DC medium supplemented with 100 ng/mL GM-CSF and 50 ng/mL IL-4. Seed 1×10^6 cells/0.5 mL in one well of a 24-well cell culture plate.
19. On day 2, feed the culture with GM-CSF and IL-4. Gently remove 250 μL of culture medium from one well. Replace with 250 μL of CellGenix DC medium supplemented with 200 ng/mL GM-CSF and 100 ng/mL IL-4 to reach final concentration of GM-CSF at 100 ng/mL and of IL-4 at 50 ng/mL.
20. Gently remove the centrifuge tube from the centrifuge and check the cell pellet. Aspirate the supernatant without disturbing the cell pellet. Using a sterile pipette, add fresh RPMI medium supplemented with 10 % of FBS, 20 μg/mL GM-CSF, and 20 μg/mL IL-4. Transfer the cell suspension back to the 10-cm cell culture dish with the adherent cells (*see* **Note 7**).
21. Incubate at 37 °C in a humidified atmosphere of 5 % CO_2 in air.
22. On day 5, harvest the cells for siRNA transduction. Using a sterile pipette, collect the supernatant containing cells. To collect the adherent cells, add 5 mL of 2 mM EDTA and incubate for 2 min at 37 °C in a humidified atmosphere of 5 % CO_2 in air. Using a sterile pipette, collect the cells and wash the dish 1× with PBS.
23. Centrifuge at 400 × *g* for 5 min at room temperature.
24. Gently remove the 50-mL conical centrifuge tube from the centrifuge and check the cell pellet. Aspirate the supernatant without disturbing the cell pellet. Resuspend the pellet in CellGenix DC medium with L-glutamine. Mix gently and thoroughly into a homogenous cell suspension.

25. Count cells using Trypan blue and a hemocytometer. Mix the cells gently but thoroughly prior to sampling for the count. Determine the cell concentration.
26. Adjust the DC culture medium volume to 2×10^6 cells/mL CellGenix DC medium supplemented with 100 ng/mL GM-CSF and 50 ng/mL IL-4. Seed 1×10^6 cells/0.5 mL in one well of a 24-well cell culture plate. The cells are ready for siRNA adenovirus transduction.

3.2.3 Ad-shRNA Transduction of Human Monocyte-Derived DC

1. On day 5 of DC culture, thaw the adenovirus particles expressing human A20 shRNA (Ad35-shA20) or control adenovirus (Ad35-control) at room temperature and keep the thawed adenovirus on ice (*see* **Note 12**). Gently mix the adenovirus stock and add the shRNA adenovirus stock into the wells containing the human monocyte-derived DC at MOI 500. For example, 0.5×10^9 virus particles are required for 1×10^6 cells in one well to reach an MOI 500. Mix by pipetting gently.
2. Incubate at 37 °C in a humidified atmosphere of 5 % CO_2 in air.
3. After 120 min, add 500 μL of CellGenix Media containing 2× concentrated cytokines and gentamicin: 10 ng/mL of IL-1β, 100 ng/mL of IL-6, 10 ng/mL of TNF-α, 1 μg/mL of PGE-2, 100 ng/mL of GM-CSF, 50 ng/mL of IL-4, and 50 μg/mL of gentamicin.
4. Incubate at 37 °C in a humidified atmosphere of 5 % CO_2 in air.
5. On day 7 of DC culture (48 h after shRNA adenovirus transduction), harvest the human DC for experimental use. Using a sterile pipette, harvest the supernatant and gently wash the plate 1× with 5 mL of pre-warmed PBS. Add 5 mL of 2 mM EDTA and incubate for 2 min at 37 °C in a humidified atmosphere of 5 % CO_2 in air. Using a sterile pipette, collect the cells and wash the dish 1× with PBS. To detect the knock down of target gene expression, use Q-PCR or Western blot analyses. The DC are also ready for antigen presentation assays.

3.3 siRNA Oligo Transduction of Human Monocyte-Derived DC

1. On day 5 of human monocyte-derived DC culture, thaw siRNA oligos for human A20 siRNA and control siRNA and keep thawed adenovirus on ice. Mix the oligos gently before use.
2. Incubate 12.5 μL of 20 μM annealed siRNA with 5 μL of Lipofectamine 2000 in a volume of 500 μL of serum-free CellGenix Media at room temperature for 20 min.
3. Add this mixture to one well of immature human monocyte-derived DC as mentioned above.
4. Incubate at 37 °C in a humidified atmosphere of 5 % CO_2 in air.
5. After 120 min, add 500 μL of CellGenix Media containing 2× concentrated cytokines and gentamicin: 10 ng/mL of IL-1β,

100 ng/mL of IL-6, 10 ng/mL of TNF-α, 1 μg/mL of PGE-2, 100 ng/mL of GM-CSF, 50 ng/mL of IL-4, and 50 μg/mL of gentamicin.

6. Incubate at 37 °C in a humidified atmosphere of 5 % CO_2 in air.
7. On day 7 of DC culture (48 h after siRNA oligo transfection), harvest the human DC for experimental use. Using a sterile pipette, harvest the supernatant and gently wash the plate once with 5 mL of pre-warmed PBS. Add 5 mL of 2 mM EDTA and incubate for 2 min at 37 °C in a humidified atmosphere of 5 % CO_2 in air. Using a sterile pipette, collect the cells and wash the dish 1× with PBS. To detect the knock down of target gene expression, use Q-PCR or Western blot analyses. The DC are also ready for antigen presentation assays.

4 Notes

1. Both C57bL/6 and Balb/C have been successfully used to generate mouse BM-DC using this protocol, although this protocol uses C57bL/6 as an example.
2. To prepare bone marrow, all muscle tissues should be removed from the femurs and tibias carefully. However, unremoved muscle tissues on the bones will not affect the process and recovery rate of bone marrow. It is also very important to process the bone quickly in order to keep the bone marrow cells in a healthy condition.
3. The bones should be processed in a sterile environment in order to prevent contamination.
4. The incubation time for red blood lysis should be less than 5 min. In general, a small number of residual red cells do not interfere with the following experiments. A second round of lysis can be performed, if required.
5. The BM-DC could be cultured in various dishes or plates. However, we have found in our experiments that seeding the bone marrow cells from one mouse in one 10-cm cell culture dish in 20 mL of conditioned medium generates large numbers of $CD11c^+$ DC.
6. This step is to enrich the cells for proliferating DC. Alternatively, bone marrow cells could be treated with a cocktail of monoclonal antibodies, including GK 1.5 anti-CD4, HO 2.2 anti-CDS, B21-2 anti-Ia, and RA3-3A1/6.1 anti-B220/CD45R and rabbit complement for 60 min at 37 °C to kill lymphocytes.
7. Although most DC are still adherent on day 3 of culture, centrifuge the supernatant so as not to lose any DC.

8. On day 7 of DC culture, the percentage of CD11c⁺ cells should be higher than 90 % as measured by FACS analysis. BM-DC are then ready for experimental use on day 7. Since it takes around 24–48 h for lentivirus to express shRNA in DC, Lv-shRNA should be transduced on day 5 of DC culture.
9. Thawed Lv-shRNA viral particles should be kept on ice. Repeated freeze-thaw cycles and prolonged exposure of the particles to ambient temperatures may result in decreased viral titers. The virus should not be used after three repeated freeze-thaw cycles.
10. The proper MOI should be determined for maximum knock-down of each target gene expression.
11. It has been reported that polybrene enhances virus infection by neutralizing charge interactions to increase binding between the pseudoviral capsid and the cellular membrane. The optimal concentration of polybrene depends on cell type and usually ranges between 2 and 10 μg/mL. Excessive exposure to polybrene (>12 h) can be toxic to some cells. In our experiments, we have found that most mouse DC cultured with polybrene overnight are healthy.
12. Thawed Ad-shRNA virus particles should be kept on ice. Repeated freeze-thaw cycles and prolonged exposure of the particles to ambient temperatures may result in decreased viral titers. The virus should not be used after three repeated freeze-thaw cycles.

Acknowledgement

This work was supported by NIH grant R01 CA148748 and DOD W81XWH-10-1-0281.

References

1. Rosenberg SA et al (2004) Cancer immunotherapy: moving beyond current vaccines. Nat Med 10:909–915
2. Iwasaki A, Medzhitov R (2004) Toll-like receptor control of the adaptive immune responses. Nat Immunol 5(10):987–995
3. Kaisho T, Akira S (2003) Regulation of dendritic cell function through Toll-like receptors. Curr Mol Med 3(4):373–385
4. Kubo T et al (2004) Regulatory T cell suppression and anergy are differentially regulated by proinflammatory cytokines produced by TLR-activated dendritic cells. J Immunol 173: 7249–7258
5. Goldstein DR (2004) Toll-like receptors and other links between innate and acquired alloimmunity. Curr Opin Immunol 16(5): 538–544
6. Pasare C, Medzhitov R (2003) Toll pathway-dependent blockade of CD4+CD25+ T cell-mediated suppression by dendritic cells. Science 299:1033–1036
7. Lee EG et al (2000) Failure to regulate TNF-induced NF-kappaB and cell death responses in A20-deficient mice. Science 289:2350–2354
8. Boone DL et al (2004) The ubiquitin-modifying enzyme A20 is required for termination of Toll-like receptor responses. Nat Immunol 5:1052–1060
9. Wertz IE et al (2004) De-ubiquitination and ubiquitin ligase domains of A20 downregulate NF-kappaB signalling. Nature 430:694–699

10. Sarma V et al (1995) Activation of the B-cell surface receptor CD40 induces A20, a novel zinc finger protein that inhibits apoptosis. J Biol Chem 270:12343–12346
11. Saitoh T et al (2005) A20 is a negative regulator of IFN regulatory factor 3 signaling. J Immunol 174:1507–1512
12. Song XT et al (2008) A20 is an antigen presentation attenuator, and its inhibition overcomes regulatory T cell-mediated suppression. Nat Med 14:258–265
13. Hong B et al (2011) Mucosal and systemic anti-HIV immunity controlled by A20 in mouse dendritic cells. J Clin Invest 121(2): 739–751
14. Song XT et al (2011) A Th1-inducing adenoviral vaccine for boosting adoptively transferred T cells. Mol Ther 19(1):211–217
15. Hong B et al (2009) Human suppressor of cytokine signaling 1 controls immunostimulatory activity of monocyte-derived dendritic cells. Cancer Res 69(20):8076–8084
16. Breckpo K et al (2009) Attenuated expression of A20 markedly increases the efficacy of double-stranded RNA-activated dendritic cells as an anti-cancer vaccine. J Immunol 182(2):860–870

Chapter 12

Fast Monocyte-Derived Dendritic Cell-Based Immunotherapy

Gamal Ramadan

Abstract

Recent reports have described a new strategy for differentiation and maturation of monocyte (Mo)-derived dendritic cells (DC) within only 48–72 h of in vitro culture (fast-DC). Mature fast-DC are as effective as mature standard-DC (generated in 7–10 days of in vitro culture) in priming and propagation of antigen-specific T-cell responses. The use of fast-DC not only reduces labor and supply cost, as well as workload and time, but also increases the DC yield from Mo, which may facilitate DC-based immunotherapy for cancer patients. Detailed protocols for generation, pulsing with different antigen sources, and transduction with adenoviral vector of Mo-derived mature fast-DC as well as using of fast-DC for priming and propagation of antigen-specific cytotoxic T-cell effectors will be described here.

Key words Adenoviral expression, Adoptive immunotherapy, Antigen-presenting cells, Dendritic cell differentiation/maturation, Dendritic cell pulsing/transduction, Fast dendritic cells, Monocyte-derived dendritic cells, Priming/expansion of T-cell effectors, Vaccination

1 Introduction

In traditional protocols, it is widely believed that the in vitro generation of human mature Mo-derived DC with full T-cell stimulatory capacity requires 5–7 days of differentiation with granulocyte-macrophage colony-stimulating factor (GM-CSF) and interleukin-4 (IL-4), followed by 2–3 days of maturation with proinflammatory cytokines and/or CD40 ligand [1–5]. However, there is increasing evidence that the time span required for in vivo DC differentiation and maturation may be shorter. Indeed, a new strategy was recently described for differentiation and maturation of human Mo-derived fast-DC with full T-cell stimulatory capacity within only 48–72 h of in vitro culture [6–8]. In this strategy, adherent blood Mo were cultured for 1 day with GM-CSF and IL-4 to generate $CD14^{-}CD1a^{+}$ immature DC (first step of fast-DC generation: differentiation). Then, they were activated and converted to $CD83^{+}$ functional antigen-presenting cells (second step

Michael J.P. Lawman and Patricia D. Lawman (eds.), *Cancer Vaccines: Methods and Protocols*, Methods in Molecular Biology, vol. 1139, DOI 10.1007/978-1-4939-0345-0_12, © Springer Science+Business Media New York 2014

of fast-DC generation: maturation) by culturing with the following proinflammatory mediators for either 1 or 2 days: tumor necrosis factor-alpha (TNF-α), interleukin-1beta (IL-1β), interleukin-6 (IL-6), and prostaglandin (PG)-E_2 [6–8]. Immature fast-DC are capable of antigen uptake and processing. After maturation, they could present the antigen and extremely increase expression of the major histocompatibility complex (MHC) and costimulatory molecules, e.g., CD86, as well as secrete large amounts of immunostimulatory cytokines such as IL-12, thus rendering them highly effective inducers of antigen-specific T-cell responses [8–11]. Moreover, fast-DC generated in only 2–3 days were capable of prime melanoma-, *Aspergillus fumigatus*-, and cytomegalovirus-specific cytotoxic T lymphocytes (CTL) as effectively as standard-DC generated in 7–10 days [8–11]. More recently, the strategy described for fast-DC generation was further modified by excluding IL-6 from the cytokines cocktail used for their maturation, which not only reduces the number of recombinant cytokines required for DC generation in vitro but may also resemble DC development in vivo more closely [12]. In this chapter, detailed protocols will be described for (1) isolation of human blood monocytes by Ficoll-Hypaque gradient centrifugation and adherence to culture flask; (2) generation, pulsing with different antigen sources (crude extract, cells lysate, cells sonicate, super-antigen, or peptides) and transduction (with adenoviral vector) of Mo-derived mature fast-DC; and (3) use of fast-DC for priming and expansion of antigen-specific CTL for clinical use. The use of fast-DC in clinical trials reduces labor, time, and cost as well as renders cells less sensitive to external disruptive factors [7, 8] and will hopefully facilitate DC-based immunotherapy and vaccination in cancer patients [9, 12].

2 Materials

Prepare all solutions using sterile cell culture grade water and analytical grade reagents. All solutions are commercially available. Diligently follow all waste disposal regulations when disposing waste materials.

2.1 Human Blood Mo Separation

1. Ca^{2+}- and Mg^{2+}-free Dulbecco's phosphate-buffered saline (DPBS): Dissolve 0.2 g of potassium chloride, 0.2 g of monobasic potassium phosphate (KH_2PO_4 anhydrous), 8 g of sodium chloride (NaCl), and 1.15 g of dibasic sodium phosphate (Na_2HPO_4 anhydrous) in 900 mL of cell culture grade water using a magnetic stirrer. Adjust pH to 7.2–7.6 by sodium hydroxide (NaOH) and then add water to 1 L. Sterilize the solution by autoclave and store at room temperature.

2. Ficoll-Hypaque gradient solution: Density 1.077 g/mL, dissolve 64.0 g of Ficoll (molecular weight 400,000) and 0.7 g of NaCl in 600 mL water using a magnetic stirrer at low speed. After adding 99.0 g of sodium diatrizoate, add water to 1 L and then mix. Sterilize the solution with a 0.22-μm filter unit. Store the solution at 4 °C away from direct light and warm it to room temperature prior to use.
3. Fetal bovine serum (FBS): Heat inactivated (by heating at 56 °C for 30 min), sterile-filtered through a 0.22-μm filter unit, and stored at 4 °C.
4. Pooled human AB serum: Heat inactivated by heating at 56 °C for 30 min, sterile-filtered through a 0.22-μm filter unit, and stored at 4 °C.
5. Roswell Park Memorial Institute (RPMI) complete medium: RPMI-1640 medium supplemented with 25 mM (4-(2-hydroxyethyl)-1-piperazineethanesulfonic acid) (HEPES), 2 mM L-glutamine, 100 U/mL of penicillin, and 100 μg/mL of streptomycin. Store the solution at 4 °C and warm it to room temperature prior to use.
6. RBC lysis solution: 8.3 g/L of ammonium chloride in 0.01 M Tris–HCl buffer, pH 7.5, sterilize the solution with a 0.22-μm filter unit. Store up to 6 months at 4 °C and warm it to room temperature prior to use.
7. 0.4 % Trypan blue solution stored at room temperature, filter through a 0.45-μm filter if reagent develops crystals.
8. Immunomagnetic beads coated with anti-human monoclonal antibodies directed against the CD34 antigen.
9. Cryopreserve solution for peripheral blood mononuclear cells (PBMC): RPMI-1640 complete medium containing 20 % pooled human AB serum and 10 % dimethyl sulfoxide (DMSO). Sterilize the solution with a 0.22-μm filter unit. Aliquot and store at ≤−20 °C, adjust to 1–6 °C at time of use.
10. Supplies: Cell scraper, cryocontainer, filter unit (0.22- and 0.45-μm filter), magnetic cell sorter separation columns, Neubauer counting chamber, polystyrene foam freezing racks, sterile conical polypropylene centrifuge tubes (15 and 50 mL), sterile cryovials, sterile pipettes (15 and 50 mL), tissue culture flasks.
11. Equipment: Autoclave, biological safety cabinet, centrifuge with 15- and 50-mL tubes carrier and culture plates carrier, humidified/37 °C/CO_2 incubator, magnetic cell sorter, magnetic stirrer, pH meter, refrigerators (4 °C, −80 °C).

2.2 Generation of Mo-Derived Mature Fast-DC

1. Pooled human AB serum.
2. RPMI-1640 complete medium.
3. 0.4 % Trypan blue solution.

4. Cytokines and proinflammatory mediators (clinical grade): GM-CSF, IL-1β, IL-4, PG-E_2, and TNF-α.
5. Antigens: 1–50 μg/mL of soluble antigens, crude antigens, culture filtrate antigens, cells lysate/sonicate, or peptides.
6. Adenoviral vector containing gene of interest.
7. Fluorescent antibodies and chemicals: fluorescein isothiocyanate (FITC)-, phycoerythrin (PE)-, peridinin chlorophyll-a protein (PerCP)-, and allophycocyanin (APC)-conjugated monoclonal antibodies to CD1a, CD14, CD40, CD45, CD83, CD86, and HLA-DR and their relevant isotype controls, 7-amino-actinomycin D.
8. Thawing solution: RPMI-1640 complete medium containing 10 % pooled human AB serum and 50 U/mL of benzonase. Sterilize the solution with a 0.22-μm filter unit. It should be prepared within 1 week of use, store at 1–6 °C.
9. Cryopreserve solution for DC: Pooled human AB serum containing 10 % DMSO and 5 % glucose. Sterilize the solution with a 0.22-μm filter unit. Aliquot and store at ≤−20 °C, adjust to 1–6 °C at time of use.
10. Supplies: Cell scraper, cryocontainer, filter unit (0.22- and 0.45-μm filter), Neubauer counting chamber, polystyrene foam freezing racks, sterile conical polypropylene centrifuge tubes (15 and 50 mL), sterile cryovials, sterile pipettes (15 and 50 mL), tissue culture flasks.
11. Equipment: Autoclave, biological safety cabinet, centrifuge with 15- and 50-mL tubes carrier and culture plates carrier, FACSCalibur flow cytometer with FCAP software package, humidified/37 °C/CO_2 incubator, refrigerators (4 °C, −80 °C), water bath (37 °C).

2.3 Priming and Expansion of Antigen-Specific CTL

1. Cryopreserve solution for PBMC.
2. FBS.
3. Pooled human AB serum.
4. RPMI-1640 complete medium.
5. Thawing solution.
6. 0.4 % Trypan blue solution.
7. Cytokines (clinical grade): IL-2, IL-12.
8. Fluorescent antibodies and chemicals: FITC-, PE-, PerCP-, and APC-conjugated monoclonal antibodies to CD3, CD4, CD8, CD19, CD56, TCR-αβ, and TCR-γδ and their relevant isotype controls, 7-amino-actinomycin D.
9. Sodium ^{51}chromate (^{51}Cr): 5 mCi/mL, store at 20–25 °C behind lead shielding.

10. 0.5 % Triton X-100: Dilute 0.5 % Triton X-100 in cell culture grade water (v/v). Make fresh on the day of use.
11. K562 erythroleukemia cells (natural killer (NK)-sensitive targets).
12. Supplies: Cell scraper, cryocontainer, filter unit (0.22- and 0.45-µm filter), Lumiplate, Neubauer counting chamber, polystyrene foam freezing racks, round-bottomed 96-well plates sterile cryovials, sterile conical polypropylene centrifuge tubes (15 and 50 mL), sterile pipettes (15 and 50 mL), tissue culture flasks, top seal A.
13. Equipment: Autoclave, biological safety cabinet, centrifuge with 15- and 50-mL tubes carrier and culture plates carrier, FACSCalibur flow cytometer with FCAP software package, humidified/37 °C/CO_2 incubator, gamma irradiator, refrigerators (4 °C, −80 °C), TopCount NXT scintillation and luminescence counter, water bath (37 °C).

3 Methods

Aseptic techniques are required for all methods described here. Carry out all procedures at room temperature unless otherwise specified.

3.1 Isolation of Human Blood Mo

1. Full heparinized blood samples (50 IU of Heparin/mL of blood) must be obtained from volunteer healthy donors or patients by venipuncture (*see* **Notes 1** and **2**).
2. Dilute the anticoagulated blood samples with Ca^{2+}- and Mg^{2+}-free DPBS in a ratio of 1:2 (*see* **Note 3**).
3. Carefully and slowly overlay 30 mL of the diluted heparinized blood on 15 mL of Ficoll-Hypaque in a 50-mL conical polypropylene centrifuge tube (*see* **Note 4**). To maintain the Ficoll-Hypaque/blood interface, it is helpful to hold the centrifuge tube at a 45° angle. If diluted specimen volume is less than 10 mL, overlay 10 mL of diluted heparinized blood on 5 mL of Ficoll-Hypaque in a 15-mL conical polypropylene centrifuge tube.
4. Centrifuge cells for 20 min at room temperature and 900 × *g* (*see* **Note 5**) without brake, since brake will disrupt the interphase.
5. After centrifugation, use a sterile pipette to gently remove the upper layer that contains the plasma and most of the platelets without disrupting the interphase. Then, transfer the PBMC, at the interphase between Ficoll-Hypaque and the plasma (Fig. 1), into new 15- or 50-mL conical polypropylene centrifuge tubes (according to the volume of the mononuclear cell layer) by using another sterile pipette. Granulocytes and erythrocytes are sedimented under Ficoll-Hypaque layer (Fig. 1).

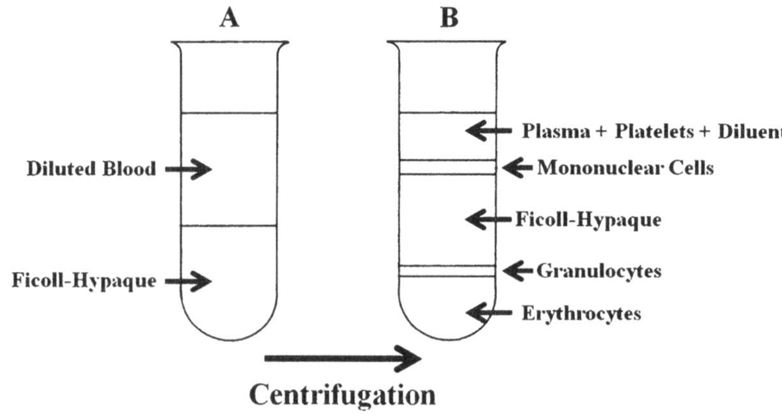

Fig. 1 Cell separation by Ficoll-Hypaque gradient centrifugation. Blood cells before centrifugation (*A*) and after centrifugation (*B*). Mononuclear cells are found at the interphase between Ficoll-Hypaque and the plasma

6. Wash PBMC by adding excess of DPBS (~3× the volume of the mononuclear cell layer) and centrifuging 10 min at 520 × *g* and room temperature. Remove supernatant, resuspend mononuclear cell pellet in DPBS, and repeat the wash 1× to remove most of the platelets (*see* **Notes 6–8**).
7. Resuspend the mononuclear cell pellet in 5–10 mL complete RPMI-1640 medium supplemented with 1 % pooled human AB serum. After performing cell count and evaluating cell viability by Trypan blue exclusion using a Neubauer counting chamber (*see* **Note 9**), cryopreserve the obtained PBMC (*see* **Note 10**) or proceed with isolation of Mo.
8. Adjust cell density at 5×10^6 PBMC/mL in RPMI-1640 complete medium containing 1 % pooled human AB serum and transfer them into an appropriate tissue culture flask (50 mL cell suspension into a 150-cm^2 tissue culture flask).
9. Let Mo adhere by incubating the culture flask horizontally for 1–2 h in 37 °C, 5 % CO_2 and humidified incubator (*see* **Note 11**).
10. After 1 h, check the cell adherence microscopically (you may increase the time of incubation for another 1 h if the cell adherence is inappropriate) and then collect the nonadherent cell fraction of PBMC (lymphocytes) by gently rinsing (2×) the culture flask with RPMI-1640 complete medium or any isotonic solution into new centrifuge tubes. Immediately count and determine the viability of the obtained lymphocytes and then cryopreserve them for future use. Thereafter, determine roughly the count of the adherent cell fraction of

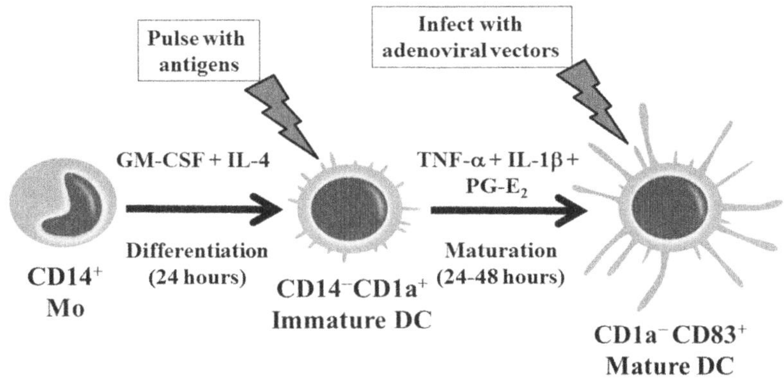

Fig. 2 Differentiation/maturation scheme of human monocyte (Mo)-derived fast-dendritic cells (fast-DC). For optimum antigen presentation and gene expression, pulsing of immature fast-DC with antigens should be performed prior to maturation, while transduction of fast-DC with adenoviral vectors containing the gene of interest should be performed post-maturation. *GM-CSF* granulocyte-macrophage colony-stimulating factor, *IL* interleukin, *PG* prostaglandin, *TNF* tumor necrosis factor

PBMC (Mo) by subtracting the number of the obtained lymphocytes from the original number of the PBMC cultured in the flask (*see* **Note 12**).

11. Add an appropriate volume of the RPMI-1640 complete medium to the flask containing the obtained Mo and proceed directly to generate Mo-derived fast-DC.

3.2 Generation, Pulsing and Transduction of Mo-Derived Mature Fast-DC

1. Incubate adherent blood Mo or frozen Mo after thawing (*see* **Notes 13** and **14**) in an appropriate culture flask at cell density $1–2 \times 10^6$ Mo/mL of RPMI-1640 complete medium containing 1 % pooled human AB serum with 800 U/mL of GM-CSF and 1,000 U/mL of IL-4 for 24 h at 37 °C, 5 % CO_2 in a humidified incubator to generate $CD14^-CD1a^+$ immature DC.
2. Then add 10 ng/mL of IL-1β, 1 μg/mL of PG-E_2, and 10 ng/mL of TNF-α to the cultures of immature fast-DC and incubate for another 24–48 h at 37 °C and 5 % CO_2 with humidity to generate $CD83^+$ mature non-pulsed fast-DC (*see* **Notes 15** and **16**) (Fig. 2).
3. To load fast-DC with antigens, add 1–50 μg/mL of either antigen preparation (soluble antigens, crude antigens, culture filtrate antigens, and cells lysate/sonicate) or peptides (*see* **Note 17**) (Table 1) to the culture of immature fast-DC (prior to maturation, Fig. 2) and incubate for 6–12 h at 37 °C and 5 % CO_2 with humidity. Then mature fast-DC as explained above.

Table 1
Examples of optimum concentrations of different antigen preparations for pulsing immature fast-dendritic cells

Antigen preparation	Optimum concentration
Cells lysate/sonicate	
Cytomegalovirus-infected fibroblast lysate	15 μg/mL [8]
Cytomegalovirus-infected fibroblast sonicate	1:500 (optimal dilution) [8]
Crude extracts	
Aspergillus fumigatus culture filtrate antigen (broth filtrate)	25–50 μg protein/mL [8, 16, 17]
Aspergillus fumigatus crude extract antigen (a mixture of broth filtrate and cytosol extract of *Aspergillus fumigatus*)	50 μg/mL [8, 17, 18]
Peptides	
Overlapping pentadecapeptides pool spanning the entire 427-amino acids coding region of *Aspergillus fumigatus* allergen-16	1 μg/mL for each peptide [10, 11, 19]
Melanoma-associated peptide (HLA-A*0201-restricted peptide Melan-A)	10 μM [9]
Human immunodeficiency virus (HIV)-associated peptide (HLA-A*0201-restricted peptide HIV-pol)	10 μM [9]
Soluble antigens	
Tetanus toxoid soluble antigen	5 μg/mL [6, 12]

4. To introduce genes into fast-DC through adenoviral transduction, infect mature fast-DC with adenoviral vector containing the gene of interest at multiplicity of infection of 150 in RPMI-1640 complete medium containing 1 % pooled human AB serum for 2 h at 37 °C and 5 % CO_2 with humidity (*see* **Note 18**) (Fig. 2). Then infected mature fast-DC are collected in appropriate polypropylene centrifuge tubes (15 or 50 mL) and washed 2× with RPMI-1640 complete medium to remove the excess of retroviral vector. After centrifugation at 300 × *g* for 10 min, remove supernatant containing excess of retroviral vector and resuspend transduced fast-DC in RPMI-1640 complete medium containing 1 % pooled human serum. Mock (medium without adenoviral vector)-transduced mature fast-DC are used as negative control.
5. Then, harvest pulsed or transduced mature fast-DC, and after determining their count and viability, cryopreserve them or proceed directly with priming antigen-specific proliferative and CTL responses (*see* **Notes 19** and **20**).

3.3 Priming and Expansion of Antigen-Specific CTL by Mo-Derived Fast-DC

1. Co-culture mature, pulsed, or transduced, gamma irradiated (25 Gy), Mo-derived fast-DC with autologous Mo-depleted PBMC (lymphocytes) at a ratio of 1:10 (stimulators to responders) in RPMI-1640 complete medium containing 10 % pooled human serum in an appropriate culture flask to generate antigen-specific CTL (*see* **Note 21**).
2. Then add 500 pg/mL of IL-12 to the culture medium, only for the first round of stimulation (*see* **Note 22**).
3. Incubate the cells in 37 °C, 5 % CO_2 and humidified incubator.
4. Feed cultures every third day with half-fresh media, RPMI-1640 complete medium containing 10 % pooled human AB serum, and 200 IU/mL of IL-2 to propagate the generated effectors.
5. Re-prime cultures with mature pulsed or transduced DC every 7 days, three to four primings at least.
6. The cultures should be routinely tested for their phenotypes (by flow cytometric analysis, *see* **Note 19**) and cytolytic reactivity (by chromium-release assay, *see* **Note 23**) 5–7 days after the third prime and onwards.
7. Propagate the generated antigen-specific CTL effectors to the number appropriate for adoptive transfer by repeating the primings (*see* **Note 24**) or harvest, and cryopreserve CTL effectors for future use (*see* **Note 10**).
8. Adjust and maintain cell density at 10^6 cells/mL throughout the culture period.

4 Notes

1. Informed consent must be obtained from all donors and patients before blood samples are collected.
2. A minimum of 10 IU/mL of heparin must be present in blood collected in citrate anticoagulants before beginning processing, because calcium in the processing reagents may cause products to clot in the absence of heparin.
3. Hank's balanced salt solution (HBSS), PBS, or normal saline (0.9 % NaCl) may be used instead of DPBS.
4. The optimal separation of bone marrow mononuclear cells (BMMC) is obtained with the same manner using different density gradient medium that has a slightly higher density than Ficoll-Hypaque (>1.080 and <1.090 g/mL as measured at 25 °C).
5. Bone marrow samples, old blood samples, and samples from patients during the first 6 months posttransplant or those receiving therapy for graft versus host disease should be centrifuged at lower centrifugal force (520 × *g*) for longer time (25–30 min) at room temperature.

6. Certain diseases associate with increased platelet concentrations (mononuclear cell to platelet cell ratio >10:1) in the peripheral blood. To remove the extra platelets in these cases, layer mononuclear cell suspension at density of $1–2 \times 10^7$ cells/mL over 3 mL of FBS in a centrifuge tube. Alternatively, carefully layer the FBS under mononuclear cell suspension, which will rise as FBS is added. Centrifuge 15 min at $200 \times g$ and room temperature. Remove the supernatant containing the platelets and resuspend mononuclear cell pellet in RPMI-1640 complete medium and proceed as in **step** 7.
7. Cord blood, and to a lesser extent peripheral blood from infants, gives a population of mononuclear cells that is contaminated with erythrocytes and their precursors. A pure mononuclear cell population is obtained either by subjecting the cells to a second cycle of Ficoll-Hypaque gradient separation as described above or by lysing the erythrocytes by RBC lysis solution as follows: add 1.0 mL of RBC lysis solution to mononuclear cell pellet, gently mix at room temperature for 1–2 min, dilute to 10 mL with DPBS, centrifuge at $300 \times g$ for 10 min, discard supernatant, resuspend mononuclear cell pellet in RPMI-1640 complete medium, and proceed as in **step** 7.
8. Mononuclear cells of cord blood, bone marrow, and apheresis samples contain many $CD34^+$ hematopoietic progenitor cells which should be removed by magnetic cell sorter using immunomagnetic beads coated with antihuman monoclonal antibodies directed against the CD34 antigen. The $CD34^-$-depleted mononuclear cells are then separated from bead-$CD34^+$ cell rosettes using an array of magnets, which are brought close to the outside of the separation chamber wall. The bead-$CD34^+$ cell rosettes are held within the magnetic field, while the $CD34^-$-depleted mononuclear cells are washed out of the chamber into a "negative fraction" container. Centrifuge the $CD34^-$-depleted mononuclear cells at $300 \times g$ for 10 min, discard supernatant, resuspend mononuclear cell pellet in RPMI-1640 complete medium, and proceed as in **step** 7.
9. Cell count/mL = Average number of cells in one large corner square × dilution factor × 10^4.

   Cell viability (%) = (Number of viable cells/total number of cells) × 100.
10. Cryopreserve PBMC (10×10^6 cells) in 1 mL of ice-cold, sterile cryopreserve solution for PBMC in a dropwise manner with gently mixing in cap cryovials. Place cryovials in cryocontainer or a polystyrene foam freezing rack in a –80 °C freezer. Transfer the vials within 3 days to long term liquid nitrogen storage ≤–135 °C.
11. Incubation at different temperature or lower percent of CO_2 induces stress to Mo and interferes with their ability to adhere.

12. You can directly collect the adherent Mo by gently scraping them from the culture flask using the cell scraper, rinsing the culture flask 2× with RPMI-1640 medium or any isotonic solution. Then count and cryopreserve them for further use, but this will decrease the number of viable cells either by the scraping process or by cryopreserving/thawing process. Some protocols allow Mo to incubate in the culture flask for 24 h in RPMI-1640 complete medium at 37 °C and 5 % CO_2 with humidity before scraping and cryopreserving. By this way, Mo become less adherent and easier to harvest, but they may start to differentiate into macrophages. Therefore, it will be better to generate fast-DC from freshly isolated Mo.
13. Thaw cryovials by partial submersion in a 37 °C water bath with gentle mixing. Uncap and transfer cells to a 15-mL centrifuge tube. Add 5 mL of thawing medium in a dropwise manner with gentle mixing, then add thawing medium to 15 mL. Afterwards, centrifuge cells at $300 \times g$ for 10 min, remove supernatant, and rewash the cells in thawing medium. Remove supernatant and resuspend cells in an appropriate volume of RPMI-1640 complete medium and then perform cell count and evaluate cell viability.
14. Before culturing the monocytes, always screen their phenotype and purity by flow cytometric analysis. In general, Mo yield obtained by the plastic adherent method is ~15–20 % of the original PBMC (purity >85 %).
15. Some protocols add 1,000 U/mL of IL-6 in addition to the mentioned proinflammatory mediators to induce maturation of fast-DC. Our recent study showed that maturation of fast-DC without IL-6 did not significantly alter the morphology, phenotype, or yield of mature DC compared with mature fast-DC generated with IL-6 [12]. Moreover, fast-DC generated without IL-6 are functional antigen-presenting cells, have the ability to induce tetanus toxoid-specific autologous T-cell proliferation, and are as suitable for gene delivery through adenoviral vector transduction as those generated with IL-6 [12].
16. Full maturation of fast-DC is induced by incubating the immature fast-DC in the presence of the proinflammatory mediators for 48 h since the cells downregulated the immature DC marker (CD1a) to 2.78 ± 0.99 % versus 11.50 ± 0.63 if fast-DC matured for only 24 h and upregulated the DC lineage marker (CD83) to 79.12 ± 2.97 % versus 63.22 ± 2.28 if fast-DC matured for only 24 h as in matured standard-DC generated in 7–10 days [8].
17. Some crude antigen preparations contain, in addition to relevant antigens, other nonantigenic components even toxins. Primary trials should be done to determine the optimum concentration for pulsing immature fast-DC with the used antigen preparation and peptides (Table 1).

18. Gene delivery into fast-DC through adenoviral vector transduction significantly increases ($P < 0.001$) if the fast-DC are transduced post-maturation compared with if they are transduced prematuration, 24.5 ± 3.8 versus 10.2 ± 3.1, respectively [12].
19. Before using pulsed or transduced mature fast-DC to prime antigen-specific proliferative and CTL responses, always screen their phenotype and purity by flow cytometric analysis. Sufficient numbers of cells (~2×10^6) are collected and immunophenotyped using a four-color direct panel including FITC-, PE-, PerCP-, and APC-conjugated monoclonal antibodies to CD1a, CD14, CD40, CD45, CD83, CD86, and HLA-DR along with the relevant isotype controls. To exclude dead cells, 7-amino-actinomycin D is added to the samples. The stained cells are acquired on a FACSCalibur flow cytometer and are analyzed from list mode data using the FCAP software package. In general, the yield of $CD83^+$ mature fast-DC obtained by the method described here is ~4–5 % of the original PBMC (viability >95 %). In addition, the mature fast-DC highly express CD40, CD45, CD86, and MHC-class II (>95 %).
20. Freeze matured DC (10×10^6 cells) in 1 mL cryopreserve solution for DC by the same manner as previously described (*see* **Note 10**).
21. Frozen mature pulsed or transduced DC as well as frozen Mo-depleted PBMC (after thawing as previously described (*see* **Note 13**)) can be also used to generate antigen-specific CTL.
22. Addition of IL-12 at the first round of priming the autologous lymphocytes with the pulsed or transduced mature fast-DC increases interferon-gamma (IFN-γ) secretion from natural killer (NK) and T-cells, which promotes the development of T-helper type-1 immune response [13, 14].
23. Cultures are tested for their cytolytic reactivity to different autologous ^{51}Cr-labelled targets. The targets are non-pulsed, antigen-pulsed, mock-infected, or adenoviral vector-infected fast-DC. ^{51}Cr-labelled K562 cells (NK-sensitive targets) are also used in the cytotoxic assay to exclude any NK-mediated cytotoxicity. All targets are incubated 2 h at 37 °C with 200 μCi ^{51}Cr. Then the targets are washed 3× with RPMI-1640 complete medium and plated at 5,000 cells/well in the cytotoxic assay plate. The ^{51}Cr-release assay is performed in triplicate, using round-bottomed 96-well plates, at effector-to-target ratios ranging from 50:1 to 6.25:1. After 4 h incubation at 37 °C in 200 μL RPMI-1640 complete medium containing 10 % FBS and 200 IU/mL IL-2, supernatants (30 μL/well) are added to a Lumiplate, and the radioactivity is measured (after drying >2 h at room temperature and covered with top seal A) in a TopCount NXT scintillation and luminescence

counter. Spontaneous release is measured using medium with targets (no effectors), and maximum release is measured using freshly prepared 0.5 % Triton X-100 with targets only. Specific lysis is calculated as [(count per minute (cpm) test − cpm spontaneous)/(cpm maximum − cpm spontaneous)] × 100.

24. At the time of propagation, the ratio of DC to CTL effectors can be reduced to 1:20 when the number of DC is limited [15].

Acknowledgements

This work was supported in part by awards from the Medical College of Wisconsin Cancer Center, the Boynton Fund of the Greater Milwaukee Foundation, the Rebecca Slye Fund, and the North-west Mutual Liberty Foundation. The author thanks Dr. Carolyn A. Keever-Taylor (Director) and all staff of BMT Processing Laboratories (Medical College of Wisconsin/Froedtert Memorial Lutheran Hospital, Milwaukee, WI, USA) for technical support and discussion. The author also thanks Dr. Gordon R. Sandford, Dr. William H Burns, Candace Krepel (Medical College of Wisconsin), and Dr. Viswanath P. Kurup (VA Medical Center, Milwaukee, WI, USA) for kindly providing the adenoviral vector, CMV Strain AD169, *Aspergillus fumigatus* conidia, *Aspergillus fumigatus* crude extract antigen, respectively.

References

1. Bender A et al (1996) Improved methods for the generation of dendritic cells from nonproliferating progenitors in human blood. J Immunol Methods 196:121–135
2. Jonuleit H et al (1997) Pro-inflammatory cytokines and prostaglandins induce maturation of potent immunostimulatory dendritic cells under fetal calf serum-free conditions. Eur J Immunol 27:3135–3142
3. Thurner B et al (1999) Generation of large numbers of fully mature and stable dendritic cells from leukapheresis products for clinical application. J Immunol Methods 223:1–15
4. Feuerstein B et al (2000) A method for the production of cryopreserved aliquots of antigen-preloaded, mature dendritic cells ready for clinical use. J Immunol Methods 245:15–29
5. Bohnenkamp HR, Noll T (2003) Development of a standardized protocol for reproducible generation of matured monocyte-derived dendritic cells suitable for clinical application. Cytotechnology 42:121–131
6. Dauer M et al (2003) Mature dendritic cells derived from human monocytes within 48 hours: a novel strategy for dendritic cell differentiation from blood precursors. J Immunol 170:4069–4076
7. Obermaier B et al (2003) Development of a new protocol for 2-day generation of mature dendritic cells from human monocytes. Biol Proced Online 5:197–203
8. Ramadan G et al (2004) Generation of *Aspergillus*- and CMV-specific T-cell responses using autologous fast DC. Cytotherapy 6: 223–234
9. Dauer M et al (2005) FastDC derived from human monocytes within 48 h effectively prime tumor antigen-specific cytotoxic T cells. J Immunol Methods 302:145–155
10. Ramadan G et al (2005) Generation of Th1 T cell responses directed to a HLA Class II restricted epitope from the *Aspergillus* f16 allergen. Clin Exp Immunol 139:257–267
11. Ramadan G et al (2005) Generation of cytotoxic T cell responses directed to human leucocyte antigen Class I restricted epitopes from the *Aspergillus* f16 allergen. Clin Exp Immunol 140:81–91

12. Ramadan G (2011) Generation of functional monocyte-derived fast dendritic cells suitable for clinical application in the absence of interleukin-6. Cytotechnology 63:513–521
13. Emtage PC et al (2003) Generating potent Th1/Tc1 T cell adoptive immunotherapy doses using human IL-12: harnessing the immunomodulatory potential of IL-12 without the *in vivo*-associated toxicity. J Immunother 26:97–106
14. Xu S et al (2003) Rapid high efficiency sensitization of $CD8^+$ T cells to tumor antigens by dendritic cells leads to enhanced functional avidity and direct tumor recognition through an IL-12-dependent mechanism. J Immunol 171:2251–2261
15. Keever-Taylor CA et al (2001) Cytomegalovirus-specific cytolytic T-cell lines and clones generated against adenovirus-pp65-infected dendritic cells. Biol Blood Marrow Transplant 7:247–256
16. Ramadan G (2008) Epstein-Barr virus-transformed B-cells as efficient antigen presenting cells to propagate *Aspergillus*-specific cytotoxic T-lymphocytes. Egypt J Immunol 15:145–157
17. Ramadan G (2012) *In vitro* expansion of human γδ and $CD56^+$ T-cells by *Aspergillus*-antigen loaded fast dendritic cells in the presence of exogenous interleukin-12. Immunopharmacol Immunotoxicol 34:309–316
18. Ramadan G (2004) The proliferative response of T cells to *Aspergillus* antigen requires prior presentation on dendritic cells. Egypt J Immunol 11:47–58
19. Zhu F et al (2008) Stimulation by means of dendritic cells followed by Epstein-Barr virus-transformed B cells as antigen-presenting cells is more efficient than dendritic cells alone in inducing *Aspergillus* f16-specific cytotoxic T cell responses. Clin Exp Immunol 151:284–296

Chapter 13

Intratumoral Injection of BCG-CWS-Pretreated Dendritic Cells Following Tumor Cryoablation

Naoshi Kawamura, Masaru Udagawa, Tomonobu Fujita, Toshiharu Sakurai, Tomonori Yaguchi, and Yutaka Kawakami

Abstract

Intratumoral administration of dendritic cells (DC) following cryoablation of tumor is one of the personalized cancer immunotherapies which is able to induce immune responses to multiple endogenous tumor antigens, including shared and unique antigens. Here we describe protocols of cryoablation of tumors, generation of cultured DC, pretreatment of DC with a Toll-like receptor (TLR)-stimulating purified component of Bacillus Calmette-Guerin cell wall fraction (BCG-CWS) and highly immunogenic keyhole limpet hemocyanin (KLH) antigen, and combined use of tumor cryoablation and intratumoral administration of BCG-CWS-pretreated DC in both a murine model and cancer patients.

Key words Dendritic cells, BCG-CWS, KLH, Cryoablation, Immunotherapy

1 Introduction

We have previously identified various human tumor antigens recognized by tumor-infiltrating T-lymphocytes using various immunological and genetic methods and evaluated immune responses to the identified tumor antigens in cancer patients [1–3]. Autologous tumor-specific unique antigens derived from genetic alterations in cancer cells were isolated from patients with favorable prognosis after immunotherapy, indicating that they were attractive targets for immunotherapy. Immunogenicity of shared antigens varies among patients depending on the expression of these antigens in cancer cells and the immunoreactivity of patients. In addition, involvement of antigen spreading to endogenous tumor antigens in in vivo tumor regression has been suggested in the vaccine trials with the identified tumor antigens. These observations indicate the importance of development of personalized immunotherapy which is able to induce immune responses against multiple tumor antigens including immunogenic shared and unique antigens such as mutated peptide antigens.

Michael J.P. Lawman and Patricia D. Lawman (eds.), *Cancer Vaccines: Methods and Protocols*, Methods in Molecular Biology, vol. 1139, DOI 10.1007/978-1-4939-0345-0_13, © Springer Science+Business Media New York 2014

Based on these observations, we have developed a personalized cancer immunotherapy involving the intratumoral administration of TLR-stimulated DC after cryoablative tumor treatment [4–6]. Cryoablation of tumor induces mainly tumor necrosis and some tumor apoptosis and results in the release of multiple endogenous tumor antigens, including shared antigens and antigens unique to the patients. Intratumoral injection of DC into cryoablated tumors results in the uptake of dead cancer cells and the release of endogenous tumor antigens by the DC. Since complete maturation of DC decreases their antigen uptake activity, cultured DC treated briefly with a TLR-stimulator such as BCG-CWS should be used. In our CT26 tumor mouse model, injected DC efficiently take up endogenous tumor antigens, move to the draining lymph nodes, and subsequently induce strong $CD8^+$ cytotoxic T Lymphocyte (CTL) specific for multiple endogenous tumor antigens.

We then performed clinical trials of the cryoablation-combined DC-based personalized immunotherapy for patients with various cancers, including melanoma, lung cancer, and colon cancer [5, 6]. DC was prepared by culturing peripheral blood $CD14^+$ monocytes isolated using the Clinimax device in the presence of granulocyte-macrophage-stimulating factor (GM-CSF) and interleukin-4 (IL4). Keyhole limpet hemocyanin (KLH) antigen was pulsed on DC to monitor the immune response to antigen expressed on the injected DC and to increase DC immunogenicity due to the strong immunogenicity of KLH. Subsequently, DC were pretreated with BCG-CWS for 2 h and injected into tumors which had been cryoablated. Cryoablation was performed by cutaneous application for melanoma, a computed tomography (CT)-guided method for lung cancer, and an ultrasound-guided method for liver metastasis of colon cancer using a specialized cryoablation device. Although clear objective tumor responses (CR/PR) were not observed, relatively good prognosis with decrease of serum tumor markers was obtained along with good immune responses to KLH measured by delayed-type hypersensitivity (DTH) skin reaction and specific IgG antibody in some patients with melanoma or lung cancer. In this chapter, we describe the protocol of this combined DC-based immunotherapy in mouse tumor models and cancer patients.

2 Materials

2.1 BCG-CWS Fractionation

1. *Mycobacterium bovis* Bacillus Calmette-Guérin.
2. Sorvall Cell Fractionator.
3. Enzymes: trypsin, chymotrypsin, and protease.
4. Saline.
5. Acetone.
6. (1:1) Diethyl ether–ethanol.

7. Chloroform.
8. (1:2) Chloroform–methanol.

2.2 Mouse Model

1. 6- to 8-week-old female BALB/c mice (H-2d).
2. CT26, a *N*-nitroso-*N*-methylurethane-induced murine colon cancer cell line.
3. Lineage Panel and Streptavidin Plus Magnetic Particles-DM (BD Biosciences, Pharmingen, San Diego, CA).
4. Murine GM-CSF (Peprotech, London, UK).
5. Dulbecco's modified essential medium (DMEM) supplemented with 10 % heat-inactivated fetal bovine serum (FBS), 100 U/mL penicillin, 100 μg/mL streptomycin.
6. CMS5a, a fibrosarcoma cell line.
7. MEM nonessential amino acids.
8. 10 mM 4-(2-Hydroxyethyl)piperazine-1-ethanesulfonic acid (HEPES) buffer.
9. 1 mM MEM sodium pyruvate.
10. Roswell Park Memorial Institute (RPMI)-1640 medium supplemented with 10 % FBS, 55 μM/L of 2-mercaptoethanol, 100 U/mL of penicillin, 100 μg/mL of streptomycin.
11. Cryomaster, which utilizes high-pressure carbon dioxide or nitrous oxide gas for freezing, is used for mouse tumor experiments and patients with melanoma in skin or lymph nodes (Keeler Ltd., Windsor, Berkshire, UK).
12. CRYOcare surgical system, which utilizes high-pressure argon gas for freezing and high-pressure helium gas for thawing, is used for patients with lung cancer and liver metastases of various cancers including colon cancer. This system automatically repeats freeze and thaw (Endo-care, Irvine, California, USA) [7, 8].

2.3 Human Studies

1. Cryomaster.
2. CRYOcare surgical system.
3. CliniMACS cell separation system (Miltenyi Inc., Gladbach, Germany).
4. rhIL-4 (R&D System Inc., Minnapolis, MN, USA).
5. rhGM-CSF (NCPG Corp., Hebei Province, P.R. China).
6. X-fold bags® (Takarabio Inc., Kyoto, Japan).
7. KLH (INTRACEL Corp., Frederick, MD, USA).
8. Influenza virus peptide (GILGFVFTL) (Multiple Peptide Systems, San Diego,CA).
9. CMV virus peptide (QYDPVAALF) (Multiple Peptide Systems, San Diego,CA).

3 Methods

3.1 BCG-CWS Fractionation

1. The cell walls are prepared from *Mycobacterium bovis* Bacillus Calmette-Guérin [9]. Disrupt the cell suspension in cold water with a Sorvall Cell Fractionator at 35,000 psi at 5–10 °C.
2. Centrifuge the disrupted product at 3,000 × *g* to remove unbroken cells and debris.
3. After depletion of cell debris, harvest the fraction by centrifugation at 20,000 × *g* for 60 min.
4. 400 mL of the "whole cell wall" fraction is then treated several times with 40 mg of trypsin, 40 mg of chymotrypsin, and 40 mg of protease and washed 3× with 1 M Tris–HCl, pH 7.2, 2× with saline and 3× with water.
5. 400 mL of the protease-treated cell wall fraction is then extracted consecutively with 200 mL diethyl ether–ethanol (1:1), 200 mL of chloroform, and 200 mL of chloroform–methanol (2:1). The cell wall residue is designated as CWS to distinguish it from "whole cell wall." The expected yield is 5–7 % of intact cells.
6. Prepare a 3 mg/mL of BCG-CWS solution as an oil-in-water emulsion for in vivo applications.
7. Prepare BCG-CWS as a 2 mg/mL of saline solution for in vitro treatment of DC.
8. Homogenize BCG-CWS with a Potter homogenizer, and heat-sterilize for 30 min at 60 °C.
9. Immature DC should be cultured with 15 mg/mL of BCG-CWS solution within 6 h to maintain phagocytic activity. The DC will gradually mature dafter in vivo administration.

3.2 Mouse Model

1. 6- to 8-week-old female BALB/c mice (H-2d) should be maintained in the specified pathogen-free conditions. The *N-nitroso-N*-methylurethane-induced murine colon cancer cell line, CT26, is cultured in DMEM supplemented with FBS and penicillin/streptomycin.
2. The fibrosarcoma cell line, CMS5a, is cultured in RPMI-1640 supplemented with FBS, 2-mercaptoethanol, and penicillin/streptomycin.

3.2.1 Generation of Murine Myeloid DC from Bone Marrow

1. Harvest femurs and tibias of mice (BALB/c for CT26 murine colon cancer cell line). Bone marrow cells (BMCs) are collected using 26 G-needle.
2. Myeloid dendritic precursors are prepared from BMCs by depleting CD3e, CD11b, Gr-1, B220, and TER119-positive cells using Lineage Panel and Streptavidin Plus Magnetic Particles-DM.

3. The myeloid DC precursors obtained are cultured in RPMI-1640 supplemented with 10 ng/mL of murine GM-CSF, 10 % FBS, 100 U/mL of penicillin, 100 μg/mL of streptomycin, 55 μM/L of 2-mercaptoethanol, 0.1 mM MEM nonessential amino acids, 10 mM HEPES buffer, and 1 mM MEM sodium pyruvate at 4×10^5/mL in 6-well plates [4].
4. On days 4 and 6, half of the medium is replaced with fresh complete medium.
5. On day 7, nonadherent cells are harvested and used as bone marrow-derived DC for subsequent experiments.

3.2.2 Mouse Tumor Model with Murine Colon Cancer Cell Line, CT26

Subcutaneously (s.c.) inoculate 5×10^5 cells in 100 μL of CT26 tumor cells into the bilateral flanks (shaved with an electric hair clippers) of the BALBc mice under anesthesia.

3.2.3 Combined Treatment of Cryoablation and Intratumoral DC Administration

1. Cryoablation of subcutaneously implanted tumor is performed 2× by touching cryoprobes connected to Cryomaster at −80 °C for 60 s (Fig. 1) (*see* **Note 1**) [4].
2. The bone marrow-derived DC are then pretreated with 15 mg/mL of BCG-CWS for 6 h. Then 2×10^5 DC in 50 μL of saline are injected into tumor site using a 27-gauge needle syringe. The second treatment can be performed 3 days after the first treatment (Fig. 2).

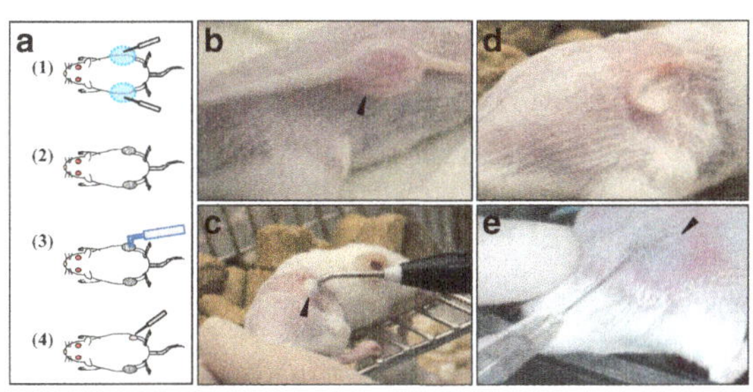

Fig. 1 Procedure of cryoablation and intratumoral DC for subcutaneously implanted murine tumor. (**a**) Schematic representation of the protocol. All drawings show dorsal views of the upper half of the mouse body. (*1*) Tumor cells are implanted on bilateral flanks at day 0. (*2*) Bilateral tumors on day 5 after implantation. (*3*) Cryoablation (freeze and thaw) of one of the implanted tumors using the cryoprobe connected to the Cryomaster. (*4*) Intratumor injection of BCG-CWS-treated DC. (**b**) Subcutaneously implanted tumor 5 days after tumor implantation (5×10^5 cells in 100 μL). *Arrowhead* shows the tumor. (**c**) Cryoablation of the tumor by touching with the cryoprobe. *Arrowhead* indicates frozen tumor. (**d**) Subcutaneous tumor after repeated cryoablation. (**e**) Injection of cultured DC (2×10^5 cells/50 μL) into cryoablated subcutaneous tumor

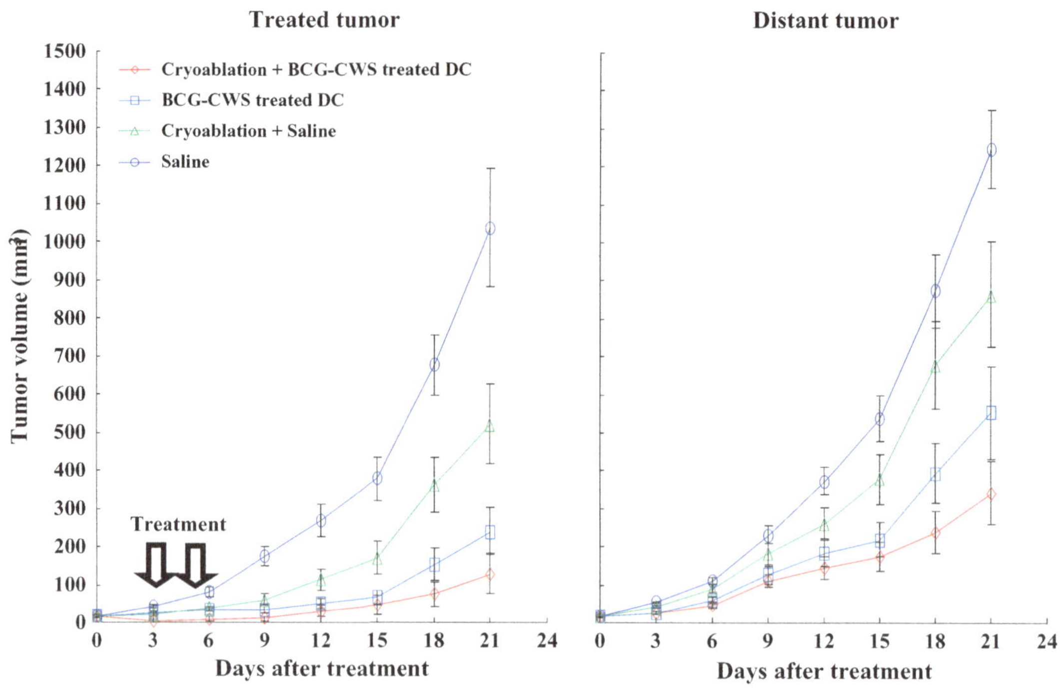

Fig. 2 Effective antitumor effects by intratumoral administration of DC following cryoablation in murine tumor model. Tumor volume was significantly decreased by combination of intratumoral administration of BCG-CWS-pretreated DC following tumor cryoablation (*open diamond*) than by either cryoablation alone (*open triangle*), BCG-CWS-treated DC alone (5×10^5 cells/mouse) (*open square*), or no treatment (*open circle*) on both treated tumor or untreated CT26 murine colon cancer cell line implanted on BALB/c mice. Cryoablation was performed 3 days after tumor implantation, and BCG-treated DC were administered intratumorally 3 and 5 days after tumor implantation

3.3 Human Studies

3.3.1 Generation of Human Monocyte-derived DC

The following protocol is based on patients with stage IV cancers including melanoma, lung cancer, esophageal cancer, and colon cancer, who were refractory to conventional therapies and had at least one tumor for cryoablation followed by administration of DC and other remote tumors for evaluation of antitumor effects, who were recruited in the Phase I/II clinical trial of immunotherapy by intratumoral administration of dendritic cells following cryoablative tumor pretreatment (approved at Keio University School of Medicine in 2005).

1. PBMC are collected from patients by using a COBE Spectra® leukapheresis device.
2. $CD14^+$ monocytes are purified from PBMC by using CliniMACS cell separation system. Aliquot the purified $CD14^+$ monocytes into the cryogenic tubes and store in the liquid nitrogen for later treatments.

3. The purified $CD14^+$ monocytes are cultured in RPMI-1640 medium supplemented with 2 % autologous serum, 100 ng/mL of rhIL-4, and 100 ng/mL of rhGM-CSF in the X-fold bags® for 6–8 days.
4. On the day prior to DC administration, KLH (for possible augmentation of immunogenicity of DC and monitoring of immune response by DC injection) is added into the bags in which the DC are cultured and incubated for 24 h.
5. Twenty-four hours after KLH addition, DC are incubated with 5 μg/mL of BCG-CWS and 1.25 μg/mL of influenza virus peptide (GILGFVFTL) for patients with HLA-A0201 or A0206, and CMV virus peptide (QYDPVAALF) for patients with HLA-A2402 or HLA-A2420 for 2 h in order to monitor the immune response (*see* **Note 2**).
6. Wash the DC 3× with saline, inject $1–2 \times 10^7$ prepared DC in saline into tumors for which cryoablative treatment has been performed.

3.3.2 Combined Treatment of Cryoablation and Intratumoral DC Administration

1. Cryoablation is performed by direct application of the cryoprobe for superficial tumors, such as skin lesions like melanoma and superficial lymph node metastases, by CT-guided application of the cryoprobe for metastases in the lung or lung cancer and by ultrasound-guided application of the cryoprobe for liver metastases of colon cancer and other cancers (see below).
2. $1–2 \times 10^7$ BCG-CWS-pretreated-KLH/virus antigen peptide-pulsed cultured DC are injected into the tumor after repeated cryoablation (repeated freeze and thaw). The same procedure is repeated for 3–4× every 1–2 weeks (Fig. 3).

3.3.3 Cryoablation of Superficial Melanoma Metastases

1. The skin over the tumor is locally anesthetized and a skin incision is made to expose the superficial tumor (subcutaneous lesions or superficial lymph node metastases) for cryoablation and DC injection without damaging skin.
2. Cryoablation is performed by touching tumors with cryoprobe of Cryomaster for at least 1 min for complete freezing and then waiting after release of cryoprobe until thawing has occurred. This procedure can be repeated 3×.

3.3.4 Cryoablation of Lung Cancer Metastases in the Lung [7, 8]

1. A 21-gauge guide needle is inserted into the tumor under fluoroscopic CT guidance under local anesthesia.
2. A stainless-steel sheath for the cryoprobe consisting of an inner guiding sheath and an external sheath is inserted over the needle. After the inner sheath is removed, a 2-mm cryoprobe is inserted through the external sheath.

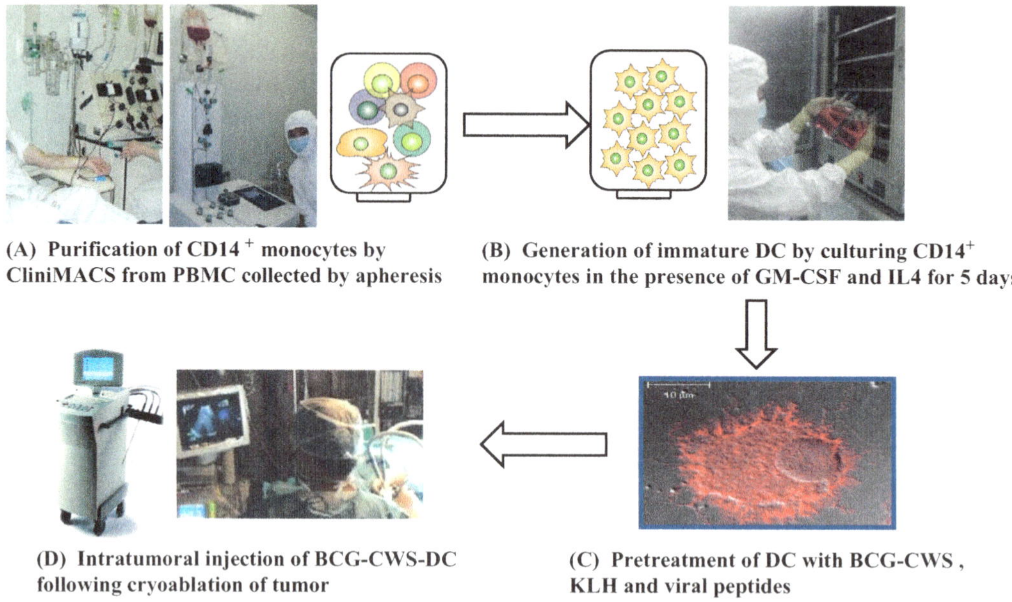

Fig. 3 Protocol for intratumoral administration of BCG-CWS-treated DC following cryoablation for patients with cancer. DC-based immunotherapy combined with tumor cryoablation is performed as follows: (**a**) Purification of $CD14^+$ monocytes by CliniMACS from patient's PBMC collected by apheresis. (**b**) Generation of immature DC by culturing $CD14^+$ monocytes in the presence of GM-CSF and IL4 for 5 days. (**c**) Pretreatment of DC with BCG-CWS, KLH, and viral peptides. (**d**) Intratumoral injection of BCG-CWS-DC following cryoablation of tumor

3. Cryoablative treatment consisting of one cycle of 5 min of freezing followed by thawing using the CRYOcare surgical system is performed. The 2-mm diameter cryoprobe freezes about 2 cm in diameter after one cycle of freezing and thawing.
4. A 21-gauge needle is then inserted and positioned adjacent to the tip of the outer sheath in the freeze-thawed tumor tissue.
5. $1–2 \times 10^7$ prepared DC are injected into three areas of the tumor through the adjacently placed needle and a needle placed through the outer sheath about 30 min after the cryoablative pretreatment.
6. After the procedure, fibrin glue is infused into the outer sheath. The outer sheath is removed, and the coagulated fibrin is filled by removing the inner sheath.

3.3.5 Cryoablation of Liver Metastases of Various Cancers

1. A 21-gauge guide needle is inserted into the tumor under ultrasound guidance under local anesthesia.
2. Utilize a similar procedure for the cryoablation as described for lung cancer for liver metastases of various cancers, including colon cancer.

4 Notes

1. In the mouse subcutaneous murine tumor model, too much cryoablation may damage the adjacent skin and decrease the immune induction. This may be due to damage of DC homing to lymph nodes.
2. Immunological monitoring can be performed by DTH skin reactions, evaluation of serum KLH-specific IgG antibody, and HLA pentamer analysis of viral specific T cells in peripheral blood. In our studies, the DTH reaction was defined positive when the diameter of erythema was more than 5 mm 48 h after intradermal injection of 1 μg of KLH or viral peptides in the patient's arm.

References

1. Kawakami Y, Rosenberg SA (1997) Human tumor antigens recognized by T-cells. Immunol Res 16:313–339
2. Kawakami Y et al (2004) Identification of human tumor antigens and its implications for diagnosis and treatment of cancer. Cancer Sci 95:784–791
3. Kawakami Y et al (2005) Immunological detection of altered signaling molecules involved in melanoma development. Cancer Metastasis Rev 24:357–366
4. Udagawa M et al (2006) Enhancement of immunologic tumor regression by intratumoral administration of dendritic cells in combination with cryoablative tumor pretreatment and Bacillus Calmette-Guerin cell wall skeleton stimulation. Clin Cancer Res 24:7465–7475
5. Kawakami Y et al (2007) Development of individualized immunotherapy based on the analysis on anti-tumor immune responses to the human tumor antigens identified using immunological and genetic methods. Gene Ther 2007:240–248
6. Kawakami Y et al (2008) Dendritic cell based personalized immunotherapy based on cancer antigen research. Front Biosci 13: 1952–1958
7. Kawamura M et al (2006) Percutaneous cryoablation of small pulmonary malignant tumors under computed tomographic guidance with local anesthesia for nonsurgical candidates. J Thorac Cardiovasc Surg 131(5):1007–1013
8. Yashiro H et al (2012) Percutaneous cryoablation of lung tumors: feasibility and safety. J Vasc Inter Radiol 23:295–302
9. Yamamura Y et al (1976) Immunotherapy of cancer with cell wall skeleton of Mycobacterium bovis-Bacillus Calmette-Guérin: experimental and clinical results. Ann N Y Acad Sci 277: 209–227

Chapter 14

Exploiting the CD1d-iNKT Cell Axis for Potentiation of DC-Based Cancer Vaccines

Roeland Lameris, Famke L. Schneiders, Tanja D. de Gruijl, and Hans J. van der Vliet

Abstract

Invariant natural killer T cells (iNKT) and dendritic cells (DC) play a central role in tumor immunity through downstream activation of immune effector cells by pro-inflammatory cytokines. Evidence is accumulating that the CD1d-iNKT cell axis can be effectively used to potentiate DC-based cancer vaccines. Here, we provide a detailed methodology for the generation of (CD1d-expressing) monocyte-derived DC (moDC) and their subsequent loading with the iNKT cell agonist α-galactosylceramide (α-GalCer) or their direct ligation by agonistic anti-CD1d monoclonal antibodies.

Key words Invariant natural killer T cells, Dendritic cells, CD1d, α-Galactosylceramide

1 Introduction

Invariant natural killer T cells (iNKT) are a unique population of lymphocytes characterized by a restricted T-cell receptor (TCR) repertoire. Unlike conventional T cells that recognize antigen (Ag) presented by polymorphic major histocompatibility complex (MHC) molecules, iNKT are confined to the recognition of (glyco) lipid Ag presented by CD1d, which is an essentially monomorphic MHC class 1-like molecule [1–3]. Interaction between Ag-presenting cells (APC), expressing (glyco)lipid-loaded CD1d, and iNKT leads to iNKT activation and the subsequent production of a wide range of cytokines, including both regulatory, e.g., interleukin (IL)-4 and IL-10, and pro-inflammatory, e.g., interferon-γ (IFN-γ) and IL-2. Hence, iNKT have been recognized for their important role in immune regulation, microbial immunity, autoimmunity, antitumor immunity, and a variety of inflammatory conditions [1, 4, 5]. Studies involving multiple tumor models elucidated the critical role of iNKT in tumor immunosurveillance

Michael J.P. Lawman and Patricia D. Lawman (eds.), *Cancer Vaccines: Methods and Protocols*, Methods in Molecular Biology, vol. 1139, DOI 10.1007/978-1-4939-0345-0_14, © Springer Science+Business Media New York 2014

[6, 7]. Notably, human observational studies demonstrated that in the presence of certain (advanced) cancers, iNKT display quantitative and qualitative defects, favoring a Th2-biased cytokine profile with decreased IFN-γ production [8–10].

iNKT research was boosted when α-galactosylceramide (α-GalCer/KRN7000), a glycolipid originally derived from the marine sponge *Agelas mauritianus*, was found to be a high-affinity ligand for iNKT [11]. α-GalCer-mediated activation of iNKT resulted in a potent antitumor immune response in multiple animal models using various tumor types [1, 12]. However, despite these promising results in animal studies, direct intravenous administration of α-GalCer in humans resulted in minimal immune activation and only in a minority of patients that had relatively normal peripheral blood iNKT frequencies. Strikingly, in "responding patients," subsequent administrations of α-GalCer resulted in blunted immune responses [13], possibly as a result of the induction of iNKT cell anergy which was also observed in mice [14].

Tumor immunity of iNKT is achieved, at least in part, through the downstream activation of effector cells such as natural killer (NK) and cytotoxic T lymphocytes (CTL), in an IFN-γ-dependent manner [1, 4]. Similar to interactions between conventional T cells and APC, interactions between CD1d-expressing APC, e.g., monocytes, B cells, DC, and iNKT, are mandatory for optimal activation of both and propagate pro-inflammatory responses through the reciprocal amplification of IL-12 and INF-γ production [1, 8]. Emerging preclinical data underscore the importance of these interactions and, more specifically, the central role of DC. In vitro treatment of iNKT cells with α-GalCer-pulsed monocyte-derived DC (moDC) resulted in potent iNKT expansion and a more consistent pro-inflammatory and cytolytic profile when compared to α-GalCer alone [15]. In addition, observed iNKT defects in cancer patients appeared to be reversible with α-GalCer-pulsed moDC and exogenous IL-12, at least in vitro [9, 16]. Clinical trials using α-GalCer-pulsed moDC, in some instances combined with adoptive transfer of enriched autologous iNKT, induced a more potent cytokine response and a tumor response in some patients [12, 17–19]. These promising results can probably be attributed to the superior ability of DC to present Ag and their expression of co-stimulatory molecules.

Here, we describe in detail how immature and mature moDC can be generated from peripheral blood and are optimally exposed to α-GalCer to allow activation and biased cytokine production in responding iNKT. Furthermore, multiple groups have targeted the CD1d molecule itself using CD1d-specific monoclonal antibodies (mAb). As it was shown that direct mAb ligation of CD1d induced a strong Th1-biased immune response, both in vitro and in vivo [20, 21], this methodology is also described.

2 Materials

2.1 Isolation of Human Peripheral Blood Mononuclear Cells (PBMC)

Store all noncellular reagents at 2–8 °C unless otherwise specified.

1. Peripheral blood sample. Keep at room temperature.
2. Phosphate-buffered saline (PBS), room temperature.
3. Lymphoprep™ (or equivalent) (p = 1.077 g/mL), kept at room temperature.
4. Shock medium: 184 mM ammonium chloride (NH_4Cl), 10 mM potassium bicarbonate ($KHCO_3$), and 0.1 mM EDTA, pH 7.0.
5. PBS-BSA buffer: 0.1 % bovine serum albumin (BSA) in PBS.

2.2 CD14+ Cell (Monocyte) Isolation and/or iNKT Isolation

1. Isolated PBMC.
2. Magnetic activated cell sorting (MACS) buffer: 0.5 % BSA, 2 mM EDTA in PBS (*see* **Note 1**).
3. For monocyte isolation: CD14 MicroBeads, human (Miltenyi Biotec Inc., Auburn, CA, USA).
4. For iNKT isolation: murine antihuman TCR Vα24 monoclonal antibodies (mAbs) (clone C15) and goat anti-mouse IgG magnetic beads, human (Miltenyi Biotec Inc., Auburn, CA, USA) (*see* **Note 2**).
5. MACS column and separator (Miltenyi Biotec Inc., Auburn, CA, USA) (*see* **Notes 3** and **4**).
6. Pre-separation filter (Miltenyi Biotec Inc., Auburn, CA, USA).

2.3 Generation of Immature moDC

1. Purified monocytes ($CD14^+$ cells).
2. PBS.
3. Cell culture medium (CCM): 10 % FBS in RPMI-1640 medium with 25 mM 4-(2-hydroxyethyl)piperazine-1-ethanesulfonic acid (HEPES), 0.05 mM beta-mercaptoethanol (β-ME), 100 IU/mL of sodium penicillin, 100 μg/mL of streptomycin sulfate, and 2.0 mM of L-glutamine (*see* **Notes 5** and **6**).
4. GM-CSF: 1,000 IU/mL of recombinant human (rh)GM-CSF.
5. IL-4: 10 ng/mL of rhIL-4.

2.4 Generation of α-GalCer-Pulsed Mature moDC

1. Immature moDC.
2. LPS: 100 ng/mL of lipopolysaccharide.
3. α-GalCer: 100 ng/mL of α-galactosylceramide (Funakoshi, Tokyo, Japan) (*see* **Note 7**).
4. EDTA: 0.5 mM EDTA.
5. CCM.

2.5 CD1d Ligation on Human moDC

1. Immature moDC.
2. PBS.
3. Anti-CD1d mAbs: 10 μg/mL of anti-CD1d mAbs (*see* **Note 8**).
4. CCM.

2.6 iNKT Expansion and Activation

1. α-GalCer-pulsed mature moDC.
2. Purified iNKT (TCR Vα24-Jα18$^+$ cells).
3. IL-2: 50 IU/mL of rhIL-2.
4. CCM.
5. Yssel's supplement: 5 % BSA in Roswell Park Memorial Institute (RPMI)-1640 medium with 25 mM HEPES, 100 IU/mL of sodium penicillin, 100 μg/mL of streptomycin sulfate, 2.0 mM of L-glutamine, 0.8 mg/mL of transferrin, 0.1 mg/mL of insulin, 0.08 μg/mL of linoleic acid, 0.08 μg/mL of oleic acid, and 0.072 μg/mL of ethanolamine.
6. Yssel's medium: RPMI-1640 with 25 mM HEPES, 100 IU/mL of sodium penicillin, 100 μg/mL of streptomycin sulfate, 2.0 mM of L-glutamine, 1 % human AB serum, and 5 % Yssel's supplement (*see* **Note 9**).
7. Feedermix: 1×10^6/mL irradiated allogeneic PBMC, 1×10^5/mL irradiated EBV-transformed B cells in Yssel's medium, supplemented with 100 ng/mL of phytohemagglutinin (PHA) and 100 IU/mL of rhIL-2.

3 Methods

Carry out all procedures at room temperature unless otherwise specified. To prevent inadequate cell resuspension after centrifugation, always resuspend the pellet in the remaining liquid (after supernatant removal) before adding any new medium (*see* **Note 10**).

3.1 Isolation of Human PBMC

1. Add the peripheral blood sample to a 50-mL tube and dilute (1:1) with PBS to a volume of 50 mL (*see* **Note 11**).
2. Gently layer 25 mL of diluted cell suspension over 15 mL of Lymphoprep™ in a 50-mL tube. Make sure that the layers do not mix (*see* **Note 12**).
3. Centrifuge at $1,000 \times g$ for 15 min at 21 °C. To prevent the layers from mixing, do *not* use brake.
4. Carefully transfer the PBMC from the mononuclear cell layer from two conical tubes to a clean 50-mL conical tube. Try to avoid aspiration of the Lymphoprep™ (*see* **Note 13**).

5. Dilute the PBMC by adding PBS-BSA buffer to a volume of 50 mL. Centrifuge at 600 × *g* for 10 min at 21 °C and discard the supernatant.
6. To lyse remaining erythrocytes, add 5–10 mL shock medium and incubate, on ice, for a maximum of 10 min. Add PBS-BSA buffer to a volume of 50 mL. Centrifuge at 530 × *g* for 5 min at 4 °C and discard the supernatant.
7. Resuspend and combine all pellets per donor. Add PBS-BSA buffer to a volume of 50 mL (*see* **Note 14**).
8. To remove platelets, centrifuge at 260 × *g* for 8 min at 4 °C and discard the supernatant. Repeat **steps** 7 and **8** three times for adequate platelet removal.
9. Resuspend the pellet in PBS-BSA buffer to a volume of 50 mL and count the PBMC.

3.2 CD14+ Cell (Monocyte) Isolation and/or iNKT Isolation (See Note 15)

1. Centrifuge the isolated PBMC at 530 × *g* for 5 min at 4 °C and discard the supernatant.
2. Resuspend the PBMC with MACS buffer to a volume of approximately 20 mL. Centrifuge at 530 × *g* for 5 min at 4 °C and discard the supernatant (*see* **Note 16**).
3. Cell isolation:
   (a) For monocyte isolation, add 20 μL of CD14 MicroBeads per 1×10^7 total cells according to manufacturer's protocol and proceed to **step 4**.
   (b) For iNKT isolation, add 1 μL of murine antihuman TCR Vα24 mAb per 2×10^6 total cells, mix thoroughly, and incubate for 30 min at 4 °C. Next, add approximately 20 mL of MACS buffer and centrifuge at 530 × *g* for 5 min at 4 °C and discard the supernatant. Add 1 μL of goat anti-mouse IgG magnetic beads per 2×10^6 total cells and proceed to **step 4**. When using anti-iNKT MicroBeads, add 100 μL per 1×10^8 total cells according to manufacturer's protocol and proceed to **step 4**.
4. Mix thoroughly and incubate for 30 min at 4 °C.
5. To wash the suspension, add 20 mL of MACS buffer, centrifuge at 530 × *g* for 5 min at 4 °C, and discard the supernatant.
6. Resuspend the cells in 1.5 mL of MACS buffer (*see* **Note 17**).
7. Place MACS columns in the magnetic field of the MACS separator and position the pre-separation filter. Now rinse columns with 1.5 mL (LS) or 0.5 mL (MS) MACS buffer. Let it pass completely and change the collecting tube.
8. Apply the cell suspension gently onto the filter and let it pass completely by gravitational force. Collect the effluent as the negative fraction (*see* **Note 18**).

9. Wash the column: Add 1.5 mL of LS or 0.5 mL of MS MACS buffer into the filter and let it pass completely by gravitational force. Repeat this step 3–4×. Again, collect the effluent as the negative fraction.
10. Remove the column from the magnetic field and place it on a collecting tube.
11. Firmly flush out the magnetically labeled cells with 3 mL of LS or 1.5 mL of MS MACS buffer into the collecting tube. This is the positive fraction.
12. Centrifuge the positive fraction at 530 × *g* for 5 min at 4 °C and discard the supernatant. Resuspend pellets in PBS-BSA buffer to a volume of 5–10 mL.
13. Determine isolated cell purity by flow cytometry. Meanwhile, keep cell suspensions at 2–8 °C. Repeat the process in case of unsatisfactory cell purity (*see* **Notes 19** and **20**).
14. Count the selected cells and proceed to Subheading 3.3 for moDC generation or to Subheading 3.6 in case of iNKT expansion (*see* **Note 21**).

3.3 Generation of Immature moDC

1. Centrifuge monocytes obtained in Subheading 3.2 at 530 × *g* for 5 min at 4 °C and discard the supernatant.
2. For every 0.5–1 × 10^6 monocytes, add 1 mL CCM and divide over culture flasks (*see* **Note 22**).
3. For immature moDC differentiation, add 1,000 IU/mL of rhGM-CSF and 10 ng/mL of rhIL-4.
4. Allow to culture at 37 °C for 5–7 days in a humidified atmosphere under 5 % CO_2 (*see* **Notes 23** and **24**). From this point, proceed to Subheading 3.4 or, in case of CD1d ligation on human moDC, to Subheading 3.5.

3.4 Generation of α-GalCer-Pulsed Mature moDC

1. To induce maturation and α-GalCer loading of immature moDC (Subheading 3.3), add 100 ng/mL α-GalCer and 100 ng/mL LPS to the culture flasks and allow maturation for 4–48 h at 37 °C in a humidified atmosphere under 5 % CO_2 (*see* **Notes 25–28**).
2. Harvest the nonadherent fraction of mature moDC and rinse the culture flask with 10 mL PBS, pool suspensions in the same tube. For the collection of the adherent fraction, add 2 mL (75-cm2 flask) or 5 mL (175-cm^2 flask) of 0.5 mM EDTA. Incubate for 5 min at 37 °C, resuspend loosened moDC in CCM, and add to the nonadherent fractions.
3. Count α-GalCer-pulsed mature moDC (*see* **Note 29**).

3.5 CD1d Ligation on Human moDC

1. Use the immature moDC from Subheading 3.3. Add 10 μg of anti-CD1d mAb per 0.5 × 10^6 cells per mL to the culture flasks and incubate for 4 h at 37 °C (*see* **Note 30**).

2. Harvest the nonadherent fraction of mature moDC and rinse the culture flask with 10 mL PBS, pool suspensions in the same tube. For the collection of the adherent fraction, add 2 mL (75-cm2 flask) or 5 mL (175-cm^2 flask) of 0.5 mM EDTA. Incubate for 5 min at 37 °C, resuspend loosened moDC in CCM and add to the nonadherent fractions.
3. Count the CD1d-ligated moDC.

3.6 Expansion and Activation of iNKT (See Note 31)

1. To increase the iNKT purity obtained in Subheading 3.2, centrifuge cells at 530×*g* for 5 min at 4 °C and discard the supernatant.
2. Resuspend cells in CCM (approximately 0.5×10^6 cells/mL) and place in appropriate well plate (*see* **Note 32**).
3. Add α-GalCer-pulsed mature moDC in a ratio of 1:5 (α-GalCer-pulsed mature moDC to iNKT fraction in CCM). Next, add 50 IU/mL of rhIL-2 (*see* **Notes 33–35**).
4. Incubate plates at 37 °C in a humidified atmosphere under 5 % CO_2 for 1 week.
5. Evaluate the iNKT purity and number weekly. If less than 90 % iNKT purity is observed, repeat from **step 1**. If iNKT purity exceeds 90 %, proceed to **step 6**.
6. Centrifuge iNKT at 530×*g* for 5 min at 4 °C, discard the supernatant, and resuspend in CCM (approximately 0.5×10^6 cells/mL).
7. For iNKT expansion, add 1 mL of feedermix per 0.5×10^6 iNKT (1 mL) and place the suspension in appropriate well plate (*see* **Notes 36** and **37**).
8. Incubate plates at 37 °C in a humidified atmosphere under 5 % CO_2 and evaluate iNKT purity and number weekly (*see* **Note 38**).
9. Repeat from **step 7** to continue iNKT expansion.

4 Notes

1. EDTA can be replaced by other anticoagulants.
2. Alternatively, murine antihuman TCR Vα24-Jα18 Abs (clone 6B11) can be used for a more specific selection of iNKT [22]. As well, MicroBeads conjugated to antihuman TCR Vα24-Jα18 mAbs (anti-iNKT MicroBeads, human (Miltenyi Biotec Inc., Auburn, CA, USA)) can be used for direct magnetic labeling.
3. Select proper size depending on obtained cell number, usually MidiMACS (LS) or MiniMACS (MS) for, respectively, a maximum of 1×10^8 and 1×10^7 labeled cells, according to manufacturers' protocol.

4. Alternatively, CliniMACS can be used for clinical scale moDC production [23].
5. Before use, thaw FBS and heat inactivate complement by incubating at 56 °C for 30 min.
6. Alternatively, 2–8 % human pooled serum (HPS) may be used.
7. For in vivo assays, dissolve α-GalCer in 5.6 % sucrose, 0.75 % L-histidine, and 0.5 % Tween 20 and heat at 60–80 °C for several minutes. For in vitro assays, dissolve α-GalCer in dimethyl sulfoxide (DMSO) at the concentration of 1 mg/mL and heat at 60–80 °C for several minutes. The solution of 1 mg/mL in DMSO can be diluted by PBS. Store at −20 °C, according to manufacturer's protocol.
8. Commercially available clones: 51.1 and 42.1.
9. Human AB serum should be pooled from >3 donors and heat inactivated before use (incubate at 56 °C for 30 min).
10. For clinical applications (adhering to cGMP guidelines), human serum albumin (HSA) and HPS or serum-free media are preferred/required rather than equivalent bovine products. NB: As described, human derived products may modify CD1d expression [24].
11. On average, a fresh peripheral blood sample contains 0.5–2.0×10^6 PBMC per mL blood. Approximately 10 % accounts for monocytes and 0.01–0.1 % for iNKT. Storing blood will decrease obtained cell numbers and quality.
12. Keep the tube as horizontal as possible and position the tip of the pipet angled against the wall of tube just above the Lymphoprep™ and add the cell suspension slowly.
13. Do not mix PBMC from different donors. This will prevent possible cell interactions.
14. In case of small pellets, 10-mL conical tubes may be used to prevent excessive cell loss. Adjust volumes adequately.
15. After $CD14^+$ cell isolation, the unlabeled fraction (containing PBL, peripheral blood lymphocytes) can be used for iNKT isolation.
16. A different technique, besides MACS isolation, used for $CD14^+$ monocyte selection, is plastic adherence. Here, 5×10^6/mL PBMC are placed in culture flasks for 1.5 h at 37 °C in a humidified atmosphere under 5 % CO_2. Monocytes will preferentially adhere to the flask. After 1.5 h, rinse flask carefully with 10 mL PBS 3×, primarily leaving the monocytes behind. Subsequently, monocytes are cultured as mentioned in the Methods section for the generation of immature moDC.
17. Resuspend cells in 0.5 mL MACS buffer when using MS-sized column. Volumes used in this and the next steps differ slightly from the manufactures' protocol.

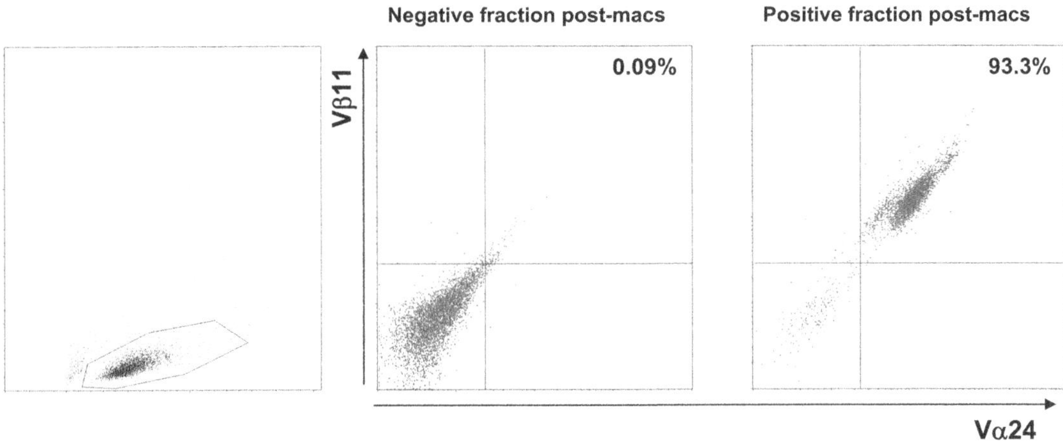

Fig. 1 Representative flow-cytometric dot plots after magnetic bead isolation of iNKT cells. The *left plot* depicts the forward and side scatter, the *middle plot* depicts the iNKT-depleted (negative) fraction, and the *right plot* depicts purified iNKT cells (positive fraction)

18. Do not allow the column to fall dry at any time during the process, including the wash steps.
19. We recommend a cell purity of >90 %. iNKT purity can be increased by repeating the magnetic separation process or by cultivation as described in Subheading 3.6.
20. To determine monocyte purity, we use CD14 (clone MφP9) with IgG1 for isotype control. For iNKT purity, we use the combination of Vα24 (clone C15) and Vβ11 (clone C21) (Fig. 1). Alternatively, tetrameric CD1d-α-GalCer complexes or murine antihuman TCR Vα24-Jα18 Abs (clone 6B11) can be used.
21. We do not recommend freezing freshly isolated iNKT.
22. Use approximately 10 mL per 75-cm^2 or 25 mL per 175-cm^2 flasks.
23. It is recommended to check the resulting immunophenotype to evaluate proper differentiation. Immature moDC will be $CD14^-$ and $CD1a^+$. We use CD14 (clone MφP9) and CD1a (clone HI149).
24. If required, immature moDC can be stored by freezing according to standard cell-freezing protocol. After thawing, allow cells to rest for 1 day in the presence of 1,000 IU/mL rhGM-CSF and 10 ng/mL rhIL-4 before use.
25. To promote distinct functional iNKT outcomes, different or altered (glyco)lipid ligands can be used [2].
26. Depending on maturation time and cytokines/agents used, different phenotypic mature moDC can be generated. As described, type 1 polarized moDC, incubated for 4 h with 100 ng/mL of α-GalCer, 100 ng/mL of LPS, and 1,000 IU/

mL of INF-γ, supported a type 1 cytokine profile in iNKT when cocultured in the presence of 10 ng/mL rhIL-15. Type 2 polarized moDC, incubated for 48 h with 100 ng/mL of α-GalCer, 100 ng/mL of LPS, and 1×10^{-7} M prostaglandin E (PGE_2), supported superior iNKT expansion and type 2 polarization when cocultured in the presence of 10 ng/mL rhIL-7 and 1×10^{-7} M dexamethasone [16].

27. If preferred, co-loading with tumor-associated antigens (TAA) can be performed here.
28. For clinical use, monophosphoryl lipid A (MPLA) may be used as an alternative for LPS as a TLR4 ligand [25]. Also, maturation cocktails can be used instead of LPS. We obtained the best results with 25 ng/mL of IL-1β, 100 ng/mL of IL-6, 75 ng/mL of TNF-α, and 1 μg/mL of PGE_2. Different cocktails have been used [18].
29. Mature moDC will be $CD83^+$. To confirm immunophenotype, we use CD83 (clone HB15a).
30. 20 ng/mL of exogenous INF-γ may be added to enhance IL-12 production [20].
31. In case of iNKT purity of >90 %, proceed to **step 6**. Otherwise, repeat **steps 1–5** until the required cell purity is reached.
32. We typically place 0.5×10^6 cells in a 24-well plate.
33. Instead of 50 U/mL of rhIL-2, a combination of 10 ng/mL of rhIL-7 and 10 ng/mL of rhIL-15 may be used [15, 16].
34. If cells are used for subsequent in vitro culture, it is advisable to irradiate α-GalCer-pulsed mature moDC with 5,000 Rad to prevent overgrowth by any remaining conventional T cells.
35. α-GalCer-pulsed mature moDC do not need to be autologous to subsequently activate or expand iNKT cells.
36. End concentration will be 50 IU/mL of rhIL-2 and 50 ng/mL of PHA.
37. Alternatively, the method described for iNKT purification (**steps 1–5**) may also be used for iNKT expansion.
38. The timing of restimulation of iNKT with feedermix is determined by their activation status. Cells can be best restimulated when they approach a "resting" state, i.e., beyond maximal proliferation. In our hands, best results are obtained with weekly restimulation.

Acknowledgements

Our work is supported by grant no. 90700309 from the Netherlands Organisation for Health Research and Development (ZonMw) and grant VU 2010–4728 from the Dutch Cancer Society (KWF).

References

1. van der Vliet HJ et al (2004) The immunoregulatory role of CD1d-restricted natural killer T cells in disease. Clin Immunol 112:8–23
2. Rossjohn J et al (2012) Recognition of CD1d-restricted antigens by natural killer T cells. Nat Rev Immunol 12:845–857
3. Godfrey DI et al (2004) NKT cells: what's in a name? Nat Rev Immunol 4:231–237
4. Godfrey DI, Kronenberg M (2004) Going both ways: immune regulation via CD1d-dependent NKT cells. J Clin Invest 114: 1379–1388
5. Wu L et al (2009) Invariant natural killer T cells: innate-like T cells with potent immunomodulatory activities. Tissue Antigens 73:535–545
6. Swann JB et al (2009) Type I natural killer T cells suppress tumors caused by p53 loss in mice. Blood 113:6382–6385
7. Bellone M et al (2010) iNKT cells control mouse spontaneous carcinoma independently of tumor-specific cytotoxic T cells. PLoS One 5:e8646
8. Exley MA et al (2011) Developing understanding of the roles of CD1d-restricted T cell subsets in cancer: reversing tumor-induced defects. Clin Immunol 140:184–195
9. Tahir SM et al (2001) Loss of IFN-γ production by invariant NK T cells in advanced cancer. J Immunol 167:4046–4050
10. Schneiders FL et al (2012) Circulating invariant natural killer T-cell numbers predict outcome in head and neck squamous cell carcinoma: updated analysis with 10-year follow-up. J Clin Oncol 30:567–570
11. Kawano T et al (1997) CD1d-restricted and TCR-mediated activation of Vα14 NKT cells by glycosylceramides. Science 278: 1626–1629
12. Schneiders FL et al (2011) Clinical experience with α-galactosylceramide (KRN7000) in patients with advanced cancer and chronic hepatitis B/C infection. Clin Immunol 140: 130–141
13. Giaccone G et al (2002) A phase I study of the natural killer T-cell ligand α-galactosylceramide (KRN7000) in patients with solid tumors. Clin Cancer Res 8:3702–3709
14. Sullivan BA, Kronenberg M (2005) Activation or anergy: NKT cells are stunned by α-galactosylceramide. J Clin Invest 115: 2328–2329
15. van der Vliet HJ et al (2001) Potent expansion of human natural killer T cells using α-galactosylceramide (KRN7000)-loaded monocyte-derived dendritic cells, cultured in the presence of IL-7 and IL-15. J Immunol Methods 247:61–72
16. van der Vliet HJ et al (2003) Polarization of Vα24+ Vβ11+ natural killer T cells of healthy volunteers and cancer patients using α-galactosylceramide-loaded and environmentally instructed dendritic cells. Cancer Res 63: 4101–4106
17. Uchida T et al (2008) Phase I study of α-galactosylceramide-pulsed antigen presenting cells administration to the nasal submucosa in unresectable or recurrent head and neck cancer. Cancer Immunol Immunother 57: 337–345
18. Chang DH et al (2005) Sustained expansion of NKT cells and antigen-specific T cells after injection of α-galactosyl-ceramide loaded mature dendritic cells in cancer patients. J Exp Med 201:1503–1517
19. Nieda M et al (2004) Therapeutic activation of Vα24+Vβ11+ NKT cells in human subjects results in highly coordinated secondary activation of acquired and innate immunity. Blood 103:383–389
20. Yue SC et al (2005) CD1d ligation on human monocytes directly signals rapid NF-κB activation and production of bioactive IL-12. Proc Natl Acad Sci USA 102:11811–11816
21. Yue SC et al (2010) Direct CD1d-mediated stimulation of APC IL-12 production and protective immune response to virus infection in vivo. J Immunol 184:268–276
22. Exley MA et al (2008) Selective activation, expansion, and monitoring of human iNKT cells with a monoclonal antibody specific for the TCR α-chain CDR3 loop. Eur J Immunol 38:1756–1766
23. Babatz J et al (2003) Large-scale immunomagnetic selection of CD14+ monocytes to generate dendritic cells for cancer immunotherapy: a phase I study. J Hematother Stem Cell Res 12:515–523
24. Gerlini G et al (2001) Cd1d is expressed on dermal dendritic cells and monocyte-derived dendritic cells. J Invest Dermatol 117: 576–582
25. Alving CR et al (2012) Adjuvants for human vaccines. Curr Opin Immunol 24:310–315

Part II

Manipulation and Modification of Immune Cells: T Lymphocytes and NK Cells

Chapter 15

Modification of T Lymphocytes to Express Tumor Antigens

Aaron E. Foster and Xiao-Tong Song

Abstract

Human T cells can be genetically modified to express tumor-associated antigens (TAA) for the induction of tumor-specific immunity, suggesting that T cells may be alternative candidates of effective antigen-presenting cells (TAPC) and may be useful in vivo as cellular cancer vaccines. The effective induction of TAA-specific T cell immune responses requires activation of T cells by CD3/CD28 antibodies and the presence of proinflammatory cytokines such as interleukin-7 (IL-7) and interleukin-12 (IL-12). Here, we describe the technique of preparing activated human TAPC pulsed with TAA peptides for the induction of tumor antigen-specific T cell immunity in vitro.

Key words TAPC, Immunotherapy, T lymphocyte, Antigen-presenting cells, Tumor-associated antigen, Peptide pulsing, T cell immunity

1 Introduction

Dendritic cells (DC) are the most potent professional antigen-presenting cells (APC) that elicit antitumor immune responses. However, the efficacy of DC-based cancer vaccines is limited by the poor viability and migration of exogenously generated DC in vivo. Alternatively, adoptively transferred T cells can proliferate exponentially and migrate between the lymphoid and vascular compartments. In addition, T cells can be modified to express tumor-associated antigens (TAA) for the induction of antigen-specific T cell immune responses, suggesting that T cells may be alternative candidates to serve as cellular vehicles for tumor antigen presentation in vivo. For example, T cells modified to express tumor antigens or viral antigens such as the influenza A matrix protein (MP1) or cytomegalovirus (CMV) pp65 could activate antigen-specific T cells in vitro or in NOD/scid xenograft experiments [1–4]. In addition, clinical trials have shown that adoptively transferred T cells that were genetically modified to express herpes simplex virus thymidine kinase (HSV-TK) induced HSV-TK-specific T cells responses, leading to their rapid elimination in vivo [5, 6].

Michael J.P. Lawman and Patricia D. Lawman (eds.), *Cancer Vaccines: Methods and Protocols*, Methods in Molecular Biology, vol. 1139, DOI 10.1007/978-1-4939-0345-0_15, © Springer Science+Business Media New York 2014

Fontana et al. also observed in their clinical trial that infusion of genetically modified lymphocytes (GML) expressing the cancer gremlin gene, MAGE-A3, induced anti-MAGE-A3 T cells in two of ten patients, which were capable of trafficking to inflamed tissues and infiltrating tumors [7]. Taken together, these data indicate that TAPC may be a useful reagent for the activation and expansion of tumor-specific T cell immunity in vitro or in vivo.

Here, we describe the protocol for preparing human TAPC for the induction of tumor-specific T cell immunity in vitro. In this protocol, human TAPC are firstly activated by CD3/CD28 antibodies followed by pulsing with model HLA-A2$^+$ peptides derived from CMVpp65, MAGE-3, and MART-1. Activated and expanded CMVpp65-, MAGE-3-, and MART-1-specific CD8$^+$ T cells will have the ability of killing either peptide-pulsed target cells or tumor cell lines. Both IL-7 and IL-12 are required for the activation of MAGE-3 and MART-1-specific CD8$^+$ T cells. These tumor-specific T cells can be further expanded to large numbers with subsequent stimulations using activated, peptide-pulsed TAPC and interleukin-2 (IL-2). Thus, effective TAPC can be successfully generated by activation by CD3/CD28 antibodies followed by pulsing with tumor antigen peptides [8, 9].

2 Materials

Diligently follow all biohazard or waste disposal regulations when disposing biohazard and waste materials.

1. Peripheral blood should be obtained with informed consent from healthy donors. Alternatively, peripheral blood or buffy coat can be purchased from Gulf Coast Regional Blood Center, Houston, TX.
2. CEM.T2 cell line (ATCC) was maintained in Roswell Park Memorial Institute (RPMI)-1640 supplemented with 2-mM GlutaMax-1 and 10 % fetal bovine serum (FBS).
3. GlutaMax-1 (Invitrogen, Carlsbad, CA, USA).
4. Fetal bovine serum (FBS).
5. Sterile cell culture grade 1× phosphate buffered saline (PBS).
6. Lymphoprep (LP) (Nycomed, Oslo, Norway).
7. 3 μg/mL β2-microglobulin.
8. OKT3 antibody (Ortho Pharmaceuticals, Raritan, NJ, USA).
9. CD28, no sodium azide (NA)/low endotoxin (NE) (Pharmingen, San Diego, CA, USA).
10. Fluorescent-labeled antibodies against CD3, CD80, CD83, CD86, and HLA-DR (Becton Dickinson, Franklin Lakes, NJ, USA).

11. Peptide/MHC I pentamers folded with NLV, FLW, or ELA peptides (ProImmune, Springfield, CA, USA).
12. CD8 microbeads and MACS columns (Miltenyi Biotech, Auburn, CA, USA).
13. Peptide HLA-A*0201 peptides derived from CMVpp65 (NLVPMVATV), MAGE-3 (FLWGPRALV), or MART-1 (ELAGIGILTV) (ProImmune, Springfield, CA, USA).
14. IL-2, IL-7 and IL-12 (Proleukin; Chiron, Emeryville, CA, USA).
15. 24-well non-tissue culture-treated plates.
16. Tissue culture-treated 24-well plates and flasks.
17. 50- and 15-mL conical centrifuge tubes.
18. Sterile pipets.

3 Methods

Unless otherwise noted, the procedure is carried out in the cell culture hood at room temperature (15–30 °C).

3.1 PBMC Processing

1. Fresh, anticoagulated whole blood specimens should be stored at room temperature and processed as soon as possible. Spray down all surfaces, racks, and reagent bottles with 70 % v/v ethanol prior to entering the cell culture hood. Measure the blood volume using a sterile pipet (*see* **Note 1**). If some of the whole blood samples contain small clots, try to remove the clots prior to processing.
2. Dilute peripheral blood 1:1 in PBS in a 50-mL conical centrifuge tubes and mix by pipetting (*see* **Note 2**). For example, using a sterile pipet, add 20 mL of PBS to each 50-mL conical centrifuge tube. Mix whole blood gently and use a sterile pipet to transfer 20 mL of whole blood into the 50-mL conical centrifuge tube. Gently mix the blood with PBS by pipetting.
3. Using a sterile pipet, add 20 or 15 mL of LP into a new 50-mL conical centrifuge tube. Carefully overlay 25 mL of diluted blood over 20 mL LP or 20 mL over 15 mL (ratio is 5:4 or 4:3, respectively) (*see* **Note 3**). Adjust the volume as necessary to utilize all the available cells.
4. Centrifuge at 400 × *g* for 40 min at room temperature with the brake off (*see* **Note 4**).
5. Gently remove the centrifuge tube from the centrifuge so as not to disturb the layers. Using a new sterile pipet, carefully harvest the cloudy white peripheral blood mononuclear cells (PBMC) band located at the interface between the plasma-PBS

fraction and the clear separation medium solution into 20 mL of PBS in a 50-mL conical centrifuge tube.

6. Centrifuge at 400 × *g* for 10 min at room temperature.
7. Gently remove the 50-mL conical centrifuge tube from the centrifuge and check for the cell pellet (*see* **Note 5**). Aspirate supernatant without disturbing the cell pellet. Resuspend the pellet in 20 mL of PBS. Mix gently and thoroughly into a homogenous cell suspension.
8. Centrifuge at 400 × *g* for 5 min at room temperature.
9. Gently remove the 50-mL conical centrifuge tube from the centrifuge and check for the cell pellet. Aspirate supernatant without disturbing the cell pellet. Resuspend the pellet in PBS. Mix gently and thoroughly into a homogenous cell suspension. If more than one tube was used for one blood sample, the cells should be combined into one tube in about 1/3 the starting blood volume of PBS.
10. Count cells using a hemocytometer. Mix cells gently but thoroughly prior to sampling for the count. Determine the cell concentration.
11. Resuspend the PBMC at 5×10^5 cells per mL in complete RPMI-1640 medium containing 10 % FBS.

3.2 Generation of TAPC

1. To generate TAPC, on day 0, coat non-tissue culture-treated 24-well plates with 1 μg/mL of OKT3 and 1 μg/mL of anti-CD28 antibody. Dilute antibodies to a final concentration of 1 μg/mL in sterile water. For example, to coat six wells, add 3 μL of OKT3 and 3 μL of anti-CD28 antibody to 3 mL of sterile water. Add 0.5 mL (=0.5 μg of each antibody) of the antibody solution into 1 well of the 24-well plate. Seal it with parafilm and incubate at 4 °C overnight.
2. On day 1, aspirate antibody solution and wash wells once with 1 mL of RPMI-1640 complete medium.
3. Aspirate medium from the antibody-coated 24-well plate and plate 1×10^6 PBMC into one well in a final volume of 2 mL of complete RPMI-1640 medium with 10 % FBS. Incubate at 37 °C overnight.
4. On day 2, aspirate and discard about 1 mL from each well and add back 1 mL of complete RPMI-1640 medium containing 200 U/mL of IL-2 to achieve a final concentration of 100 U/mL. Return to incubator.
5. On day 3, harvest the cells from the wells using a sterile pipet. Pool cell suspension in 50-mL conical centrifuge tubes.
6. Centrifuge at 400 × *g* for 5 min at room temperature. Gently remove the tube from the centrifuge and check for the cell pellet.

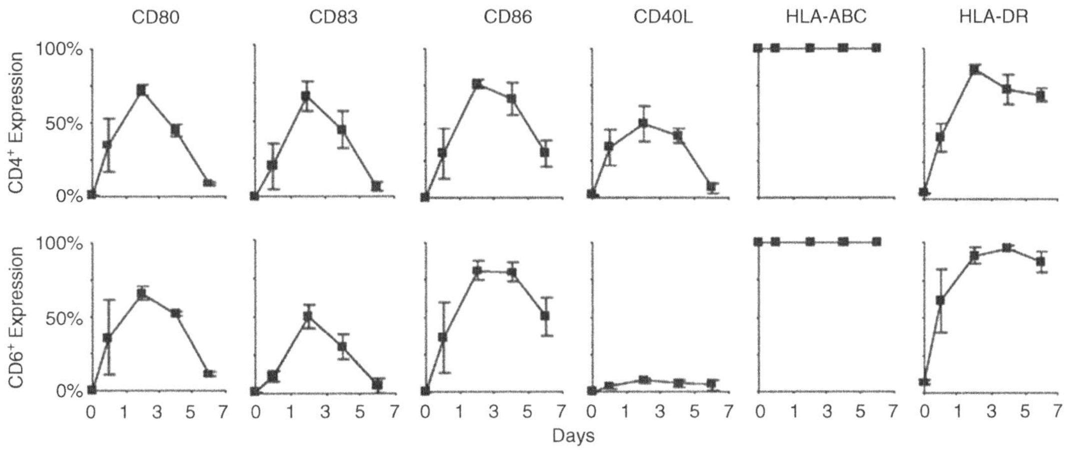

Fig. 1 Characteristics of TAPC. T cells were measured for expression of surface molecules by flow cytometry after activation by CD3 and CD28 stimulation. Expression of CD80, CD83, CD86, CD40L, HLA-ABC, and HLA-DR and was measured for CD4 (*top*)- and CD8 (*bottom*)-gated lymphocytes in combination with CD3 gating strategy (reproduced from [6] with permission from Elsevier)

Aspirate supernatant without disturbing the cell pellet. Resuspend the pellet in a volume of complete medium estimated to give 1×10^6 cells per mL. Mix gently and thoroughly into a homogenous cell suspension.

7. Count cells using a hemocytometer. Mix cells gently but thoroughly prior to sampling for the count. Determine the cell concentration.
8. Adjust the medium volume to achieve a cell concentration at 1×10^6 cells per mL by adding complete medium or by centrifugation and resuspension. The harvested human T cells are ready for use as TAPC (*see* **Note 6**). TAPC should be cultured and expanded in 100 U/mL IL-2 containing RPMI medium with 10 % FBS.
9. Prior to use as TAPC, remove an aliquot of $0.5–1 \times 10^6$ cells to verify APC capability by measuring expression of CD80, CD83, and CD86. Stain the cells with antibodies against CD3, CD80, CD83, CD86, or HLA-DR. Analyze the cells with flow cytometry (Fig. 1) (*see* **Note 7**).

3.3 Generation of TAA-Specific Cytotoxic T Lymphocytes (CTL)

1. To prepare responder CTL, isolate $CD8^+$ T cells from PBMCs by MACS column and suspend at 1×10^6 cells per mL in complete RPMI-1640 medium with 10 % FBS.
2. To pulse TAPC with peptides, harvest TAPC and plate at 1×10^6 cells per mL in a 24-well plate and pulse with 5 μg/mL HLA-A*0201 peptides derived from CMVpp65 (NLVPMVATV), MAGE-3 (FLWGPRALV), or MART-1

(ELAGIGILTV) in combination with 3 μg/mL β2-microglobulin for 2 h at 37 °C.

3. Harvest TAPC into a 15-mL conical centrifuge tube. Adjust the medium volume to 5 mL by adding fresh complete RPMI-1640 medium. Irradiate peptide-pulsed TAPC (30 Gy).
4. Centrifuge the irradiated peptide-pulsed TAPC at 400 × *g* for 5 min at room temperature. Gently remove the tube from the centrifuge and check for the cell pellet. Aspirate the supernatant without disturbing the cell pellet. Resuspend the pellet in 20 mL of PBS. Mix gently and thoroughly into a homogenous cell suspension. Count cells using a hemocytometer. Mix cells gently but thoroughly prior to sampling for the count. Determine the cell concentration. Adjust TAPC concentration to 1×10^5 cells per mL.
5. Using a sterile pipet, add 1 mL of TAPC (1×10^5 cells) into a well of a 24-well plate. Using another sterile pipet, add 1 mL of $CD8^+$ responder T cells (1×10^6 cells) into the same well containing TAPC, so the ratio of peptide-pulsed TAPC to $CD8^+$ responder cells is 1:10. Supplement culture with 100 U/mL of Il-2 and 10 ng/mL each of IL-7 and IL-12 during the first stimulation.
6. Feed with 100 U/mL IL-2 every 2–3 days. To do so, aspirate and discard about 1 mL from each well and add back 1 mL of complete RPMI-1640 medium containing 200 U/mL of IL-2 to achieve a final concentration of 100 U/mL. Return to incubator.
7. After 1 week, restimulate CTL cultures with activated, peptide-pulsed TAPC in medium containing 50 U/mL of IL-2.
8. Feed with 100 U/mL of IL-2 every 2–3 days. To do so, aspirate and discard about 1 mL from each well and add back 1 mL of complete RPMI-1640 medium containing 200 U/mL of IL-2 to achieve a final concentration of 100 U/mL. Return to incubator.
9. On day 14, harvest the cells and analyze for specificity by pentamer analysis or CTL assay (Fig. 2). The cells could be also frozen back for future experiments.

4 Notes

1. To determine the usable blood volume, the whole blood can be transferred to conical tubes by using a sterile pipet. The volume can be determined as it is pipetted or read from the tubes.
2. The maximum ratio of blood to PBS should be approximately 2:1. Use 1× 50-mL tube for each 20–25 mL of adult whole blood or 1× 15-mL tube for each 5–7.5 mL of pediatric whole blood.

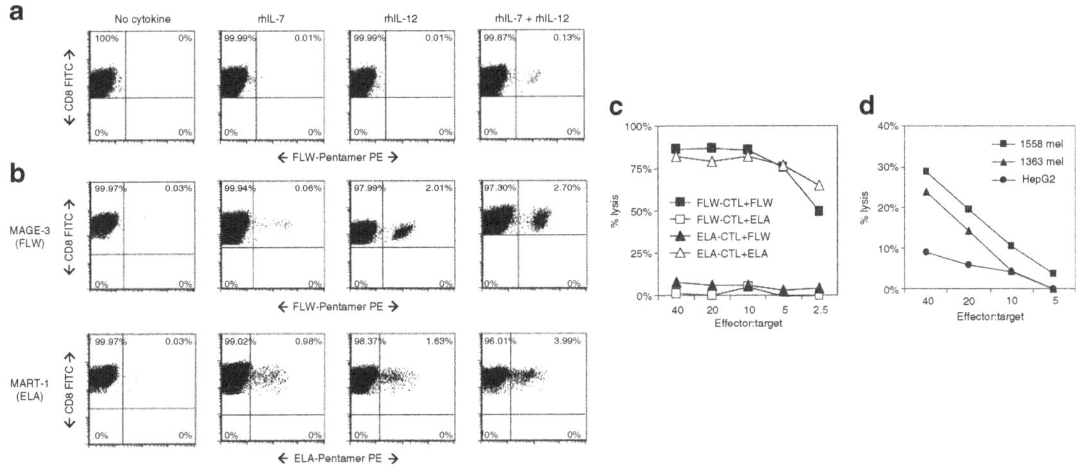

Fig. 2 Stimulation of TAA-specific T cells by TAPC requires IL-7 and IL-12. (**a**) To determine whether IL-7, IL-12, or both cytokines were necessary for induction of TAA-specific T cell responses, TAPC were loaded with FLW peptide and used to stimulate autologous CD8$^+$ T cells without cytokines (*far left*), 10 ng/mL of IL-7 (*middle left*), 10 ng/mL of IL-12 (*middle right*), or both cytokines (*right*). FLW-specific T cell expansion was then measured by flow cytometry using FLW HLA-A2-restricted pentamers. (**b**) T cell cultures stimulated with TAPC pulsed with either FLW (*top row*) or ELA (*bottom row*) were stimulated on a weekly basis in the presence of IL-2 after the initial stimulation in the presence of IL-7 and IL-12. Expansion and specificity were calculated after measurement by flow cytometry using FLW or ELA HLA-A2-restricted pentamers. TAPC stimulation generates functional TAA-specific CTL. (**c**) FLW- and ELA-specific CTL generated by TAPC stimulation retain the ability to lyse CEM.T2 cells pulsed with cognate peptide but do not lyse cells bearing control peptide. (**d**) FLW-specific CTL generated by TAPC loaded with FLW peptide were used in a ^{51}Cr-release assay against the HLA-A*0201 cell lines 1363mel, 1558mel, and HepG2. Both 1363mel and 1558mel express MAGE-3 and are killed by FLW-specific CTL, whereas the MAGE-3-negative cell line, HepG2, is not killed (reproduced from [6] with permission from Elsevier)

Use as many tubes as required to distribute all of the whole blood for each donor.

3. The separation steps should be performed as quickly as possible since Lymphoprep is toxic to cells.
4. Ensure the brake is off so that the acceleration and deceleration do not disrupt the density gradient and the gradients do not mix.
5. If the cell pellet is not visible, make sure that the centrifuge is operating properly. Recentrifuge the 50-mL conical centrifuge tube. If the cell pellet is still not visible after recentrifuging, recentrifuge at 1,000 ×g in order to improve cell separation.
6. If frozen TAPC are used as APC, TAPC should be reactivated on CD3/CD28-coated plates for 48 h.
7. One of the important things we found was that restimulation of TAPC prior to use upregulated the expression of co-stimulatory molecules such as CD80, CD86, CD83, and HLA-DR and made them better APC. Usually, we reactivated with CD3/CD28 for 24–48 h prior to peptide pulsing.

References

1. Cooper LJ et al (2005) Enhanced anti-lymphoma efficacy of CD19-redirected influenza MP1-specific CTLs by co-transfer of T cells modified to present influenza MP1. Blood 105:1622–1631
2. Naota H et al (2006) Generation of peptide specific CD8+ T cells by phytohemagglutinin-stimulated antigen mRNA-transduced CD4+ T cells. J Immunol Methods 314:54–66
3. Atanackovic D et al (2003) Monitoring $CD4^+$ T cell responses against viral and tumor antigens using T cells as novel target APC. J Immunol Methods 278:57–66
4. Melenhorst JJ et al (2006) Robust expansion of viral antigen-specific $CD4^+$ and $CD8^+$ T cells for adoptive T cell therapy using gene-modified activated T cells as antigen presenting cells. J Immunother 29:436–443
5. Berger C et al (2006) Analysis of transgene specific immune responses that limit the in vivo persistence of adoptively transferred HSV-TK-modified donor T cells after allogeneic hematopoietic cell transplantation. Blood 107: 2294–2302
6. Riddell SR et al (1996) T-cell mediated rejection of gene-modified HIV-specific cytotoxic T lymphocytes in HIV-infected patients. Nat Med 2:216–223
7. Fontana R et al (2008) Peripheral blood lymphocytes genetically modified to express the self/tumor antigen MAGE-A3 induce antitumor immune responses in cancer patients. Blood 113(8):1651–1660, 19
8. Foster AE et al (2007) Autologous designer antigen-presenting cells by gene modification of T lymphocytes blasts with IL-7 and IL-12. J Immunother 30:506–516
9. Kaka AS et al (2009) Genetic modification of T cells with IL-21 enhances antigen presentation and generation of central memory tumor-specific cytotoxic T lymphocytes. J Immunother 32:726–736

Chapter 16

Genetic Modification of Mouse Effector and Helper T Lymphocytes Expressing a Chimeric Antigen Receptor

Liza B. John, Tess M. Chee, David E. Gilham, and Phillip K. Darcy

Abstract

Genetic modification of primary mouse T cells with chimeric antigen receptors (CAR) has emerged as an important tool for optimizing adoptive T cell immunotherapy strategies. However, limitations in current protocols for generating highly pure and sufficient numbers of enriched effector and helper CAR$^+$ T cell subsets remain problematic. Here, we describe a new retroviral transduction protocol for successfully generating transduced CD8$^+$ and CD4$^+$ T lymphocytes for in vitro and in vivo characterization.

Key words Murine T lymphocytes, Chimeric antigen receptor, Enrichment, Transduction, T cell polarization

1 Introduction

Adoptive cell therapy (ACT) involving the transfer of gene-modified T cells expressing antigen-specific chimeric antigen receptors (CAR) has emerged as a promising approach for the treatment of cancer [1–3]. ACT has traditionally utilized either enriched CD8$^+$ T cells or unfractionated T cells, comprising predominantly of CD8$^+$ T cells, in both mouse models and human trials. However, recent reports including a study from our laboratory have demonstrated an important role for CD4$^+$ T cells in adoptive immunotherapy [4, 5].

CD4$^+$ T cells are comprised of varying subsets that include T helper 1 (Th1), T helper 2 (Th2), T helper 9 (Th9), T helper 17 (Th17), and T regulatory cells (Treg). The roles of Th1 and Th2 CD4$^+$ cell subsets are well characterized. Th1 cells typically secrete interferon-γ (IFN-γ), tumor necrosis factor (TNF), and interleukin-2 (IL-2) and have been associated with improved patient outcomes and reduced tumor burden [6, 7]. In contrast, Th2 cells secrete interleukin-4 (IL-4), interleukin-5 (IL-5), and interleukin-13 (IL-13) which have long been associated with allergy and, in a cancer context, with poor patient outcomes [8]. However, other studies

Michael J.P. Lawman and Patricia D. Lawman (eds.), *Cancer Vaccines: Methods and Protocols*, Methods in Molecular Biology, vol. 1139, DOI 10.1007/978-1-4939-0345-0_16, © Springer Science+Business Media New York 2014

have demonstrated that Th2 cells can contribute to antitumor responses [6, 8]. Th9 cells, Th17 cells, and Treg have been associated with playing a role in establishing a tumor-promoting environment [9–12]. Th9 cells are the most recently discovered $CD4^+$ T cell subset that secretes interleukin-9 (IL-9) and are strongly implicated in allergic responses [13]. Th17 cells are known to secrete interleukin-17A (IL-17A) and interleukin-17F (IL-17F), as well as interleukin-21 (IL-21) and interleukin-22 (IL-22) [14], while Treg secrete interleukin-10 (IL-10) and transforming growth factor-β (TGF-β), which have been associated with poor patient prognosis and reduced survival [12]. Further understanding the role of these different T cell subsets in the context of cancer may significantly enhance the effectiveness of ACT and other immune-based therapies.

Previous protocols for generating enriched mouse T cell subsets expressing CAR have utilized coculture methods involving retrovirus-producing packaging cells for transduction of $CD8^+$ and $CD4^+$ T lymphocytes with the scFv-anti-erbB2-CD28-ζ receptor [5]. However, a number of constraints encountered using this technique include poor viability and low yield of transduced $CD8^+$ and $CD4^+$ T cells, making in vivo studies more difficult.

In this chapter, we describe a new technique for generating transduced mouse $CD8^+$ and polarized $CD4^+$ T helper subsets (Th1 and Th2) using a combination of immunomagnetic enrichment and retroviral transduction that overcomes problems with poor viability and yield. We include the description of a functional cytokine assay for measuring antigen-specific responses of these transduced T cell subsets. Collectively, this new protocol provides a practical and simple approach for enabling characterization of the contribution of gene-modified T cell subsets in ACT.

2 Materials

1. Dissection equipment: scissors and forceps, sterilized.
2. 10-cm culture dishes.
3. Roswell Park Memorial Institute (RPMI)-1640 complete medium: RPMI-1640 supplemented with 10 % (vol/vol) heat-inactivated fetal bovine serum (FBS), 2 mM glutamine, 1 mM sodium pyruvate, 0.1 mM nonessential amino acids, 100 U/mL of penicillin, and 100 μg/mL of streptomycin.
4. 5-mL and 60-mL syringes.
5. 70-μm nylon sieve.
6. Falcon 50-mL polypropylene tubes.
7. ACK lysis buffer: 0.15 M NH_4Cl (8.29 g), 1.0 mM $KHCO_3$ (1.0 g), 0.1 mM Na_2EDTA (37.2 mg) made up to 800 mL with distilled water and pH adjusted to 7.4 with 1 M HCl,

then topped up to 1 L with more distilled water, sterilized through a 0.2-μm filter, and stored at room temperature.

8. 6-well and 24-well tissue culture plates, treated and untreated.
9. Mouse anti-CD3e (clone 145-2C11) and anti-CD28 (clone 37.51) purified antibodies.
10. Recombinant human IL-2 (rhIL-2) stock at 5×10^6 IU/mL.
11. Recombinant mouse IL-7.
12. Ficoll-Paque.
13. 1× phosphate-buffered saline (PBS).
14. Magnetically activated cell sorting (MACS) buffer: 1× PBS with 1 % 0.5 M EDTA and 1 % FBS.
15. MACS Dynabeads: anti-mouse CD4 antibody-conjugated beads and anti-mouse CD8 antibody-conjugated beads (Miltenyi Biotec, Bergisch Gladbach, Germany).
16. Dynal MPC-50 magnet.
17. LS column (Miltenyi Biotec).
18. VarioMACS Separator (Miltenyi Biotec).
19. Murine ecotropic GP+E86 retroviral-producing packaging cell line containing pLXSN vector alone or scFV anti-Her2 receptor construct.
20. 75-cm^2 filtered tissue culture flasks.
21. RetroNectin.
22. 0.45-μm filter for syringes.
23. Mouse anti-c-myc tag conjugated to Alexa (AF) 488.
24. Mouse anti-IgG2a AF488 isotype antibody.
25. Anti-mouse CD8-PeCy7, CD4 Pacific Blue, CD62L-APC, CD44-PE, NK1.1-PE, CD11b-APC, CD11c Pacific Blue, and F4/80-Pe-Cy7 antibodies.
26. FACS buffer: 1× PBS with 2 % FBS.
27. Propidium iodide (PI) viability stain.
28. Polarization reagents: anti-IL-4 monoclonal antibody (mAb), recombinant IL-12, recombinant IL-4, and anti-IFN-γ mAb.
29. Tumor target cells (24JK and 24JK-Her-2 C57BL/6 mouse sarcomas) (NIH, Bethesda, MD, USA and Peter MacCallum Cancer Centre, Australia, respectively).
30. Purified anti-c-myc tag antibody and a corresponding purified IgG2a isotype antibody.
31. F96 Maxisorp immuno plate.
32. Purified "capture" antibody and secondary biotinylated "detection" antibody.

33. Wash solution: 0.5 mL of Tween 20 in 1 L of 1× PBS.
34. Blocking solution: 1× PBS with 2 % FBS.
35. Cytokine standards of known quantity.
36. Streptavidin-horseradish peroxidase (HRP) conjugate.
37. 3,3′, 5,5′-Tetramethylbenzidine (TMB) tablets.
38. Citrate phosphate buffer (10× stock): 18.24 g Na_2HPO_4, 12.77 g citric acid made up to 250 mL with distilled water and pH adjusted to 5.0: 1× working stock diluted 1:10.
39. 30 % hydrogen peroxide (H_2O_2).
40. 1 M sulfuric acid (H_2SO_4).
41. Benchmark microplate reader (Bio-Rad, Hercules, CA, USA).
42. SoftMax Pro software (Molecular Devices, Sunnydale, CA, USA).

3 Methods

3.1 Retroviral-Mediated Transduction of Enriched Mouse Lymphocytes

3.1.1 Enrichment of Splenic Mouse T Lymphocytes

1. To isolate mouse splenocytes, dissect the spleen(s) from syngeneic donor mice, transfer to a sterile 10-cm culture dish containing RPMI-1640 complete medium, and homogenize under manual force (*see* **Note 1**).
2. Strain the cell suspension through a 70-μM nylon sieve into a 50-mL Falcon tube to produce a single cell suspension and wash culture dish with medium, again transferring through sieve into collecting tube. Centrifuge at 187 × *g* for 5 min to pellet cells.
3. Resuspend pellet in 3 mL of hypotonic ACK lysis buffer per spleen to deplete the red blood cells present in the suspension and rock at room temperature for 3–5 min, then neutralize with an equivalent volume of complete medium and centrifuge at 187 × *g* for 5 min.
4. Resuspend pelleted cells at 2.5×10^7/well in 5 mL of complete medium in a 6-well plate and add 500 ng/mL of anti-CD3, 500 ng/mL of anti-CD28, 100 U/mL of rhIL-2, and 2 ng/mL of mIL-7 (*see* **Note 2**) to activate T lymphocytes, then place plate in a 37 °C incubator overnight (day 0).

3.1.2 Isolation of Mouse $CD8^+$ and $CD4^+$ T Lymphocytes

1. For negative selection, harvest unfractionated activated T lymphocytes after overnight activation into a 50-mL Falcon tube and add 10 mL of Ficoll-Paque to separate live cells from dead cells (*see* **Note 3**), then centrifuge at 388 × *g* for 10 min at room temperature with acceleration/deceleration at 6 (Eppendorf 5810 R) (day 1).
2. Using a 1-mL pipette, harvest live cells on interface layer (between Ficoll and medium) to a new 50-mL Falcon tube

and resuspend in fresh complete medium (*see* **Note 4**). Dead cells will pellet at the bottom of the Ficoll tube. Centrifuge live cells at 187 × *g* for 5 min at room temperature and resuspend pellet in magnetically activated cell sorting (MACS) buffer at 90 μL of buffer per 10^7 total cells.

3. To generate enriched mouse $CD8^+$ or $CD4^+$ T cells, add 10 μL of either anti-mouse CD4 antibody-conjugated beads or anti-mouse CD8 antibody-conjugated beads, respectively, per 10^7 total cells and incubate at 4 °C for 15 min.
4. Following incubation, wash the cells with 10 mL of MACS buffer and centrifuge at 187 × *g* for 5 min at room temperature, and then resuspend pellet in 3 mL of MACS buffer and transfer into an LS column mounted on a VarioMACS separator to isolate desired T cell population (*see* **Note 5**). Wash the column 2× with 5 mL of MACS buffer.
5. Repeat enrichment (**step 3** onwards) for $CD4^+$ T cell population 2× in total (*see* **Note 6**).
6. Perform cell count of fractionated T cells and centrifuge at 187 × *g* for 5 min at room temperature prior to retroviral transduction (day 1). Purity of isolated T cell subsets can be verified at this stage by flow cytometry; *see* Subheading 3.2.

3.1.3 Retroviral Transduction of Enriched Mouse T Lymphocyte Population

1. Seed out 6×10^6 GP + E86 retroviral-producing packaging cells (*see* **Note 7**) containing the transgene of interest, e.g., scFv-anti-Her2 receptor construct or control (empty) vector alone, into a 75-cm^2 flask and coat six-well polystyrene treated plate(s) with 10 μg/mL RetroNectin (*see* **Note 8**) for incubation overnight at 37 and 4 °C, respectively (day 0).
2. Collect viral supernatant and pass through a 0.45-μm filter into a 50-mL Falcon tube to discard any nonadherent packaging cells. Add filtered supernatant at 2.5 mL/well to pre-coated RetroNectin plate(s), and then centrifuge at 1,200 × *g* for 30 min at room temperature (day 1). Centrifugation enhances RetroNectin-assisted transduction. Replace complete medium in flasks containing retroviral-producing packaging cells and re-incubate for use the next day.
3. Resuspend fractionated $CD8^+$ and $CD4^+$ T cells (*see* Subheading 3.1.2, **step 6**) in 5 mL of viral supernatant at 1×10^7 cells/well (*see* **Note 9**) and add to virus-/RetroNectin-coated plates with 100 U/mL rhIL-2 and 2 ng/mL mIL-7 following centrifugation above. Centrifuge plates at 1,200 × *g* for 90 min at room temperature, and then incubate plate(s) overnight at 37 °C.
4. On day 2, harvest retrovirally transduced fractionated $CD8^+$ and $CD4^+$ T cell subsets into 50-mL Falcon tubes and centrifuge at 187 × *g* for 5 min at room temperature to pellet the

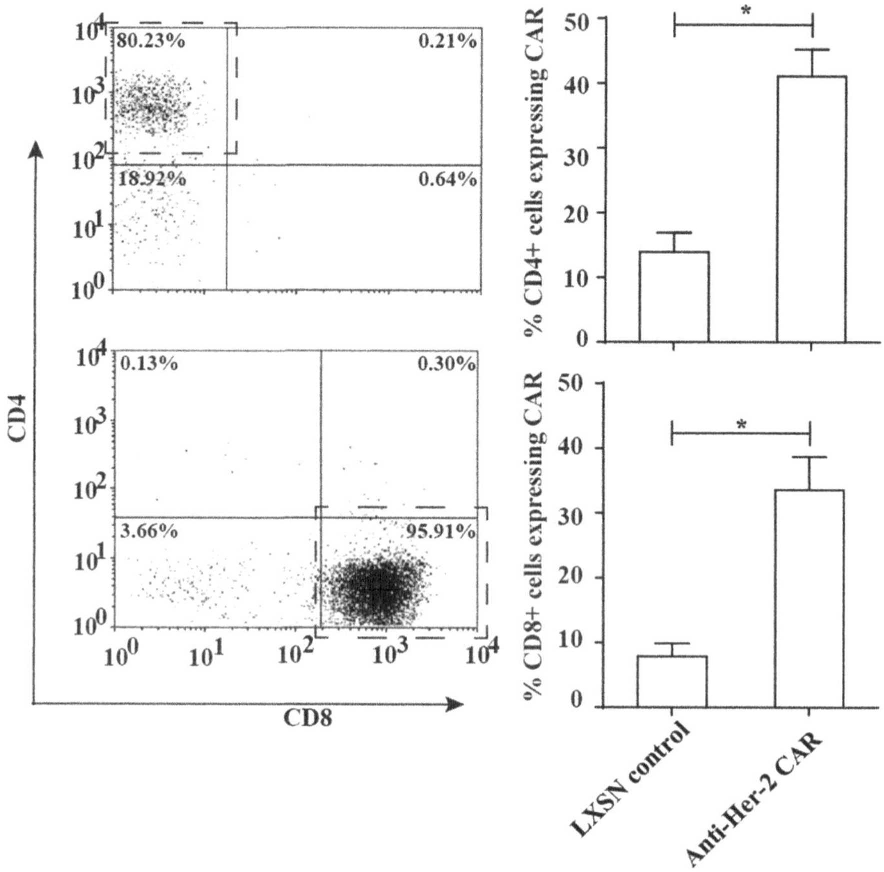

Fig. 1 Enrichment and generation of transduced $CD8^+$ and $CD4^+$ T cells expressing the anti-Her-2 CAR. (* $p < .05$, as determined by mean-whitney test)

cells. Repeat **steps 2** and **3**, resuspending fractionated T cells in the same volume of viral supernatant as for day 1.

5. Following centrifugation, incubate plate(s) for 4 h at 37 °C prior to harvesting the transduced $CD8^+$ and $CD4^+$ T cell subsets and culturing at 1×10^7 cells/well into 6-well tissue culture plate(s) containing 5 mL/well of complete medium supplemented with 100 U/mL of rhIL-2 and 2 ng/mL of mIL-7.
6. On day 4, add 5 mL/well of complete medium supplemented with 100 U/mL of rhIL-2 and 2 ng/mL of mIL-7.
7. The efficiency of retrovirus transduction and purity of T cell populations can then be determined by flow cytometry (Fig. 1).

3.2 Analysis of Transduction Efficiency and T Cell Purity

The most optimal approach to determining transduction efficiency of the fractionated mouse $CD8^+$ and $CD4^+$ T lymphocytes is by direct identification of the CAR. This may include staining for the presence of the scFv or novel regions, e.g., CD8 hinge, within the

CAR. Alternatively, a specific mAb directed against a tag epitope that has been incorporated at the extracellular region of the CAR transgene may be used. Transduced T cells can also be effectively identified through the incorporation of other marker genes, e.g., eGFP and tCD34 [15].

1. We use a c-*myc* tag antibody purified from supernatants of mouse 9E10 cells and conjugated to Alexa (AF) 488 fluorochrome to determine the level of CAR transgene expression on transduced T lymphocytes by flow cytometry, compared to background fluorescence using an IgG2a AF488 isotype antibody (Fig. 1).
2. The purity of $CD8^+$ and $CD4^+$ T cell populations (Fig. 1), as well as the effector status of the transduced cells, can then be determined by flow cytometry using anti-mouse CD8, CD4, CD62L, and CD44 cell surface markers. Cell surface markers for NK (NK1.1), myeloid (CD11b), and dendritic cells (CD11c), as well as macrophages ($CD11b^+$ $F4/80^+$), can also be measured to exclude the presence of these other populations in the samples. Collectively, this involves staining up to 1×10^6 transduced T lymphocytes with 50 μL of diluted antibody at 4 °C for 25 min, washing 2× in FACS buffer, and resuspending cells in 0.3 mL of FACS buffer containing PI viability stain. The phenotype of the cell population can then be determined by flow cytometry.

3.3 Polarization of $CD4^+$ T Cells into Th1 and Th2 Subsets

1. To polarize transduced $CD4^+$ T cells to a Th1 or Th2 subset, on day 4 of retroviral transduction, add a combination of 1 μg/mL of anti-IL-4 mAb and at least 0.1 pg/mL of rIL-12 to generate a Th1 $CD4^+$ T cell subset. Add at least 1 pg/mL of rIL-4 and 2 μg/mL of anti-IFN-γ mAb to generate a Th2 $CD4^+$ T cell subset.
2. Incubate plates for 72 h at 37 °C prior to in vitro functional assays.

3.4 Determining Antigen-Specific Cytokine Secretion by Transduced T Cell Subsets

3.4.1 Coculture of Cells

1. In order to coculture unfractionated $CD8^+$ and polarized $CD4^+$ Th1 and Th2 cells with antigen-positive and antigen-negative target cells, on day 7 post-transduction, culture tumor cells (antigen positive or negative) in 24-well tissue culture plates at 1×10^6 cells/well. Incubate at 37 °C, 5 % CO_2 for 1–2 h to allow cells to adhere to the plate.
2. For positive controls, include anti-CD3/anti-CD28 antibody-coated wells at final a concentration of 500 ng/mL in PBS. In addition, coat single wells with purified anti-c-*myc* tag antibody diluted 1/1,000 in 1 mL PBS and a corresponding purified IgG2a isotype antibody at final a concentration of 500 ng/mL in PBS as a positive and negative control, respectively, for T cells transduced with the chimeric antigen receptor. Incubate at 37 °C, 5 % CO_2 for 1–2 h.

3. Following this incubation, aspirate the supernatant from all the wells and wash 3× in PBS.
4. Add 1×10^6 gene-modified or control T cells per well onto the target cells (1:1 ratio) or immobilized antibody-coated wells (1 mL total volume/well). Add T cells alone to a single well as a further negative control.
5. Coculture T cells and target cells overnight at 37 °C, 5 % CO_2.
6. The following day, spin the 24-well plates at 187 × *g* for 5 min at room temperature. Collect the supernatants (~800 μL) from the wells using a 1-mL pipette and filter tips and transfer to another 24-well tissue culture plate in preparation for analysis by enzyme-linked immunosorbent assay (ELISA) (*see* **Note 10**).

3.4.2 ELISA for Assessing Cytokine Secretion

1. Coat a 96-well ELISA plate (NUNC F96 Maxisorp immuno plate) with purified "capture" antibody diluted in PBS and incubate at 4 °C overnight (*see* **Note 11**). Wash the plate 3× with wash solution.
2. Block the plate with 200 μL/well of blocking solution and incubate at room temperature for 1 h. Wash the plate 5× with wash solution.
3. Serially dilute standards (twofold) in blocking buffer and add 100 μL/well in duplicate wells to the plate. For blank wells, add 100 μL/well of blocking buffer alone in duplicate.
4. Add T cell supernatant samples (derived in Subheading 3.4.1) to appropriate wells of the plate in duplicate at the following dilutions: neat, diluted 1:10 in medium and diluted 1:100 in medium (*see* **Note 12**).
5. Incubate the plate with standards and T cell supernatant samples loaded, at room temperature for 2–4 h. Wash the plate 6× with wash solution and tap the plate dry onto a paper towel.
6. Dilute the secondary biotinylated "detection" antibody in blocking buffer and add 100 μL/well to the plate. Incubate at room temperature for 1 h. Wash the plate 6× with wash solution and tap the plate onto a paper towel.
7. Dilute the streptavidin-HRP conjugate 1/500 in blocking buffer, and add 100 μL/well to the plate. Incubate at room temperature for 30 min. Wash the plate 8× with wash solution and tap the plate onto a paper towel.
8. Dilute a single TMB substrate tablet in 10 mL of citrate phosphate buffer and wait until completely dissolved before adding 2 μL hydrogen peroxide solution (*see* **Note 13**). Add 100 μL/well TMB substrate solution and incubate at room temperature until blue color develops (5–15 min).

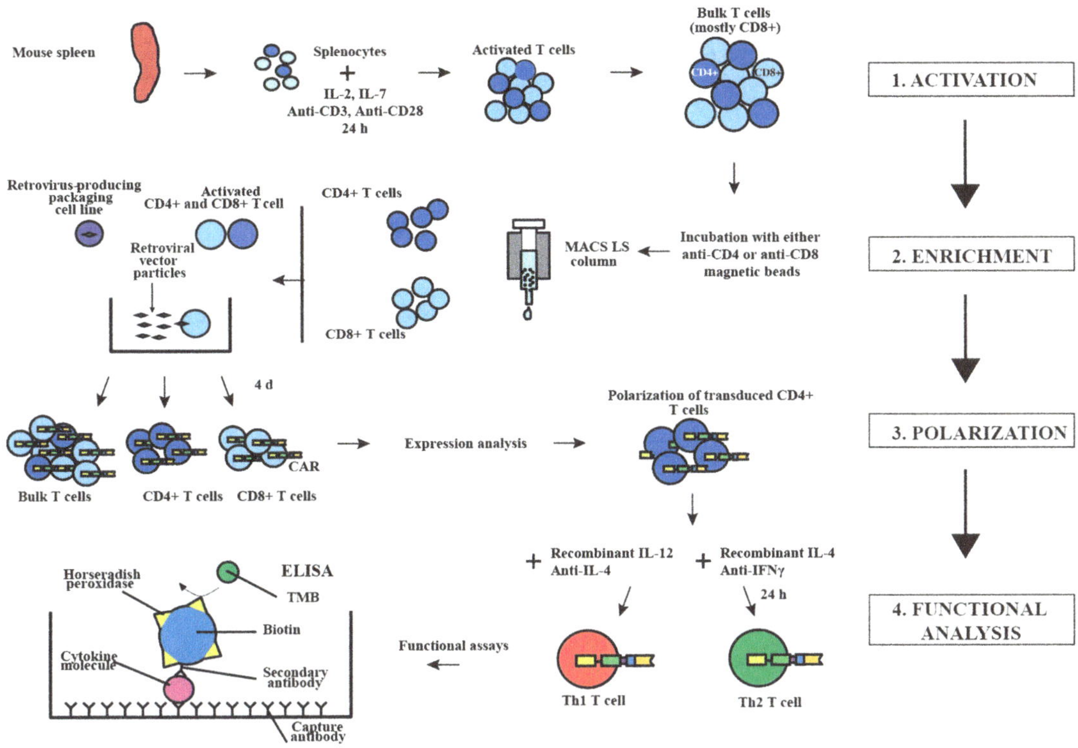

Fig. 2 Generation of gene-modified effector and helper T cells

9. Stop the reaction with 50 μL/well 1 M H_2SO_4 (turns the color of the reaction yellow). Read the optical density (OD) of the wells using a plate reader and SoftMax Pro software at 450 nm wavelength.
10. Analyze and calculate levels of Th1 (IFN-γ) and Th2 (IL-4) cytokine secreted using equation generated from the linear portion of the standard curve.

A schematic summarizing the methods described in Subheadings 3.1–3.4 is presented in Fig. 2.

4 Notes

1. When asserting manual force to homogenize isolated spleen, use plunger end of a 5-mL syringe (~1×10^8 cells/spleen).
2. IL-7 is required to maintain the viability of T cells during enrichment and retroviral transduction.

3. For optimal Ficoll separation, harvest unfractionated T lymphocytes to a maximum volume of 30 mL/Falcon tube and add 10 mL of Ficoll on gravity speed.
4. After centrifugation, aspirate and discard some medium to enable use of a 1-mL pipette to harvest live cells on interface layer. Alternatively, disposable Pasteur pipettes can be used.
5. Stand-alone MACS columns can also be used for obtaining enriched $CD8^+$ or $CD4^+$ T cells.
6. Repeat enrichment step for $CD4^+$ T cell population to achieve optimal level of purity.
7. It is important to seed GP + E86 retroviral-producing packaging cells at $\sim 6 \times 10^6$ the day before transduction which results in ~70–80 % cell confluency and production of high-titer virus supernatant.
8. RetroNectin can be used up to 2× between consecutive retroviral transductions and used stocks can be stored at 4 °C for up to 1 month at 10 μg/mL.
9. We found that seeding fractionated $CD8^+$ and $CD4^+$ T cells at 1×10^7cells/well, rather than 5×10^6 cells/well as previously done with bulk unfractionated T cells, in viral supernatant enhanced their viability and expansion following transduction.
10. Supernatants may be frozen at −20 °C and analyzed at a later time point.
11. Purified "capture" antibody must be diluted in PBS and not blocking buffer; otherwise, the assay will not work.
12. Further dilutions can be used as absolute values should not be extrapolated outside of the standard curve if the OD values for samples lie outside the limits of the standards.
13. TMB substrate solution is best made fresh, no more than 20 min prior to use. The addition of H_2O_2 is essential for the color reaction to occur.

References

1. Pham CD, Mitchell DA (2012) Chasing cancer with chimeric antigen receptor therapy. Immunotherapy 4(4):365–367
2. Rosenberg SA (2012) Raising the bar: the curative potential of human cancer immunotherapy. Sci Transl Med 4(127):127ps8
3. Curran KJ et al (2012) Chimeric antigen receptors for T cell immunotherapy: current understanding and future directions. J Gene Med 14(6):405–415
4. Xie Y et al (2010) Naive tumor-specific CD4+ T cells differentiated in vivo eradicate established melanoma. J Exp Med 207(3):651–667
5. Moeller M et al (2005) Adoptive transfer of gene-engineered $CD4^+$ helper T cells induces potent primary and secondary tumor rejection. Blood 106(9):2995–3003
6. Tosolini M et al (2011) Clinical impact of different classes of infiltrating T cytotoxic and helper cells (Th1, Th2, Treg, Th17) in patients with colorectal cancer. Cancer Res 71(4):1263–1271
7. Moeller M et al (2007) Sustained antigen-specific antitumor recall response mediated by gene-modified CD4+ T helper-1 and CD8+ T cells. Cancer Res 67(23):11428–11437

8. Ellyard JI et al (2007) Th2-mediated anti-tumour immunity: friend or foe? Tissue Antigens 70(1):1–11
9. Noelle RJ, Nowak EC (2010) Cellular sources and immune functions of interleukin-9. Nat Rev Immunol 10(10):683–687
10. Sfanos KS et al (2008) Phenotypic analysis of prostate-infiltrating lymphocytes reveals Th17 and Treg skewing. Clin Cancer Res 14(11):3254–3261
11. Chen D et al (2012) Increased IL-17-producing $CD4^+$ T cells in patients with esophageal cancer. Cell Immunol 272(2):166–174
12. Oleinika K et al (2013) Suppression, subversion and escape: the role of regulatory T cells in cancer progression. Clin Exp Immunol 171(1):36–45
13. Kaplan MH (2013) Th9 cells: differentiation and disease. Immunol Rev 252(1):104–115
14. Korn T et al (2009) IL-17 and Th17 Cells. Annu Rev Immunol 27(1):485–517
15. Cheadle EJ et al (2010) Natural expression of the CD19 antigen impacts the long-term engraftment but not antitumor activity of CD19-specific engineered T cells. J Immunol 184(4):1885–1896

Chapter 17

Genetic Modification of Cytotoxic T Lymphocytes to Express Cytokine Receptors

Serena K. Perna, Barbara Savoldo, and Gianpietro Dotti

Abstract

Adoptive transfer of tumor-infiltrating lymphocytes (TIL) or antigen-specific cytotoxic T lymphocytes (CTL) is safe and can be effective in cancer patients. Achievement of clinical responses in these patients is associated with the in vivo expansion and persistence of the transferred T lymphocytes. For this reason, recombinant human interleukin-2 (IL-2) is frequently used to support the in vivo survival of T lymphocytes infused into patients. However, IL-2 also causes important side effects. Thus, alternative strategies are highly demanded to limit cytokine-related off-target effects and to redirect the responsiveness of specific T-cell subsets to selected cytokines. Interleukin-7 (IL-7) is a promising alternative cytokine as it possesses the above mentioned properties. However, because its receptor is downregulated in ex vivo-expanded T cells, methods are required to restore their responsiveness to this homeostatic cytokine. In this chapter, we describe the methodology to obtain the ectopic expression of IL-7 receptor alpha (IL-7Rα) in antigen-specific CTL, using Epstein–Barr virus-specific CTL (EBV-CTL), as a model.

Key words Immunotherapy, Cytotoxic T lymphocytes, Cytokine receptors, Interleukin-2, Interleukin-7, Adoptive transfer of T lymphocytes

1 Introduction

Adoptive transfer of tumor-infiltrating lymphocytes (TIL) or antigen-specific cytotoxic T lymphocytes (CTL) expanded ex vivo has proven safe and effective for the treatment of melanoma and virus-associated malignancies, such as Epstein–Barr virus-mediated posttransplant lymphomas (PTLD), and EBV-associated Hodgkin's lymphomas and nasopharyngeal carcinomas [1–4].

A prerequisite for the adoptive transfer of TIL or antigen-specific CTL is the ex vivo expansion of specific T-cell precursors from tumor biopsies (in case of TIL) or from peripheral blood (in case of antigen-specific CTL) of cancer patients. Despite the variety of protocols available for the ex vivo expansion of TIL and antigen-specific CTL, a common element is the use of gamma-chain (γc) cytokines such as IL-2, IL-7, and interleukin-15 (IL-15)

Michael J.P. Lawman and Patricia D. Lawman (eds.), *Cancer Vaccines: Methods and Protocols*, Methods in Molecular Biology, vol. 1139, DOI 10.1007/978-1-4939-0345-0_17,

in the culture media to obtain robust numeric expansions of T lymphocytes [5–7]. At the end of the ex vivo culture, both TIL and antigen-specific CTL show potent effector function, but they remain highly dependent from exogenous cytokines for their continuous growth. Unfortunately, γc cytokines, such as IL-2 and IL-15, are usually unavailable at the tumor site at the doses used in culture conditions, so that transferred TIL and CTL are rapidly starved from these crucial survival factors in vivo.

Several strategies have been explored to sustain the in vivo proliferation and persistence of adoptively transferred TIL and CTL. One approach relies on the administration of the recombinant IL-2. For a long time, this cytokine, which mediates its effects through the binding with a heterotrimeric receptor complex composed of the IL-2Rα, IL-2Rβ, and common γ-chain (γc) [8], has been considered the ideal T-cell growth factor despite the fact that it causes an array of adverse effects resulting from the capillary leak syndrome and lymphoid infiltration in many organs [9, 10]. More recently however, it has become evident that because of the broad expression of its receptor, IL-2 can also promote the expansion of regulatory T cells, a subset of T cells that impairs the function of antigen-specific T lymphocytes, including TIL and CTL [11]. Thus, evidences in the field of adoptive immunotherapy are accumulating suggesting that IL-2 may not be the most favorable γc cytokine to sustain the expansion and persistence of adoptively transferred TIL and CTL in vivo.

IL-7 and IL-15 are other crucial homeostatic cytokines, and the recombinant forms of these proteins have been recently introduced in the clinical arena. IL-7 seems well tolerated in preliminary clinical studies and supports the proliferation of both CD4 and CD8, naïve and memory T cells, and immature B cells [12]. However, the utility of this cytokine in supporting adoptively transferred T cells is questionable since a key component of its receptor, the alpha subunit (IL-7Rα or CD127), is usually downregulated in TIL and CTL expanded ex vivo, so that these cells are impaired in their capacity to use either the IL-7 physiologically available in the circulation or in lymphodepleted conditions or the administrated recombinant protein. IL-15 shows promising results in preclinical studies in nonhuman primates, as it can induce the expansion of natural killer cells, CD8 and CD4 from both central-memory and effector-memory compartment [13]. Importantly, even if TIL and CTL do not express the high-affinity receptor for IL-15 (IL-15Rα), IL-15 may still support the growth of TIL and CTL as the recombinant cytokine can simply function by engaging the β and γc chains of the IL-2 receptor complex. However, it remains to be defined whether IL-15 is safe in human subjects or if it shares some of the toxic effects observed with IL-2.

Considering the limitations associated with the systemic administration of γc cytokines, several strategies have been exploited to reduce the toxicity and the off-target effects of these cytokines. The genetic manipulation of T lymphocytes offers the unique opportunity to restore the capacity of these cells to produce their own cytokines or to express cytokine receptors aimed at creating responsiveness to homeostatic cytokines or cytokines aberrantly expressed by tumor cells. The transgenic expression of cytokines such as IL-2 and IL-15 by ex vivo-expanded antigen-specific T cells has been extensively evaluated in preclinical models and reached the clinical application [14–17].

This chapter focuses on an alternative genetic approach: the ectopic expression of cytokine receptors or growth factor receptors in antigen-specific T cells. This effect is accomplished through the expression of chimeric cytokine receptors (CCR) that are fusion proteins in which the signaling domains of the β and γc chains of the IL-2 receptor complex are fused with the extracellular portion of receptors for cytokines that physiologically do not support the growth of T cells. For example, the extracellular portions of the granulocyte–macrophage colony-stimulating factor (GM-CSF) and erythropoietin (Epo) have been fused with IL-2βγc to create GM-CSF/IL-2βγc [18] and Epo/IL-2βγc [19] chimeric receptors, respectively. T cells expressing GM-CSF/IL-2βγc become therefore responsive to GM-CSF, locally produced by activated T cells or administered as a recombinant protein. Similarly, T cells expressing the Epo/IL-2βγc become responsive to Epo, which can be administered as a recombinant protein. CCR can similarly be used to redirect the responsiveness of T cells toward inhibitory cytokines, thus converting a negative signal into a positive signal. An example of this strategy is represented by the fusion IL-4Rα/IL-2βγc chimeric receptor to combine the extracellular domain of the IL-4 receptor with the signaling domains of IL-2βγc [20, 21]. As a result, these genetically modified T cells proliferate in response to the inhibitory cytokine IL-4, often released within the tumor microenvironment. Although very promising in preclinical models, these approaches may have significant limitations in cancer patients. For example, the release of GM-CSF by activated T cells may be insufficient to support their own growth. Similarly, IL-4 is detected at significant levels (superimposable to that achieved in vitro cultures) only in patients with advanced stage tumors who usually do not benefit from T-cell-based therapies. Finally, the doses of recombinant GM-CSF and Epo required in vivo to support the growth of T cells may induce significant expansion of cell subsets physiologically responding to these growth factors and thus induce significant side effects.

The approach that we describe here is based on the constitutive expression of IL-7Rα—the key receptor for IL-7—by antigen-specific CTL [22]. IL-7 is a nonredundant cytokine involved in primary T- and B-cell development. It is produced by stromal cells, keratinocytes, and gut epithelial cells and is continuously available in secondary lymphoid organs to support the survival of naïve T cells and memory cells. Furthermore, IL-7 levels in the plasma are inversely correlated with the number of T cells, so that IL-7 is the main cytokine driving the immune reconstitution in lymphopenic conditions [23]. Several studies have shown that CTL and TIL used for adoptive cell therapy lack the expression of IL-7Rα and thus do not respond to IL-7. Restoring the expression of IL-7Rα by these cells, through gene transfer, results in their proliferation in response to IL-7 without modifications of their antigen specificity. This proposed strategy appears advantageous as compared to other approaches since it restores the responsiveness of ex vivo-expanded CTL and TIL to a cytokine that physiologically controls the homeostasis of T cells, allowing their favorable expansion in lymphodepleted hosts and upon administration of recombinant IL-7 that was well tolerated in phase I clinical studies [12].

In this chapter, we describe the protocol optimized to efficiently transduce antigen-specific CTL with a retroviral vector encoding the IL-7Rα, to selectively expand them, and to test their function.

2 Materials

2.1 Genetic Modification of EBV-Specific CTL (EBV-CTL)

1. Peripheral blood mononuclear cells (PBMC) from EBV-seropositive donors.
2. EBV-immortalized lymphoblastoid cell lines (EBV-LCL), cultured in Roswell Park Memorial Institute (RPMI)-1640 medium, supplemented with 10 % fetal bovine serum (FBS), 2 mM L-glutamine, 100 IU/mL of penicillin, and 100 mg/mL of streptomycin.
3. CTL medium: 45 % RPMI-1640 medium, 45 % Click's Medium supplemented with 10 % FBS, glutamine, and penicillin–streptomycin.
4. Recombinant human (rh) IL-2. Reconstitute in medium at 200 U/mL. Store at −80 °C. A single aliquot can be used up to 5×.
5. rhIL-7: Reconstitute in medium at 10 ng/mL. Store at −80 °C. A single aliquot can be used up to 5×.
6. 24-well non-tissue culture-treated plates.
7. 24-well tissue culture-treated plates.
8. Recombinant fibronectin fragment: RetroNectin (FN CH-296) (Takara Shuzo, Otsu, Japan). Reconstitute in water at 1 mg/mL and store aliquots at −20 °C. A single aliquot can be used up to 3×.

9. IL-7Rα retroviral supernatant (Vector Production Facility, Baylor College of Medicine, Houston, TX). Store at −80 °C. Do not refreeze.
10. Enzyme-free cell dissociation solution.
11. Trypan blue.

2.2 Immunophenotyping

1. Monoclonal antibodies conjugated with different fluorochromes: CD3-APC, CD4-PERCP, CD8-APC, CD127-PE.
2. 5-mL polystyrene tubes.
3. FACS wash buffer: 1 % FBS in phosphate-buffered saline (PBS).
4. FACSCalibur system equipped with the filter set for quadruple fluorescence signals and CellQuest software.

2.3 STAT5 Phosphorylation

1. 5-mL polystyrene tubes.
2. rhIL-2.
3. rhIL-7.
4. FACS buffer.
5. Fixation buffer: 2 % paraformaldehyde in PBS.
6. Permeabilization buffer: 90 % methanol in water.
7. Alexa Fluor 647 mouse anti-STAT5 (pY694) (BD Phosflow Reagents, San Jose, CA, USA).

2.4 Cytotoxicity Assay

1. 100 μC ^{51}Chromium (MP Biomedicals, Solon, OH, USA).
2. 96-well V-bottom plates.
3. Triton-X: Dilute in water to a final concentration of 1 % and store at room temperature.
4. Packard Cobra Quantum gamma counter (Packard Instrument Company, Downers Grove, IL, USA).
5. Target cells: Autologous LCL, HLA-mismatched LCL (negative control to exclude alloreactivity), and K562 (negative control to exclude NK activity). These cells are maintained in culture in T75 flasks in RPMI-1640, supplemented with 10 % FBS, glutamine, penicillin, and streptomycin at 37 °C, 5 % CO_2.

2.5 Coculture Assay

1. CTL medium.
2. rhIL-2.
3. rhIL-7.
4. 24-well tissue culture-treated plates.

3 Methods

3.1 Genetic Modification of EBV-CTL

Here, we describe the generation of EBV-CTL and their transduction with a retroviral vector.

1. Thaw PBMC, wash, count, and resuspend at 2×10^6/mL in complete medium. Irradiate autologous EBV-LCL at 40 Gy, wash, count, and resuspend at 5×10^4 cell/mL in complete medium. Incubate in 24-well plates at 1 mL/well of PBMC and 1 mL/well of irradiated EBV-LCL (40:1 effector to target ratio).
2. After 10–12 days, collect EBV-CTL, wash, count, and resuspend at 1×10^6/mL in complete medium. Irradiate autologous EBV-LCL at 40 Gy, wash, count, and resuspend at 2.5×10^5 cell/mL in complete CTL medium. In a 24-well plate, cocultivate 1 mL/well of PBMC and 1 mL/well of irradiated EBV-LCL (4:1 effector to target ratio).
3. After 3–4 days, remove 1 mL of medium and replace with complete medium containing 50 U/mL of IL-2.
4. After 3 days, collect CTL, wash, count, resuspend them at 1×10^6 cells/mL, and aliquot 1 mL/well in 24-well tissue culture plate; add 1 mL of irradiated autologous EBV-LCL (40 Gy) resuspended at 2.5×10^5 cell/mL in complete medium containing 50 U/mL of IL-2.
5. On day 3, coat the required number of wells of a non-tissue culture-treated 24-well plate with RetroNectin at a concentration of 7 μg/mL of PBS/well and incubate at 4 °C for 16–24 h.
6. On day 4, remove the RetroNectin-coated plate from 4 °C, aspirate RetroNectin, and wash the plate with 1 mL of complete medium for 10–30 min.
7. Add 0.5 mL/well of the retroviral supernatant and incubate for 20 min in the biosafety cabinet. Aspirate and add another 0.5 mL of retroviral supernatant for 20 min (*see* **Note 1**).
8. Aspirate and add 1.5 mL of retroviral supernatant and 0.5 mL of T cells resuspended at the concentration of 1×10^6/mL in complete medium containing 100 IU/mL rhIL-2 (*see* **Note 2**).
9. Spin plate at $1{,}000 \times g$ for 30 min and incubate at 37 °C for 72 h.
10. After 72 h of incubation, harvest the cells from each well and remove eventual adherent cells by using 0.5 mL cell dissociation medium per well, 5 min incubation and restimulate 1×/week for 2 weeks with irradiated (40 Gy) autologous EBV-LCL (4:1 effector to target ratio), with the addition of 2.5 ng/mL of exogenous rhIL-7 or 50 U/mL of rhIL-2 (*see* **Note 3**).
11. Assess transduction efficiency of EBV-CTL by FACS analysis using CD127-PE antibody (*see* Subheading 3.2).

3.2 Testing the Transduction Efficiency

Expression of the CD127, assessed by FACS analysis, is used to evaluate the transduction efficiency of EBV-CTL.

1. Collect control non-transduced (NT) and IL-7Rα[+] EBV-CTL, wash, count them, and resuspend at the concentration of 1×10^6/mL in FACS wash buffer.
2. Aliquot 0.2 mL of cells in polystyrene tubes.
3. Add 1 μL of CD127-PE to each tube.
4. Optional: Add 1 μL of other monoclonal antibodies, like differently conjugated CD3 and CD4 and CD8 to assess the expression of CD127 by the different T cells.
5. Incubate at 4 °C, in the dark for 30 min.
6. Wash with 2 mL of FACS buffer, spin, and decant. Resuspend in 0.2 mL of FACS buffer.
7. Assess the transduction efficiency at the FACS as shown in Fig. 1.

3.3 Testing Functionality of the IL-7Rα

3.3.1 Expansion of IL-7Rα[+] EBV-CTL Is Determined by Cell Count of Viable Cells

1. Collect and count EBV-CTL using a 1:1 dilution with Trypan blue to determine viability of CTL; resuspend CTL in CTL medium at the concentration of 1×10^6/mL and aliquot at 1 mL/well.
2. Add 1 mL of irradiated autologous EBV-LCL (40 Gy) resuspended at 2.5×10^5/well in complete medium with 2.5 ng/mL of exogenous rhIL-7.
3. Incubate at 37 °C, 5 % CO_2.
4. On day 4, remove 1 mL of medium and replace with fresh medium, with the addition of 2.5 ng/mL of exogenous rhIL-7.
5. Incubate at 37 °C, 5 % CO_2.
6. On day 7, collect and count EBV-CTL using Trypan blue to determine their viability.
7. Repeat weekly stimulation, from **steps 1** to **6**.

3.3.2 STAT5 Phosphorylation Is Used to Assess the Signaling of the Receptor

1. Collect NT and IL-7Rα[+] EBV-CTL, wash, count them, and resuspend at the concentration of 1×10^6/mL in complete medium. Aliquot cells in 5-mL polystyrene tubes to a concentration of 1×10^6/tube.
2. Add 2.5 ng/mL of exogenous rhIL-7 or 50 U/mL of rhIL-2.
3. Incubate for 15 min at 37 °C, 5 % CO_2.
4. Wash with 2 mL of FACS buffer, spin, and decant.
5. Add 1 mL of the fixation buffer, incubate for 10 min at 37 °C, spin, and decant.
6. Add 1 mL of permeabilization buffer, incubate for 30 min on ice, spin, and decant.

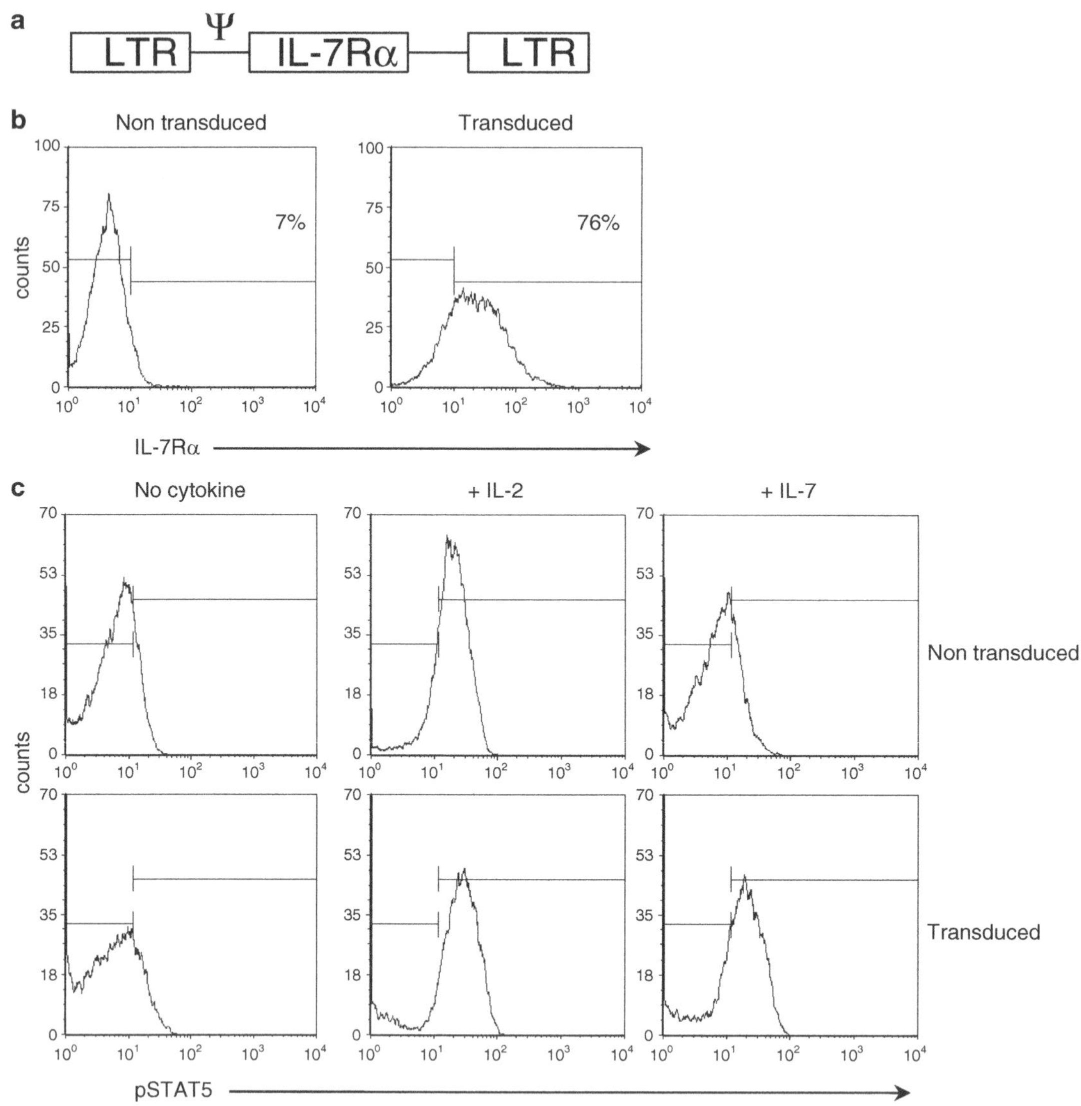

Fig. 1 Transduction efficiency of genetically modified EBV-CTL and assessment of the functionality of the IL-7Rα transgene. Panel (**a**) shows the schema of the gamma-retroviral vector used to transduce the EBV-CTL. Panel (**b**) shows the transduction efficiency of one representative EBV-CTL line. CTLs were transduced with the IL-7Rα vector and the expression of the transgene was measured on the cell surface by FACS analysis. Panel (**c**) shows the phosphorylation of STAT5 in response to IL-2 or IL-7 in control non-transduced (NT) and transduced EBV-CTL. STAT5 is phosphorylated in both NT and transduced EBV-CTL in response to IL-2, but it is phosphorylated only in IL-7Rα^{+} EBV-CTL in response to IL-7

7. Wash with FACS buffer 2×.
8. Add 10 μL of Alexa Fluor 647 mouse anti-STAT5, and incubate for 1 h at room temperature, in the dark.
9. Wash and proceed with the FACS acquisition.

3.3.3 Short-Term Cytotoxicity Assay

This short-term assay is used to ensure that EBV-CTL retain their ability to lyse their native target cells.

1. Collect and pellet at least 5×10^6 target cells (*see* **Notes 4** and **5**).
2. Resuspend target cells by finger-clicking and perform radiolabeling by adding 100 μCi of ^{51}Chromium in a radioactive safety cabinet. Labeled cells are then incubated for 1 h at 37 °C, with a gentle finger flicking every 15 min.
3. Wash ^{51}Chromium-labeled target cells by centrifugation at $400 \times g$ for 3 min using 5 mL of complete medium; count cells after the fourth wash, and then resuspend them at the concentration of 5×10^4/mL in complete medium.
4. Collect transduced EBV-CTL cultivated with rhIL-2 or rhIL-7, wash, count them, and resuspend at the concentration of 2×10^6/mL in complete medium. Aliquot cells in a 96-well V-bottom plate. Perform serial dilutions (1:2) to obtain triplicates of wells containing cell numbers ranging from 2×10^5/well to 2.5×10^4/well.
5. Add 100 μL of the appropriate target cells to the wells containing 100 μL of the diluted EBV-CTL, 100 μL of medium only (spontaneous release), or 100 μL of 1 % Triton-X (maximum release).
6. Incubate the plates for 4–5 h at 37 °C, 5 % CO_2.
7. Spin plate at $400 \times g$ for 3 min, collect 100 μL of supernatant, transfer in appropriate tubes, and read using the γ-counter (*see* **Note 6**).
8. The percent of killing is calculated as follows:
   [cpm from experimental wells (target + CTL) − cpm of target cells in the presence of medium only (spontaneous release)/ cpm of target cells in the presence of 1 % Triton-X (maximum release) − cpm of target cells in the presence of medium only (spontaneous release)] × 100.

3.3.4 Coculture Assay

This assay is used to ensure that EBV-CTL retain their ability to eliminate from the culture their native target cells in a long-term assay.

1. Collect autologous EBV-LCL, wash, count them, and resuspend at the concentration of 2×10^6/mL in complete medium. Aliquot cells in a 24-well tissue culture-treated plate to a concentration of 1×10^6/well.
2. Collect NT and IL-7Rα$^+$ EBV-CTL, wash, count them, and resuspend at the concentration of 0.5×10^6/mL in complete medium. Aliquot cells in a 24-well tissue culture-treated plate to a concentration of 0.5×10^6/well.
3. Add 2.5 ng/mL of exogenous rhIL-7 or 50 U/mL of rhIL-2.

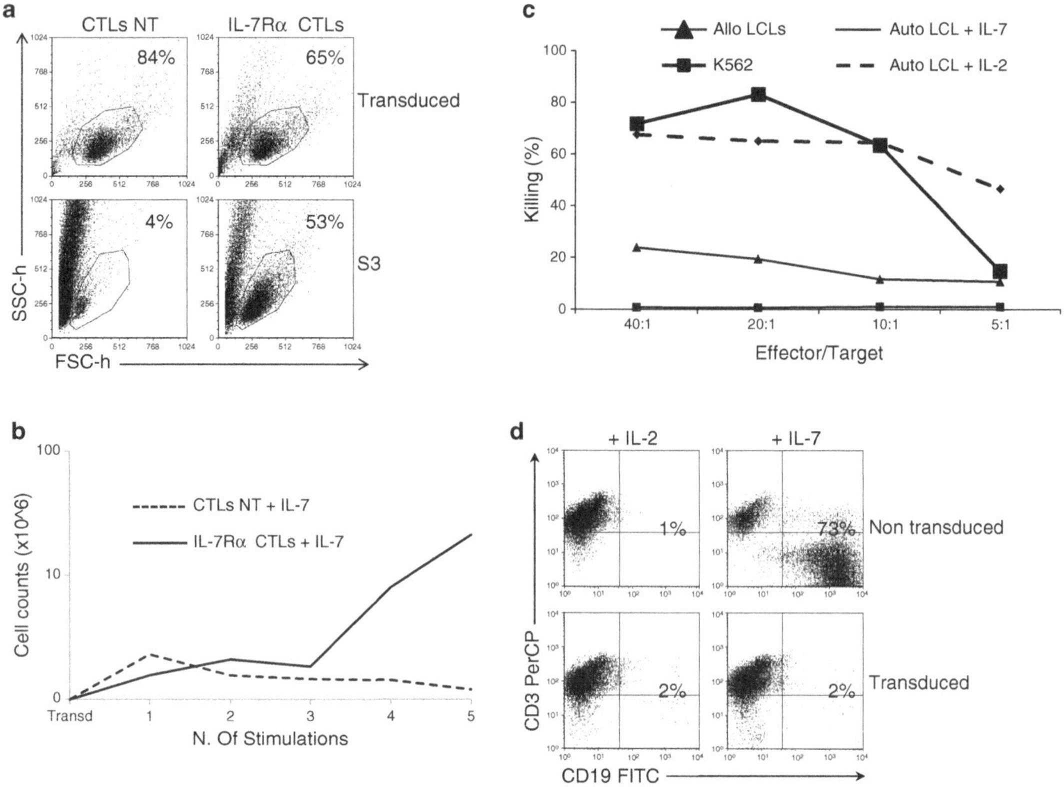

Fig. 2 Functional characterization of genetically modified EBV-CTL. Panel (**a**) shows the viable gating assessing the physical parameters by FACS analysis in control NT and IL-7Rα⁺ EBV-CTL. EBV-CTL viability was assessed immediately after the transduction and after 3 weeks of culture in which EBV-CTL were weekly stimulated with the antigen and in the presence of IL-7. NT EBV-CTL do not survive in culture since they do not respond to IL-7, while IL-7Rα⁺ EBV-CTL remain viable when stimulated with the antigen in the presence of IL-7. Panel (**b**) shows that IL-7Rα⁺ EBV-CTL but not control NT cells expand in vitro when stimulated weekly with autologous EBV-LCL in the presence of IL-7. Panel (**c**) shows the results of a representative ^{51}Chromium-release assay. IL-7Rα⁺ EBV-CTL induce comparable lysis of the autologous EBV-LCL when cultivated in IL-2 or IL-7, confirming retained killing activity against the native target antigen. The lysis of allogeneic EBV-LCL, regardless of whether CTL are grown in IL-2 or IL-7, is negligible, confirming retained MHC restriction. No significant reactivity (<10 %) is observed against the K562 cell lines. Panel (**d**) shows the plot of a representative coculture experiment of EBV-CTL and autologous EBV-LCL. The ratio EBV-CTL to EBV-LCL was 1:2. Residual EBV-LCL were quantified by day 7 of culture based on their CD19 expression by FACS analysis. Control NT and IL-7Rα⁺ EBV-CTL eliminated equally well EBV-LCL in the presence of IL-2. By contrast, only IL-7Rα⁺ EBV-CTL eliminated EBV-LCL in the presence of IL-7

4. Incubate for 7 days at 37 °C, 5 % CO_2.
5. Assess cytotoxic activity of NT or IL-7Rα⁺ EBV-CTL by FACS analysis using anti-CD3-PerCP and anti-CD19-FITC antibodies as shown in Fig. 2.

4 Notes

1. Avoid multiple thawing and freezing of the supernatants.
2. Keep some non-transduced (NT) CTL as controls. These cells will need to be plated at the same concentration in complete medium containing 2.5 ng/mL of rhIL-7 in a 24-well tissue culture-treated plate.
3. The cell count of the transduced EBV-CTL is expected to drop during the first 2 weeks in culture in the presence of rhIL-7 due to the selection of the IL-7Rα^+ EBV-CTL.
4. Do not provide the culture with IL-7 for at least 3 days before testing the expression of IL-7Rα to avoid significant underestimation of the receptor expression.
5. To evaluate EBV-CTL specificity, autologous EBV-LCL, HLA class I and II mismatched EBV-LCL, and K562 cell lines are used as target cells. If CTL are antigen specific, only autologous EBV-LCL are expected to be significantly lysed.
6. Wear appropriate radioprotection equipment and monitor the work area using a survey meter. Label and dispose of radioactive waste according to approved guidelines. Personnel monitoring with a thermoluminescence dosimeter is recommended.

References

1. Rosenberg SA et al (1994) Treatment of patients with metastatic melanoma with autologous tumor-infiltrating lymphocytes and interleukin 2. J Natl Cancer Inst 86:1159–1166
2. Straathof KC et al (2005) Treatment of nasopharyngeal carcinoma with Epstein-Barr virus-specific T lymphocytes. Blood 105:1898–1904
3. Bollard CM et al (2007) Complete responses of relapsed lymphoma following genetic modification of tumor-antigen presenting cells and T-lymphocyte transfer. Blood 110:2838–2845
4. Heslop HE et al (2010) Long-term outcome of EBV-specific T-cell infusions to prevent or treat EBV-related lymphoproliferative disease in transplant recipients. Blood 115:925–935
5. Rooney CM et al (1995) Use of gene-modified virus-specific T lymphocytes to control Epstein-Barr-virus-related lymphoproliferation. Lancet 345:9–13
6. Quintarelli C et al (2008) Cytotoxic T lymphocytes directed to the preferentially expressed antigen of melanoma (PRAME) target chronic myeloid leukemia. Blood 112:1876–1885
7. Dudley ME et al (2003) Generation of tumor-infiltrating lymphocyte cultures for use in adoptive transfer therapy for melanoma patients. J Immunother 26:332–342
8. Overwijk WW, Schluns KS (2009) Functions of gammaC cytokines in immune homeostasis: current and potential clinical applications. Clin Immunol 132:153–165
9. Schwartzentruber DJ (2001) High-dose interleukin-2 is an intensive treatment regardless of the venue of administration. Cancer J 7: 103–104
10. Acquavella N et al (2008) Toxicity and activity of a twice daily high-dose bolus interleukin 2 regimen in patients with metastatic melanoma and metastatic renal cell cancer. J Immunother 31:569–576
11. Ahmadzadeh M, Rosenberg SA (2006) IL-2 administration increases CD4+ CD25(hi) Foxp3+ regulatory T cells in cancer patients. Blood 107:2409–2414
12. Sportes C et al (2008) Administration of rhIL-7 in humans increases in vivo TCR repertoire diversity by preferential expansion of naive T cell subsets. J Exp Med 205:1701–1714
13. Berger C et al (2009) Safety and immunologic effects of IL-15 administration in nonhuman primates. Blood 114:2417–2426

14. Liu K, Rosenberg SA (2001) Transduction of an IL-2 gene into human melanoma-reactive lymphocytes results in their continued growth in the absence of exogenous IL-2 and maintenance of specific antitumor activity. J Immunol 167:6356–6365
15. Heemskerk BL et al (2008) Adoptive cell therapy for patients with melanoma, using tumor-infiltrating lymphocytes genetically engineered to secrete interleukin-2. Hum Gene Ther 19:496–510
16. Quintarelli C et al (2007) Co-expression of cytokine and suicide genes to enhance the activity and safety of tumor-specific cytotoxic T lymphocytes. Blood 110:2793–2802
17. Hoyos V et al (2010) Engineering CD19-specific T lymphocytes with interleukin-15 and a suicide gene to enhance their anti-lymphoma/leukemia effects and safety. Leukemia 24: 1160–1170
18. Evans LS et al (1999) Expression of chimeric granulocyte-macrophage colony-stimulating factor/interleukin 2 receptors in human cytotoxic T lymphocyte clones results in granulocyte-macrophage colony-stimulating factor-dependent growth. Hum Gene Ther 10:1941–1951
19. Minamoto S et al (1995) Acquired erythropoietin responsiveness of interleukin-2-dependent T lymphocytes retrovirally transduced with genes encoding chimeric erythropoietin/interleukin-2 receptors. Blood 86:2281–2287
20. Wilkie S et al (2010) Selective expansion of chimeric antigen receptor-targeted T-cells with potent effector function using interleukin-4. J Biol Chem 285:25538–25544
21. Gasser S et al (2000) Constitutive expression of a chimeric receptor that delivers IL-2/IL-15 signals allows antigen-independent proliferation of $CD8^{+}$CD44high but not other T cells. J Immunol 164:5659–5667
22. Vera JF et al (2009) Genetic manipulation of tumor-specific cytotoxic T lymphocytes to restore responsiveness to IL-7. Mol Ther 17: 880–888
23. Ma A et al (2006) Diverse functions of IL-2, IL-15, and IL-7 in lymphoid homeostasis. Annu Rev Immunol 24:657–679

Chapter 18

Monitoring the Frequency and Function of Regulatory T Cells and Summary of the Approaches Currently Used to Inhibit Regulatory T Cells in Cancer Patients

Chiara Camisaschi, Marcella Tazzari, Licia Rivoltini, and Chiara Castelli

Abstract

Regulatory T cells (Treg) are a subset of T lymphocytes that in humans represent less than the 10 % of circulating CD4$^+$ T cells. Treg are specialized in the inhibition of the immune responses and play a crucial role in the maintenance of immunological tolerance. Several lines of evidence clearly documented the role of Treg in restraining antitumor immune responses. For this reason, antitumor immunotherapy approaches have been recently associated with drug treatments aimed at depleting Treg or blocking their functions. A summary of the currently used in vivo approaches to limit Treg expansion in cancer patients is here provided.

A comprehensive phenotypic and functional monitoring of Treg is crucial for the precise assessment of the effects that these different drug treatments exert on Treg. In this chapter, we will provide guidelines for an accurate ex vivo identification of human Treg. Due to the phenotypic and functional heterogeneity, intrinsic plasticity, and the lack of a unique marker exclusively expressed by human Treg, the clear-cut identification of this T cell subset requires the expert usage of multiparametric flow cytometry analysis (FACS). In this view, a combination of phenotypic and functional assessment of Treg is mandatory. In this chapter, we will describe the most reliable methods to identify and monitor the modulation of human Treg in patients undergoing immunological or drug-based treatments. Protocols to measure ex vivo the suppressive functions of Treg are also provided.

Key words Regulatory T cells, CFSE, Multiparametric FACS analysis, Intracellular staining, Immunomagnetic isolation, Suppression assay, Treg depletion

1 Introduction

1.1 Strategies Currently Used to Block or Inhibit Treg

Many recent studies suggest that the induction or presence of Treg might account for the failure of cancer immunotherapy. Therefore, consistent with the concept that effective cancer therapies are multimodal, the association of treatments aimed at modulating Treg frequency or functions with active cancer immunotherapeutic interventions represents an attractive perspective. The advantage and the possible success of these combinatorial treatments are well supported by abundant data achieved in preclinical murine models

Michael J.P. Lawman and Patricia D. Lawman (eds.), *Cancer Vaccines: Methods and Protocols*, Methods in Molecular Biology, vol. 1139, DOI 10.1007/978-1-4939-0345-0_18,

Table 1
Strategies to inhibit Treg in humans

Strategies		Setting	Reference
Treg depletion			
Chemotherapy	Cyclophosphamide (CTX)	Metastatic melanoma Metastatic breast cancer	[3, 4] [5]
CD25 targeting/depletion of CD25+ cells	Anti-CD25 mAb (daclizumab) Denileukin diftitox (ONTAK®) Anti-CD25 immunotoxin	Metastatic melanoma Metastatic breast cancer Metastatic melanoma Metastatic renal cell carcinoma Metastatic melanoma	[6] [7] [8–10] [11] [12, 13]
Blockade of Treg function			
CTLA-4 targeting	Anti-CTLA-4 (ipilimumab, tremelimumab)	Melanoma advanced gastric and esophageal	[14] [15]
Anti-angiogenic molecules	Sunitinib malate Sorafenib Imatinib mesylate	Metastatic renal cell carcinoma Metastatic renal cell carcinoma Gastrointestinal stromal tumors	[16, 17] [18] [19]
Blockade of Treg recruitment			
Chemokine receptor inhibitors (temozolomide/carmustine)	CCR4/CCL22	Glioblastoma multiforme (GBM)	[20]

[1, 2] and by some recent human clinical trials. Table 1 summarizes strategies used for Treg inhibition in humans [3–20].

Many strategies are currently used to manipulate Treg, including Treg depletion, inhibition of Treg function, or blockade of Treg trafficking into lymph nodes or tumors. The approach of Treg depletion adopted in clinical trials includes the usage of molecules targeting CD25 (daclizumab, denileukin diftitox [ONTAK], anti-CD25 immunotoxin) or the administration of cyclophosphamide (*N*,*N*-bis (2-chloroethyl)-1,3,2-oxazaphosphinan-2-amine 2-oxide, the generic name for Cytoxan (CTX), Endoxan). However, CD25 is also expressed by activated effector T cells, and therefore, administration of anti-CD25 molecules could possibly limit positive antitumor responses. Importantly, transient depletion of Treg during priming of antitumor immunity, rather than chronic depletion of Treg, should be considered to avoid the development of autoimmune side effects. So far, the use of antibodies that target molecules constitutively expressed by Treg, i.e., CTLA-4, GITR, or OX-40, leading to their functional inhibition is extensively investigated. Moreover, various drugs originally developed for other therapeutic indications, e.g., anti-angiogenic molecules, tyrosine kinase inhibitors, etc., have recently been discovered to inhibit Treg.

It should be highlighted that, in some cases, conflicting results on the biological effects of these treatments in limiting Treg have been reported. This could be due to different patients' tumor stages or administration schedules. However, difficulties in the interpretation of data could also stem from the multiplicity of methods used to detect Treg ex vivo in treated patients. Thus, in our view, it is mandatory to define a consensual method to identify human Treg by ex vivo analysis.

1.2 Complexity of Treg Studies: Advantage of Multiparametric FACS Analysis and Ex Vivo Functional Assays

Naturally occurring $CD4^+$ Treg in humans are a heterogeneous population characterized by the high expression level of CD25 (α-chain of IL-2 receptor) and the positivity for the intracellular transcription factor, forkhead box P3 (Foxp3) [21]. However, these proteins are not exclusively expressed by Treg, being also detectable, although at different intensity, on activated conventional CD4 T cells. The introduction of the CD127 (α-chain IL-7 receptor) surface marker amplified the Treg definition [22], and Treg have been also defined as $CD4^+$ T cells expressing intermediate-to-high levels of CD25 and negative/low levels of CD127. Since these are cell surface markers, this alternative identification method has been mainly applied for sorting/enriching a population with Treg features.

However, in our experience, the $CD127^{low/neg}$ fraction also includes a limited number of $CD25^{int}$ T cells expressing a low level of Foxp3 intensity. Since $CD25^{int}$ and $Foxp3^{low}$ are also shared by conventional T cells [23], the $CD4^+$ population gated as $CD25^+$ $CD127^{low/neg}$ cannot be considered as pure Treg.

A more accurate analysis of human Treg is achieved by the simultaneous staining for CD4, CD25, Foxp3, and CD45RA. This combination of markers allows the identification of two different subsets of Treg, namely, activated Treg and resting Treg. Most importantly, it allows the discrimination of Treg from conventional activated, not suppressive T cells [24]. Thus, combining the most recent information on human Treg phenotype, the following scenario should be considered when monitoring Treg frequency (Fig. 1):

1. $CD4^+CD25^{hi}Foxp3^+CD45RA^{neg}$ T cells: activated Treg, ready to exert their suppressive functions

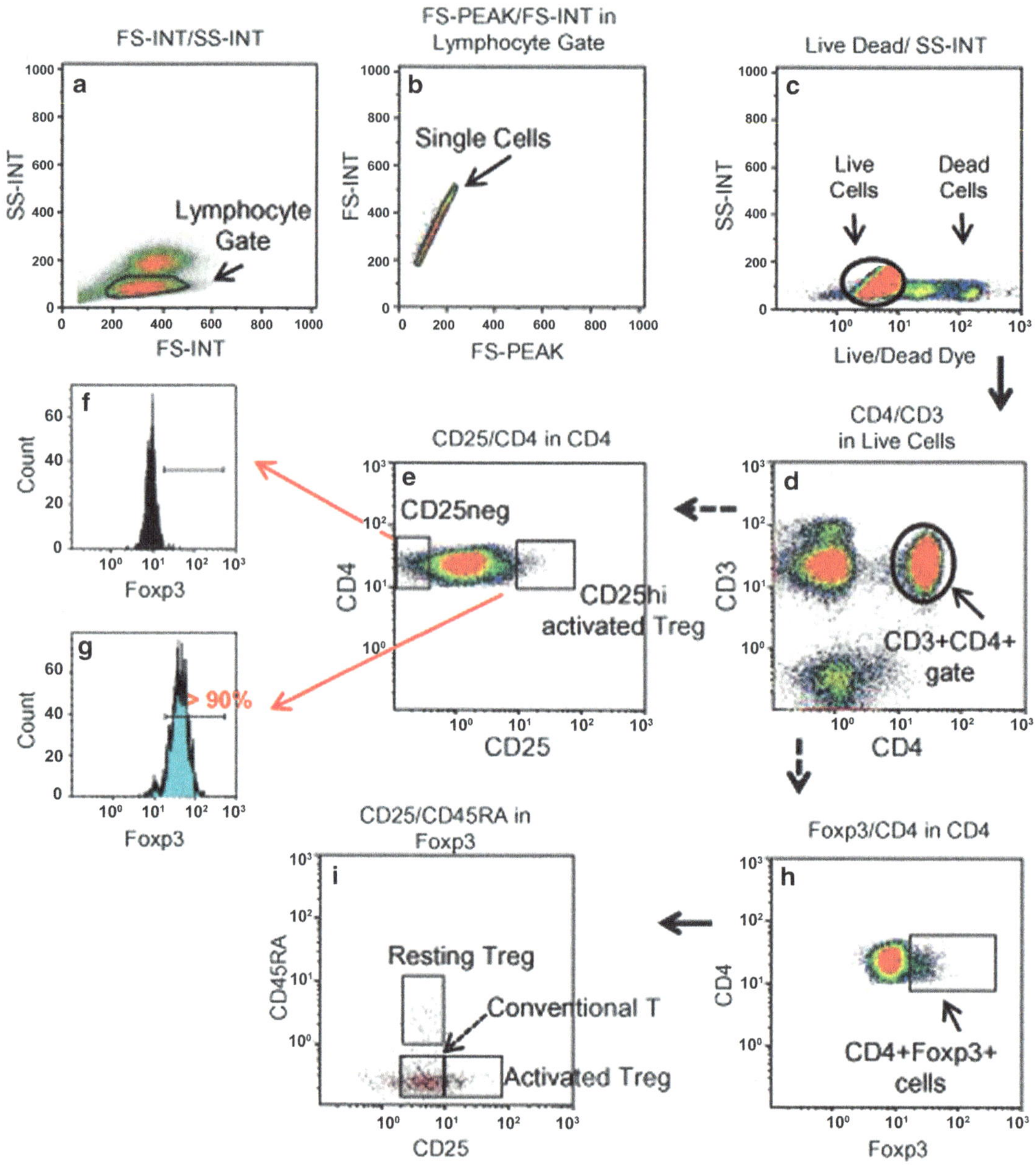

Fig. 1 Gating strategy for Treg analysis. PBMC were stained with LIVE/DEAD dye; anti-CD3, CD4, CD25, and CD45RA superficial monoclonal antibodies (mAbs); and the intracellular anti-Foxp3. Lymphocytes are identified based on the physical parameters (**a**). In the lymphocyte population, single cells are gated for the subsequent analysis, while cell duplets excluded (**b**). Live cells are gated for their negative expression of the LIVE/DEAD dye (**c**) and the $CD4^+$ lymphocytes are detected as cell double positive for CD3 and CD4 (**d**). In the CD4 vs. CD25 dot plot of $CD4^+CD3^+$ cells, the $CD25^{neg}$ population is gated (**e**) and used to set the negative Foxp3 marker as reported in (**f**); the $CD25^{hi}$ region is then set to obtain Foxp3 positivity higher than 90 %, as shown in (**g**). In the CD4 vs. Foxp3 dot plot of $CD4^+CD3^+$ cells, the $Foxp3^+$ cells are gated for the subsequent analysis (**h**). CD25 vs. CD45RA dot plot of the $Foxp3^+$ cells is shown in (**i**). Three different subsets are defined: the activated Treg ($CD45RA^{neg}CD25^{hi}$), the resting Treg ($CD45RA^+CD25^{int}$), and the conventional T cells ($CD45RA^{neg}CD25^{int}$). The marker for CD25 and CD45RA positivity is set based on the isotype control, while the $CD25^{hi}$ marker is defined in (**e**)

2. $CD4^+CD25^{int}Foxp3^{low}CD45RA^+$ T cells: resting Treg, which are suppressive and ready to convert to activated Treg in vivo and in vitro
3. $CD4^+CD25^{int}Foxp3^{low}CD45RA^{neg}$ T cells: not suppressive, conventional activated T cells

Therefore, at present, the more comprehensive method to characterize Treg should also include the usage of the CD45RA marker. Concerning CD127, this cell surface protein certainly discriminates all $Foxp3^+$ cells, and in combination with CD45RA, it can be used to sort out a pure Treg population that will include both resting and activated suppressive cells.

In addition to molecules constitutively expressed by human Treg such as CTLA-4, GITR, CD27, CD28, OX-40, and CD62L, the expression of major histocompatibility (MHC) class II, CCR7, CD147, CD39, GARP, and co-stimulatory molecule as ICOS and LAG-3 [25–31] identifies different Treg subsets, highlighting the wide heterogeneity of this population. Furthermore, recent studies provide evidence not only for functional heterogeneity but also for high lineage plasticity. Treg can indeed differentiate into IL-17-producing Th17, acquiring RORγt expression with or without losing Foxp3 expression [32, 33], or in the presence of IL-12, they can acquire a Th1 phenotype secreting IFN-γ and expressing T-bet, without losing Foxp3 [34].

Recently, a highly conserved CpG-enriched element, located in the 5′ untranslated region (5′UTR) of *foxp3*, has been identified as the Treg-cell-specific demethylated region (TSDR) [35]. This region is constantly and steadily demethylated in Treg, but not in non-suppressive T cells that transiently express Foxp3 after activation. Thus, the usage of methylation-specific qPCR is considered a precise technique to identify Treg [35, 36]. However, although this method has been successfully used to measure the frequency of circulating Treg in vaccinated cancer patients [37], its applicability is restricted to pure lymphocyte samples and cannot be used to detect Treg in tumor tissue [38]. Most importantly, it cannot be associated with any other ex vivo analysis of Treg aimed at defining their functional features.

To date, the in vitro suppressive assay is the most reliable method to assess the functional activity of Treg. This assay measures the Treg ability to suppress the proliferation of target cells, usually represented by autologous $CD4^+CD25^-$ T cells. We found that in some particular conditions, Treg purified by FACS sorting or by immunomagnetic isolation display a certain degree of proliferation. In this condition, the carboxyfluorescein diacetate succinimidyl ester (CSFE)-based proliferation assay should be used instead of the [^{3}H] thymidine incorporation assay, since it detects only the proliferation activity of the CSFE-labeled target cells. Since Treg functions are multiple, the production of immunosuppressive cytokines, such as IL-10 and TGF-β, is also crucial in defining active Treg [31, 39]. This ex vivo functional assay can be directly combined with the Treg phenotypic analysis, and thus, it can be performed when the limited availability of patients' T cells compromises the possibility to set up in vitro immunosuppressive assays.

In conclusion, lacking a unique specific marker to define Treg in humans, the multiparametric FACS analysis is required to identify Treg ex vivo. Notably, this analysis allows the definition of the functional properties of the different Treg subsets, thus providing additional information on their activation status and homing capacity.

2 Materials

1. Ficoll-Paque™ endotoxin-tested solution (<0.12 EU/mL) (density 1,077 g/L) stored at room temperature.
2. Roswell Park Memorial Institute (RPMI)-1640 medium.
3. Heat-inactivated fetal bovine serum (FBS).
4. Heat-inactivated human serum (HS).
5. ACK Lysing Buffer: 8.29 g of NH_4Cl (0.15 M), 1 g of 10 mM $KHCO_3$, 37.2 mg of 0.1 mM Na_2EDTA in 800 mL of H_2O and adjust pH to 7.2–7.4 with 1 N HCl. Add H_2O to 1 L, filter sterilize through a 0.2-μm filter, and store at 4 °C.
6. Complete RPMI-1640 medium: RPMI-1640 supplemented with 180 U/mL each of penicillin and streptomycin and 2 mM glutamine.
7. Trypan blue solution.
8. Phosphate-buffered saline (PBS).
9. LIVE/DEAD Fixable Staining Kit (Molecular Probes, Eugene, OR, USA). The kit includes five vials of reactive dye and one vial of dimethyl sulfoxide (DMSO). Both reactive dye and anhydrous DMSO should be brought to room temperature. Reconstitute one vial of dye with 50 μL of DMSO and mix well. Once reconstituted, store it at −20 °C and protect it from light. To avoid repeated freezing and thawing, we recommend storing it in aliquots once reconstituted.
10. Foxp3 Staining Buffer Set (eBioscience, San Diego, CA, USA). All reagents should be stored at 4 °C. The kit includes 4× eBioscience Fix/Perm Concentrate, eBioscience Fix/Perm Diluent, and 10× eBioscience Permeabilization Buffer. Dilute 1 part Fix/Perm Concentrate with 3 parts Fix/Perm Diluent. Pre-warm the Permeabilization Buffer and dilute to 1× with deionized/distilled H_2O and store at 4 °C. Prepare immediately before use. This buffer should not be stored more than 1 day.

Table 2
Column characteristics

Column	Max. number of labeled cells	Max. number of total cells
LD	10^8	5×10^8
MS	10^7	2×10^8
LS	10^8	2×10^8

11. Treg culture medium: X-VIVO 15 medium supplemented with 10 % heat-inactivated FBS, 1 % heat-inactivated HS, 2 mM glutamine, and 180 U/mL each of penicillin and streptomycin [40].
12. Anti-CD3/CD28 beads (DynaBeads® CD3/CD28 T cell Expander) (Dynal Biotech, Oslo, Norway), stored at 4 °C and vortexed prior to use.
13. GolgiStop protein transport inhibitor containing monensin (or GolgiPlug protein transport inhibitor containing brefeldin A) (BD Biosciences, San Jose, CA, USA).
14. Cytofix/Cytoperm Fixation/Permeabilization Kit (BD Biosciences). All reagents should be stored at 4 °C. The kit includes fixation/permeabilization solution and Perm/Wash buffer (10× concentrate containing FBS and saponin). Pre-warm Perm/Wash buffer and dilute to 1× with deionized/distilled water prior to use. This kit is used for staining intracellular cytokines with fluorochrome-conjugated anti-cytokine antibodies.
15. $CD4^+CD25^+$ Regulatory T Cell Isolation Kit, human, (Miltenyi Biotec, Bergisch Gladbach, Germany). All reagents should be stored at 4 °C. The kit includes a cocktail of biotinylated antibodies and Anti-Biotin MicroBeads for depletion of non-$CD4^+$ T cells and Anti-Biotin MicroBeads and CD25 MicroBeads for subsequent positive selection of the $CD4^+CD25^+$ cells. The $CD4^+CD25^+$ Regulatory T Cell Isolation Kit (Miltenyi Biotec) was developed for the isolation of $CD4^+CD25^+$ T cells from peripheral blood mononuclear cells (PBMC).

    Reagents not included: MACS buffer (prepare a solution with 1× PBS, 1 mM ETDA, and 1 % FCS; filter and keep cold (2–8 °C)) (*see* **Note 1**). Pre-separation filters, 30 μm (Miltenyi Biotec), and columns (Miltenyi Biotec) (Table 2).
16. DynaBeads® CD3/CD28 T cell Expander.
17. CellTrace™ CFSE Cell Proliferation Kit for flow cytometry includes CellTrace™ CFSE (Component A), ten vials, each containing 50 μg of lyophilized powder, and DMSO (Component B), one vial containing 0.5 mL of high-quality DMSO. Store desiccated at ≤−20 °C until required for use.

Avoid repeated freezing and thawing. Before opening the vial, allow the product to warm to room temperature. Briefly, CFSE passively diffuses into cells. It is colorless and not fluorescent until the acetate groups are cleaved by intracellular esterases to yield highly fluorescent CFSE. The succinimidyl ester group reacts with intracellular amines, forming fluorescent conjugates that are well retained and can be fixed with aldehyde fixatives. The label is inherited by daughter cells after either cell division or cell fusion and is not transferred to adjacent cells in a population.

3 Methods

3.1 Isolation of Human PBMC by Ficoll-Paque™ Gradient Centrifugation

The following protocol has been optimized for the purification of PBMC from peripheral blood samples:

1. Place fresh blood (*see* **Note 2**) into 50-mL conical tubes and dilute 1:2 with RPMI-1640 medium.
2. Slowly layer 30–35 mL of diluted blood over 15 mL of Ficoll-Paque™ in a 50-mL conical tube.
3. Centrifuge at 350–400 × *g* for 35 min at 20 °C without applying the brake.
4. Aspirate the upper layer, containing the plasma and most of the platelets, leaving the mononuclear cell layer (lymphocytes, monocytes, and thrombocytes) undisturbed at the interphase.
5. Using another pipette, carefully transfer the mononuclear cell layer to new 50-mL centrifuge tubes (*see* **Note 3**).
6. Wash cells by filling the conical tube with RPMI-1640 medium and centrifuge at 400 × *g* for 10 min at 4 °C, with the brake. Carefully remove the supernatant.
7. For removal of platelets, resuspend the cells in RPMI-1640 medium and centrifuge at 200 × *g* for 10 min.
8. If the mononuclear cell layer is contaminated with red blood cells, a lysing step with ACK Lysing Buffer may be required. Resuspend cell pellet in 10 mL of ACK Lysing Buffer and incubate on ice for no longer than 8 min (*see* **Note 4**).
9. Wash with complete RPMI-1640 medium supplemented with 10 % heat-inactivated HS. Centrifuge for 10 min at 400 × *g* and discard supernatant.
10. Resuspend the cell pellet in complete RPMI-1640 medium plus 10 % HS.
11. Count the cells and determine viability by Trypan blue exclusion (*see* **Note 5**).

3.2 Staining and Gating Strategy for Data Analysis

The following section describes how to perform both surface and intracellular staining of key molecules that allow the monitoring of Treg in human PBMC.

3.2.1 Cell Staining

All staining should be performed at 4 °C with minimal exposure to light.

1. Add a cell suspension of PBMC or tumor-infiltrating lymphocytes (TIL) (*see* Subheading 3.1) containing 10^6 cells to each tube.
2. Wash the cells with cold PBS (*see* **Note 6**). Discard the supernatant by rapid inversion of the tubes.
3. Resuspend the cells in 1 mL of PBS.
4. Add 1 μL of reconstituted viability dye (LIVE/DEAD Violet Fixable Staining Kit).
5. Incubate on ice for 30 min. Tubes must be kept in the dark.
6. Wash cells with cold PBS to remove the excess of reactive dye.
7. Centrifuge samples at 300–400 × *g* at 4 °C for 8 min, and discard supernatant.
8. Start staining procedures to the remaining volume of cell suspension. Leave one sample unstained; this will be used to define the background fluorescence. Prepare single-stain "compensation controls" for each fluorochrome used in the experiment (*see* **Note 7**). To determine the degree of background caused by nonspecific binding of the heavy chain of the antibody, stain one sample with appropriate intra- and extra-isotype controls. Add directly conjugated primary antibody for surface markers: anti-CD3, anti-CD4, anti-CD25, and anti-CD45RA according to manufacturer's instructions (*see* **Notes 8–11**).
9. Incubate for 30 min in the dark.
10. Wash cells with cold PBS.
11. Resuspend the cell pellet with pulse vortex and add 1 mL of freshly prepared fixation/permeabilization working solution to each sample. Pulse vortex again.
12. Incubate at 4 °C for 40 min in the dark.
13. Centrifuge 8 min at 400 × *g* at 4 °C.
14. Wash 1× by adding 4 mL of 1× Permeabilization Buffer followed by centrifugation and decanting of supernatant.
15. Add anti-human Foxp3 (clone PCH101, eBioscience) antibody or the corresponding isotype control (Rat IgG2a), vortex, and incubate at 4 °C for 30 min in the dark.
16. Wash cells with 4 mL of 1× Permeabilization Buffer. Centrifuge and decant supernatant.

17. Resuspend stained cells in 250 μL of cold PBS. Keep cell suspension at 4 °C in the dark until analyzed by flow cytometry. Fixed cells should be read within 24 h.

3.2.2 Flow Cytometry Acquisition

1. For cytometer setup, run the unstained fixed sample and adjust forward scatter (FS) and side scatter (SS) parameter voltages to clearly visualize the lymphocytes population (*see* **Note 12**).
2. Gate the lymphocyte population.
3. On the unstained sample, establish levels of background fluorescence (autofluorescence) by adjusting the voltages such that the unstained cells appear in the first decade of a logarithmic scale for each fluorochrome to be measured.
4. To determine compensation values, spectral overlap values are measured for all fluorophores via single-sample controls in every detector. To measure spectral overlap values, run single-color tubes where cells are stained with each fluorochrome-labeled CD4 separately (or single-stained BD CompBeads™) (*see* **Note 7**).
5. Once FS/SS voltages are set and compensation samples are run; the experimental samples can be collected and analyzed.

3.2.3 Gating Strategy for Data Analysis

This section describes how to perform analysis of the compensated data collected for human Treg identification. For this purpose, we use the FlowJo™ data analysis package (http://www.Treestar.com) or Kaluza software (Beckman Coulter). Figure 1 shows an example of the 5-color stain combination and the recommended gating strategy.

1. Start with gating the lymphocyte population (a).
2. Remove large clumps of cells (cell duplets) visualizing the gated lymphocytes on an FS-INT/FS-PEAK dot plot (b).
3. Gate out dead cells identifying them on an SS-INT/LIVE/DEAD dye dot plot (c). Dead cells nonspecifically trap fluorochrome-conjugated antibodies. Therefore, it is imperative to include stains that enable elimination of dead cells during FACS analysis. The LIVE/DEAD viable dye is based on the covalent reaction of the fluorescent reactive dye with cellular proteins. Since the dye cannot penetrate the cell membrane in viable cells, only the surface proteins are available to react with the dye, while in case of damaged membranes, it stains both the interior of the cell and the cell surface. This will result in a difference in fluorescence intensity between live (weak staining) and dead cell (bright staining) allowing their simultaneous discrimination. This discrimination is completely preserved following sample fixation.
4. Within the live cells, create a gate for the $CD3^+CD4^+$ population (d).

5. Set the CD25^{neg} population based on the CD4 vs. CD25 expression (e).
6. Set the negative Foxp3 marker in the gated CD25^{neg} population (f).
7. Use this marker to detect the percentage of the Foxp3 population in CD25^{hi} (g) (*see* **Note 13**). Based on this marker, set the CD25^{hi} region in order to achieve a positivity of Foxp3 expression more than >90 % (e).
8. Visualize the CD4 vs. Foxp3 dot plot within CD3^{+}CD4^{+} cells and gate the Foxp3^{+} cells (h).
9. In the selected Foxp3^{+} cells, analyze the CD25 vs. CD45RA expression defining three different subsets (i): the activated Treg (CD45RA^{neg}CD25^{hi}), the resting Treg (CD45RA^{+}CD25^{int}), and the conventional T cells (CD45RA^{neg}CD25^{int}). Set the marker for CD25 and CD45RA positivity based on the isotype control and the CD25^{hi} marker as defined in (e).

3.3 Functional Assessment of Treg

3.3.1 Intracellular Staining for Immunosuppressive Cytokines Production (Stimulation)

1. Resuspend isolated Treg (see Subheading 3.4) or PBMC in Treg medium and seed them in 48-well plates at a concentration of 10^6/mL.
2. Add 1 μL/mL of anti-CD3/CD28 beads (DynaBeads® CD3/CD28 T cell Expander) and mix thoroughly.
3. After 1–2 h of stimulation, add 0.7 μL/mL of GolgiStop protein transport inhibitor and mix thoroughly (*see* **Note 14**).

3.3.2 Intracellular Staining for Immunosuppressive Cytokines Production (Staining)

1. Harvest and wash cells with cold PBS (*see* **Note 6**), and pellet by centrifugation for 8 min at 250×*g* at 4 °C.
2. Place 10^6 cells/tube and stain them with LIVE/DEAD dye; *see* Subheading 3.2.1.
3. Stain surface molecules with anti-CD3, anti-CD25, anti-CD4, anti-CD45RA, or isotype controls according to manufacturer's instruction (*see* **Note 10**).
4. Wash with cold PBS and pellet by centrifugation for 8 min at 250×*g* at 4 °C.
5. Decant the supernatant and resuspend cells in 250 μL of BD Cytofix/Cytoperm solution for 20 min at 4 °C.
6. Wash cells 2× in 1 mL of 1× BD Perm/Wash solution.
7. Resuspend fixed/permeabilized cells in 50 μL of BD Perm/Wash solution containing a fluorochrome-conjugated anti-cytokine antibody or isotype controls (IL-10, TGFβ1) according to manufacturer's instructions (*see* **Notes 15** and **16**).
8. Incubate at 4 °C for 30 min protected from light.

9. Wash cells in 1 mL of 1× BD Perm/Wash solution and resuspend in 200 μL of PBS prior to flow cytometric analysis (for Treg gating strategy, follow the instructions described in Subheading 3.2.3 and analyze the cytokines expression within the gated Treg population).

3.4 Immuno magnetic Treg Isolation

Cell sample: PBMC isolated by human peripheral blood are used as starting material.

The isolation of $CD4^+CD25^+$ Treg is performed in a 2-step procedure: negative selection of $CD4^+$ (Subheadings 3.4.1 and 3.4.2) and positive selection of $CD25^+$ cells (Subheadings 3.4.3 and 3.4.4) using the human $CD4^+CD25^+$ Regulatory T Cell Isolation Kit. Work fast, keep cells cold, and use precooled solutions.

3.4.1 Magnetic Labeling of Non-$CD4^+$ Cells

1. Determine cell number (*see* **Notes 3** and **17**).
2. Centrifuge cell suspension at 300 × *g* for 10 min at 4 °C.
3. Pipette off supernatant completely.
4. Resuspend the cell pellet in 90 μL of MACS buffer per 10^6 cells.
5. Add 10 μL of Biotin-Antibody Cocktail per 10^6 cells.
6. Mix well and incubate for 10 min at 4 °C in the dark.
7. Add 20 μL of Anti-Biotin MicroBeads per 10^6 cells.
8. Mix well and incubate for an additional 15 min at 4 °C in the dark.
9. Wash cells by adding 10–20× labeling volume of buffer and centrifuge at 300 × *g* for 10 min at 4 °C.
10. Resuspend the cell pellet in 500 μL of MACS buffer per10^7 cells.
11. Proceed to magnetic separation.

3.4.2 Magnetic Separation of the $CD4^+$ Fraction

1. Place column (MS or LS, based on the cells number) (Table 2) in the magnetic field of the MACS separator and prepare the column by rinsing with the appropriate volume of MACS buffer (*see* **Note 18**).
2. Apply the cell suspension onto the prepared column.
3. Wash column 3× with 3 mL of MACS buffer to collect total unlabeled effluent cell fraction.
4. Collect unlabeled $CD4^+$ cells which pass through in a separate tube.
5. Rapidly count cells and pellet them by centrifugation at 300 × *g* for 10 min.
6. Resuspend the cell pellet in 500 μL of MACS buffer per 10^7 cells.

7. Place LD column in the magnetic field and prewash column with 1 mL of MACS buffer.
8. Apply cell suspension onto the prepared column.
9. Wash column 2× with 1 mL of MACS buffer to collect total unlabeled effluent cell fraction (*see* **Note 19**).
10. Collect unlabeled CD4 cells which pass through.

3.4.3 Positive Selection of $CD4^+CD25^+$ Regulatory T Cells

1. Determine cell number (*see* **Note 20**).
2. Centrifuge cell suspension at 300×g for 10 min.
3. Pipette off supernatant completely.
4. Resuspend cell pellet in 90 μL of buffer per 10^6 cells.
5. Add 10 μL per 10^6 cells of CD25 MicroBeads. Mix well and incubate for 15 min at 4 °C in the dark.
6. Wash cells by adding 10–20× labeling volume of buffer and centrifuge at 300×g for 10 min at 4 °C.
7. Resuspend the cell pellet in 500 μL of MACS buffer (500 μL/10^7 cells).
8. Proceed to magnetic separation.

3.4.4 Magnetic Separation of the $CD4^+CD25^+$ Fraction

1. Place MS column in the magnetic field of the MACS separator and prepare the column by rinsing with 0.5 mL of MACS buffer.
2. Apply cell suspension onto the prepared column.
3. Wash column 3× with 0.5 mL of MACS buffer to collect total unlabeled effluent cell fraction.
4. Collect unlabeled $CD4^+CD25^-$ cells which pass through in a separate tube.
5. Remove column from the separator and place it on a new collection tube.
6. Pipette 1 mL of MACS buffer onto the column and immediately flush out fraction with the magnetically labeled cells by firmly applying the plunger supplied with the column (these cells are the $CD4^+CD25^+$ fraction).
7. Place a new MS column and repeat the same procedure described above with the $CD4^+CD25^+$ fraction (*see* **Note 21**).
8. To enrich the $CD25^{neg}$ fraction, allow it to pass through onto a new LD column; see Subheading 3.4.2, steps 7–9.
9. Collect unlabeled $CD4^+CD25^-$ cells which pass through in a separate tube (*see* **Notes 21** and **22**).

3.4.5 Check the Purity of the $CD4^+CD25^+$ and $CD4^+CD25^-$ Fractions

1. Stain:
   (a) 50,000 cells with isotype controls to set physical parameter and negative fluorescence

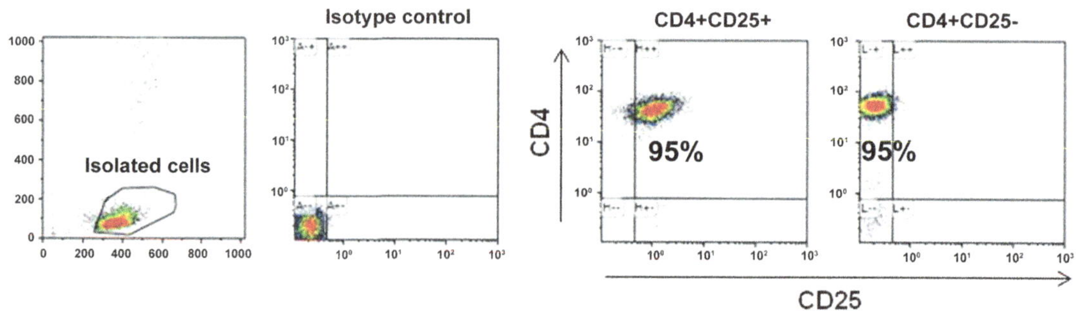

Fig. 2 Purity check after immunomagnetic separation. CD4$^+$CD25$^+$ regulatory T cells were isolated from human PBMC using the CD4$^+$CD25$^+$ Regulatory T Cell Isolation Kit. Both the CD25$^+$ and CD25^{neg} fraction were stained with anti-CD4 and CD25 mAbs and analyzed by FACS. Cell debris and dead cells are excluded from the analysis based on scattered signals. The marker for CD25 and CD4 positivity is set based on the isotype control. The *percentages* reported in graph indicate cell purity

(b) 50,000 CD25$^-$ fraction with anti-CD4 and anti-CD25 antibodies

(c) 50,000 CD25$^+$ fraction with the same combination of anti-CD4 and anti-CD25 antibodies (*see* **Note 23**).

2. Set FACS and start acquisition (expected purity ≥95 %) (Fig. 2).

3.5 In Vitro Inhibition Assays for Treg Functions: CFSE Staining Procedure

3.5.1 CFSE Staining

1. Prepare a 5 mM stock solution immediately prior to use by dissolving the content of a CFSE vial (Component A) in 18 μL of DMSO (Component B). CellTrace™ CFSE Cell Proliferation Kit for flow cytometry.
2. Dilute CFSE at a final concentration of 50 μM (1:100) in complete RPMI-1640 medium with 5 % FBS.
3. Resuspend CD25$^-$ lymphocytes in a 50-mL conical bottom tube at 10^6/mL (minimum volume 1 mL, scale up in case of higher cell number) in complete RPMI-1640 medium with 5 % FBS and label them with CFSE at a final concentration of 5 μM (1:10). Gently vortex (*see* **Note 24**).
4. Incubate the cells at 37 °C for 15 min (*see* **Note 25**).
5. Block immediately with the same volume of cold FBS and spin with complete RPMI-1640 medium with 10 % FBS by filling the conical tube.
6. Centrifuge the cells 5 min at 300 × *g*. Discard supernatant and vortex pellet to obtain single cell suspension. Wash at least 2× (*see* **Note 26**).
7. Check the staining by microscopy using standard fluorescein filter or flow cytometer (488-nm excitation source) (Ex/Em of CFSE 492/517 nm) and resuspend cells in Treg culture medium (*see* **Note 27**).

8. Set up in vitro cell cultures under appropriate conditions (*see* **Note 28**).
9. Harvest cells and stain for other markers if necessary (*see* **Note 29**).
10. Analyze using a flow cytometer with 488-nm excitation and emission filters appropriate for fluorescein.

3.5.2 Immuno-suppression Assay

1. Label responder cells (autologous-isolated $CD4^{+}CD25^{-}$ or total PBMC) with CFSE.
2. Seed cells in a round bottom 96-well plate, at least in triplicates:
   (a) Effector cells: seed sorted $CD4^{+}CD25^{+}$ Treg in decreasing number (ratio to 1:1 until at least 1:32 responder to effector cells), volume 90 μL/well.
   (b) Responder cells: seed the same number of cells in each well, generally 50,000 cells in a volume of 90 μL/well.
   (c) Stimulate with anti-CD3/CD28 beads. Prepare a working dilution (mix 14.5 μL in 2 mL of Treg medium) and add 20 μL/well.
   (d) Final volume of 200 μL in Treg medium.

   Recommended controls:
   (a) Responder cells only: 50,000 cells in 90 μL plus 110 μL of medium, both labeled and unlabeled.
   (b) Responder cells: 50,000 cells in 90 μL plus 90 μL of medium, both labeled and unlabeled, plus 20 μL of anti-CD3/CD28 working dilution.
   (c) (Optional) Responder T cells: 50,000 cells in 90 μL plus 90 μL of medium, both labeled and unlabeled, plus 20 μL of anti-CD3/CD28 working dilution plus 100 UI/mL of IL-2 (*see* **Note 30**).
3. After 3–5 days, when stimulated control responder cells have proliferated, harvest cells and analyze them directly by flow cytometry. Cells can be analyzed in their culture medium without washing. If fluorescent antibody staining is required, perform this as normal (*see* **Note 31**).

3.5.3 FACS Acquisition and Analysis

CFSE has to be read as FITC, 488 nm excitation (*see* Fig. 3).

1. Adjust FS/SS settings to clearly see the lymphocyte gate.
2. Visualize unstimulated CFSE-labeled responder cells between the 10^2 and 10^3 decade of Log on the X-axis. These cells provide a fluorescence measurement of nondividing lymphocytes.
3. Set the negative/autofluorescence of the activated lymphocytes population with unlabeled stimulated $CD25^{neg}$ or $CD25^{+}$ when available (*see* **Note 32**).

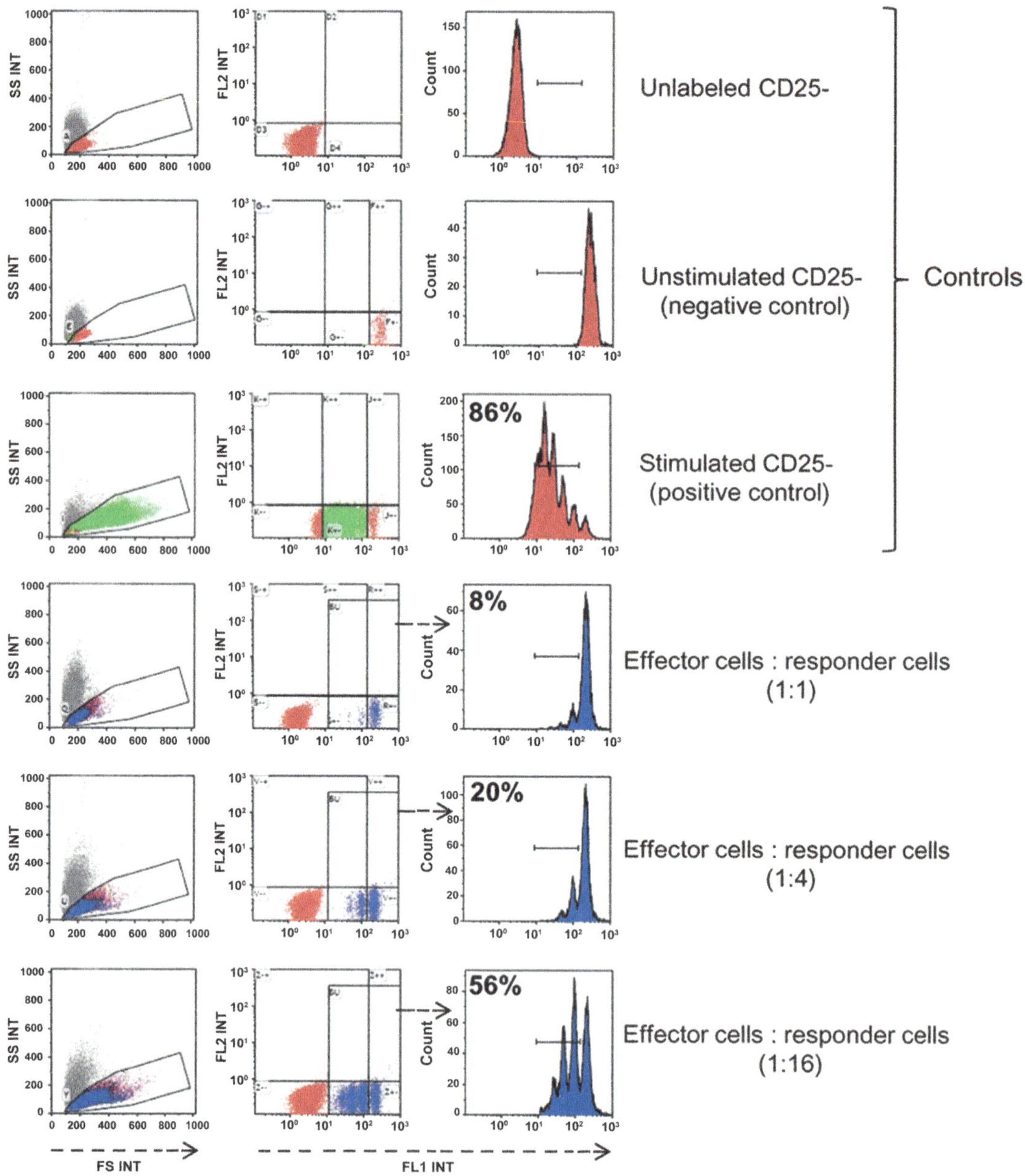

Fig. 3 CFSE FACS analysis. CFSE-labeled $CD4^+CD25^-$ T cells were stimulated with anti-CD3/CD28 beads and assessed for proliferative capacity after 72 h in the presence of autologous Treg. The *upper histograms* represent the controls: unlabeled $CD4^+CD25^{neg}$ T cells, CFSE-labeled unstimulated $CD4^+CD25^{neg}$ T cells, and CFSE-labeled stimulated $CD4^+CD25^{neg}$ T cells. The *lower histograms* show the proliferation of CFSE-labeled $CD4^+CD25^{neg}$ T cells (responder cells) in the presence of different ratio of autologous Treg (effector cells). Gating strategy: gate lymphocytes, and then, based on the CFSE-positive and CFSE-negative expression, exclude the Treg (unlabeled effector cells), and gate the CFSE-positive cells (responder cells). Their proliferation percentage is calculated inside this gate. The marker is drawn between the first pick on the *right* (not proliferated cells, negative control) and the end of the maximum cell proliferation (positive control)

4. Acquire all samples.
5. The total number of responder cells that have undergone divisions can be calculated by a curve-fitting software or as % of positive cells gated between un-proliferated (step 2) and unlabeled (step 3) markers. The percentage of inhibition of proliferation is calculated as follows:

   % of inhibition = 100 × [1 − (mean proliferation (responder and effectors)/mean proliferation (responder only with beads))] (*see* **Note 33**).

4 Notes

1. Buffer content has been changed to improve cell viability.
2. This protocol is intended to use for patient or healthy donor (HD) blood samples; however, it could be also adapted for the purification of PBMC from buffy coat. Blood samples should be stored at room temperature (18–25 °C) before processing.
3. Be aware that you do not aspirate the Ficoll-Paque™ PLUS solution at this step. Ficoll contamination could interfere with secondary immunomagnetic purification of Treg.
4. The volume of ACK Lysing Buffer should be decided on the basis of pellet dimension/cell number.
5. Viability of the cell suspension is better maintained by keeping cells in a container with crushed ice. This will also reduce loss of cells that have a tendency to "stick" to plastic.
6. If using a viability dye, avoid buffers or solutions containing sodium azide or extraneous proteins, i.e., serum, for cell suspension or washing.
7. We usually perform single-stain samples using anti-CD4 antibodies for each fluorochrome that allow detecting both a negative and a bright positive signal within the lymphocyte gate. However, to optimize fluorescence compensation settings, you can also use BD CompBeads™. The advantage is that the spectral overlap determination can be performed using antibodies identical to those used in the experiments or the corresponding isotype controls. In fact, BD CompBeads™ are beads that have been coupled to an antibody specific for the kappa light chain of Ig from rat or mouse. These beads are easy to stain and have a robust fluorescence signal regardless to the kappa antibody conjugate, thus ensuring a good spectral overlap determination.
8. We highly recommend performing titration of antibodies for optimal staining in your own assay system.
9. This 4-color surface staining combination may be implemented by adding other surface markers that have been related to the Treg phenotype, such as CD127 or co-stimulatory

molecules (for more details, see the Introduction) or intracellular cytokines (*see* **Note 16**).

10. We recommend choosing the appropriate fluorochrome based on the level of antigen expression. You should prefer brighter fluorochrome for dimly expressed antigen or for antigens expressed only on rare cell population.

11. You may also need to include a fluorescence-minus-one (FMO) control, particularly when dimly fluorescing antigens have to be detected within the Treg subset. The FMO control reveals the maximum fluorescence expected for a given subset in a given channel when the reagent used in the channel is omitted from the stain set. In fact, defining the boundary between positive and negative cells has always been a challenge when dully staining subsets need to be resolved. Thus, this control allows a simple decision as to where to place the upper boundary for nonstaining cells in the channel.

12. The light-scatter profiles of the cells on the flow cytometer will change considerably after the permeabilization step; thus, it is important to treat all tubes (controls and samples) in the same way. The permeabilization step will also lead to a loss of discrimination between live and dead cells. Therefore, a viability dye is fundamental to identify dead cells by fluorescence staining and exclude them in FACS analysis.

13. We suggest that biological comparison controls, such as Foxp3 expression within the CD25^{neg} population vs. CD25^{pos} one, are usually the most relevant control for determining positivity of the subpopulation of interest. This is because the internal biological control accounts for spillover effects on the channel of interest by including all of the antibody conjugates present in the sample. And, like an isotype control, it accounts for nonspecific staining in the channel of interest.

    In the context of stimulation assays (*see* Subheading 3.3.1), the unstimulated (or irrelevantly stimulated) sample could be used to distinguish positive from negative events beside the appropriate isotype control tube.

14. Be careful in choosing GolgiStop (monensin) or GolgiPlug (brefeldin A) based on the cytokines to be studied; monensin is recommended for IL-10.

15. For the detection of other cytokines, for example, IL-2, IFN-γ, and IL-17 (for more details, see Introduction), use the same protocol described.

16. If Foxp3 monoclonal antibody will be added, use the eBioscience buffers and protocol. The anti-cytokine antibody and anti-Foxp3 antibody can be added together; *see* Subheading 3.3.2.

17. It is very important that cells do not contain platelets and that the correct starting number is determined.

18. Use pre-separation filters to remove cell clumps that could affect cell separation purity and recovery.
19. This second passage on LD column allows a better purity of the recovered $CD4^+$ T cells.
20. It is crucial to precisely count the $CD4^+$ cells. To use the right volume of MACS buffer and CD25 MicroBeads, we highly recommend considering 10 % more than the counted cell number.
21. This second passage has been added to increase cell purity.
22. Another method to isolate Treg for further analysis consists in the use of a flow cytometer able to physically sort cells based on the combination of different fluorochrome-conjugated antibodies. This technique allows the addition of further superficial markers other than CD4 and CD25.
23. It is highly recommended to choose fluorochromes that do not need to be compensated; otherwise, use single-color controls or BD CompBeads™ to set the compensation.
24. Do not label with more than 5 μM CFSE if you want to look at cell division after 1–2 days. For longer time points, you can increase the CFSE concentration up to 10 μM. Usually, to inhibit CD25 proliferation, Treg take 3–5 days.
25. Gently vortex cells for 5 min; it is very important to have a uniform cell labeling.
26. Washing the cells more than 2× helps to produce a tighter initial CFSE peak.
27. It is important to count cells after coloration. Do not allow the labeled cells to stay without light protection or you will lose the sharpness of the staining.
28. Set immediately the test to avoid that $CD25^-$ could start to proliferate.
29. Positive and negative controls in the test are mandatory to choose the convenient time to harvest the cells; see suppression assay for details.
30. When cell number is not limited, set the same controls also with effector cells, especially to check their viability.
31. Since during prolonged culture periods, cells could die, to assess cell death, add viability dye (*see* Subheading 3.2.1) compatible with fluorescent antibody staining.
32. If cells have to be stained with other antibodies, it is important to have CFSE cultures without antibody as well as unlabeled cultures with antibody to be able to set the correct compensations, especially between FL-1 (CFSE)- and PE-labeled antibody (FL-2); in fact, CFSE has a strong peak

fluorescence intensity at 517 nm, which precludes the use of similar fluorescent conjugates.

33. If last cell divisions are hardly detectable because labeled cells appear above the autofluorescence of unlabeled cells, the amount of CFSE used should be increased in order to maximize the number of detectable cell divisions.

References

1. Ghiringhelli F et al (2004) $CD4^+CD25^+$ regulatory T cells suppress tumor immunity but are sensitive to cyclophosphamide which allows immunotherapy of established tumors to be curative. Eur J Immunol 34:336–344
2. Lutsiak M et al (2005) Inhibition of $CD4^+25^+$ T regulatory cell function implicated in enhanced immune response by low-dose cyclophosphamide. Blood 105:2862–2868
3. Ghiringhelli F et al (2007) Metronomic cyclophosphamide regimen selectively depletes $CD4^+CD25^+$ regulatory T cells and restores T and NK effector functions in end stage cancer patients. Cancer Immunol Immunother 56:641–648
4. Slingluff CL et al (2011) Randomized multicenter trial of the effects of melanoma-associated helper peptides and cyclophosphamide on the immunogenicity of a multipeptide melanoma vaccine. J Clin Oncol 29:2924–2932
5. Ge Y et al (2012) Metronomic cyclophosphamide treatment in metastasized breast cancer patients: immunological effects and clinical outcome. Cancer Immunol Immunother 61:353–362
6. Jacobs JF et al (2010) Dendritic cell vaccination in combination with anti-CD25 monoclonal antibody treatment: a phase I/II study in metastatic melanoma patients. Clin Cancer Res 16:5067–5078
7. Rech AJ, Vonderheide RH (2009) Clinical use of anti-CD25 antibody daclizumab to enhance immune responses to tumor antigen vaccination by targeting regulatory T cells. Ann N Y Acad Sci 1174:99–106
8. Mahnke K et al (2007) Depletion of $CD4^+CD25^+$ human regulatory T cells in vivo: kinetics of treg depletion and alterations in immune functions in vivo and in vitro. Int J Cancer 120:2723–2733
9. Attia P et al (2005) Inability of a fusion protein of IL-2 and diphtheria toxin (denileukin diftitox, DAB389IL-2, ONTAK) to eliminate regulatory T lymphocytes in patients with melanoma. J Immunother 28:582–592
10. Morse MA et al (2008) Depletion of human regulatory T cells specifically enhances antigen-specific immune responses to cancer vaccines. Blood 112:610–618
11. Dannull J et al (2005) Enhancement of vaccine-mediated antitumor immunity in cancer patients after depletion of regulatory T cells. J Clin Invest 115:3623–3633
12. Powell DJ et al (2007) Administration of a CD25-directed immunotoxin, LMB-2, to patients with metastatic melanoma induces a selective partial reduction in regulatory T cells in vivo. J Immunol 179:4919–4928
13. Powell DJ et al (2008) Partial reduction of human $FOXP3^+$ CD4 T cells in vivo after CD25-directed recombinant immunotoxin administration. J Immunother 31:189–198
14. Menard C et al (2008) Ctla-4 blockade confers lymphocyte resistance to regulatory T-cells in advanced melanoma: surrogate marker of efficacy of tremelimumab? Clin Cancer Res 14:5242–5249
15. Ralph C et al (2010) Modulation of lymphocyte regulation for cancer therapy: a phase II trial of tremelimumab in advanced gastric and esophageal adenocarcinoma. Clin Cancer Res 16:1662–1672
16. Finke JH et al (2008) Sunitinib reverses type-1 immune suppression and decreases T-regulatory cells in renal cell carcinoma patients. Clin Cancer Res 14:6674–6682
17. Adotevi O et al (2010) A decrease of regulatory T cells correlates with overall survival after sunitinib-based antiangiogenic therapy in metastatic renal cancer patients. J Immunother 33:991–998
18. Desar I et al (2011) Sorafenib reduces the percentage of tumour infiltrating regulatory T cells in renal cell carcinoma patients. Int J Cancer 129:507–512
19. Balachandran VP et al (2011) Imatinib potentiates antitumor T cell responses in gastrointestinal stromal tumor through the inhibition of ido. Nat Med 17:1094–1100

20. Jordan JT et al (2008) Preferential migration of regulatory T cells mediated by glioma-secreted chemokines can be blocked with chemotherapy. Cancer Immunol Immunother 57:123–131
21. Baecher-Allan C et al (2005) Functional analysis of highly defined, FACS-isolated populations of human regulatory CD4+ CD25+ T cells. Clin Immunol 115:10–18
22. Liu W et al (2006) CD127 expression inversely correlates with FoxP3 and suppressive function of human CD4+ T reg cells. J Exp Med 203:1701–1711
23. Allan SE et al (2007) Activation-induced FOXP3 in human T effector cells does not suppress proliferation or cytokine production. Int Immunol 19:345–354
24. Miyara M et al (2009) Functional delineation and differentiation dynamics of human CD4+ T cells expressing the FoxP3 transcription factor. Immunity 30:899–911
25. Tosello V et al (2008) Differential expression of CCR7 defines two distinct subsets of human memory CD4+CD25+ Tregs. Clin Immunol 126:291–302
26. Baecher-Allan C et al (2006) MHC class II expression identifies functionally distinct human regulatory T cells. J Immunol 176:4622–4631
27. Ito T et al (2008) Two functional subsets of FOXP3+ regulatory T cells in human thymus and periphery. Immunity 28:870–880
28. Solstad T et al (2011) CD147 (Basigin/Emmprin) identifies FoxP3+CD45RO+CTLA4+-activated human regulatory T cells. Blood 118:5141–5151
29. Borsellino et al (2007) Expression of ectonucleotidase CD39 by Foxp3+ Treg cells: hydrolysis of extracellular ATP and immune suppression. Blood 110:1225–1232
30. Tran DQ et al (2009) GARP (LRRC32) is essential for the surface expression of latent TGF-beta on platelets and activated FOXP3+ regulatory T cells. Proc Natl Acad Sci USA 106:13445–13450
31. Camisaschi C et al (2010) LAG-3 expression defines a subset of CD4(+)CD25(high)Foxp3(+) regulatory T cells that are expanded at tumor sites. J Immunol 184:6545–6551
32. Bovenschen HJ et al (2011) Foxp3+ regulatory T cells of psoriasis patients easily differentiate into IL-17A-producing cells and are found in lesional skin. J Invest Dermatol 131:1853–1860
33. Raffin C et al (2011) Ex vivo IL-1 receptor type I expression in human CD4+ T cells identifies an early intermediate in the differentiation of Th17 from FOXP3+ naive regulatory T cells. J Immunol 187:5196–5202
34. Dominguez-Villar M et al (2011) Identification of T helper type 1-like, Foxp3+ regulatory T cells in human autoimmune disease. Nat Med 17:673–675
35. Baron U et al (2007) DNA demethylation in the human FOXP3 locus discriminates regulatory T cells from activated FOXP3(+) conventional T cells. Eur J Immunol 37:2378–2389
36. Wieczorek G et al (2009) Quantitative DNA methylation analysis of FOXP3 as a new method for counting regulatory T cells in peripheral blood and solid tissue. Cancer Res 69:599–608
37. de Vries IJ et al (2011) Frequency of circulating Tregs with demethylated FOXP3 intron 1 in melanoma patients receiving tumor vaccines and potentially Treg-depleting agents. Clin Cancer Res 17:841–848
38. Lucas S et al (2012) Demethylation of the FOXP3 gene in human melanoma cells precludes the use of this epigenetic mark for quantification of Treg in unseparated melanoma samples. Int J Cancer 130:1960–1966
39. Zheng SG et al (2004) Natural and induced CD4+CD25+ cells educate CD4+CD25- cells to develop suppressive activity: the role of IL-2, TGF-beta, and IL-10. J Immunol 172:5213–5221
40. Levings MK et al (2001) Human CD25(+)CD4(+) T regulatory cells suppress naive and memory T cell proliferation and can be expanded in vitro without loss of function. J Exp Med 193:1295–1302

Chapter 19

Cytokine Activation of Natural Killer Cells

Syh-Jae Lin, Pei-Tzu Lee, and Ming-Ling Kuo

Abstract

$CD3^-CD56^+$ natural killer (NK) cells can kill various tumors in a non major histocompatibility complex (MHC)-restricted fashion. Recent advances have been made in the application of NK cells for the treatment of patients with acute myelogenous leukemia (AML). Allogeneic donor-derived NK cells can be activated in vitro and infused into patients receiving stem cell transplants. We describe in this chapter the method to activate NK cells with cytokines and to ascertain their degree of activation.

Key words Natural killer cells, Cytokines, Interleukin-15

1 Introduction

Natural killer (NK) cells are a distinct lineage of lymphoid cells defined as membrane $CD3^-$, $CD16^+$, and/or $CD56^+$, which exert spontaneous cytotoxicity against a broad range of malignancies [1, 2] and are promising candidates for adoptive immunotherapy [3, 4]. Conventional NK activation protocols using interleukin-2 (IL-2) caused significant systemic toxicities, thus hampered their therapeutic applications [5]. Interleukin-15 (IL-15) is an IL-2-like gamma-chain signaling cytokine with the unique ability to not only enhance NK function but also promote NK differentiation and survival [6, 7]. IL-15 appears to be less toxic than IL-2 [8] and can prevent NK cell apoptosis [9]. In animal studies, IL-15 promoted a graft-versus-leukemia effect and immune reconstitution following bone marrow transplantation [10]. Therefore, IL-15 seems to be a valuable growth factor to support the generation of NK cells for cancer therapy. In this chapter, we describe the isolate and stimulate NK cells using cytokines.

Michael J.P. Lawman and Patricia D. Lawman (eds.), *Cancer Vaccines: Methods and Protocols*, Methods in Molecular Biology, vol. 1139, DOI 10.1007/978-1-4939-0345-0_19, © Springer Science+Business Media New York 2014

2 Materials

2.1 NK Cell Separation

1. Heparinized whole blood obtained using a vacutainer.
2. Ficoll-Hypaque (GE Healthcare Bio-Sciences AB, Uppsala, Sweden).
3. Hank's balanced salt solution (HBSS).
4. Dulbecco's phosphate-buffered saline (DPBS) at 4 °C.
5. Roswell Park Memorial Institute (RPMI)-1640 medium.
6. Fetal bovine serum (FBS).
7. Penicillin and streptomycin.
8. NK isolation buffer: phosphate-buffered saline (PBS), pH 7.2 containing 0.5 % BSA and 2 mM EDTA.
9. MACS NK cell isolation kit (Miltenyi Biotec, Bergisch Gladbach, Germany).
10. MACS LS separation columns (Miltenyi Biotec).
11. MACS separators (Miltenyi Biotec).
12. RBC lysis solution: 0.15 M NH_4Cl, 1.0 mM $KHCO_3$, and 0.1 mM Na_2-EDTA.

2.2 NK Cell Activation

1. Human recombinant IL-2 (PeproTech, Rocky Hill, NJ, USA).
2. Human recombinant IL-15 (PeproTech).

2.3 NK Cell Cytotoxic Activity

1. Target cell: K-562 (ATCC: CCL-243) or Daudi (ATCC: CCL-213).
2. Sodium chromate (^{51}Cr) (The Radiochemical Centre, Uppsala, Sweden).
3. RPMI-1640 medium.
4. Fluorescein isothiocyanate (FITC)-labeled anti-CD45 monoclonal antibodies (BD Biosciences, San Diego, CA, USA).
5. Propidium iodide (PI).
6. 12×75-mm round bottom polystyrene tubes.
7. TopCount NXT (Packard, Meriden, CT, USA).
8. FACSCanto II flow cytometry (BD Biosciences, San Jose, CA, USA).
9. 3 % Triton-X-100.

3 Methods

3.1 Peripheral Blood Mononuclear Cells (PBMC) Isolation

1. Transfer 10 mL fresh whole blood (*see* **Note 1**) from heparinized syringe to a 50-mL Falcon tube.
2. Add an equal volume of HBSS into the 50-mL Falcon tube containing whole blood. Mix by pipetting.

3. Add 10 mL Ficoll-Hypaque solution to a new 50-mL Falcon tube.
4. Gently layer 20 mL of the diluted blood sample onto Ficoll-Hypaque-containing tube.
5. Centrifuge at 1,000 × *g* for 15 min at 18–22 °C with the centrifuge brake off.
6. Draw off the upper layer using a clean dropper and transfer to a new 50-mL tube. Then, add HBSS to 40 mL in the tube (*see* **Note 2**).
7. Centrifuge at 400 × *g* for 5 min at room temperature.
8. Remove supernatant, then add 5 mL RBC lysis solution to the pellet, and mix by pipetting for 5 min (*see* **Note 3**).
9. Centrifuge at 400 × *g* for 5 min at room temperature.
10. Remove supernatant, and resuspend cells in 30 mL HBSS for wash.
11. Centrifuge at 400 × *g* for 5 min at room temperature.
12. Repeat **steps 10** and **11** for final wash.
13. Remove supernatant, and resuspend cells in complete RPMI-1640 medium. Count the cells [11–13].

3.2 NK Cell Separation

1. Separate PBMC from whole blood by Ficoll-Hypaque centrifugation.
2. Resuspend cell pellet in 40 μL of NK isolation buffer per 10^7 cells (*see* **Note 4**).
3. Add 10 μL of NK Cell Biotin-Antibody Cocktail (T cells, B cells, stem cells, dendritic cells, monocytes, granulocytes, and erythroid cells are indirectly magnetically labeled by using of biotin-conjugated antibodies) for 10^7 cells.
4. Mix well and refrigerate for 10 min at 4 °C.
5. Add 20 μL of NK Cell Biotin-Antibody Cocktail for 10^7 cells.
6. Mix well and refrigerate for an additional 15 min at 4 °C.
7. Wash cells by adding 1–2 mL of buffer per 10^7 total cells and centrifuge at 400 × *g* for 5 min at 4 °C.
8. Resuspend up to 10^8 cells in 500 μL of buffer.
9. Place the column in the magnetic field of a suitable MACS separator.
10. Rinse the column 2× with 3 mL of buffer.
11. Apply cell suspension onto the column.
12. Collect the unlabeled cells that pass through the column and wash the column 3× with ice-cold buffer.
13. Count the unlabeled cells. The purified NK cells are maintained in RPMI-1640 medium containing 10 % FBS. Analyze the purity of the NK cells by flow cytometry (Fig. 1) (*see* **Note 5**).

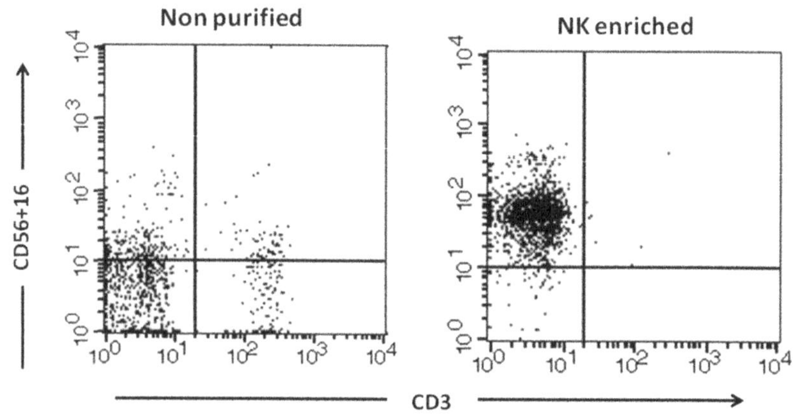

Fig. 1 Purified NK cell population by negative selection: Using magnetic beads through a series of negative selection process (to avoid inadvertent activation), we are successful in obtaining a highly purified (>90 %) NK cell (CD3$^-$/CD16 or 56$^+$) population from PBMC

3.3 NK Cell Activation

1. PBMC and purified NK cells were maintained in RPMI-1640 medium containing 10 % FBS (*see* **Note 6**).
2. 1×10^7/mL of PBMC and purified NK cells were incubated with 10 ng/mL IL-2 or 10 ng/mL IL-15 for 18 h (short term) or 1–4 weeks (long term) at 37 °C in a CO_2 incubator.
3. In long-term cultures, cytokines should be added every other day. Cells should be harvested and half of the medium may be replaced every 3 days (*see* **Note 7**).
4. Analyze the percentage of NK cells in PBMC cultures. Assess the functional marker on NK cells by flow cytometry [14–16] (*see* **Note 8**).

3.4 Assessment of NK Cell Cytotoxicity ^{51}Cr-Release Assay

1. 2×10^6/mL of K562 or Daudi target cells are suspended in PBS and incubated with 100 μCi of ^{51}Cr in a 37 °C water bath for 2 h with mixing every 15–20 min.
2. After 2 h, the chromated cells are washed 3× with RPMI-1640 medium containing 10 % FBS and resuspended at a concentration of 1×10^5/mL.
3. To achieve a 10:1 effector to target (E:T) ratio, 10^4 target cells in 100 μL (final concentration 5×10^4/mL) and 10^5 effectors are added to each well; 5×10^4/mL effectors are added for a 5:1 ratio; 10^4 effectors are added for a 1:1 ratio. The final volume is 0.2 mL for each well.
4. The plates containing target cells and effectors are centrifuged at 100 × g for 3–5 min and then incubated at 37 °C in a CO_2 incubator.

5. After 4 h, plates are centrifuged at 400 × g for 5 min. The culture supernatants are harvested and the ^{51}Cr release assessed using a TopCount NXT γ-scintillation counter.
6. Maximum release is determined by incubating target cells with 3 % Triton-X-100 and spontaneous release is determined by incubating the targets in medium alone [17–19].
7. The percent-specific lysis is calculated as follows:

$$\% \, lysis = 100 \times \frac{Mean\ experimental\ cpm - Mean\ spontaneous\ release\ cpm}{Mean\ maximal\ release\ cpm - Mean\ spontaneous\ release\ cpm}$$

3.5 Assessment of NK Cell Cytotoxicity by Flow Cytometric Analysis

1. 1×10^6/mL of K-562 target cells and 5×10^6/mL of NK effectors cells are resuspended with RPMI-1640 medium containing 10 % FBS in a 12 × 75-mm round bottom polystyrene tube.
2. To achieve a 5:1 effector to target (E:T) ratio, 2×10^5 target cells in 200 μL and 1×10^6 effectors are added to each tube; 5×10^5 effectors are added for a 2.5:1 ratio and 2×10^5 for a 1:1 ratio. The final volume is 0.4 mL for all tubes. Tubes are mixed by gently tapping and incubated at 37 °C in a CO_2 incubator.
3. Control tubes containing only target or effector cells are set up as background.
4. After incubation, 10 μL of FITC-CD45 are added to each tube. The tubes are then mixed gently and incubated for 20 min on ice.
5. Add PBS and wash 1×, and centrifuge at 400 × g for 5 min.
6. Remove the supernatant.
7. 20 μL of 1 μg/mL of PI is added to each tube 10 min before acquisition [20] (Fig. 2).

4 Notes

1. The blood samples should be stored at room temperature and processed within 24 h in the dark.
2. Resultant layers are approximately (from top to bottom): plasma—platelets—mononuclear cells—Ficoll—RBC (with granulocytes).
3. One may omit this step if the pellet looks clean. But if the cell pellet has a lot of RBC, RBC lysis buffer could be used until the pellet is clear.
4. Make sure the elution buffer is ice-cold throughout the process. The procedure of NK cell separation is following using the MACS NK isolation kit data sheet.

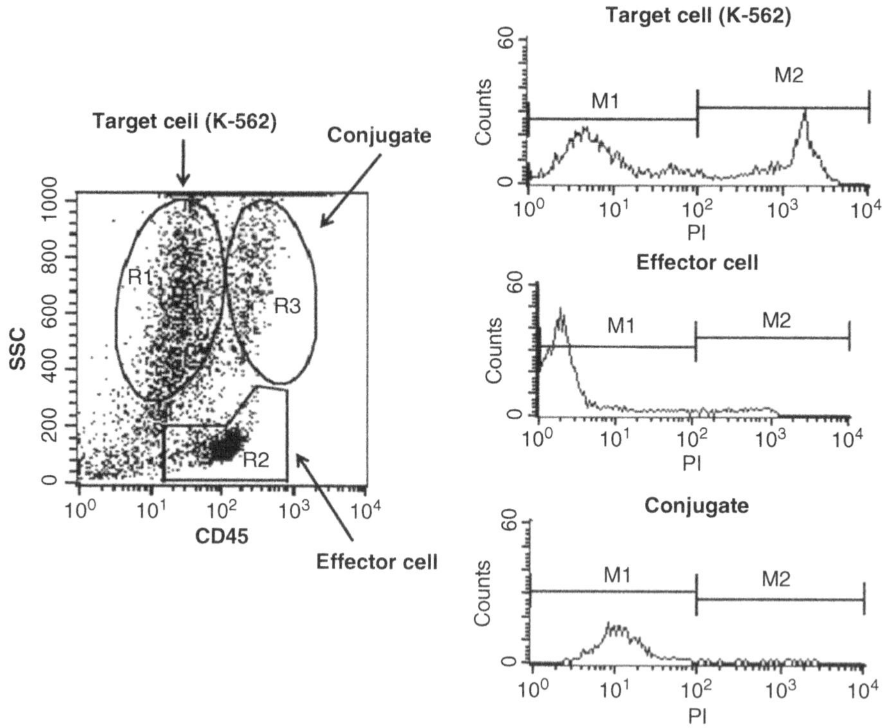

Fig. 2 Flow cytometric measurement of K-562 cytotoxicity of enriched NK cells using FITC-conjugated anti-CD45 staining and side scatter profiles to identify different cell populations and propidium iodide (PI) to detect dead cells. Target cells, NK cells, and NK-K-562 conjugates are identified by R1, R2, and R3. Percentages of dead cells in different regions are calculated from histograms showing PI uptake. *SSC* side scatter

5. The cells are stained with FITC- or phycoerythrin (PE)-conjugated mouse antihuman mAbs, anti-CD3/CD16+CD56, and assessed by flow cytometry.
6. We can also stimulate PBMC with cytokines to generate lymphokine-activated killer (LAK) cells, which are a mixture of T cells and NK cells displaying MHC-nonrestricted cytotoxicity.
7. The timing is arbitrary. It is advisable to change the media once it turns yellow.
8. The percentage of $CD3^{-}CD56^{+}$ NK cells in PBMC will increase upon cytokine stimulation. The activation marker of NK cells includes CD25, CD69, CD94, NKG2D, activating receptors, perforin, and granzyme.

References

1. Farag SS, Caligiuri MA (2006) Human natural killer cell development and biology. Blood Rev 20:123–137
2. Lin SJ, Kuo ML (2011) Cytotoxic function of umbilical cord blood natural killer cells: relevance to adoptive immunotherapy. Pediatr Hematol Oncol 28:640–646
3. Suck G (2006) Novel approaches using natural killer cells in cancer therapy. Semin Cancer Biol 16:412–418

4. McKenna DH et al (2007) Good manufacturing practices production of natural killer cells for immunotherapy: a six-year single-institution experience. Transfusion 47:520–528
5. Rosenberg SA et al (1989) Experience with the use of high-dose interleukin-2 in the treatment of 652 cancer patients. Ann Surg 210:474–484
6. Grabstein KH et al (1994) Cloning of a T cell growth factor that interacts with the beta chain of the interleukin-2 receptor. Science 264:965–968
7. Lin SJ et al (2008) Role of interleukin-15 in umbilical cord blood transplantation. Int Rev Immunol 27:518–531
8. Munger W et al (1995) Studies evaluating the antitumor activity and toxicity of interleukin-15, a new T cell growth factor: comparison with interleukin-2. Cell Immunol 165:289–293
9. Lin SJ, Kuo ML (2008) Effect of cyclosporin-A on interleukin-15 activated umbilical cord blood natural killer cell function. Cytotherapy 10:397–405
10. Alpdogan O, Eng JM et al (2005) Interleukin-15 enhances immune reconstitution after allogeneic bone marrow transplantation. Blood 105:865–873
11. Timonen T, Saksela E (1980) Isolation of human NK cells by density gradient centrifugation. J Immunol Methods 36:285–289
12. Boyum A (1968) Isolation of mononuclear cells and granulocytes form human blood. Scand J Clin Lab Invest 21(s97):77–89
13. Boyum A (1976) Isolation of lymphocytes, granulocytes and macrophages. Scand J Immunol 5(s5):9–15
14. Melder RJ et al (1991) Adhesion characteristics of human interleukin-2-actviated natural killer cells. Cell Immunol 132:177–192
15. Whiteside TL (1997) Isolation of human NK cells and generation of LAK activity. Curr Protoc Immunol 2:Unit 7.7
16. Grimm EA et al (1982) Lymphokine-activated killer cell phenomenon. Lysis of natural killer-resistant fresh solid tumor cells by interleukin 2-activated autologous human peripheral blood lymphocytes. J Exp Med 155: 1823–1841
17. Whiteside TL (1997) Measurement of cytotoxic activity of NK/LAK cells. Curr Protoc Immunol 2:Unit 7.18
18. Lin SJ et al (2000) Effect of interleukin-15 and Flt3-ligand on natural killer cell expansion and activation: umbilical cord vs. adult peripheral blood mononuclear cells. Pediatr Allergy Immunol 11:168–174
19. Oner O, Savasan S (2005) Combinational IL-2/IL-15 induction dose not future enhance IL-15-induced lymphokine-activated killer cell cytotoxicity against human leukemia/lymphoma cells. Clin Immunol 115:240–249
20. Lin SJ et al (2004) Evaluation of cytotoxic function and apoptosis in interleukin (IL)-12/ IL-15-treatedumbilical cord or adult peripheral blood natural killer cells by a propidium-iodide based flow cytometry. Pediatr Allergy Immunol 15:79–85

Part III

Manipulation and Modification of Tumor Cells

Chapter 20

Loading of Acute Myeloid Leukemia Cells with Poly(I:C) by Electroporation

Eva Lion, Charlotte M. de Winde, Viggo F.I. Van Tendeloo, and Evelien L.J.M. Smits

Abstract

In this chapter, we describe the technique of electroporation as an efficient method to load primary leukemic cells with the double-stranded RNA (dsRNA) analogue, polyriboinosinic polyribocytidylic acid (poly(I:C)), and detail on the delicate freezing and thawing procedure of primary leukemic cells.

Electroporation is a non-viral gene transfer method by which short-term pores in the membrane of cells are generated by an electrical pulse, allowing molecules to enter the cell. RNA electroporation, a technique developed in our laboratory, is a widely used and versatile transfection method for efficient introduction of both coding RNA (messenger RNA) and non-coding RNA, e.g., dsRNA and small interfering (siRNA), into mammalian cells. Accurate cell processing and storage of patient material is essential for optimal recovery and quality of the cell product for downstream applications.

Key words Electroporation, RNA, Poly(I:C), Adjuvant, Cancer cells, Patient specific

1 Introduction

Cancer cells express tumor-associated antigens (TAA). Nonetheless, in general, cancer cells can escape immune control. This can be partly explained by the lack of specific danger signals that trigger innate immune reactions via pattern recognition receptors (PRR), nor do cancer cells secrete inflammatory cytokines, such as tumor necrosis factor-alpha or type I interferons (IFNs), to alert immune cells of their presence. Enabling them to trigger PRR and/or to produce inflammatory cytokines can contribute to induction of effective anticancer immune responses and is therefore a promising strategy in cancer immunotherapy [1]. Bringing TAA in close proximity to danger signals might be a way to induce protective adaptive immune responses that target cancer cells, in this way breaking their immune escape.

Michael J.P. Lawman and Patricia D. Lawman (eds.), *Cancer Vaccines: Methods and Protocols*, Methods in Molecular Biology, vol. 1139, DOI 10.1007/978-1-4939-0345-0_20, © Springer Science+Business Media New York 2014

Several studies have underscored the potential role of PRR ligands and, in particular, synthetic double-stranded RNA (dsRNA) analogue polyriboinosinic polyribocytidylic acid (poly(I:C)), as a critical cancer vaccine component as it was shown to exert several antitumor functions. Poly(I:C) is a well-described danger signal (viral mimetic) that is able to trigger cell death and induce the production of proinflammatory cytokines, including type I IFNs in various cell types. Under defined conditions, poly(I:C) is a powerful natural killer (NK) cell activation signal [2–10], and it has been shown to efficiently activate and mature dendritic cells (DC) [11–16] and stimulate NK-DC interactions [2, 17, 18]. The synthetic dsRNA was also demonstrated to directly [19–22] and indirectly [23–26] promote cross-presentation of antigens by DC. However, a recent study reported an opposite inhibitory effect on cross-presentation [27]. Interestingly, different mouse in vivo and human in vitro studies demonstrated that tumor cell-associated poly(I:C) induced strong antitumor activity [23, 26, 28–30].

Macromolecules can be efficiently transferred into a cell through electroporation, a non-viral gene transfer method generating short-term pores in the cell membrane by an electrical pulse; *see* Fig. 1. Messenger RNA (mRNA) electroporation, a technique developed in our laboratory [31, 32], is now widely used and implemented as a transfection method, especially to load dendritic cells ex vivo with antigens and immunostimulatory molecules [33–38]. Moreover, this technique also allows the efficient introduction of non-coding RNA, e.g., dsRNA and siRNA, into cells [26, 39, 40]. The success of RNA transfection stems from its superior cytoplasmic expression efficiency, its simplicity over viral transduction protocols, and its clinical safety profile because of a strictly transient expression profile and the inability to integrate into the host genome [35].

We have demonstrated that electroporation with the dsRNA analogue poly(I:C) induces highly immunogenic cell death of acute myeloid leukemia (AML) cells, evidenced by their enhanced capacity to activate DC and NK cell functions [39–41]. AML is the most common type of acute leukemia in adults yet continues to have the lowest survival rate of all leukemias [42]. AML harbors a number of mechanisms to evade immune surveillance resulting in dysfunctional antileukemic immune responses unable to control tumor outgrowth [43]. The challenge in treating AML patients brought into complete remission by polychemotherapy is to clear low levels of persistent residual leukemia (stem) cells that are the central cause of relapse of the disease after standard chemotherapy. In this regard, immunotherapy is now being thoroughly investigated for its potential to fight residual leukemic cells [44, 45]. Here, we describe electroporation as an efficient method to load primary human AML cells with poly(I:C) and detail on the delicate freezing and thawing procedure of primary leukemic cells.

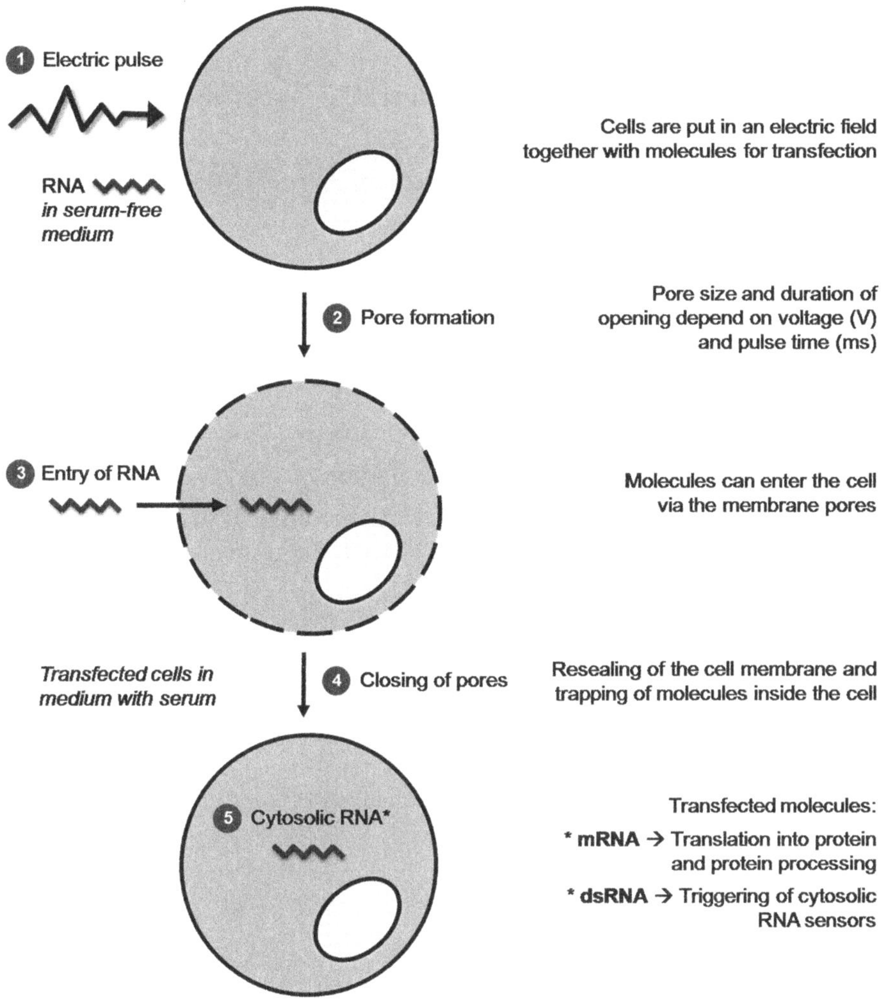

Fig. 1 Schematic overview of RNA electroporation

2 Materials

2.1 Freezing Primary AML Cells

1. Peripheral blood mononuclear cells (PBMC) isolated by gradient separation (*see* **Note 1**) from fresh heparinized blood collected from patients diagnosed with AML, i.e., primary AML cells.
2. Fetal bovine serum (FBS) (*see* **Note 2**).
3. Cryopreservation medium consisting of 80 % FBS + 20 % dimethylsulfoxide (DMSO) stored at 4 °C.
4. 2 mL cryopreservation tubes.
5. Cryofreezing container (cryo 1 °C freezing container, rate of cooling −1 °C/min).
6. Ficoll-Paque Plus (Amersham Biosciences, Uppsala, Sweden).

2.2 Thawing Primary AML Cells

1. 37 °C water bath.
2. Pre-warmed (37 °C) thawing medium: Iscove's modified Dulbecco's medium (IMDM) supplemented with 40 % FBS.
3. DNase.
4. Pre-warmed culture medium: IMDM supplemented with 10 % FBS.
5. 50-mL tubes.

2.3 Electroporation of Primary AML Cells with Poly(I:C)

1. Gene Pulser XCell Electroporation System for eukaryotic cells (includes a main unit, the CE module, and the ShockPod cuvette chamber (Bio-Rad, Hercules, CA, USA)).
2. 4-mm electroporation cuvette (1 per electroporation).
3. Serum-free IMDM medium.
4. Serum-free Opti-MEM medium without phenol red (Gibco, Life Technologies, Ghent, Belgium).
5. 1 μg/μL poly(I:C) working solution in RNase-free water (*see* **Note 3**) (InvivoGen, Toulouse, France).
6. Filter tips (*see* **Note 3**).
7. 50-mL tubes.
8. Transfer pipettes.
9. IMDM culture medium supplemented with 10 % FBS.

3 Methods

Carry out all procedures at room temperature unless specified otherwise. In order to maintain cell sterility, all procedures should be carried out in a laminar flow biosafety cabinet.

3.1 Freezing Primary AML Cells

1. Count the total primary AML cell (PBMC) number for cryopreservation.
2. Calculate the volume of cryopreservation medium required to give a final freezing density of 5×10^6 cells/mL up to 50×10^6 cells/1.5 mL.
3. Centrifuge cells once for 5 min at $450 \times g$.
4. Carefully take off the supernatant with a pipette without disturbing the cell pellet (*see* **Note 4**).
5. Resuspend the pellet in cold FBS (4 °C) in half the volume of cryopreservation medium calculated in **step 2**.
6. Dilute the cell suspension 1:1 with cold cryopreservation medium (80 % FBS + 20 % DMSO). Add the medium dropwise, gently stirring the tube.
7. Aliquot the cell suspension into sterile labeled cryopreservation tubes (*see* **Note 5**). Transfer the tubes to a cryofreezing

container and immediately store at −80 °C (*see* **Note 6**). Subsequently, transfer vials the next day in the damp phase of a liquid nitrogen freezer until further use.

3.2 Thawing Primary AML Cells

1. Quickly thaw primary AML cells (PBMC) in a 37 °C water bath with constant, moderate agitation (<1 min) until ice in the ampule is no longer visible. Dilute the thawed cells slowly, using pre-warmed thawing medium (IMDM + 40 % FBS) in a 50-mL tube.
2. Add 40 U/mL of DNase and incubate on a roller for 15 min.
3. Centrifuge the cells for 5 min at 480 × *g*.
4. Carefully remove the supernatant with a pipette without disturbing the cell pellet (*see* **Note 4**).
5. Resuspend the pellet in pre-warmed thawing medium (IMDM + 40 % FBS).
6. Centrifuge cells 1× for 5 min at 480 × *g*.
7. Carefully remove the supernatant (*see* **Note 4**).
8. Resuspend the pellet in pre-warmed culture medium (IMDM + 10 % FBS).
9. Let cells rest for 2–4 h at 37 °C prior to use (*see* **Note 7**).

3.3 Electroporation of Primary AML Cells with Poly(I:C)

Cell numbers and volumes of reagents mentioned are for a single electroporation. A schematic overview of the electroporation technique is given in Fig. 1.

1. Wash 5–10 × 10^6 primary AML cells once with 10–20 mL serum-free IMDM medium and once with 5 mL serum-free Opti-MEM medium. Centrifuge cells for 5 min at 480 × *g* (*see* **Note 8**).
2. Carefully remove the supernatant (*see* **Note 4**).
3. Prepare a 50-mL collection tube with 15 mL of culture medium (IMDM + 10 % FBS).
4. Adjust the parameters of the Gene Pulser XCell for electroporation of leukemic cells using the "time constant protocol" (*see* **Note 9**) applying a voltage of 300 V and a pulse time of 7 ms (*see* **Note 10**). For electroporation of eukaryotic cells, electroporation cuvettes with an electrode distance of 4 mm are routinely used.
5. Resuspend the washed primary AML cells in 200 μL of Opti-MEM medium per electroporation, and transfer the cell suspension into a 4-mm cuvette (*see* **Note 11**).
6. Add 10–20 μg of poly(I:C) (maximum volume of 20 μL) to the cell suspension (*see* **Notes 12** and **13**).
7. Insert the cuvette into the ShockPod cuvette chamber (*see* **Note 14**), and trigger the pulse by pushing the zap button.

8. Immediately after the electroporation, transfer the cell suspension to the collection tube (pre-warmed IMDM + 10 % FBS) with a transfer pipette, and rinse the cuvette once with culture medium from the same collection tube.
9. Optionally: to remove the excess of extracellular poly(I:C), centrifuge the cells for 5 min at 480 × *g*, and carefully discard the supernatant.
10. Resuspend the cells to a concentration of 1–5 × 10^6 cells/mL, and incubate for at least 30 min (typically 2–3 h) at 37 °C.
11. After this recovery phase, electroporated AML cells can be collected and/or resuspended for downstream immune assays.

4 Notes

1. Density gradient separation is performed with Ficoll-Paque Plus, and approximately 20–50 mL of fresh heparinized blood is processed.
2. In order to avoid clotting of proteins in the FBS, it can be passed through a 100-μm nylon cell strainer and aliquoted in sterile 50-mL tubes.
3. Working with RNA-based adjuvants requires avoiding contact with RNAses. It is important to wear gloves and use filter tips throughout the experimental procedure. It is important to sufficiently concentrate the poly(I:C) stock solution, e.g., 1 μg/μL in RNase-free water, in order to keep the poly(I:C) volume to a minimum (maximum 20 μL for standard electroporation in 200 μL electroporation buffer). Otherwise, there is a risk of osmotic shock and cell damage prior to the electroporation.
4. Cell pellets from patient-derived material after centrifugation are relatively loosely attached to the tube; therefore, do not decant post-centrifugation, but carefully remove the supernatant with a pipette.
5. Prior to filling, label each vial with cell type, cell number, date, and initials of the operator.
6. DMSO is cytotoxic for cells at room temperature. Therefore, it is important to perform freezing of cells quickly and to place the freezing container at −80 °C immediately after loading with the filled cryovials.
7. Determine viability and cell number of thawed cells prior to use. Typically, thawed PBMC of AML patients are >60 % viable (negative for propidium iodide), and >50 % of the frozen cells can be recuperated.
8. In case UV- or γ-irradiation of tumor cells is required, it is advisable to schedule the irradiation prior to electroporation procedure [40].

9. The same electroporation procedure can also be performed with human or murine leukemic cell lines [39, 40], cultured DC [32, 36–38], and stem cells [46]. For other primary cells or cell lines, electroporation settings might require optimization.
10. Alternatively, an "exponential protocol" with voltage, 300 V; capacitance, 150 μF; resistance (Ω), infinite (∞); and cuvette, 4 mm, can be used. Using these settings, a similar pulse time of around 7 ms should be achieved. Overall, to minimize cell damage, it is important that the pores induced by the electrical pulse do not last longer than 10 ms.
11. During the electroporation procedure, it is important to work quickly to reduce the exposure time of cells to serum-free medium and to resuspend the cells after shocking as soon as possible in serum-containing medium to speed up the resealing process of the membrane pores.
12. It has been reported in the literature that simian kidney epithelial Vero cells electroporated with 10 μg poly(I:C) using a similar procedure retained 11 ng poly(I:C), which was sufficient to cause biological effects such as DC activation and cross-priming [26].
13. Instead of poly(I:C), other RNA reagents can be electroporated, such as mRNA, siRNA, or the Toll-like receptor 7/8 ligand R-848 (47). Notably, the immunogenicity of AML cells by R-848 was more pronouncedly increased by passive pulsing of R-848 as compared to R-848 electroporation [47].
14. In order to secure a sterile working environment, the ShockPod cuvette chamber can be placed in the laminar flow hood.

Acknowledgements

This work was supported in part by research grants of the University of Antwerp (BOF-KP and Prize Rosa Blanckaert), Research Foundation Flanders (FWO Vlaanderen), Foundation against Cancer (Stichting tegen Kanker), the Methusalem program of the Flemish Government, and the Hercules Foundation, Belgium. E.S. is a postdoctoral fellow of the Research Foundation Flanders. E.L. is a holder of an Emmanuel Van der Schueren scholarship of the Vlaamse Liga tegen Kanker (VLK).

References

1. Goutagny N et al (2012) Targeting pattern recognition receptors in cancer immunotherapy. Target Oncol 7:29–54
2. Akazawa T et al (2007) Antitumor NK activation induced by the Toll-like receptor 3-TICAM-1 (TRIF) pathway in myeloid dendritic cells. Proc Natl Acad Sci U S A 104: 252–257
3. Girart MV et al (2007) Engagement of TLR3, TLR7, and NKG2D regulate IFN-gamma secretion but not NKG2D-mediated cytotoxicity by human NK cells stimulated with

suboptimal doses of IL-12. J Immunol 179: 3472–3479
4. Lauzon NM et al (2006) The direct effects of Toll-like receptor ligands on human NK cell cytokine production and cytotoxicity. Cell Immunol 241:102–112
5. McCartney S et al (2009) Distinct and complementary functions of MDA5 and TLR3 in poly(I:C)-mediated activation of mouse NK cells. J Exp Med 206:2967–2976
6. Perrot I et al (2010) TLR3 and Rig-like receptor on myeloid dendritic cells and Rig-like receptor on human NK cells are both mandatory for production of IFN-gamma in response to double-stranded RNA. J Immunol 185: 2080–2088
7. Pisegna S et al (2004) p38 MAPK activation controls the TLR3-mediated up-regulation of cytotoxicity and cytokine production in human NK cells. Blood 104:4157–4164
8. Salem ML et al (2006) The adjuvant effects of the toll-like receptor 3 ligand polyinosinic-cytidylic acid poly (I:C) on antigen-specific $CD8^+$ T cell responses are partially dependent on NK cells with the induction of a beneficial cytokine milieu. Vaccine 24:5119–5132
9. Schmid KN et al (2004) APC-independent activation of NK cells by the Toll-like receptor 3 agonist double-stranded RNA. J Immunol 172:138–143
10. Sivori S et al (2004) CpG and double-stranded RNA trigger human NK cells by Toll-like receptors: induction of cytokine release and cytotoxicity against tumors and dendritic cells. Proc Natl Acad Sci U S A 101:10116–10121
11. Adams M et al (2003) Dendritic cell (DC) based therapy for cervical cancer: use of DC pulsed with tumour lysate and matured with a novel synthetic clinically non-toxic double stranded RNA analogue poly [I]:poly [C(12) U] (Ampligen R). Vaccine 21:787–790
12. Benwell RK et al (2010) Double stranded RNA-relative to other TLR ligand-activated dendritic cells induce extremely polarized human Th1 responses. Cell Immunol 264:119–126
13. Boullart AC et al (2008) Maturation of monocyte-derived dendritic cells with Toll-like receptor 3 and 7/8 ligands combined with prostaglandin E2 results in high interleukin-12 production and cell migration. Cancer Immunol Immunother 57:1589–1597
14. Lore K et al (2003) Toll-like receptor ligands modulate dendritic cells to augment cytomegalovirus- and HIV-1-specific T cell responses. J Immunol 171:4320–4328
15. Strowig T et al (2008) Tonsilar NK cells restrict B cell transformation by the Epstein-Barr virus via IFN-gamma. PLoS Pathog 4:e27
16. Verdijk RM et al (1999) Polyriboinosinic polyribocytidylic acid (poly(I:C)) induces stable maturation of functionally active human dendritic cells. J Immunol 163:57–61
17. Moretta A et al (2008) NK cells at the interface between innate and adaptive immunity. Cell Death Differ 15:226–233
18. Zanoni I et al (2007) Self-tolerance, dendritic cell (DC)-mediated activation and tissue distribution of natural killer (NK) cells. Immunol Lett 110:6–17
19. Datta SK et al (2003) A subset of Toll-like receptor ligands induces cross-presentation by bone marrow-derived dendritic cells. J Immunol 170:4102–4110
20. Durand V et al (2004) Shaping of adaptive immune responses to soluble proteins by TLR agonists: a role for IFN-alpha/beta. Immunol Cell Biol 82:596–602
21. Fujimoto C et al (2004) Polyriboinosinic polyribocytidylic acid [poly(I:C)]/TLR3 signaling allows class I processing of exogenous protein and induction of HIV-specific CD8+ cytotoxic T lymphocytes. Int Immunol 16:55–63
22. Jongbloed SL et al (2010) Human CD141+ (BDCA-3)+dendritic cells (DCs) represent a unique myeloid DC subset that cross-presents necrotic cell antigens. J Exp Med 207: 1247–1260
23. Cui Z et al (2007) Learning from viruses: the necrotic bodies of tumor cells with intracellular synthetic dsRNA induced strong anti-tumor immune responses. Pharm Res 24:1645–1652
24. Cui Z, Qiu F (2006) Synthetic double-stranded RNA poly(I:C) as a potent peptide vaccine adjuvant: therapeutic activity against human cervical cancer in a rodent model. Cancer Immunol Immunother 55:1267–1279
25. Salio M, Cerundolo V (2005) Viral immunity: cross-priming with the help of TLR3. Curr Biol 15:R336–R339
26. Schulz O et al (2005) Toll-like receptor 3 promotes cross-priming to virus-infected cells. Nature 433:887–892
27. Frleta D et al (2009) Influenza virus and poly(I:C) inhibit MHC class I-restricted presentation of cell-associated antigens derived from infected dead cells captured by human dendritic cells. J Immunol 182:2766–2776
28. Kovalcsik E et al (2011) Poly(I:C)-induced tumour cell death leads to DC maturation and Th1 activation. Cancer Immunol Immunother 60:1609–1624
29. Kubler K et al (2011) Immunogenic cell death of human ovarian cancer cells induced by cytosolic poly(I:C) leads to myeloid cell maturation and activates NK cells. Eur J Immunol 41: 3028–3039

30. McBride S et al (2006) Cell-associated double-stranded RNA enhances antitumor activity through the production of type I IFN. J Immunol 177:6122–6128
31. Ponsaerts P et al (2002) mRNA-electroporated mature dendritic cells retain transgene expression, phenotypical properties and stimulatory capacity after cryopreservation. Leukemia 16:1324–1330
32. Van Tendeloo VF et al (2001) Highly efficient gene delivery by mRNA electroporation in human hematopoietic cells: superiority to lipofection and passive pulsing of mRNA and to electroporation of plasmid cDNA for tumor antigen loading of dendritic cells. Blood 98:49–56
33. Smits EL et al (2009) Dendritic cell-based cancer gene therapy. Hum Gene Ther 20:1106–1118
34. Van Nuffel AM et al (2010) Immunotherapy of cancer with dendritic cells loaded with tumor antigens and activated through mRNA electroporation. Methods Mol Biol 629:405–452
35. Van Tendeloo VF et al (2007) mRNA-based gene transfer as a tool for gene and cell therapy. Curr Opin Mol Ther 9:423–431
36. Van Tendeloo VF et al (2010) Induction of complete and molecular remissions in acute myeloid leukemia by Wilms' tumor 1 antigen-targeted dendritic cell vaccination. Proc Natl Acad Sci U S A 107:13824–13829
37. Anguille S et al (2012) Interleukin-15-induced CD56(+) myeloid dendritic cells combine potent tumor antigen presentation with direct tumoricidal potential. PLoS One 7, e51851
38. Anguille S et al (2009) Short-term cultured, interleukin-15 differentiated dendritic cells have potent immunostimulatory properties. J Transl Med 7:109
39. Lion E et al (2009) Acute myeloid leukemic cell lines loaded with synthetic dsRNA trigger IFN-gamma secretion by human NK cells. Leuk Res 33:539–546
40. Smits EL et al (2007) Proinflammatory response of human leukemic cells to dsRNA transfection linked to activation of dendritic cells. Leukemia 21:1691–1699
41. Lion E et al (2011) Poly(I:C) enhances the susceptibility of leukemic cells to NK cell cytotoxicity and phagocytosis by DC. PLoS One 6:e20952
42. Deschler B, Lubbert M (2006) Acute myeloid leukemia: epidemiology and etiology. Cancer 107:2099–2107
43. Lion E et al (2012) Natural killer cell immune escape in acute myeloid leukemia. Leukemia 26(9):2019–2026
44. Smits EL et al (2009) Immunotherapy of acute myeloid leukemia: current approaches. Oncologist 14:240–252
45. Smits EL et al (2011) Clinical evaluation of cellular immunotherapy in acute myeloid leukaemia. Cancer Immunol Immunother 60:757–769
46. Smits E et al (2004) RNA-based gene transfer for adult stem cells and T cells. Leukemia 18:1898–1902
47. Smits EL et al (2010) The Toll-like receptor 7/8 agonist resiquimod greatly increases the immunostimulatory capacity of human acute myeloid leukemia cells. Cancer Immunol Immunother 59:35–46

Chapter 21

Autologous Tumor Cells Engineered to Express Bacterial Antigens

Vijayakumar K. Ramiya, Maya M. Jerald, Patricia D. Lawman, and Michael J.P. Lawman

Abstract

Cancer immunotherapies are emerging as promising treatment modalities in the management of the disease. As a result, cancer vaccines are considered to be immensely crucial in preventing recurrence, a well-known nemesis in cancer patients because they have the potential to activate memory antitumor immunity. Due to poor antigenicity and self-tolerance, most tumor antigens require interventional vaccine therapies to provide an adequate "danger" signal to the immune system in order to activate a robust, clinically meaningful antitumor immunity. It has been postulated that this requirement may be achieved by providing bacterial and/or viral immunogens to prime this type of immune response. Briefly, we provide here a method of transfecting whole tumor cells with plasmid DNA encoding an immunogenic bacterial protein such as Emm55, which was derived from *Streptococcus pyogenes* (*S. pyogenes*). Subsequent inactivation of the transfected cells by irradiation (100 Gray) prevents replication. This type of whole-cell vaccine, e.g., ImmuneFx™, has demonstrated activity in a murine neuroblastoma model, in canine lymphoma patients with naturally occurring disease, and in many cancer types in companion animals. The protocols described in this chapter provide the necessary materials and methodologies to manufacture such a vaccine.

Key words *Streptococcus pyogenes*, Emm55, Autologous, Tumor cells, ImmuneFx™, Canine lymphoma

1 Introduction

Since William Coley's usage of bacterial extracts in patients with sarcomas to induce antitumor immunity nearly 120 years ago [1], enormous progress has been achieved in tumor biotechnology. The demonstration that immunization with influenza virus-infected tumor cell lysates could induce clinically efficacious antitumor immunity in murine models provided a basis for modern-day autologous/genetically altered tumor cell vaccines [2]. Whole-tumor-cell vaccines have the advantage of being applied to many different types of cancer and can thus be multi-indication cancer vaccines.

Michael J.P. Lawman and Patricia D. Lawman (eds.), *Cancer Vaccines: Methods and Protocols*, Methods in Molecular Biology, vol. 1139, DOI 10.1007/978-1-4939-0345-0_21, © Springer Science+Business Media New York 2014

The whole-cell vaccine also has the advantage of activating antitumor CD8⁺ T cells via direct and indirect (cross-priming) pathways [3]. Unlike other forms of vaccines, i.e., idiotype, protein, and peptide, whole-tumor-cell vaccines present a plethora of tumor antigens (known and unknown) to the immune system via epitope spreading. Therefore, in theory, whole-cell vaccines should increase clinical efficacy by educating the adaptive immune response to attack tumor cells throughout the body with fewer tumor cells escaping recognition. In support of this contention, an overview of metastatic colon cancer immunotherapy trials demonstrated a higher clinical benefit rate with whole-cell vaccine (46 %) compared to dendritic cell (17 %)-, peptide (13 %)-, or idiotype antibody-based (3 %) vaccines [4]. In a meta-analysis of tumor vaccines encompassing multiple cancers, Neller and colleagues concluded that whole-cell tumor vaccines provided objective clinical responses in 8.1 % of patients compared to that of 3.6 % with defined antigens [5]. Due to the nature of most tumor antigens, being self-proteins, they are generally not immunogenic and hence not able to mount an efficient antitumor immunity. To augment antitumor immune responses, it is critical, therefore, to introduce a "danger signal" to the tumor cells, which will enable induction of a robust antitumor response. One approach has been to mix whole tumor cells with mycobacteria, bacilli Calmette–Guerin (BCG), e.g., CanVaxin™ for melanoma and Oncovax™ for colon cancer. Another has been to modify whole tumor cells with bacterial genes, e.g., ImmuneFx™. This chapter describes the transfection-mediated modification of autologous tumor cells with genes encoding immunogenic bacterial proteins, such as Emm55, and subsequent inactivation of the transfected cells by irradiation.

Preclinical data from studies in dogs with lymphoma (Table 1) [6] and a variety of tumors in multiple canine and feline breeds (Table 2) demonstrate the clinical usage to date of this multi-indication approach in animals. A Phase 1b clinical study with asymptomatic human patients with indolent non-Hodgkin lymphoma is planned.

2 Materials

2.1 Purification of Plasmid DNA

1. EndoFree™ Qiagen plasmid purification kit (Mega kit) with all buffers and accessories along with DNA columns, Buffers P1, P2, P3, FWBR, ER, QBT, QN, QC, TE buffer, Nuclease free water to make 70 % EtOH, RNase and Lyse blue vials (Qiagen, Valencia, CA, USA) (*see* **Note 1**).
2. Nuclease-free 1.5-mL Eppendorf microfuge tubes.
3. 15- and 50-mL polystyrene tubes.
4. 0.5-, 10-, 20-, 200-, and 1,000-μL pipette tips.

Table 1
The summary of data collected from a canine lymphoma preclinical study using the autologous whole-cell ImmuneFx™ cancer vaccine which uses the *emm55* gene derived from *S. pyogenes*

Canine breed	Age	Sex	Biopsy	Electroporation time (ms)	Electroporation volts (KV)	Transfection (%)	Expression post G418 (%)	Biopsy to vaccination (days)
Labrador	NK	M	Aspirate	0.40	0.348	10–15	>60	ND
Mix breed	10	M	Aspirate	0.40	0.342	8–12	>50	ND
Mix breed	10	M	Aspirate	0.40	0.350	11–14	>70	ND
Retriever	12	M	Aspirate	0.40	0.196	9–12	>55	ND
Shih Tzu	9	F	Aspirate	0.40	0.380	10–14	>65	ND
Doberman	NK	M	Aspirate	0.40	0.380	10–16	>65	ND
Irish Wolf Hound	7	M	Tissue	0.58	0.530	10–16	>65	23
Golden Retriever	6	F	Tissue	0.40	0.352	15–20	60	ND
Braid	5	F	Tissue	0.40	0.348	20	>65	ND
Labrador Mix	8	M	Tissue	0.56	0.520	16	70	ND
Doberman	8	F	Tissue	0.40	0.36	19	65	14
Labrador Retriever	7	M	Tissue	0.58	0.520	20	75	ND
Bulldog	6	M	Aspirate	0.40	0.352	10–14	>75	24
Golden Retriever	12	F	Tissue	0.58	0.530	15–18	>75	16
Dachshund	7	M	Aspirate	0.58	0.530	9–15	>60	15
Vizsia	4	M	Tissue	0.58	0.530	15–18	>50	21
Greyhound	10	F	Tissue	0.60	0.520	15–20	>75	18
Weish Corgi	11	M	Aspirate	0.56	0.520	10–13	>65	33

(continued)

Table 1
(continued)

Canine breed	Age	Sex	Biopsy	Electroporation time (ms)	Electroporation volts (KV)	Transfection (%)	Expression post G418 (%)	Biopsy to vaccination (days)
Chow Chow	12	M	Tissue	0.58	0.500	9–13	>55	26
Tibetan Spaniel	9	M	Tissue	0.58	0.530	22	>60	30
Standard Poodle	8	M	Tissue	0.58	0.530	25	>70	61
Labrador Mix	6	M	Tissue	0.60	0.530	27	>65	23
B. Collie Mix	7	M	Tissue	0.56	0.500	19	>75	21
Standard Poodle	9	M	Tissue	0.61	0.520	21	65	18
Aus. Shepherd	6	M	Tissue	0.58	0.520	24	70	18
Airedale	11	M	Tissue	0.60	0.540	27	75	14
Boykin Spaniel	7	M	Tissue	0.41	0.340	10–12	>70	14
English Bulldog	5	M	Tissue	0.45	0.346	13–14	>80	12
Labrador Mix	5	M	Tissue	0.56	0.510	21	>70	14
Boxer	6	M	Tissue	0.46	0.520	17	>70	14
Golden Retriever	7	F	Tissue	14.6	0.076	ND	ND	13
German Shepherd	6	M	Tissue	13.4	0.1	ND	ND	6

The majority of dogs received pcDNA/*emm55* plasmid DNA, while the last two received the pAc/*emm55* plasmid. A variety of breeds, sexes, and ages were treated in this study The average vaccine regimen consisted of 4-weekly and 4-monthly doses of 1×10^7 irradiated cells with a minimum of 10 % transfected cells in a given dose. No patient exhibited any side effects or other illnesses related to this vaccine therapy. An overall improved survival of 222 days over historical (untreated) control of 60 days has been observed in canine lymphoma

Table 2
Autologous whole-cell ImmuneFx™ cancer vaccine therapy has been utilized in several cancer types in both canine and feline species

Cancer types	Canine	Feline
Lymphoma	31	1
Squamous cell carcinoma	2	0
Fibrosarcoma	2	3
Transitional cell carcinoma	1	0
Osteosarcoma	1	0
Hemangiopericytoma	3	0
Histiocytic sarcoma	1	0
Cutaneous T-cell lymphoma	1	0
Sebaceous gland carcinoma	1	0
Chondrosarcoma	0	1

5. Isopropanol.
6. 70 % molecular grade ethanol.
7. Molecular grade water.
8. 250-mL conical centrifuge tubes.
9. Luria-Bertani (LB) agar plates and broth with 50 μg/mL kanamycin (*see* **Note 2**).

2.2 Culture Media for Solid Tumors

1. Dulbecco's minimal essential medium (DMEM) supplemented with the following: 10 % heat-inactivated fetal bovine serum (FBS) (DMEM–10 % FBS), 1× MEM nonessential amino acid solution, 1× penicillin–streptomycin solution, 1 μg/mL hydrocortisone.
2. Wash medium for solid tumors: DMEM medium supplemented with 2× penicillin–streptomycin solution.

2.3 Culture Media for Lymphoma Tumors

1. X-Vivo™ 20 medium supplemented with the following: 10 % heat-inactivated FBS (X-Vivo–10 % FBS).
2. Wash medium for lymphoma or liquid tumors: X-Vivo™ medium supplemented with 2× penicillin–streptomycin.

2.4 Tissue Processing of Solid and Lymphoma Tumors

1. Sterile scissors and forceps.
2. 50-mL conical tubes.
3. 15-mL conical tubes.
4. 70 % ethanol.

5. Collagenase/hyaluronidase.
6. T75 tissue culture flasks.
7. Sterile distilled water.
8. DNase I.
9. 0.4 % Trypan blue.
10. Sterile 100 × 20-mm tissue culture Petri dishes.
11. 2-mL cryogenic vials.
12. Recovery cell culture freezing medium (Invitrogen, Life Technologies, Carlsbad, CA, USA).
13. 5-, 10-, 25-mL sterile pipettes.
14. 0.22- and 0.45-μm syringe filters.
15. 12-mL syringes and sterile 20 mL luer-lock syringes.
16. 0.25 % Trypsin–EDTA solution. Bring to room temperature in the hood prior to use.
17. Hanks' Balanced Salt Solution (HBSS).
18. RBC Lysis buffer.
19. Fico/Lite-LymphoH.
20. Sterile 18 G × 1.5 in. needles.
21. Sterile 100 × 20 mm tissue culture Petri dishes.
22. T175 tissue culture flasks.
23. 2-mL cryogenic vials.

2.5 Transfection of Plasmid DNA into Tumor Cells

1. Purified plasmid DNA.
2. 50-mL conical tubes.
3. Mirus electroporation buffer.
4. Recovery cell culture freezing medium.
5. 1.5-mL Eppendorf tubes.
6. Gene Pulser 0.4-cm cuvettes.
7. 0.4 % Trypan blue.
8. 2-mL cryogenic vials.
9. 10- and 200-μL pipettes.
10. 10- and 200-μL barrier pipette tips.
11. T175 tissue culture flasks.
12. CellRad irradiation device (Faxitron, Tucson, AZ, USA).

2.6 Immunofluorescence Assay for Transfected Cells

1. Dulbecco's PBS (DPBS).
2. Heat-inactivated FBS.
3. 4 % formaldehyde: 1 mL of formaldehyde in 8 mL of DPBS (can be stored at room temperature in the dark).

4. Staining buffer: 2.5 mL of FBS in 47.5 mL of DPBS (5 % FBS) and 50 mg of sodium azide (0.1 %).
5. Permeabilization buffer: 10 mg of saponin in 10 mL of staining buffer.
6. FITC-conjugated mouse IgG isotype control.
7. FITC-conjugated anti-CD45 monoclonal antibodies (*see* **Note 3**).
8. Monoclonal antibodies against the bacterial protein of interest.
9. 5-mL tubes.
10. 200-μL pipette tips.
11. 5-mL pipettes.
12. Prolong® Gold anti-fade reagent with DAPI.
13. Cytocentrifuge Cytospin 3.

3 Methods

3.1 Extraction of Endotoxin-Free Plasmid DNA

1. The following steps are to be carried out after overnight culture of plasmid DNA-transformed *Escherichia coli* in LB broth at 37 °C in a shaker incubator. Just before Mega kit plasmid extraction, as described by the kit manufacturer, follow these steps:
   (a) Add RNase A solution to Buffer P1.
   (b) Check Buffer P2 for any SDS precipitation.
   (c) Pre-chill Buffer P3 to 4 °C.
   (d) Optional: Add LyseBlue reagent to Buffer P1.
2. Collect 500 mL of bacterial culture, and pellet the bacteria in 250-mL conical tubes by centrifuging at 6,000 × *g* for 15 min at 4 °C. Remove all traces of supernatant by inverting the open centrifuge tube until all medium has been drained. Dispose of the supernatant after autoclaving. Resuspend the bacterial pellet in 50 mL of Buffer P1.
3. Add 50 mL of Buffer P2, mix thoroughly by inverting 6× and incubate for 5 min at room temperature.
4. During the incubation time, screw the QIAfilter Cartridge onto a glass bottle with a 45-mm neck and connect it to a vacuum source.
5. Add 50 mL of pre-chilled Buffer P3, and mix thoroughly by inverting 6×.
6. Pour the lysate into the QIAfilter Cartridge, and incubate for 10 min. Pull the liquid through by applying vacuum. Add 50 mL of Buffer FWB2 to the QIAfilter Cartridge, and gently stir the precipitate using a sterile spatula or a 5-mL pipette. Apply vacuum again until all the liquid has completely passed through.

7. Add 12.5 mL of Buffer ER to the filtered lysate, mix by inverting the bottle approximately 10× and incubate on ice for 30 min. Equilibrate a QIAGEN-tip 2500 by applying 35 mL of Buffer QBT, and allow the column to empty by gravity flow.
8. Apply the filtered lysate from **step 7** to the QIAGEN-tip, and allow it to enter the tip. Wash the QIAGEN-tip with 200 mL of Buffer QC.
9. Elute the bound DNA with 35 mL of Buffer QN.
10. Precipitate the DNA by adding 24.5 mL (0.7 volume) of room-temperature isopropanol to the eluted DNA. After mixing thoroughly, centrifuge at 6,000 × *g* for 60 min at 4 °C to pellet the DNA.
11. Wash the DNA pellet with 7 mL of endotoxin-free 70 % ethanol (kept at room temperature) and centrifuge at 6,000 × *g* for 60 min at 4 °C. Carefully decant the supernatant without disturbing the pellet.
12. Air-dry the pellet in a sterile hood for 10–20 min, and dissolve the plasmid DNA in either endotoxin-free TE Buffer or water.
13. Prior to use in transfecting patient tumor cells, each lot of plasmid must be certified according to established criteria. The following are the specifications we use:
    (a) Quantification of plasmid (1 mg/mL).
    (b) Gel electrophoresis (>50 % supercoiled DNA).
    (c) Restriction enzyme digestion and agarose gel (to document the presence of the gene insert).
    (d) Endotoxin (<100 EU/mg plasmid DNA).
    (e) Sterility test (should be negative).
    (f) Sequencing (must match the reference sequence).

3.2 Processing Solid Tumors

1. Wear protective clothing—lab coat, gloves, and face mask.
2. Most of the procedure should be performed under a laminar flow hood.
3. Spray specimen container with 70 % ethanol, and place solid tumor tissue sample under the hood.
4. Place sterile scissors and forceps in individual 50-mL tubes containing 40 mL of 70 % ethanol, and let tubes stand upright in a 50-mL tube rack.
5. Drain forceps by holding them vertically over a clean paper towel. Avoid touching the paper towel.
6. Use forceps to collect tumor from specimen container, and place it in a 100 × 20-mm Petri dish with 5–10 mL of wash medium. Replace forceps in ethanol.
7. Using sterile scissors, mince the tissue into approximately 1.0 mm^3 pieces.

8. Place all minced tissue pieces in a 50-mL conical tube(s), secure cap, and invert 3–5 times.
9. Pulse centrifuge at 680 × *g*. Once the speed reaches 680 × *g*, stop the centrifugation. Repeat this process 3–5× until the medium appears clear.
10. Prepare 10 mL of culture medium containing collagenase/hyaluronidase (2–3× concentration depending on the texture of the tissue) and 50 μg/mL of DNase I (*see* **Note 4**). Filter solution through the 0.45-μm syringe filter and then through a 0.22-μm syringe filter into a sterile 15-mL conical tube.
11. Discard the supernatant, add the filtered collagenase/hyaluronidase solution to the pellet, and place the tube into a 37 °C water bath.
12. Gently swirl the tube every 15–30 min for cell release, and determine viability. A total of 2–4 h may be needed to digest 5 mL of minced tissue pellet, depending on the texture and type of tissue. It is difficult to digest the entire tissue. Some will remain as undigested pieces. Carefully collect the collagenase/hyaluronidase solution containing single cells, leaving the undigested tissue sections undisturbed. Continue digesting partially digested pieces to attain a sufficient number of cells. If necessary, use fresh enzymes (*see* **Note 4**).
13. Place single-cell suspension in a 50-mL conical tube and add 30–40 mL of wash medium. Also, add 30–40 mL of wash medium to the undigested tissue sections.
14. Centrifuge both tubes at 680 × *g* for 8 min.
15. Repeat washing the "single"-cell pellet and undigested tissue pieces two additional times.
16. Determine cell viability and total cell number.
17. Resuspend the single-cell pellet and undigested tissue pieces in 10 mL of DMEM–10 % FBS culture medium each.
18. Seed the cells in 1 or multiple T75 tissue culture flasks at a concentration of $1–10 \times 10^5$ cells per flask in 15–25 mL of medium.
19. Incubate the flasks at 37 °C in humidified atmosphere of 5 % CO_2.
20. Monitor cultures daily for cell growth. Solid tumor cells adhere to the flasks.
21. When the tumor cells are 80 % confluent, prepare for splitting the culture by trypsinization.
22. Expand the cells to reach the desired cell number. Every solid tumor type varies in expansion capabilities (*see* **Note 5**).
23. When sufficient cells are attained, proceed to transfection.

3.3 Trypsinization of Adherent Cells

1. Under a laminar flow hood, remove the spent medium, and dispose of it in 10 % bleach. Add 15 mL of HBSS to gently wash the flask, and discard the medium.
2. Add 5 mL of 1× trypsin to each T75 flask (*see* **Note 6**).
3. Place the flasks at 37 °C for 5–10 min.
4. Remove the flasks and shake for 30 s with gentle tapping with the palm of hand.
5. Observe under a microscope to ascertain that cells are in suspension.
6. Add 10 mL of sterile DMEM–10 % FBS to the flask and mix gently by using a 10-mL pipette.
7. Transfer the cells to a 50-mL conical tube, add an additional 15 mL of DMEM with 10 % FBS, and centrifuge at 680 × *g* for 10 min. Discard the supernatant.
8. Wash the cell pellet at least two more times with 10 mL of DMEM–10 % FBS.
9. Determine cell viability, and continue cell expansion until the required cell number is achieved.

3.4 Processing Lymphoma Tumor Specimens

1. Wear protective clothing—lab coat, gloves, and face mask. And perform the procedures under a laminar flow hood.
2. Spray the specimen container with 70 % ethanol and place under the hood.
3. Place sterile scissors and forceps in individual 50-mL tubes containing 40 mL of 70 % ethanol. Let tubes stand upright in a 50-mL tube rack.
4. Drain forceps by holding them vertically over a paper towel. Avoid touching the paper towel.
5. Gently collect the lymph node (LN) from the container and place in a 100 × 20-mm Petri dish. Replace the forceps in the ethanol.
6. Attach an 18 G luer-lock needle to a 20-mL syringe.
7. Using a 25-mL sterile pipette, add 20 mL of X-Vivo™ wash medium to a Petri dish with the LN.
8. Aspirate the medium into the 20-mL syringe. Holding the LN with the forceps, make several holes in the LN by gently inserting the needle through the LN capsule and inject medium into the LN. The suspended LN cells will exit through the holes.
9. Repeat this aspiration/injection process using X-Vivo™ wash medium until most of the cells have been released. Collect the cell-containing medium in fresh 50-mL conical tubes.
10. Centrifuge the cells at 680 × *g* for 8 min.

11. If applicable, combine all cell pellets into one 50-mL tube and centrifuge at 680 × *g* for 8 min.
    (a) Discard the supernatant. Examine cell pellet, and determine the degree of contamination with RBC. If significant RBC are present, remove using RBC lysis buffer. Depending on the size of pellet, add 5–10 mL lysis buffer to the cell pellet mixing gently with a pipette for 3–5 min. Add 20–30 mL X-Vivo™ wash medium to the cell suspension. Centrifuge the cell suspension at 680 × *g* for 8 min. Discard the supernatant. The cell pellet should appear white.
    (b) Resuspend cell pellets in X-Vivo™ wash medium, and determine cell density and viability. If viability is poor (<60 %), use a one-step Ficoll gradient to enrich viable cells. This step also removes RBC. Depending on cell concentration, resuspend the LN cells in 10 mL aliquots. Using a 10-mL pipette carefully float the cell suspension onto 10 mL of Ficoll. Centrifuge the Ficoll gradient at 1,890 × *g* for 25 min at 20 °C. Locate the band of cells at the interface of the X-Vivo™ culture medium and Ficoll. Using a 5-mL pipette, carefully remove these cells and place in a clean 50-mL tube. The majority of dead cells will form a pellet at the bottom of the Ficoll layer along with RBC. Add 20 mL of X-Vivo™ wash medium to the viable cells, and centrifuge at 680 × *g* for 8 min. Discard the supernatant, resuspend the pellet in 20 mL of X-Vivo™ wash medium, and repeat cell viability count.
12. Seed T175 tissue culture flasks with a lymphoma cell concentration of $10–20 \times 10^7$ cells per flask. Add fresh X-Vivo™ medium with 10 % FBS to give a total volume of 45 mL/flask.
13. If sufficient cells are available, proceed to transfection.

3.5 Transfection of Plasmid DNA into Tumor Cells

1. Using trypan blue, determine the viable number of tumor cells.
2. Reconstitute the cells in a sterile 50-mL conical tube to a final cell concentration $10–20 \times 10^6$ cells/300 μL of Mirus buffer for lymphoma cells or 5×10^6 cells/300 μL of Mirus buffer for solid tumor cells.
3. Add 5–20 μg of plasmid DNA per 300 μL of Mirus buffer reaction (*see* **Note 7**).
4. Mix the cell/plasmid mixture using a barrier pipette tip, and transfer the mixture to a 0.4-cm sterile gene pulsing cuvette in Mirus buffer.
5. Pulse samples at 240 V and 750 μF (*see* **Note 7**). This will vary for different cell types and may depend on the equipment. A balance has to be reached between transfection efficiency and cell death.

6. Transfer the cells from each cuvette into T175 flasks containing 30–40 mL of culture medium. For small cell concentrations, $\leq 1 \times 10^6$, use T25 flasks.
7. Place the flasks in a 37 °C incubator in a humidified atmosphere of 5 % CO_2.
8. Allow cells to express the protein of interest by culturing for 48 h.
9. After 48 h, collect $10–15 \times 10^6$ cells/mL for γ-irradiation (100 Gray) (*see* **Note 8**).
10. Following irradiation, wash the cells with culture medium, adjust the cell concentration, and aliquot in cryogenic vials at cell concentrations appropriate for vaccine applications, e.g., 1×10^7/mL with recovery cell culture freezing medium.
11. Store at −80 °C for 24 h in a freezing container (*see* **Note 9**), and then transfer to a liquid nitrogen dewar for long-term storage of transfected tumor cells in the vapor phase of liquid nitrogen.

3.6 Immunofluorescence Assay for Transfected Cells

1. Resuspend cells in 5-mL tubes in 3 mL of staining buffer and centrifuge at $680 \times g$ for 5 min.
2. Discard the supernatant. Resuspend the cell pellet in 100 μL of 4 % formaldehyde to fix the cells.
3. Incubate at 4 °C for 20 min in the dark.
4. Wash the cells 2× in 3 mL of staining buffer.
5. Resuspend the pellet in 100 μL of staining buffer. Add 10 μL of isotype antibody to one tube and a combination of 5 μL of anti-"protein of interest antibody" to another tube. Incubate for 30 min at 4 °C in the dark.
6. Wash the cells 2× in 3 mL of staining buffer.
7. Resuspend the cells, isotype, and protein of interest tubes in 100 μL of permeabilization buffer. Add the combination of 5 μL of anti-protein of interest antibodies. Incubate for 30 min at 4 °C in the dark.
8. Wash the cells 2× in 3 mL of staining buffer.
9. Resuspend the cells in 500 μL of staining buffer.
10. Prepare slide-absorbent filter pad-adaptor assembly for cytocentrifugation.
11. Add 100 μL of cells into each slide assembly.
12. Spin the slides at $300 \times g$ for 3 min.
13. Once cytocentrifugation is complete, allow the slides to dry for 5 min.
14. Over the cell spot on the slide, add 25 μL of anti-fade reagent, and gently place a cover slip over the anti-fade reagent (Fig. 1).

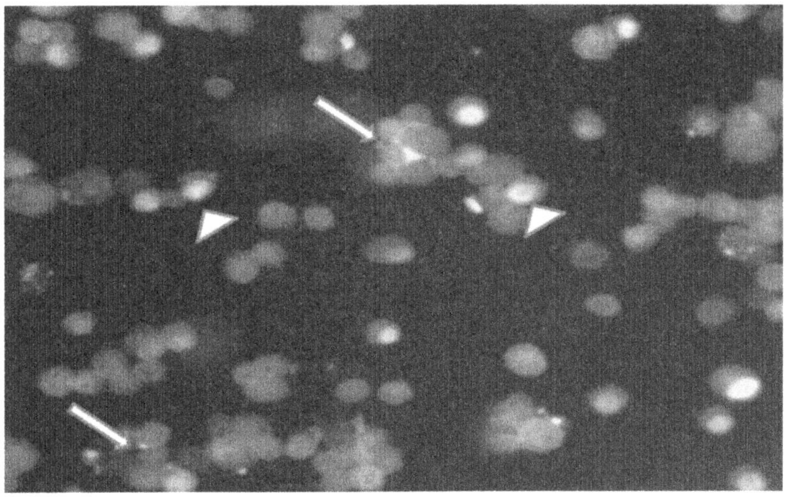

Fig. 1 A representative immunofluorescence of T lymphoma cells transfected with pAc/*emm55* plasmid. Expression of Emm55 protein is identified using a combination of two monoclonal antibodies directed against Emm55. Both cytoplasmic (*arrow head*) and surface expression (*arrows*) can be seen

15. Observe the fluorescence using an FITC filter.
16. Save images of cells, both under phase contrast regular lighting and with FITC filter, for each field. Have at least 200 cells from different fields of view for estimating efficacy.
17. Once images are saved, count the total number of cells under phase contrast regular lighting and the number of cells exhibiting fluorescence under FITC.
18. The transfection efficiency is calculated as follows:

$$\frac{\textit{Number of cells fluorescing}}{\textit{Total number of cells in the same field}} \times 100$$

4 Notes

1. Endotoxin-free plasmid extraction is crucial in therapies intended for clinical trials. Although autologous whole-cell ImmuneFx™ cancer vaccine therapy does not involve direct plasmid DNA injection into patients, our plasmid specification accepts only <100 EU/mg of plasmid.
2. The usage of ampicillin may not be acceptable in clinical trials. Therefore, it is recommended that penicillin and other beta-lactam antibiotics be avoided during production due to the risk of serious hypersensitivity reactions in patients and conferring unnecessary risk of antibiotic resistance to environmental microbes [7].

3. Mouse anti-canine CD45 antibody, clone CD12.10C12, recognizes the canine homolog of CD45, a glycoprotein of approximately 200 kDa which is expressed by cells of hematopoietic origin. This antibody serves as a positive control for lymphoma cells in our immunofluorescence assay.
4. The DNAse is added to prevent clumping of the cells, and it also helps to reduce viscosity resulting from DNA released from damaged cells. The collagenase/hyaluronidase enzyme mixture is supplied as a 10× solution, and it is optimized for overnight digestion of mouse mammary tissue by the manufacturer. We have used the enzyme mixture in at least eight different types of canine solid tumors (Table 2). Depending on tumor texture, 2–3× concentrations have been used and digestion duration varied from 2 to 4 h. In some instances, the partially digested pieces of tumor tissue required a second helping of fresh enzymes. Due to our processing requirements, no overnight digestion is carried out.
5. The rate of growth of solid tumor cells in vitro is substantially different among tumor types and among the tumor masses of the same tumor type in different patients. While chondrosarcoma, hemangiopericytoma, and fibrosarcoma cells exhibit fast growth, all epithelial tumors we have processed have provided few cells following digestion and slower growth rates in cultures.
6. While fibroblastic sarcoma, hemangiopericytoma, and chondrosarcoma cells lift off the plate with 1× trypsin, most epithelial cells require 2–3× trypsin to detach from the plastic surface. This property of epithelial cells has been utilized in eliminating fibroblast cells from epithelial cell cultures, i.e., differential trypsinization.
7. The electroporation parameters described here are for BioRad Genepulser II. Depending on the electroporation equipment used, the parameters have to be optimized. Besides the equipment, the optimization protocols should consider factors such as cell type, cell number, plasmid dose per reaction, electroporation buffer, and the percent transfection desired. A balance has to be achieved between attaining a desirable transfection level and the resulting cell death due to the parameters set.
8. A cellular vaccine such as ImmuneFx™ must be inactivated prior to administration into patients to avoid replication of tumor cells. In order to determine the optimal radiation dose with CellRad (an X-ray-based irradiation device), a range of doses (50, 100, and 150 Gray) with primary tumor cells and a lymphoma cell line were studied and a dose of 100 Gray was found to be optimal by AlamarBlue assay.
9. It is critical that the cell cryo-storage protocol include a freezing container with isopropyl alcohol (maintained at room tem-

perature when not in use) as it enables a decrease of −1 °C per minute in a −80 °C freezer. This prevents ice crystal formation within the cells and thereby protects cells from a loss of integrity and reduction in viability.

Acknowledgement

The development of the protocols and preclinical studies were funded by Morphogenesis, Inc.

References

1. Coley W (1893) The treatment of malignant tumors by repeated inoculations of Erysipelas: with a report of ten original cases. Am J Med 105:487–511
2. Lindenmann J, Klein PA (1967) Viral oncolysis: increased immunogenicity of host cell antigen associated with influenza virus. J Exp Med 126: 93–102
3. Wolkers MC et al (2001) Redundancy of direct priming and cross-priming in tumor-specific $CD8^+$ T cell responses. J Immunol 167: 3577–3584
4. Nagorsen D, Thiel E (2006) Clinical and immunological responses to active specific cancer vaccines in human colorectal cancers. Clin Cancer Res 12:3064–3069
5. Neller MA et al (2008) Antigens for cancer immunotherapy. Semin Immunol 20:286–295
6. Lawman ML et al (2008) Anti-tumor response induced by autologous cancer vaccine in canine lymphoma. Cancer Ther 6:827–840
7. Guidance for human somatic cell therapy and gene therapy. Food and Drug Administration, Center for Biologics Evaluation and Research, 1998

Chapter 22

Tumor Cell Transformation Using Antisense Oligonucleotide

Mohamed R. Akl and Nehad M. Ayoub

Abstract

Major histocompatibility complex (MHC) Class II-positive, invariant chain (Ii)-suppressed tumor cells induce both T helper and cytotoxic T lymphocytes' responses. Genetically controlled immunotherapy could be utilized for prophylactic vaccination of tumor-free individuals who are at high risk of developing tumor and can be therapeutic for treating established tumors that are nonresponsive to existing therapies. In this chapter, we provide practical methods to create a potent in vivo tumor cell vaccine by inducing MHC Class II and Ii using MHC Class II transactivator (CIITA) or interferon-gamma (IFN-γ) and subsequently inhibiting Ii by antisense oligonucleotides. We also describe the development of an adenoviral vector.

Key words Tumor cell vaccine, Antisense oligonucleotides, MHC Class II+/Ii− phenotype, $CD4^+$ T helper cells, $CD8^+$ cytotoxic T lymphocytes

1 Introduction

Cancer immunotherapy is thought to work by overcoming the ability of cancer cells to escape immune surveillance by using methods that are capable of boosting the immune response against that cancer. Several mechanisms have been proposed by which tumor cells become non-immunogenic [1–3]. Therefore, researchers have spent many years studying ways to trigger or enhance a patient's inadequate immune response to their specific tumor. Tumor cell-based immunotherapy is considered to be one of the more promising techniques to coerce tumor cells to present their own antigens to the immune system [4]. Most tumors are MHC Class I positive but negative for MHC Class II [5]. MHC Class I molecules are expressed on all nucleated cells of the body. $CD4^+$ T helper cells recognize antigenic peptides presented by MHC Class II molecules on antigen-presenting cells (APC). MHC Class II molecules are composed of α and β chains that assemble in the endoplasmic reticulum (ER) into an αβ heterodimer. A third chain, the invariant chain or Ii, interacts with this heterodimer to form a heterotrimer. Subsequently, a trimer of this heterotrimer is formed,

Michael J.P. Lawman and Patricia D. Lawman (eds.), *Cancer Vaccines: Methods and Protocols*, Methods in Molecular Biology, vol. 1139, DOI 10.1007/978-1-4939-0345-0_22, © Springer Science+Business Media New York 2014

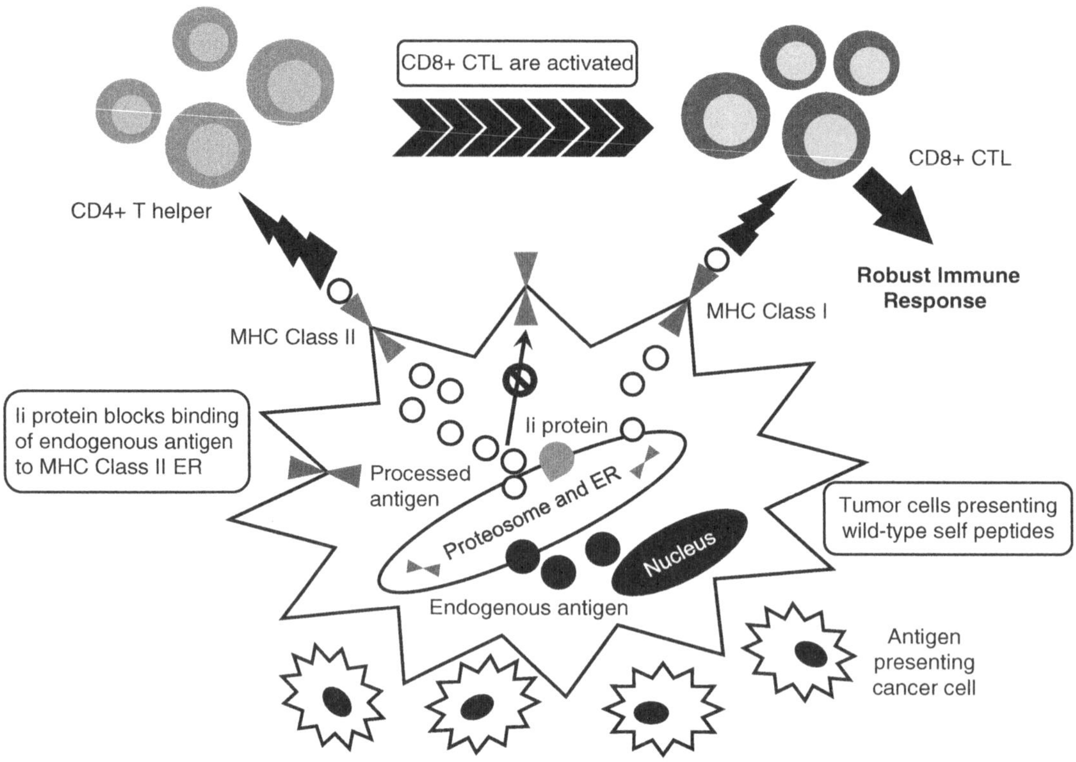

Fig. 1 Presentation of endogenous antigens by antigen-presenting tumor cells

resulting in a nonameric complex. Ii acts as a pseudo-substrate by allowing a small segment, called CLIP for Class II-associated Ii peptide, to enter the peptide-binding groove of MHC Class II [6]. Ii, an integral membrane glycoprotein, promotes the proper folding of MHC Class II molecules in the ER, facilitating their efficient transport from this compartment through the Golgi complex to endosomes and preventing Class II molecules from loading peptides intended for binding to MHC Class I molecules in the ER [6, 7].

Normally, only exogenous antigens are processed for MHC Class II presentation to CD4$^+$ T helper cells. Activated CD4$^+$ T helper cells help the full activation of CD8$^+$ cytotoxic T lymphocytes (CTL). Without the help from CD4$^+$ T helper cells, recognition of MHC CI/peptide complex by CD8$^+$ CTL will fail, resulting in CTL anergy. MHC Class II molecules on APC do not normally bind the ambient peptides of the ER at the time of their synthesis. This is because Ii protein blocks endogenous antigenic peptide binding sites in the ER from being presented by MHC Class II molecules (Fig. 1) [8–10]. Thus, under normal conditions, Ii protein expression is always co-regulated with MHC Class II molecules. Accordingly, suppression of Ii protein in the ER allows nascent MHC Class II molecules to bind peptides transported there for binding to MHC Class I molecules. This enables CD8$^+$

CTL to kill tumor cells directly upon recognition of peptide epitopes expressed on MHC Class I molecules (Fig. 1) [4]. Tumor cells which express varying levels of MHC Class II molecules often upregulate the expression of the Ii protein [10–12]. Earlier findings showed that superinduction of Ii protein renders tumor cells unrecognized by $CD4^+$ T cells, facilitating tumor cell escape from immune surveillance, even if MHC Class I recognition occurred [4]. In addition, tumors expressing MHC Class II molecules without the Ii protein are expected to present endogenous tumor antigenic peptides to $CD4^+$ T cells that are transported into the ER destined for MHC Class I presentation [4]. $CD4^+$ T cells specific for endogenous tumor antigens are thus activated and a robust antitumor immune response can be induced (Fig. 1) [5]. Ultimately, the induction of MHC Class II+/Ii− tumor cell phenotype will enhance these tumor cells to present their own tumor antigens, via MHC Class II, leading to the activation of $CD4^+$ T helper cells and finally resulting in a potent tumor cell immune response. Induction of MHC Class II molecules in tumor cells by transfecting genes encoding the MHC Class II transactivator (CIITA) or interferon-gamma (IFN-γ) is not an efficient method for inducing an antitumor immune response. However, suppression of the co-induced immunoregulatory protein, Ii, using antisense methodologies resulted in more efficient antitumor immunity [4].

Antisense oligonucleotides have been used for a number of years to modify the expression of specific genes both in vivo and in vitro [13]. Oligonucleotides are unmodified or chemically modified single-stranded DNA molecules. In general, they are relatively short (13–25 nucleotides) and hybridize to a unique sequence complementary to a specific mRNA, thus inhibiting its expression and inducing a blockade in the transfer of genetic information from DNA to protein [14]. Here, we demonstrate practical methods to create potent in vivo tumor cell vaccine by the induction of MHC Class II and Ii using CIITA or IFN-γ and subsequently inhibiting Ii by antisense oligonucleotides. We also describe a method for creating a recombinant adenovirus construct.

2 Materials

1. SaI murine sarcoma cell line (MHC Class I^+, MHC Class II^-, Ii $protein^-$).
2. SaI-CIITA subline stably transfected with human MHC Class II transactivator cDNA.
3. SaI-INF-γ subline stably transfected with the mouse *INF-γ* gene.
4. Renca cells, a murine renal carcinoma cell line.
5. Iscove's modified Dulbecco's medium (IMDM) supplemented with 5 % fetal bovine serum (FBS), 2 mM L-glutamine,

200 U/mL penicillin, and 200 mg/mL of streptomycin for maintenance of SaI and SaI-CIITA.

6. Dulbecco's modified Eagle medium (DMEM) supplemented with FBS (10 %) for maintenance of Renca cells.
7. Roswell Park Memorial Institute (RPMI)-1640 medium.
8. Hanks' balanced salts solution (HBSS).
9. Antibodies: anti-murine MHC Class II monoclonal antibody (mAb) M5/114.15.2. Anti-murine Ii mAb can be used as a supernatant from the hybridoma In.1. In.1 is a rat anti-mouse hybridoma cell line that is used to raise monoclonal antibodies against constant regions of murine histocompatibility antigens.
10. Adenoviral DNA and necessary reagents for making recombinant adenoviruses (Quantum Biotechnology, Montreal, Canada).
11. Ribomax™ large-scale RNA production system (Promega, Madison, WI, USA).
12. *E. coli* RNase H.
13. ^{32}P-labeled mouse Ii RNA.
14. Electroporation cuvettes.
15. Trypan blue dye.
16. Formaldehyde.
17. 1 M glycine.
18. 0.2 % saponin.
19. Oligonucleotides.
20. Trypsin.

3 Methods

3.1 Assessment of the In Vivo Activities of Ii Antisense Oligonucleotide: Immunoprevention

The goal of the following experiment is to evaluate the use of antisense oligonucleotides to suppress the expression of the Ii protein in SaI cells transfected with either CIITA or INF-γ genes resulting in the expression of MHC Class II molecules [15].

3.1.1 Choice of Antisense Oligonucleotide Using RNase H Activation Assay

1. Mouse Ii RNA probe can be prepared by in vitro transcription of Ii cDNA using T7-Ribomax™ large-scale RNA production system.
2. Mix 5×10^5 cpm ^{32}P-labeled mouse Ii RNA with 2 μg of yeast tRNA in 1× RNase H buffer; heat at 70 °C for 3 min then cool slowly to room temperature.

3. Add 0.2 pM of each oligodeoxynucleotide to be tested, and incubate at 70 °C for 3 min before addition of 0.5 U of *E. coli* RNase H in final reaction volume of 10 μL.
4. RNase H digestion can be carried out at 37 °C for 10 min to stop the digestion; add 8 μL of loading buffer, and heat the sample at 90 °C for 5 min. Afterwards, store the sample on ice.
5. 5 μL of each sample can be separated by electrophoresis using a polyacrylamide gel.

3.1.2 Electroporation of Antisense Oligonucleotides

1. Trypsinize SaI cells and sublines, and then wash 2× with serum-free RPMI-1640 medium, and resuspend in 0.5 mL of serum-free RPMI-1640 medium.
2. Add 2×10^6 cells in 500 μL medium containing various concentrations of oligonucleotides to a 4-mm-gap electroporation cuvette.
3. Place the cuvette containing sample in ice for 10 min, and then subject it to electroporation (1,200 μF/200 V) with an Electro Cell Manipulator 600 system.
4. After electroporation, keep the sample cuvette at room temperature for another 10 min.
5. Re-culture the electroporated cells in 6-well plates with complete IMDM medium, and double the amount of supplements for 1–3 days.
6. Afterwards, analyze the SaI cells and sublines for the expression of MHC Class II molecules and Ii protein.
7. Measure cell viability by Trypan blue dye exclusion (*see* **Note 1**).

3.1.3 Immunofluorescent Staining of Cultured Sal Cells

1. For cell surface staining of MHC Class II molecules, wash $0.5–1 \times 10^6$ cells with HBSS, and incubate the cells with 20 μg/mL of M5/114.15.2 antibody in a total volume of 200 μL for 45 min on ice at room temperature.
2. Wash the cells 2× with HBSS followed by incubation with fluorescein-conjugated secondary antibody for 30 min at room temperature.
3. Wash the cells 3× with HBSS and fix them with 2 % formaldehyde for 15 min on ice.
4. For intracellular staining of Ii protein, wash $0.5–1 \times 10^6$ cells with HBSS, and fix using 2 % formaldehyde at room temperature for 15 min.
5. Wash the cells with 1 mL of 1 M glycine at room temperature for 5 min (*see* **Note 2**).
6. Permealize the cells with 0.2 % saponin, and incubate with 200 μL of Ii mAb In.1 for 60 min on ice.

7. Wash the cells, and label with fluorescein-conjugated secondary antibody for 30 min at in 0.2 % saponin for 30–45 min at room temperature.
8. Wash the cells and fix them again with 2 % formaldehyde for 15 min.
9. Analyze the cells using FACS for the expression of MHC Class II molecules and Ii protein.

3.1.4 In Vivo Immunization and Tumor Challenge

All murine studies involving in vivo challenges must be preapproved by your Institution's IACUC committee.

1. Treat SaI-CIITA and SaI-INF-γ cells with Ii antisense, sense, or mismatch oligonucleotide controls for various lengths of time in order to generate different experimental groups.
2. Wash the cells and resuspend in HBSS.
3. Fix the cells with 0.15 % formaldehyde or irradiate them with 50 Gy before immunization.
4. Inject mice with various numbers of cells, intraperitoneally (IP), with 0.5 mL of cell suspension (*see* **Note 3**).
5. Acclimate the immunized mice for 4 weeks prior to challenging them by IP injections of varying concentrations of SaI cells.
6. Monitor growth of peritoneal (ascitic) tumors every other day from day 7 following challenge for 1 week and every other day thereafter.
7. Humane euthanasia procedures should be carried out on animals with at least 2 mL of ascites fluid.

3.2 Therapeutic Vaccine by Intratumoral DNA Injection: Immunotherapy

The Ii-RGC Ii antisense reverse gene construct will transform only a fraction of the cells in a treated nodule; in order to establish a potent, systemic immune response capable of eradicating nontransduced tumor cells, we use recombinant adenoviruses (rAV) [16, 17].

3.2.1 Generation of rAV

1. Generate *Ii* fragments by PCR with appropriate oligonucleotide primers using either a murine genomic *Ii* gene or a murine *Ii* cDNA gene as templates.
2. Using sequencing, confirm that the fragments generated are correct *Ii* constructs.
3. Create Ii-RGC which inhibits Ii protein e*xp*ression in various cell lines in vitro.
4. Create rAV containing 1 gene or gene combinations, e.g., *CIITA*, *INF-γ*, and *Ii-RGC*.
5. All gene(s) or gene combinations, along with their promoters and poly A signals, should be PCR excised and cloned into the pQBI/BN vector by standard molecular biology methods.

6. Transfect the vectors into 293A adenoviral packaging cells with Cla1-digested adenoviral DNA according to the manufacturer's instructions.
7. At 3 weeks after co-transfection, screen resulting plaques by PCR to ensure the presence of the *CIITA*, *IFN-γ*, and *Ii-RGC* genes along with their promoters.
8. Expand and titrate the virus according to the manufacturer's instructions (*see* **Note 4**).

3.2.2 Infection of Renca Cells with Recombinant Adenoviruses

1. Plate Renca cells at 5×10^4 cells per well in 24-well plates 18–24 h before infection.
2. Add the viruses (constructions of rAV containing CIITA and INF-γ) at different multiplicity of infection (MOI).
3. Replace the culture medium every 24 h with 2 mL of fresh medium.
4. Harvest cells at different times starting at 6 h postinfection to 96 h, and assay for the expression of MHC Class II molecules with FACS analysis following staining with anti-mouse I-E^k mAb (M5/114.15.2) (*see* **Note 5**).

3.2.3 Transfection of Renca Cells with Ii-RGC Using Electroporation

1. After rAV infection, trypsinize Renca cells, and wash 2× with serum-free RPMI-1640 medium, and resuspend in 0.5 mL of serum-free RPMI-1640 medium.
2. Transfer the cells to a 4-mm-gap electroporation cuvette with 25 μM of antisense, sense, or mismatch oligonucleotides, and mix.
3. Place the cuvette on ice for 10 min, and then subject it to electroporation (1,250 μF/250 V) with an Electro Cell Manipulator 600.
4. Keep the cuvette at room temperature for another 10 min, and then re-culture the cells in a 6-well plate with complete DMEM medium until the cells are analyzed for the expression of MHC Class II molecules and Ii protein (*see* **Note 6**).

3.2.4 Immunostaining of Cultured Cells

1. Stain the cells using mAb for MHC Class II molecules and Ii protein.
2. For cell surface staining of MHC Class II molecules, wash the cells with HBSS, and incubate them with M5/114.15.2 mAb in a total volume of 200 μL for 45 min at room temperature.
3. Wash the cells, and incubate them with fluorescein-conjugated secondary antibody for 30 min at room temperature.
4. Wash the cells and fix them with 10 % formaldehyde for 10 min.
5. For intracellular staining of Ii protein, wash the cells with HBSS, and fix them with 2 % formalin at room temperature for 10 min.

Table 1
In vivo experimental groups

Control + ad-empty
rAV-IL-2
rAV-CIITA/INF-γ
rAV-CIITA/INF-γ + Ad-IL-2
rAV-CIITA/ INF-γ + Ad-IL-2 + Ad-Ii-RGC

6. Wash the cells with 1 mL of 1M glycine at room temperature for 5 min.
7. Permealize the cells with 0.2 % saponin, and incubate with 200 μL of Ii mAb In.1 for 60 min on ice.
8. Wash the cells, and label them with fluorescein-conjugated secondary antibody in 0.2 % saponin for 30–45 min at room temperature.
9. Wash the cells and fix them again with 10 % formaldehyde for 10 min.
10. Analyze the cells using FACS for the expression of MHC Class II molecules and Ii protein.

3.2.5 Intra-tumoral Treatment with Adenoviral Vectors

1. Inject Balb/c mice (~10 animals per group) subcutaneously (SC) with Renca cells at 2×10^5 cells in 0.1 mL HBSS (*see* **Note 7**).
2. On day 8 post cell injection, treat mice with established tumors of about 0.3 cm in diameter with intra-tumoral injections of rAVs mixtures (in situ) by a dose of individual rAV particles which is known to induce MHC Class II expression in >95 % of cells in vitro.
3. Randomly assign animals to different experimental groups as listed in Table 1.
4. To ensure the suppression of Ii induced by CIITA and IFN-γ, a tenfold dose of previously determined effective MOI in in vitro assays for rAV/Ii-RGC can be used, and a subtherapeutic dose of particles for rAV-IL-2 can be used.
5. Inject 50 μL of rAV particles in each tumor using 0.3-mL insulin syringes (*see* **Note 8**).
6. Inject the mice with corresponding rAV particles for 5 consecutive days, and monitor them for tumor growth.
7. Measure the tumors 3× a week using calipers.

8. Monitor animals for delayed tumor growth, complete or partial tumor regression.
9. Continue animal observation for 60 days. Animals which develop large tumors (~1.5–2 cm^3) should be sacrificed (*see* **Notes 9–12**).

4 Notes

1. Since electroporation kills about 50 % of cells, consider increasing the number of treated cells in case the final number of viable cells after electroporation is very low.
2. Glycine is used to neutralize excess formaldehyde. Efficient washing of cells with HBSS or phosphate-buffered saline can be effective for formaldehyde neutralization as well.
3. Both fixed and irradiated cells can be used to immunize mice. Irradiated cells are apparently more potent and provide long-lasting immunity.
4. Suppression of Ii protein may depend on the Ii-RGC:CIITA ratio. In case of subeffective suppression of Ii protein, consider increasing the ratio of Ii-RGC:CIITA.
5. In case no viral plaques are observed following transfection in 293 cells, assure that plasmid DNA preparation is optimal. Make sure that 293 cells are healthy and that concentrations of plasmids are optimal. Assure that 293 cells are used at an early passage level or utilize fresh stocks of cells.
6. If the efficiency of the transient transfection is not high enough, improve the transfection efficiency by optimizing the conditions or using different types of transfection reagents. Make sure to include positive controls.
7. Clean and sterilize the inoculation area of the mice with ethanol. Assure minimal bleeding from tumor site upon injection, and avoid repeated injections into the same site.
8. Administration of IL-2 plasmid is recommended to enhance immune response in animals.
9. Measure tumor volumes using the following formula:

$$\left(mm^3\right):\frac{\left[\left(width\right)^2 \times length\right]}{2}$$

10. Tumor regression is considered complete if the tumor burden has become unpalpable. Tumor regression is considered partial if tumor volume dropped to less than 50 % of the tumor volume at the start of treatment.

11. Monitor animals for signs of toxicity or infections.
12. Calculate mouse body weight change using the formula:

$$\frac{(\textit{Mouse weight on day } x - \textit{Mouse weight on day } 1)}{\textit{Mouse weight on day } 1} \times 100$$

A weight loss of ≥15 % of the initial body weight is considered toxic.

References

1. Restifo NP et al (1993) Molecular mechanisms used by tumors to escape immune recognition: immunogenetherapy and the cell biology of major histocompatibility complex class I. J Immunother 14:182–190
2. Costello RT et al (1999) Tumor escape from immune surveillance. Arch Immunol Ther Exp (Warsz) 47:83–88
3. Garcia-Lora A et al (2003) Tumour immunology, vaccination and escape strategies. Eur J Immunogenet 30:177–183
4. Humphreys RE et al (2004) Forcing tumor cells to present their own tumor antigens to the immune system: a necessary design for an efficient tumor immunotherapy. Cell Mol Immunol 1(3):180–185
5. Hillman GG et al (2004) Turning tumor cells in situ into T-helper cell-stimulating, MHC Class II tumor epitope-presenters: immuno-curing and immuno-consolidation. Cancer Treat Rev 30(3):281–290
6. Marsman M et al (2005) Chaperoning antigen presentation by MHC Class II molecules and their role in oncogenesis. Adv Cancer Res 93: 129–158
7. Castellino F et al (1997) Antigen presentation by MHC class II molecules: invariant chain function, protein trafficking, and the molecular basis of diverse determinant capture. Hum Immunol 54(2):159–169
8. Bertolino P, Rabourdin-Combe C (1996) The MHC Class II-associated invariant chain: a molecule with multiple roles in MHC class II biosynthesis and antigen presentation to $CD4^+$ T cells. Crit Rev Immunol 16:359–379
9. Kropshofer H et al (1996) Editing of the HLA-DR-peptide repertoire by HLA-DM. EMBO J 15:6144–6154
10. Xu M et al (2000) Genetic modulation of tumor antigen presentation. Trends Biotechnol 18:167–172
11. Spiro RC et al (1984) The Ii nature of p35 on hairy leukemic cells. Semin Oncol 11:427–432
12. Baskar S et al (1994) MHC class II-transfected tumor cells induce long-term tumor-specific immunity in autologous mice. Cell Immunol 155:123–133
13. Scanlon KJ et al (1995) Oligonucleotide-mediated modulation of mammalian gene expression. FASEB J 9:1288–1296
14. Dias N, Stein CA (2002) Antisense oligonucleotides: basic concepts and mechanisms. Mol Cancer Ther 1(5):347–355
15. Qiu G et al (1999) Cancer immunotherapy by antisense suppression of Ii protein in MHC-class-II-positive tumor cells. Cancer Immunol Immunother 48(9):499–506
16. Lu X et al (2003) Tumor immunotherapy by converting tumor cells to MHC class II-positive, Ii protein-negative phenotype. Cancer Immunol Immunother 52(10):592–598
17. Hillman GG et al (2003) Generating MHC Class II+/Ii− phenotype after adenoviral delivery of both an expressible gene for MHC Class II inducer and an antisense Ii-RNA construct in tumor cells. Gene Ther 10(17):1512–1518

Chapter 23

The Direct Display of Costimulatory Proteins on Tumor Cells as a Means of Vaccination for Cancer Immunotherapy

Haval Shirwan, Esma S. Yolcu, Rajesh K. Sharma, Hong Zaho, and Orlando Grimany-Nuno

Abstract

Therapeutic vaccines against cancer are at their prime, owing to our comprehensive understanding of immune effector responses generated against tumor and the mechanisms employed by the progressing tumor to evade the immune system. The immune system is primed by tumor-associated antigens (TAA) that are perceived as foreign. Therefore, the identification of TAA led to the development of subunit vaccine formulations comprising defined TAA as stand-alone vaccines or in combination with immune adjuvants. Inasmuch as cancer cells express a diverse set of TAA, novel immunomodulatory approaches that not only use tumor cells as a source of diverse TAA but also convert them into competent antigen-presenting cells have significant therapeutic potential as cell-based vaccines. Toward this end, we have developed a novel protein display approach designated as ProtEx™ as a safe and efficient alternative to DNA-based gene expression to generate novel immunomodulatory molecules and display them on tumor cells for the development of cancer vaccines. This chapter describes the ProtEx™ technology and its application to the generation of tumor cell-based cancer vaccines.

Key words ProtEx™, LIGHT, 4-1BBL, CD137, SA-4-1BBL, Cancer vaccine, Costimulation

1 Introduction

Cancer is the leading cause of death in the United States and many developed countries. There is currently no clinically proven regimen to permanently eradicate malignant tumors. Therapeutic vaccines have potential to serve as an attractive alternative to standard treatments because of their specificity, safety, and long-term immunological memory, which is critical for controlling micrometastases that are the primary cause of recurrences and cancer-related mortality. Various vaccine strategies have been developed including the use of specific tumor-associated antigens (TAA) in conjunction with nonspecific or specific adjuvants; whole tumor cell lysates; tumor cells genetically modified to express costimulatory molecules, cytokines, or chemokines; DC pulsed with tumor

Michael J.P. Lawman and Patricia D. Lawman (eds.), *Cancer Vaccines: Methods and Protocols*, Methods in Molecular Biology, vol. 1139, DOI 10.1007/978-1-4939-0345-0_23, © Springer Science+Business Media New York 2014

antigens or transfected with tumor RNA or DNA; and intratumoral injection of various vectors encoding a range of immunostimulatory molecules [1–5].

The use of whole tumor cells or lysates from such cells is a scientifically sound approach for the development of therapeutic cancer vaccines as vaccination with whole tumor cells or cell lysates appears to be more effective in eradicating disseminated cancer in animal models than individual TAA-based vaccines [1–3, 6]. Tumor cells may serve as depots for all TAA and, as such, possess the ability to activate diverse immune responses, leading to improved therapeutic efficacy. This approach also safeguards against various immunoevasive mechanisms, such as antigenic drift and tolerance to these antigens acquired during the course of tumor progression [7, 8]. Inasmuch as $CD8^+$ T cells serve as an important effector of the immune system against tumors [9], and these cells recognize endogenous tumor antigens presented by class I MHC molecules, immunization with whole tumor cells modified to acquire the capacity of serving as antigen-presenting cells (APC) represents an important vaccine strategy. In particular, direct presentation of antigens by tumor cells to $CD8^+$ T cells and their activation, differentiation, and acquisition of effector functions within the tumor microenvironment will override various limitations faced by other tumor antigen-based cancer vaccine approaches, the most obvious ones being inefficient presentation of exogenous antigens via a class I pathway and inability of activated T cells to traffic into the tumor site [10].

Immune responses mediated by T cells play a critical role in the prevention and eradication of cancer [2, 11, 12]. A productive T cell response, however, requires three distinct signals: (1) T cell receptor interaction with MHC/peptide complex, (2) costimulation via CD28 and tumor necrosis factor receptor superfamily, and (3) cytokines elaborated by activated lymphocytes and professional APC, such as macrophages and dendritic cells [13–17]. Although tumors employ several different mechanisms to evade the immune system [2, 3, 12, 18], the lack of costimulation is the most commonly used mechanism [19, 20]. Tumor cells manipulated via gene transfer approaches to express costimulatory molecules were, therefore, shown to generate effective antitumor immune responses when used as vaccines [20–22]. From the perspective of therapeutic cancer vaccines, gene transfer approaches are laborious, not applicable to certain tumors, and may also involve safety concerns. Therefore, we developed a method, ProtEx™, that allows for rapid, durable, and efficient display of exogenous proteins on tumor cells without the complication of gene transfer approaches. This technology involves (1) generation of a chimeric protein consisting of core streptavidin (SA) and functional domains of a desired protein (Fig. 1), (2) modification of the cell membrane with biotin, and

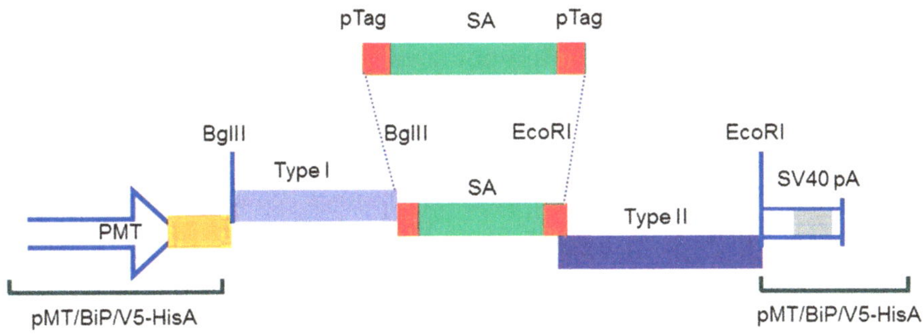

Fig. 1 Generation of SA chimeric proteins. Schematic diagram of cloning strategies for type I and type II proteins to generate chimeric molecules with streptavidin (SA) using pMT/BiP/V5-HisA vector for expression in *Drosophila* Schneider 2 cells

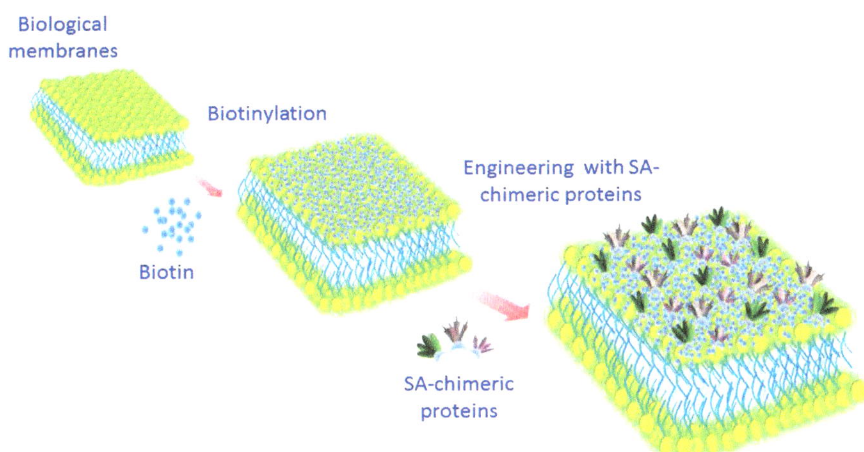

Fig. 2 Schematic diagram of ProtEx™ technology. Any biological membrane can be modified with biotin followed by engineering with SA chimeric proteins singly or in combination within 3 h under physiological conditions

(3) engineering of the biotinylated cells with the chimeric protein under physiological conditions without any deleterious effect to the target cell viability and function (Fig. 2). Inasmuch as receptor-ligand interactions on the surface of immune cells are critical to immune responses and these interactions do not need to be extensive in duration [23], transient display of exogenous immunological ligands on the cell surface provides a powerful approach to immunomodulation [24–27].

The direct display of SA chimeric proteins with defined immunological functions on biological membranes as described in this chapter has significant potential as a practical (performed on established and primary cells within 3 h), efficient (~100 % of targeted cells), and safe alternative to DNA-based gene expression for immunomodulation to treat immune-based disorders. Importantly, this technology allows for the display of multiple proteins simultaneously and at desired levels on biological membranes. The codisplay of immunological ligands with complementary and/or synergistic functions has significant potential for the development of combinatorial immunomodulatory approaches for effective immune therapies. Furthermore, the transient display of proteins with pleiotropic effects overcomes the unwanted effects associated with continuous expression of proteins using DNA-based gene therapy. Although we present examples of engineering isolated primary or tumor cells with various SA chimeric proteins, this approach can also be applied to engineering of tissues or organs, providing a platform with broad applications in the field of immunomodulation.

2 Materials

The following materials are used for the expression of costimulatory molecules and engineering of tumor cells and their use as cell-based vaccines against cancer in mice:

1. Cellfectin® II Reagent.
2. DES®–Inducible Kit with pCoHygro.
3. Chelating Sepharose Fast Flow.
4. Phosphate-buffered saline (PBS).
5. Deionized water (endotoxin-free, Millipore filtered, autoclaved).
6. 0.5 M sodium chloride (NaCl), filtered.
7. 20 mM ethylenediaminetetraacetic acid (EDTA) in PBS and pH 8.0, filtered.
8. Imidazole in 50 mM Tris–HCl, pH 8.0 and 10 mM in 50 mM Tris–HCl, pH 8.0.
9. 10 % Pluronic F-68 solution.
10. Cupper (II) sulfate pentahydrate ($CuS0_4{\cdot}5H_2O$).
11. 20 % ethanol.
12. SA forward primer: 5′AGATCTCATCATCACCA TCACC ATATCACCGGCACC.
13. SA reverse primer: 5′GAATTCGGAGGCGGCGGACGGCT.
14. 4-1BBL forward primer: 5′ATCGAATTCCGCACCGAGCC TCGGCCAGCG.
15. 4-1BBL reverse primer: 5′GGACTCGAGCATAGCAGCTT GAGGACTTAGC.
16. EZ-Link Sulfo-NHS-SS-biotin.
17. LAL Chromogenic Endotoxin Quantitation Kit.

18. TC-1 cell line.
19. *Streptomyces avidinii* genomic DNA.
20. PCR2.1TOPO vector.
21. pMT/BiP/V5-His vector.
22. Schneider 2 cells.
23. Schneider 2 medium.
24. Restriction enzymes *BglII, EcoRI,* and *Xho*I.
25. Lipopolysaccharide (LPS).
26. Kimwipes.
27. 15-mL Falcon tubes.
28. BCA protein assay.
29. T75 flasks.
30. Fetal bovine serum (FBS).
31. 10-kDa Centricons.

3 Methods

Good laboratory practices with respect to the cell culture, protein expression, and purification need to be exercised. Extreme caution needs to be practiced to prevent cell contamination, and as such, all equipment and solutions used for cell culture and protein expression must be sterile and endotoxin-free. Protein purification needs to be performed in a cold room for the most optimum outcome, and purified protein needs to be aliquoted and stored in –80 °C until use. Inasmuch as the primary focus of this chapter is on the ProtEx™ technology, we will refrain from detailed protocols related to molecular cloning and transfection and maintenance of S2 cells. All animals in past experiments were cared for in accordance with the University of Louisville Institutional and NIH guidelines.

3.1 Cloning of Streptavidin

1. 0.2 μg of *S. avidinii* genomic DNA is used as template for amplification in PCR using core streptavidin-specific forward and reverse primers (*see* **Note 1**).
2. The PCR product is run on an agarose gel, purified, and restricted with *Bgl* II and *Eco* RI.
3. The restriction enzyme digestion is repurified using a PCR purification kit and used for cloning into *Bgl* II- and *Eco* RI-restricted pMT/BiP/V5-His $CuSO_4$-inducible DES expression vector.
4. After transformation of competent cells, a colony containing the recombinant plasmid with streptavidin is identified and used for large-scale plasmid preparation.

3.2 Construction of SA-4-1BBL

1. Mouse splenocytes are stimulated with 5 μg/mL LPS for 2 days to upregulate the expression of 4-1BBL on antigen-presenting cells.
2. Total RNA is isolated from activated cells using a standard protocol.
3. Two micrograms of RNA is converted into the first-strand cDNA in 20 μL of total reaction mixture using oligo(dT).
4. Two microliters of the first-strand cDNA reaction is used as template in RT-PCR with forward and reverse primers specific for the extracellular domain of 4-1BBL.
5. The PCR product is then cloned into the PCR2.1TOPO vector.
6. A single clone containing the accurate sequence for 4-1BBL is digested with *Eco* RI and *Xho* I and subcloned into pMT/BiP/V5-HisA expression vector containing the 6×His Tag core SA sequence (described in Subheading 3.1) and restricted with the same enzymes (*see* **Note 2**) (Fig. 1).
7. A clone containing the chimeric gene can be identified by sequencing and used for transfection of S2 cells and protein expression.

3.3 Reviving and Maintaining the S2 Cells

1. Take out a vial of S2 cells from liquid nitrogen.
2. Thaw it by warming up the vial in a 37 °C water bath until 50 % of the vial content is thawed (*see* **Note 3**).
3. Rinse the vial with 70 % ethanol; wipe and dry the outside of vial using Kimwipes before transferring the content into a 15-mL Falcon tube.
4. Bring up the volume to 14 mL with complete S2 cell medium and Schneider's medium supplemented with 10 % FBS (*see* **Note 4**).
5. Centrifuge the cells at 328 × *g* (Beckman GS-6KR centrifuge) for 7 min at 4 °C to collect cells.
6. Decant the supernatant and resuspend the cells in 10 mL of complete S2 cell medium.
7. Transfer the cells into a T75 flask for culturing in a 27 °C non-humidified incubator without CO_2.
8. Change the medium the next day and add 10 mL of fresh complete S2 medium.
9. Maintain the cells by counting every other day until the cell concentration reaches 20×10^6 cells/mL.
10. Collect the cells by tapping the flask several times to dislodge cells.

11. Transfer the cell suspension into a sterile conical tube and centrifuge as in **step 5**.
12. Split the cells by seeding at a density of 5×10^5 viable cells/mL (*see* **Note 5**).

3.4 Transfection of Drosophila S2 Cells

1. S2 cells are co-transfected with pMT/BiP/V5-His containing the chimeric SA-4-1BBL plasmid and pCoHygro selection vector at 19:1 ratio.
2. Stable transfectants are established using hygromycin B selection medium (*see* **Note 6**).

3.5 Expression and Purification of SA-4-1BBL

1. Seed S2 cells at 5×10^6 cells/mL and viability of >95 % in 200 mL of complete S2 cell medium in a 500-mL shake flask.
2. Incubate the flask at 27 °C with a constant stirring rate of 90–105 rpm until cell density reaches ~20–30 × 10^6 cells/mL with >95 % viability.
3. Transfer the cell suspension into a sterile conical tube and centrifuge as in Subheading 3.3, **step 5**.
4. Resuspended the cells at 20×10^6 cells/mL in 250 mL of Schneider's medium without serum in a 500-mL shake flask.
5. Add $CuSO_4$ at a final concentration of 1 mM.
6. Incubate the flask at 22 °C with a constant stirring rate of 90–105 rpm for 3 days (*see* **Note 7**).
7. Transfer the cell suspension into a sterile conical tube, and collect the supernatant following centrifugation at 328 × *g* for 10 min at 4 °C.
8. Transfer supernatant to fresh centrifuge tube(s) and repeat centrifugation one more time at 2,053 × *g* for 10–15 min at 4 °C.
9. Pass the supernatant through 0.2-μm Nalgene sterile filters, and store at 4 °C until purification (*see* **Note 8**).

3.6 Purification Using Immobilized Metal Ion Affinity Chromatography

1. Mix filtered supernatant with 5 mM imidazole and rotate for 1 h at 4 °C (*see* **Note 9**).
2. Wash a 150-mL column with deionized water.
3. Mix Sepharose Fast Flow by gently shaking or inverting the bottle several times.
4. Pack 20 mL of Sepharose Fast Flow into the column, and wash packed matrix with 200 mL of sterile deionized H_2O.
5. Close the bottom valve and load 500 mL of SA-4-1BBL supernatant.
6. Open the valve and collect the flow through at a rate of 8 mL/min.

7. Wash the column with 100 mL of PBS at a flow rate of 12 mL/min.
8. Wash the column with 50 mL of 0.5 M NaCl at a flow rate of 12 mL/min.
9. Wash the column with 50 mL of 5 mM imidazole at a flow rate of 12 mL/min.
10. Wash the column with 10 mL of 10 mM imidazole at a flow rate of 12 mL/min.
11. Elute SA-4-1BBL protein with 20 mL of 100 mM imidazole at a flow rate of 3 mL/min.
12. Collect elution as 3-mL fractions.
13. Strip the column with 40 mL of 20 mM EDTA at a flow rate of 10 mL/min, and collect the first 10 mL of elution (*see* **Note 10**).
14. Run 20 μL from each fraction on an SDS-PAGE to check the presence and purity of SA-4-1BBL protein.
15. Pool and dialysate the fractions containing SA-4-1BBL against PBS.
16. Concentrate the protein by passing through a 10-kDa Centricon.
17. Measure the protein concentration using BCA protein assay.
18. Test for endotoxin using LAL Chromogenic Endotoxin Quantitation Kit.
19. Aliquot the protein solution and keep in −80 °C for long-term storage.

3.7 Reviving and Maintaining the TC-1 Cells

1. Remove a vial of TC-1 cells from liquid nitrogen.
2. Thaw the cells by warming the vial in a 37 °C water bath until 50 % of the vial contents are thawed (*see* **Note 3**).
3. Rinse the vial with 70 % ethanol; wipe and dry outside of vial using Kimwipes before damping the content into a 15-mL Falcon tube containing 7 mL of RPMI 1640 medium.
4. Bring up the volume to 14 mL.
5. Pellet the cells at 328 × *g* (Beckman GS-6KR centrifuge) for 7 min at 4 °C.
6. Decant the supernatant and resuspend the cells in 10 mL of complete TC-1 medium (RPMI 1640 supplemented with 2 mMl-glutamine, 4.5 g/L of glucose, 10 mM HEPES, 1.0 mM sodium pyruvate, 2 mM nonessential amino acids, and 10 % FBS) (*see* **Note 11**).
7. Transfer the cells into a T75 flask for culturing overnight.
8. Change the media next day and add 10 mL of fresh TC-1 medium.

3.8 Splitting the TC-1 Cells

1. Split the cells when the culture reaches 90 % confluency (*see* **Note 12**); aspirate off the old medium and wash the flask with 10 mL of RPMI 1640.
2. Add 3–5 mL of trypsin and incubate the flask for 3–5 min at 37 °C.
3. When the cells start coming off the flask surface, immediately add 1 mL of FBS, and shake flask gently to block the trypsin.
4. Add 9 mL of RPMI 1640 and pipette up and down to make a single cell suspension.
5. Transfer the cells into a 15-mL Falcon tube.
6. Centrifuge cells at 328 × *g* for 7 min at 4 °C to collect the cell pellet.
7. Decant the medium and resuspend the cells in 2–3 mL complete TC-1 medium.
8. Count the viable cells using a hemocytometer.
9. Transfer 1.5–2×10^6 TC-1 cells into a T75 flask containing 10 mL of TC-1 medium.
10. Change the medium every other day, and use the cells for tumor challenge or preparation of the vaccine as described below.

3.9 Vaccine Preparation

1. Trypsinize 80–90 % confluent TC-1 cells and collect in a 50-mL Falcon tube as described above.
2. Count the cells and determine their viability (*see* **Note 13**).
3. Centrifuge the tube at 328 × *g* for 7 min at 4 °C to collect the cells.
4. Decant the medium and resuspend the cell pellet in 50 μM EZ-Link Sulfo-NHS-SS-biotin (50,000 cells/mL), and incubate for 30 min at room temperature on a rotating shaker (*see* **Note 14**).
5. Wash the cells by adding 30 mL of PBS followed by centrifugation at 328 × *g* for 7 min at 4 °C.
6. Resuspend the cells in 5 mL of PBS; transfer to a 15-mL Falcon tube and count.
7. Irradiate the biotinylated cells at 15,000 cGy using a gamma irradiator.
8. Divide the cells into three fractions containing the appropriate number of cells to be co-engineered with recombinant proteins or left un-engineered to be used as control to assess biotinylation levels.
9. Collect cell pellet by centrifuging at 328 × *g* for 7 min at 4 °C.
10. Resuspend the cells in PBS containing 2 μg of each SA-LIGHT and SA-4-1BBL protein/1×10^6 TC-1 cells/100 μL. Use equal molar amounts of SA (~100 μg/1×10^6 cells) as a control.

11. Incubate for 30 min at 4 °C on a rotating shaker.
12. Add 10 mL of PBS and wash the cells by centrifugation at $328 \times g$ for 7 min at 4 °C.
13. Resuspend the engineered cells in an appropriate volume of PBS; count, and aliquot 2×10^6 cells in 200 μL in 1.5-mL sterile Eppendorf tubes for vaccination. Keep the cells on ice until use.
14. Take an aliquot of LIGHT/4-1BBL or SA-engineered cells, and stain with appropriate fluorochrome-conjugated antibodies (Abs) against LIGHT, 4-1BBL, and SA, and analyze using flow cytometry to assess the levels of each protein on the cell surface. Biotinylated cells without protein engineering (*see* **step 8**) should be stained with APC-SA to confirm biotinylation levels (*see* **Notes 15, 16**).

3.10 TC-1 Tumor Inoculation

1. Aliquot 1×10^5 TC-1 cells per 1.5-mL sterile Eppendorf tube containing 200 μL of PBS on ice.
2. Once in the vivarium, fingertip the vial to mix TC-1 cells, and aspirate all the volume into 1-mL syringe with a 27-gauge needle.
3. Inject the cells subcutaneously (SC) into C57BL/6 mice in the middle of right flank (*see* **Note 17**).

3.11 Vaccination with LIGHT/4-1BBL-Engineered TC-1 Cells

1. Label 1.5-mL sterile Eppendorf tubes with the corresponding animal numbers, 1 tube per mouse.
2. Dispense 200 μL of sterile PBS containing 2×10^6 LIGHT/4-1BBL-engineered cells into each tube.
3. Similarly, dispense 200 μL of sterile PBS containing 2×10^6 SA-engineered cells into each tube.
4. Transfer tubes on ice into the vivarium and perform vaccination using a 27-gauge needle SC in close proximity to the site of challenge with the live TC-1 cells.
5. Monitor tumor growth 2× a week using digital calipers. Mice with tumors of 15 mm in diameter or poor health conditions should be euthanized per Institutional Animal Care and Use Committee guidelines (*see* **Note 18**).

4 Notes

1. The 5′-primer include sequences for *Bgl* II and 6 His residues to allow cloning in frame with the *Drosophila* secretion signal (BiP) for expression as a secreted protein and purification using Ni-affinity columns.

2. In designing the gene for the chimeric proteins, we clone type I proteins N-terminus and type II proteins C-terminus to the SA to facilitate the generation of functional chimeric immunological ligands with respect to binding to biotin and counter immune receptors (Fig. 2).
3. Do not let the cells thaw completely at 37 °C as the recovery after culturing will be slow.
4. This medium is used for maintaining cells, but not for protein expression as biotin in FBS may compete with biotin on cell surface for engineering.
5. Refer to Invitrogen DES expression system protocol for extensive information for the growth, maintenance, and induction of S2 cells.
6. Refer to Invitrogen DES expression system protocol for extensive information on transfection of S2 cells and the establishment of stable transfectants.
7. Monitor the cell growth by taking samples on daily basis. Cells should expand slightly for the first 24 h followed by a steady decrease in viability. Harvest the medium for protein purification if the cell numbers drop below 10×10^6 cells/mL.
8. Supernatant can be frozen at −80 °C for long-term storage.
9. This process blocks the low-binding Drosophila proteins rich in histidine to the column.
10. Re-equilibrate the column with 200 mL of deionized sterile water, and store the packed column in 0.01 M NaOH in cold room.
11. Refer to ATCC for the TC-1 cell product description for complete information on the growth and maintenance of this cell line in culture.
12. Do not let cells reach beyond 90 % confluency as such cells may change their growth characteristics and expression of TAA.
13. The use of cells with less than 85 % viability may compromise their growth in vivo, and such cells may further undergo death in vivo.
14. Biotinylation of the cell membrane is an important and critical step in the process of displaying SA chimeric exogenous proteins on the cell surface. We have historically used EZ-Link™ Sulfo-NHS-LC-Biotin from Pierce for biotinylation. However, there are numerous forms of biotin with various spacer arms available commercially that can be used for this purpose. Although we have not performed a systematic analysis of biotin with various spacer arms, it intuitively makes sense that biotin with longer spacer arms may have better efficacy in binding to

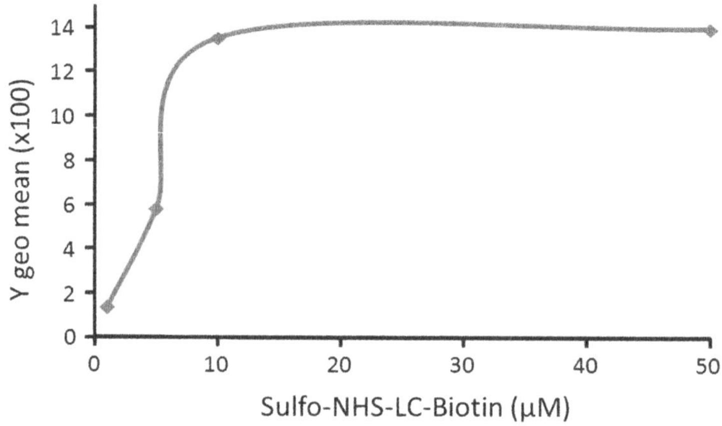

Fig. 3 Concentration-dependent display of biotin on the cell surface. 2.5×10^6 mouse splenocytes were biotinylated using various concentrations of Sulfo-NHS-LC-Biotin. The cell surface presence of biotin was assessed using APC-labeled SA and analysis using flow cytometry. Geometric mean fluorescence intensity (Y geo mean) is graphed as a function of biotin concentrations

SA chimeric protein by avoiding potential steric hindrance due to the size and conformation of the chimeric protein. We have tested various biotin concentrations for cell surface modification to determine an optimal platform that allows simultaneous display of several SA chimeric proteins without compromising the cell survival or function. Sulfo-NHS-LC-Biotin concentrations varying from 1 to 50 μM were tested. There was a direct correlation between the biotin concentration and the level of biotin detected on the cell surface (Fig. 3). However, we have been using 5 μM Sulfo-NHS-LC-Biotin for applications aimed at displaying a single SA chimeric protein on tumor or primary cells for systemic immunomodulation [26, 27]. However, this concentration can further be increased to 10–50 μM if more than one chimeric proteins are aimed for simultaneous display on the cell surface without compromising the viability and function of the cell.

15. Using various SA chimeric proteins, we demonstrated efficient cell surface display of these proteins irrespective of the nature of the target cells, which included established rodents and human tumor cells of various origins [19, 25, 29] as well as primary cells, including endothelial cells, splenocytes, and bone marrow cells [26, 28, 30]. At a given biotin concentration used for the cell surface modification, there was a direct correlation between the concentration of an SA chimeric protein and the numbers of such protein being displayed on the cell surface (Fig. 4).
16. We have demonstrated that multiple proteins can be simultaneously displayed at the surface of primary cells, such as

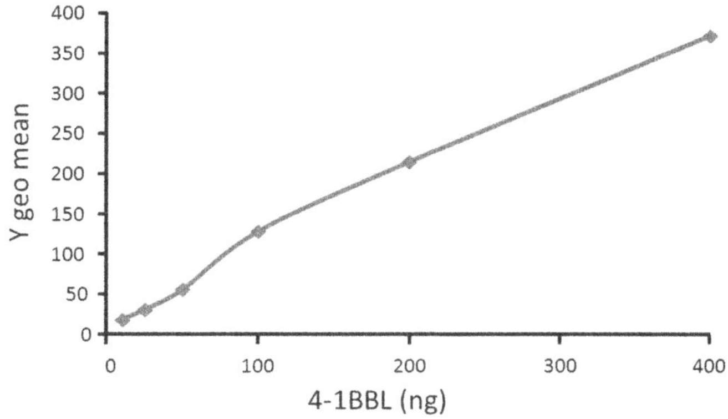

Fig. 4 Dose-dependent display of SA chimeric proteins on the cell surface. 1×10^6 mouse splenocytes were biotinylated using Sulfo-NHS-LC-Biotin (5 μM) and engineered with various concentrations of 4-1BBL. Cells were stained using an anti-4-1BBL Ab and analyzed in flow cytometry. Geometric mean fluorescence intensity (Y geo mean) is graphed as a function of protein concentrations

splenocytes, or tumor cells without compromising the viability and function of the cells. For example, biotinylated (15 μM) TC-1 tumor cells (Fig. 5) or splenocytes (Fig. 6) co-displayed 2 SA chimeric costimulatory proteins, 4-1BBL and LIGHT, on their surface with equal efficiency. The in vitro kinetics of turnover on the surface of splenocytes was rather slow and protein dependent, 4-1BBL having faster kinetics ($t_{1/2}$~5 days) than LIGHT ($t_{1/2}$>8 days) (Fig. 6). Importantly, TC-1 cells modified with a higher concentration of biotin (50 μM) and engineered with 2 μg of each 4-1BBL and LIGHT proteins could be further engineered with SA as a third protein. As shown in Fig. 7, all the cells had the three proteins displayed on their surface, suggesting that this platform may allow simultaneous display of more than three proteins on the cell surface with equal efficiency and levels.

17. A bulb under the skin should be obvious if the injection is performed accurately.
18. Table 1 shows the efficacy of vaccination with TC-1 cells co-engineered with SA-4-1BBL and SA-LIGHT costimulatory molecules.

Acknowledgement

This study was funded in parts by Kentucky Lung Cancer Research Program, the W.M. Keck Foundation, and the Commonwealth of Kentucky Research Challenge Trust Fund.

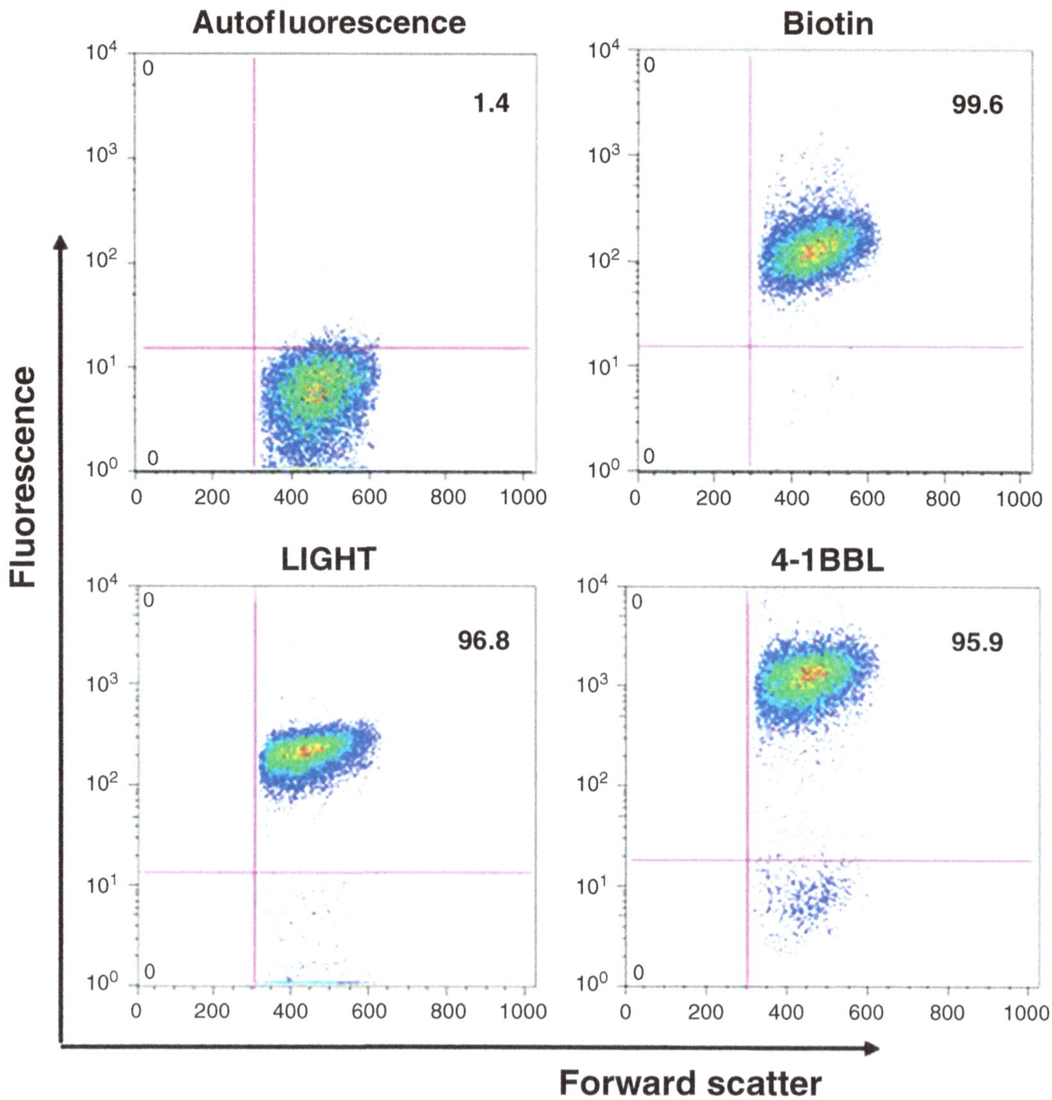

Fig. 5 Engineering of TC-1 tumor cells with 2 SA chimeric proteins simultaneously. TC-1 cells were biotinylated using 15 μM of Sulfo-NHS-LC-Biotin and engineered with chimeric LIGHT and 4-1BBL proteins at 200 ng/protein/10^6 cells. Cells were stained with Abs against SA (LIGHT) and 4-1BBL molecules and analyzed using flow cytometry

Conflict of interest disclosure: The ProtEx™ technology described herein is licensed from University of Louisville by ApoVax, Inc. for which H. Shirwan serves as CSO and Member of the Board, and H. Shirwan and E.S. Yolcu have significant financial interest in the Company. All the other authors declare no conflicts of interest.

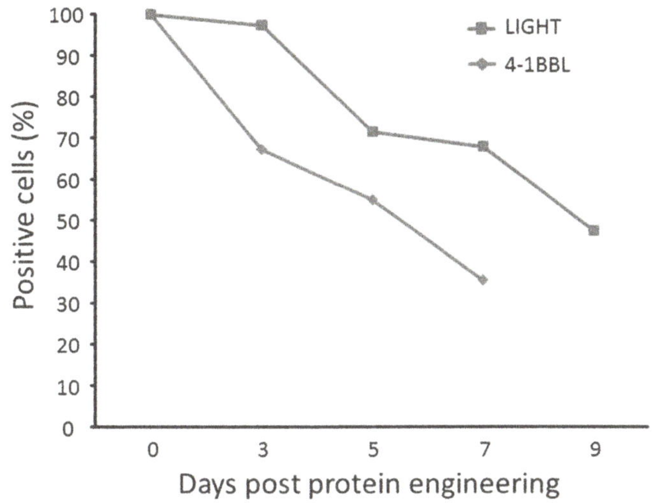

Fig. 6 Turnover kinetics of SA chimeric proteins from the cell surface in vitro. Mouse splenocytes were biotinylated (15 μM) and engineered with chimeric LIGHT and 4-1BBL proteins at 200 ng/protein/10^6 cells. Cells were stained with Abs against SA (LIGHT) and 4-1BBL molecules and analyzed using flow cytometry at the indicated times to determine the loss of proteins from the surface of more than 50 % of cells

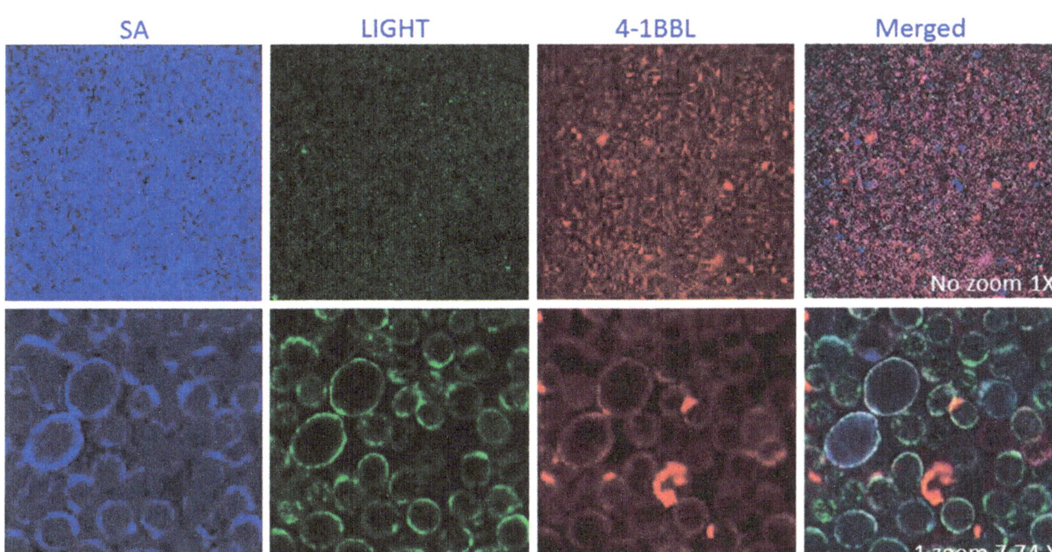

Fig. 7 Engineering TC-1 tumor cells to simultaneously display on their surface multiple proteins. TC-1 cells were biotinylated using 50 μM EZ-Link Sulfo-NHS-SS-biotin followed by incubation of 10^6 cells with 2 μg of chimeric 4-1BBL and 2 μg of LIGHT proteins. The cell surface presence of chimeric proteins was detected using Abs against 4-1BBL (*red*) or SA portion of LIGHT (*green*). Fluorochrome-labeled streptavidin (SA, *blue*) was used as a third protein to assess the presence of free biotin remaining on the cell surface after engineering with the chimeric proteins

Table 1
Vaccination with TC-1 cells co-engineered with both SA chimeric LIGHT and 4-1BBL proteins prevents tumor growth in a therapeutic setting[a]

Vaccination	Tumor growth	Survival (%)
None	20/20	0
SA-TC-1	6/6	0
LIGHT/4-1BBL-TC-1	4/7	~57

[a]Naïve C57BL/6 mice were challenged SC on the right flank with 1×10^5 live TC-1 cells followed by vaccination SC with 2×10^6 irradiated TC-1 cells engineered using 50 μM biotin and 2 μg of each LIGHT and 4-1BBL protein per 10^6 cells on the same day. Mice without vaccination or those vaccinated with TC-1 cells engineered with equimolar amount of SA protein was used as controls. Mice were monitored for tumor development for 60 days

References

1. Berzofsky JA et al (2004) Progress on new vaccine strategies for the immunotherapy and prevention of cancer. J Clin Invest 113: 1515–1525
2. Finn OJ (2003) Cancer vaccines: between the idea and the reality. Nat Rev Immunol 3: 630–641
3. Platsoucas CD et al (2003) Immune responses to human tumors: development of tumor vaccines. Anticancer Res 23:1969–1996
4. Dougan M, Dranoff G (2009) Immune therapy for cancer. Annu Rev Immunol 27:83–117. doi:10.1146/annurev.immunol.021908.132544
5. Schlom J (2012) Therapeutic cancer vaccines: current status and moving forward. J Natl Cancer Inst 104:599–613
6. Keenan BP, Jaffee EM (2012) Whole cell vaccines—past progress and future strategies. Semin Oncol 39:276–286
7. Hazelbag S et al (2002) Transforming growth factor-beta1 induces tumor stroma and reduces tumor infiltrate in cervical cancer. Hum Pathol 33:1193–1199
8. Terabe M, Berzofsky JA (2004) Immunoregulatory T cells in tumor immunity. Curr Opin Immunol 16:157–162
9. Srivastava AK et al (2012) Prime-boost vaccination with SA-4-1BBL costimulatory molecule and survivin eradicates lung carcinoma in CD8[+] T and NK cell dependent manner. PLoS One 7:e48463
10. Ochsenbein AF et al (2001) Roles of tumour localization, second signals and cross priming in cytotoxic T-cell induction. Nature 411: 1058–1064
11. Antonia SJ et al (2004) Current developments of immunotherapy in the clinic. Curr Opin Immunol 16:130–136
12. Pardoll DM (2002) Spinning molecular immunology into successful immunotherapy. Nat Rev Immunol 2:227–238
13. Gimmi CD et al (1993) Human T-cell clonal anergy is induced by antigen presentation in the absence of B7 costimulation. Proc Natl Acad Sci USA 90:6586–6590
14. Anderson RC et al (2007) Lack of B7 expression, not human leukocyte antigen expression, facilitates immune evasion by human malignant gliomas. Neurosurgery 60:1129–1136
15. Azuma M et al (1993) B70 antigen is a second ligand for CTLA-4 and CD28. Nature 366: 76–79
16. Allison JP, Krummel MF (1995) The Yin and Yang of T cell costimulation. Science 270: 932–933
17. Grossman Z et al (2004) Concomitant regulation of T-cell activation and homeostasis. Nat Rev Immunol 4:387–395
18. Chen L (2004) Co-inhibitory molecules of the B7-CD28 family in the control of T-cell immunity. Nat Rev Immunol 4:336–347
19. Singh NP et al (2003) A novel approach to cancer immunotherapy: tumor cells decorated with CD80 generate effective antitumor immunity. Cancer Res 63:4067–4073
20. Townsend SE, Allison JP (1993) Tumor rejection after direct costimulation of CD8+ T cells

by B7-transfected melanoma cells. Science 259:368–370

21. Antonia SJ et al (2002) Phase I trial of a B7-1 (CD80) gene modified autologous tumor cell vaccine in combination with systemic interleukin-2 in patients with metastatic renal cell carcinoma. J Urol 167:1995–2000
22. Horig H et al (2000) Phase I clinical trial of a recombinant canarypoxvirus (ALVAC) vaccine expressing human carcinoembryonic antigen and the B7.1 co-stimulatory molecule. Cancer Immunol Immunother 49:504–514
23. Kaech SM et al (2002) Effector and memory T-cell differentiation: implications for vaccine development. Nat Rev Immunol 2:251–262
24. Yolcu ES et al (2011) Pancreatic islets engineered with SA-FasL protein establish robust localized tolerance by inducing T regulatory cells in mice. J Immunol 187: 5901–5909
25. Sharma RK et al (2010) Tumor cells engineered to codisplay on their surface 4-1BBL and LIGHT costimulatory proteins as a novel vaccine approach for cancer immunotherapy. Cancer Gene Ther 17:730–741
26. Yolcu ES et al (2008) Induction of tolerance to cardiac allografts using donor splenocytes engineered to display on their surface an exogenous fas ligand protein. J Immunol 181: 931–939
27. Yolcu ES et al (2002) Cell membrane modification for rapid display of proteins as a novel means of immunomodulation: FasL-decorated cells prevent islet graft rejection. Immunity 17:795–808
28. Askenasy N et al (2003) Display of Fas ligand protein on cardiac vasculature as a novel means of regulating allograft rejection. Circulation 107:41–47
29. Singh NP et al (2006) Primary tumor cells from cancer patients decorated with a novel form of CD80 protein serve as effective antigen-presenting cells for the induction of autologous T-cell immune responses ex vivo. Hum Gene Ther 17:334–346
30. Pearl-Yafe M et al (2007) Fas-ligand enhances hematopoietic cell engraftment through abrogation of alloimmune responses and nonimmunogenic interactions. Stem Cells 25(6): 1448–1455

Part IV

Manipulation of Immune/Tumor Interactions

Chapter 24

Cloning Variable Region Genes of Clonal Lymphoma Immunoglobulin for Generating Patient-Specific Idiotype DNA Vaccine

Soung-chul Cha, Hong Qin, Ippei Sakamaki, and Larry Kwak

Abstract

Available therapies for lymphoplasmacytic lymphoma (LPL) provide no survival advantage if started before signs or symptoms of end-organ damage develop; hence, current recommendations are to follow a program of observation while patients are in the asymptomatic phase of disease. We hypothesize that using idiotypic determinants of a B-cell lymphoma's surface immunoglobulin as a tumor-specific marker, we can develop patient-specific chemokine-idiotype fusion DNA vaccines that induce an immune response against LPL. By activating the host immune system against the tumor antigen, we postulate that disease control of asymptomatic phase lymphoplasmacytic lymphoma can be maintained. These chemokine-idiotype fusion DNA vaccines provide protection in a lymphoma mouse model and have recently entered clinical trials. Herein, we describe procedures for the generation of therapeutic vaccines, particularly "second-generation" recombinant vaccines. Specifically, in the Methods section we describe how to identify lymphoma-associated immunoglobulin V (IgV) genes from patient biopsy and how to assemble these genes as single-chain variable gene fragment (scFv) in-frame with MIP-3α to generate novel DNA fusion vaccines.

Key words DNA vaccines, Lymphoplasmacytic lymphoma, Chemokine, Idiotype, Single-chain variable gene fragment

1 Introduction

Immunoglobulin (Ig) molecules are composed of heavy and light chains, which possess highly specific variable regions at their amino termini. The variable regions of heavy and light chains combine to form the unique antigen-recognition site of the Ig protein. These variable regions contain determinants that can themselves be recognized as antigens, or *idiotypes*. B-cell malignancies are composed of a clonal proliferation of mature resting and reactive lymphocytes that synthesize a single Ig molecule with unique heavy and light chain variable regions on their cell surface. The idiotypic determinants of the surface Ig of a B-cell lymphoma can thus serve as a tumor-specific marker for the malignant clone.

Michael J.P. Lawman and Patricia D. Lawman (eds.), *Cancer Vaccines: Methods and Protocols*, Methods in Molecular Biology, vol. 1139, DOI 10.1007/978-1-4939-0345-0_24,

In a recently completed randomized, double-blind, controlled, multicenter phase III clinical trial, patient-specific tumor-derived idiotype (Id) protein was conjugated with a carrier protein, keyhole limpet hemocyanin (KLH), and administered together with an adjuvant, granulocyte-macrophage colony-stimulating factor (GM-CSF), to patients with advanced stage, previously untreated follicular lymphoma (FL), in complete remission following standard induction chemotherapy. Vaccination with Id-KLHCSF significantly prolonged disease-free survival (DFS), when compared with the control group that received a nonspecific immune stimulant (KLHCSF) [1]. However, Id vaccines are "custom" made for each patient by generating and screening Id-secreting hybridomas. This process is usually time-consuming and laborious for most B-cell malignancies.

An alternative to idiotype protein vaccination is to use DNA vaccines. Recent achievements in antibody engineering and delivery are making it possible to overcome these obstacles and simplify production of more efficient custom-made idiotypic vaccines. Any delivery system that does not require protein expression holds tremendous potential for the goal of streamlining vaccine production. Immunoglobulin variable genes specific for the B-cell malignancies can be readily cloned and combined into single-chain variable fragment (scFv) format encoding a single polypeptide consisting solely of V_H and V_L genes linked together in-frame by a short, 15-amino acid linker. Preliminary studies in mice and humans showed that the DNA vaccines are weakly immunogenic in most cases and need to be used together with adjuvants to render them immunogenic. Our group showed that the efficiency of DNA vaccination in vivo could be greatly increased by encoding a fusion protein consisting of idiotype (scFv) fused to a proinflammatory chemokine moiety that facilitates targeting of antigen-presenting cells for chemokine receptor-mediated binding, uptake, and processing of scFv antigen for subsequent presentation to $CD4^+$ or $CD8^+$ T cells or both [2, 3]. Specifically, mice immunized by gene gun with plasmids encoding monocyte chemotactic protein 3 (MCP-3) or interferon-inducible protein 10 (IP-10)-scFv fusions, but not scFv alone, induced protective antitumor immunity against a large tumor challenge, i.e., 20× the minimum lethal dose. Furthermore, the level of protection was equivalent or superior to that of the prototype Id-KLH protein vaccine. According to current guidelines for management of LPL, observation is recommended for patients who are asymptomatic of their disease [4, 5]. We plan to investigate the safety and feasibility of using a novel DNA vaccine encoding a MIP-3α fused lymphoma idiotype in single chain format in patients who are in the asymptomatic phase of LPL before symptoms develop.

Neoplastic B cells are encountered in biopsy specimens at various frequencies, but generally exceed 30 % of the total

B-lymphocyte population [4]. Accordingly, the lymphoma-associated IgV gene is expected to be repeated in this population at a similarly high frequency. Identification of the lymphoma-associated IgV gene is based on the clonal multiplication of a VH-DH-JH sequence, as opposed to what is seen in normal B cells. We employ a 2-part IgV gene fingerprinting strategy to establish a method for identification of the lymphoma-associated IgV gene from the lymphoma biopsy specimen. First, the distribution of the lymphoma biopsy V gene subset was analyzed by semiquantitative touch-down reverse transcriptase-polymerase chain reaction (RT-PCR)-based assay using specific primers; see Primer Preparation. The second part of this protocol shows how to identify the unique recurring nucleotide sequence among the VH-DH-JH sequence present in the more robustly amplified PCR product.

2 Materials

2.1 Identification of Lymphoma-Associated Immunoglobulin Variable Gene

1. Roswell Park Memorial Institute (RPMI)-1640 medium.
2. Dimethyl sulfoxide (DMSO).
3. B-cell isolation kit II (Miltenyi Biotec, Auburn, CA, USA).

2.1.1 Preparation of Patient's Sample

2.1.2 RNA Extraction and cDNA Synthesis

1. Qiagen RNeasy Mini Kit (Qiagen, Valencia, CA, USA).
2. QIAshredder homogenizer (Qiagen).
3. Absolute ethanol, 200 proof molecular biology grade.
4. β-Mercaptoethanol.
5. Diethylpyrocarbonate (DEPC)-treated water.
6. Superscript III First-strand synthesis system for RT-PCR (Invitrogen, Life Technologies, Carlsbad, CA, USA).

2.1.3 Primer Preparation

1. PCR grade water.
2. Oligonucleotide/primer 25-nM scale.
   R = A or G; S = C or G; Y = C or T.

2.1.4 Amplification and Cloning of V Genes from Primary Cells

1. Phusion High-Fidelity PCR Master Mix with HF Buffer (New England Biolabs, Ipswich, MA, USA).
2. PCR grade water.
3. Zymoclean Gel DNA Recovery Kit (Zymo Research, Irvine, CA, USA).
4. StrataClone Ultra Blunt PCR Cloning Kit (Stratagene, La Jolla, CA, USA).
5. Miniprep DNA Extraction Kit (Qiagen).

2.2 Synthesis and Cloning of the scFv Gene in Chemokine-scFv DNA Vaccine Plasmid

1. pVax-n7 vector (modified from pUMVC3).
2. *Xho* I, *Eco* RI, and *Not* I restriction enzymes.
3. XL1-Blue Supercompetent cells.
4. Luria Bertani (LB) medium with 100 μ/mL of ampicillin.
5. MegAlign software (DNA-STAR, Madison, WI, USA).

3 Methods

3.1 Identification of Lymphoma-Associated Immunoglobulin Variable Gene

3.1.1 Preparation of Patient's Sample

A 15-mL bone marrow aspirate sample is collected from the contralateral side for vaccine production and to bank additional tumor cells for immunologic assays. Patients must provide a bone marrow aspiration sample providing at least 2 million $CD20^+$ and/or $CD38^+$ cells (approximately 10 mL) using the B-cell isolation kit. The cells are centrifuged at 300 × *g* at room temperature. Bone marrow mononuclear cells can at this stage be directly stored at −80 °C prior to use. Cell storage medium comprises 50:40:10 (v/v/v) RPMI-1640 medium, FBS, and DMSO, and cells are typically frozen at a concentration of 2×10^6/mL.

3.1.2 RNA Extraction

1. If required, pellet the cells by centrifuging for 7 min at 250 × *g* in a centrifuge tube. Aspirate the supernatant and discard (*see* **Note 1**).
2. Flick the tube to loosen the cell pellet. Add 350 μL (for $<5 \times 10^6$ cells) or 600 μL (for $>5 \times 10^6$ cells) of Buffer RLT, and vortex or pipet to mix (*see* **Note 2**).
3. Pipet the lysate into a QIAshredder spin column placed in a 2-mL collection tube, and centrifuge for 2 min at full speed (8,000 × *g*). Use the homogenized lysate in the collection tube for further processing. Discard the QIAshredder spin column.
4. Add 1 volume of 70 % ethanol to the homogenized lysate in the collection tube, and mix well by pipetting.
5. Transfer up to 700 μL of the sample to an RNeasy spin column placed in a 2-mL collection tube supplied in the kit. With the lid of the tube closed, centrifuge for 30 s at ≥8,000 × *g* and discard the flow-through. Do NOT throw away the collection tube. Repeat this step if sample volume exceeds 700 μL, discarding the flow-through each time.
6. Add 700 μL Buffer RW1 to the RNeasy spin column. Close the lid and centrifuge for 30 s at ≥8,000 × *g*. Discard the flow-through. Do not throw away the collection tube (*see* **Note 3**).
7. Add 500 μL Buffer RPE to the RNeasy spin column. Close the lid and centrifuge the column for 30 s at ≥8,000 × *g* to wash the spin column membrane. Discard the flow-through.

8. Add 500 μL Buffer RPE to the RNeasy spin column. Close the lid and centrifuge for 2 min at ≥8,000 × *g*. This step is essential for removing all the ethanol from the collection tube (*see* **Note 4**).
9. Place the RNeasy spin column in a new 1.5-mL RNase-free collection tube provided in the kit. Add 30–50 μL RNase-free water directly to the spin column membrane. Close the lid and centrifuge for 1 min at ≥8,000 × *g* to elute the RNA.
10. Optional: If the expected RNA yield is >30 μg, repeat the previous step using the same collection tube. Alternately, if a higher RNA concentration is desired, then pass the eluate from the previous step through the column a second time.
11. Remove an aliquot to perform UV spectrophotometry to evaluate quality and concentration. Optional: In addition to UV spectrophotometry, perform agarose gel electrophoresis of the extracted RNA.
12. The manager or designee should review the data and approve the acceptance criteria (*see* **Note 5**).

3.1.3 cDNA Synthesis

1. Briefly centrifuge each component at 3,000 × *g* before use.
2. Add the following components to a nuclease-free 0.2-mL microcentrifuge tube:

Up to 5 μg RNA	*n* μL
50 ng/μL random hexamers	1 μL
10 mM dNTP mix	1 μL
RNase-free water	to 10 μL

3. Incubate at 65 °C for 5 min.
4. Place on ice for at least 1 min.
5. Prepare cDNA synthesis mix by adding the following components in the indicated order:

10× RT Buffer	2 μL
25 mM $MgCl_2$	4 μL
0.1 M DTT	2 μL
RNase OUT (40 U/μL)	1 μL
200 U/μL Superscript III RT	1 μL

6. Add 10 μL of cDNA synthesis mix to the RNA/primer mix prepared in **step 2**. Mix gently and quick spin.
7. Incubate at 25 °C for 10 min, followed by incubation at 50 °C for 50 min.

8. Terminate the reaction by incubating at 85 °C for 5 min. Chill on ice.
9. Quick spin the tube(s) and add 1 μL of RNase H.
10. Incubate at 37 °C for 20 min.
11. Transfer the cDNA to a larger tube, e.g., 1.5-mL microcentrifuge tube. Label the tube with processing label and sample identity.
12. Label and store the tube at −20 °C.

3.1.4 Primer Preparation

1. Prepare 100 μM primer stock solutions in water for each lyophilized primer. Use the nanomolar data provided on the certificate of analysis to calculate the required volume of DEPC water to prepare the stock solution (*see* **Note 6**).
2. Prepare 10 μM working stocks for the primers by making a 1:10 dilution of the 100 μM stock solution.
3. Store the stock and working stock primer solutions at −20 °C. Thaw and use as needed for PCR amplification.

3.1.5 Amplification and Cloning of V Genes from Primary Cells

For identification of lymphoma-associated V_H from an FL patient biopsy, cDNA samples are amplified in four separate reactions ($V_H1/2$, V_H3, $V_H4/6$, and V_H5) with 5′ leader region primers specific for each of the 6 human VH families and a Cγ primer [6]. In previous studies, an analysis of the amplification products from these reactions showed that although all primer pairs resulted in a specific band of the appropriate size, the primer specific for V_H3 generated a more robust band. The bands resulting from the rest of the V_H primers are presumably from the V_H gene of normal B cells in the biopsy specimen. In contrast, for samples from a normal healthy donor, the intensity of amplification products from all the V_H gene subsets was of similar intensities (Fig. 1c). Contamination from extraneous DNA was excluded by negative controls in which cDNA was not added to the PCR reaction (Fig. 1a). For V_L analysis of tumors, only the monotypic light chain known to be present from the cell phenotype was investigated. The Vκ or Vλ primers were used with the appropriate J primers. A similar pattern of amplification was seen with kappa chain primers. The primer specific for $V_κ1/2$ resulted in a more robust band than the primers for the other $V_κ$ subsets (Fig. 1a).

1. Thaw on ice the Phusion High-Fidelity PCR Master Mix with HF Buffer, cDNA template, and primer stocks.
2. Briefly centrifuge at 3,000 × *g* before use.
3. Use a new aliquot of water for each PCR setup.
4. Perform the cDNA dilution and PCR reaction setup in a biological safety cabinet.

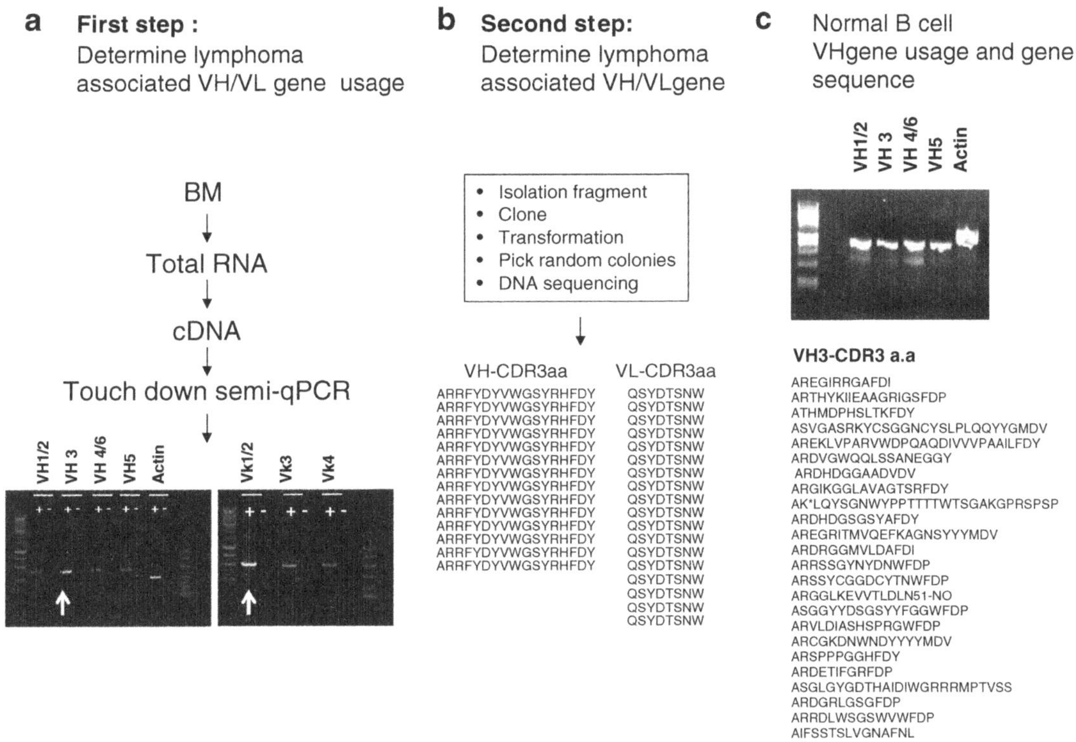

Fig. 1 Molecular cloning of lymphoma-associated VH and VL gene. (**a**) Identification of lymphoma-associated VH and VL genes by semiquantitative RT-PCR: The patient B-cell tumor cDNA was amplified with 5′ primers specific for each of the VH and VL family genes, along with a 3′-μ chain constant region primer using touch-down RT-PCR. Reactions with no cDNA served as the negative controls. The amplified PCR products were analyzed on a 1 % agarose gel. (**b**) Determination of lymphoma-associated VH and VL genes: Gel-purified PCR products were ligated into the pSC-B vector and transformed into *Escherichia coli* cells. Following transformation, 24 individual clones from VH and VL were randomly selected and sequenced. All sequences from any given Ig class within a patient biopsy were aligned, and the number of identical sequences was determined. The V segment of any clone was identified as its closest match in the Vbase2 (http://www.vbase2.org) and IMGT/V-QUEST (http://www.imgt.org) database. (**c**) Heavy chain gene sequences from normal B cells. B cells isolated from a normal healthy donor's PBMC were processed in the same manner as identifying lymphoma-associated VH/VL gene

5. Dilute the cDNA 1:5 (cDNA:PCR grade water) for use as template in the PCR reaction.
6. Prepare PCR reactions for primer pairs listed in Table 1. Prepare the reactions according to **steps a–d** below, adding the reaction components in the indicated order. Each time a PCR reaction is set up, include the beta-actin control and the no template control (NTC) for each primer pair.

Table 1
Primers for PCR amplification of VH and VL genes

Heavy chain forward primers	
5′ L-VH 1	ACAGGTGCCCACTCCCAGGTGCAG
5′ L-VH 3	AAGGTGTCCAGTGTGARGTGCAG
5′ L-VH 4/6	CCCAGATGGGTCCTGTCCCAGGTGCAG
5′ L-VH 5	CAAGGAGTCTGTTCCGAGGTGCAG
Heavy chain reverse primer	
3′ Cμ CH1	GGGAATTCTCACAGGAGACGA
Lambda light chain forward primers	
5′ L VL 1	GGTCCTGGGCCCAGTCTGTGCTG
5′ L VL 2	GGTCCTGGGCCCAGTCTGCCCTG
5′ L VL 3	GCTCTGTGACCTCCTATGAGCTG
5′ L VL 4/5	GGTCTCTCTCSCAGCYTGTGCTG
5′ L VL 6	GTTCTTGGGCCAATTTTATGCTG
5′ L VL 7	GGTCCAATTCYCAGGCTGTGGTG
5′ L VL 8	GAGTGGATTCTCAGACTGTGGTG
Lambda light chain reverse primer	
3′ Cλ	CACCAGTGTGGCCTTGTTGGCTTG
Kappa light chain forward primers	
PR5′ L Vκ 1/2	ATGAGGSTCCCYGCTCAGCTGCTGG
PR5′ L Vκ 3	CTCTTCCTCCTGCTACTCTGGCTCCCAG
PR5′ L Vκ 4	ATTTCTCTGTTGCTCTGGATCTCTG
Kappa light chain reverse primer	
3′ Cκ 494	GTGCTGTCCTTGCTGTCCTGCT
Actin forward primer	
Actin F1379	AGCGAGCATCCCCCAAAGTT
Actin reverse primer	
Actin R1663	GGGCACGAAGGCTCATCATT

(a) Variable heavy chain:

	Sample (μL)	NTC (μL)
cDNA (1:5 diluted)	1	–
PCR grade water	7	8
10 μM 5′ VH primer	1	1
10 μM 3′ Cμ CH1	1	1
2× Phusion Master Mix	10	10
Total	20	20

(b) Variable kappa light chain:

	Sample (μL)	NTC (μL)
cDNA (1:5 diluted)	1	–
PCR grade water	7	8
10 μM 5′ Vκ primer	1	1
10 μM 3′ Cκ 494	1	1
2× Phusion Master Mix	10	10
Total	20	20

(c) Variable lambda light chain:

	Sample (μL)	NTC (μL)
cDNA (1:5 diluted)	1	–
PCR grade water	7	8
10 μM 5′ Vλ primer	1	1
10 μM 3′ Cλ	1	1
2× Phusion Master Mix	10	10
Total	20	20

(d) Control actin:

	Sample (μL)	NTC (μL)
cDNA (1:5 diluted)	1	–
PCR grade water	7	8
10 μM 5′ actin F1379	1	1
10 μM 3′ actin R1663	1	1
2× Phusion Master Mix	10	10
Total	20	20

7. Mix reaction components and briefly centrifuge at 3,000 × *g*. Label and record each reaction with a PCR number. The PCR number is a consecutive numerical number proceeding from the last PCR number used.
8. Program a standard thermocycler to run the reaction using the following condition and annealing temperatures according to Table 2 (*see* **Note 7**). The annealing temperature must be set based on the primer pair used for amplification *see* Table 2.

Table 2
PCR amplification cycles and annealing temperatures/conditions

	Forward primer	Reverse primer	*Annealing temp. for the first 10 cycles (°C)	**Annealing temp. for 21 cycles (°C)
Heavy chain	5′ L-VH1	3′ CμCH1	64–59	59
	5′ L-VH3	3′ CμCH1	64–59	59
	5′ L-VH4/6	3′ CμCH1	64–59	59
	5′ L-VH5	3′ CμCH1	64–59	59
Kappa chain	5′ L-Vκ1/2	3′ Cκ494	72–67	67
	5′ L-Vκ3	3′ Cκ494	70–65	65
	5′ L-Vκ4	3′ Cκ494	70–65	65
Lambda chain	5′ L-VL1	3′ Cλ	71–66	66
	5′ L-VL2	3′ Cλ	71–66	66
	5′ L-VL3	3′ Cλ	67–62	62
	5′ L-VL4/5	3′ Cλ	71–66	66
	5′ L-VL6	3′ Cλ	63–58	58
	5′ L-VL7	3′ Cλ	67–62	62
	5′ L-VL8	3′ Cλ	63–58	58
Beta-actin	Actin F1379	Actin R1663	–	–

* See table 2 for annealing temperature of primer pair used
** See table 2 for annealing temperature of primer pair used

1 cycle	98 °C denature, 3 min
10 cycles of	98 °C denature, 10 s *64–59 °C (drop 0.5 °C each cycle) annealing, 10 s 72 °C extension, 10 s
21 cycles of	98 °C denature, 10 s **59 °C annealing, 10 s
72 °C extension, 10 s	
1 cycle	72 °C, 5 min final extension 4 °C hold

* See table 2 for annealing temperature of primer pair used
** See table 2 for annealing temperature of primer pair used

9. Remove an aliquot of each PCR reaction, and verify PCR products by agarose gel electrophoresis (*see* **Note 8**).
10. High-intensity PCR product bands with correct sizes are excised, 450 bp. Use the Zymoclean Gel DNA Recovery Kit to purify the bands. Insert purified PCR fragments into pSC-B vector system according to manufacturer's instruction. Twenty-four colonies are picked and cultured individually in 3 mL of

LB with ampicillin for approximately 16–24 h. Bacteria are harvested and extracted for plasmid DNA using Qiagen's protocol. Digest with *Eco* RI (flanks the insert in pSC-B vector), analyze the size of the insert on agarose gel, and sequence the insert.

3.1.6 DNA Sequence Analysis

The second part of this survey attempts to identify the unique recurring nucleotide sequence among the V_H-D_H-J_H sequence present in the high-intensity PCR product band. Neoplastic B cells are encountered in biopsy specimens at various frequencies, but generally exceed 30 % of the total B-lymphocyte population [7]. Accordingly, the lymphoma-associated V gene is expected to be repeated in this population at a similarly high frequency. Identification of the lymphoma-associated V gene is based on the clonal multiplication of a V_H-D_H-J_H sequence, as opposed to what is seen in normal B cells. Thus, the lymphoma-associated V gene is identified by a unique signature CDR3 motif in both V_H and V_L. All sequences from any given Ig class within a biopsy are aligned by MegAlign software, and the number of identical sequences is determined. The V segment of any clonal, lymphoma-associated V transcript is identified as its closest match in the Vbase (http://www.vbase2.org) and IMGT/V-QUEST (http://www.imgt.org/IMGT_vquest/vquest?livret=0&Option=humanIg) (*see* **Note 9**).

3.2 Gene Assembly of scFv and Cloning of scFv in Chemokine-scFv DNA Vaccine Plasmid

3.2.1 Expression Vector: Chemokine-scFv DNA Vaccine Plasmid

For our clinical trial DNA vaccine plasmid construction, human MIP-3α, including the secretion leader sequence, was cloned in-frame with FL patient-derived sFv and a separately introduced HA tag to monitor expression of sFv by Western blotting (*see* **Note 9**) and called pVax-N7 (Fig. 2a). The pUMVC3 is a derivative of a pUC19-based plasmid and contains the cytomegalovirus immediate early promoter-enhancer with a partially deleted intron A and rabbit β-globin polyadenylation signal flanking a polylinker for insertion of heterologous open reading frames, as well as the kanamycin resistance gene. This vector was generated by the University of Michigan for human gene therapy studies. DNA vaccines constructed with this vector have been approved by FDA for human studies [8, 9].

3.2.2 Synthesis of scFv DNA Sequences

The synthetic gene is designed based on the VH and VL gene from patients with a flexible $(G_4S)_3$ linker between VH and VL genes. This gene carried an *Xho* I restriction site at its 5′-end and a *Not* I site at the 3′-end. Gene synthesis is performed by BIOMATIK. The synthetic gene pattern is CTCGAG—[FR1-CDR1-FR2-CDR2-FR3-CDR3-FR4]—GGT GGT GGT GGT TCT GGC GGC GGC GGC AGC GGT GGC GGT GGG AGC—[FR1-CDR1-FR2-CDR2-FR3-CDR3-FR4]—gGC GGC CGC. The synthetic gene is cloned into pBluescript II SK (+) by BIOMATIK (Fig. 2b).

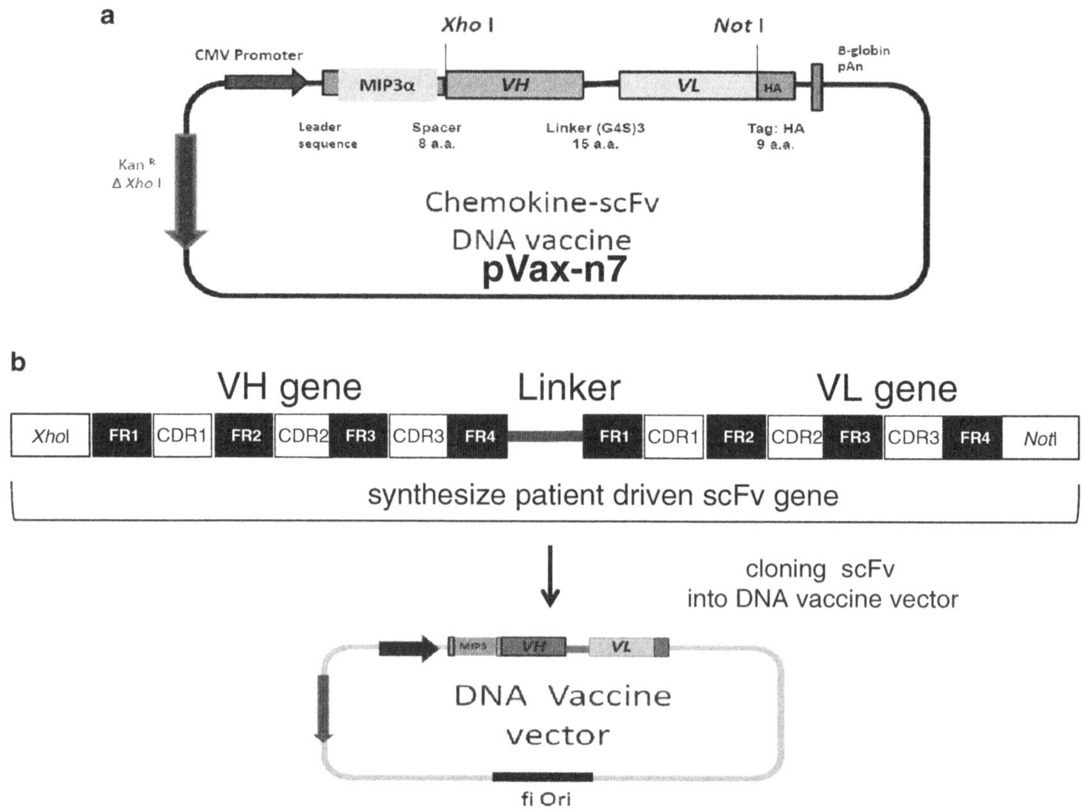

Fig. 2 Chemokine fusion patient-specific scFv DNA vaccine. (**a**) The expression vector is a modified pUMVC3 vector from University of Michigan. Prior to cloning the patient scFv, the vector was linearized by digesting with *Xho* I and *Not* I. A MIP3α chemokine gene, along with its own signal leader sequence, was fused in-frame with patient scFv to aid the secretion of a fusion protein in mammalian cells. A spacer consisting of eight amino acids was introduced between the chemokine and the scFv. The vector was further modified by introducing a Kozak sequence (CCACC) at the 5′-end (immediately preceding the start codon) and a human influenza hemagglutinin (HA) tag (as an epitope) at the 3′-end of the MIP3α-scFv fusion gene. (**b**) Scheme of patient-specific lymphoma-associated scFv gene: The synthetic gene was designed based on the VH and VL gene sequences obtained from patients while introducing a flexible (G4S)3 linker between VH and VL genes, with a *Xho* I restriction site at the 5′-end and *Not* I site at the 3′-end. These restriction sites were used for cloning the synthetic scFv gene into the DNA vaccine vector. **Leader sequence**: MIP-3α secretion leader sequence amino acid. **VH**: Patient specific Immunoglobulin Variable Heavy Chain; **VL**: Patient specific Immunoglobulin Variable Light Chain. **Kan^R Δ *Xho* I**: Introducing silent mutations *Xho* I restrict enzyme site in the Kanamycin resistant coding gene. **CDR1**, **CDR2**, and **CDR3**: complementarity-determining regions. **FR1**, **FR2**, and **FR3**: Framework regions

3.2.3 Assembly by Cloning

1. Prepare pBluescript II SK-patient scFv gene from 5 mL of overnight bacterial cultures grown in LB with 100 μg/mL of ampicillin using QIAprep Spin Miniprep Kit as described.
2. For ligation of insert into the 3.9 kb pVax-n7, double digest pBluescript II SK-scFv with *Xho* I and *Not* I and gel-purify.

Use a 2:1 molar ratio of insert to pVax-n7; mix the following in a microcentrifuge tube and incubate overnight at 16 °C:

Component	Volume (μL)
15 ng insert DNA (scFv), *Xho* I and *Not* I digested	2
50 ng vector DNA (pVax-n7) *Xho* I and *Not* I digested	3
T4 ligase buffer, 10×	2
3 U/μL T4 ligase	1
Nuclease-free water	20

3. Heat inactivate the ligase at 65 °C for 10 min, and transform 5 μL of ligase reaction into XL-1 Blue-competent bacterial cells following standard protocols.
4. Between 5 and 10 colonies are randomly selected and amplified by overnight culture using ampicillin selection. Plasmid DNA is purified by the miniprep method.
5. Digest with *Xho* I and *Not* I and check the size on an agarose gel.
6. Verify the sequence of the entire gene by DNA sequencing to make sure that the synthetic scFv gene did not introduce mutations, and ensure that the cloning sites are in-frame with the upstream MIP-3α/VH and downstream HA tag gene. For sequencing, the forward primer is based on MIP-3α (5′-ATG TGC TGT ACC AAG AGT TTG CTC CTG G), and the reverse primer is based on the β-globin poly (A) tail sequence (5′-CCC ATA TGT CCT TCC GAG TGA GAG).

4 Notes

1. Patient tumor samples should yield at least 1 million cells for identification of lymphoma-associated VH/VL genes. Perform this procedure in the designated work area. Always use appropriate precautions to avoid RNase contamination when preparing and handling RNA. Perform all steps of the procedure, including centrifugation, at room temperature. During the procedure, work quickly.
2. Buffer RLT may form a precipitate upon storage. If necessary, redissolve by warming and then place at room temperature. Add 10 μL of β-ME per 1 mL Buffer RLT prior to use.
3. While removing the spin column to discard the flow-through, be careful that the column does not touch the flow-through, and empty the collection tube completely.

4. Buffer RPE is supplied as a concentrate. Before using for the first time, add 4 volumes of ethanol (96–100) as indicated on the bottle to obtain a working solution.
5. RNA extraction results acceptance criteria:
   (a) UV spectrophotometer A260/280 = 1.8–2.1
   (b) Agarose gel: (1) 2 distinct visible bands of sizes ~1.9 kb and ~5.0 kb and (2) no visual appearance of RNA degradation.
6. Prepare 100 μM primer stock solutions in water for each lyophilized primer. Use the nmoles data provided on the specification sheet to calculate the volume of DEPC water required to prepare the stock solution:

   For example, if the nmoles of the primer = 25.1 nmoles
   To make a 100 μM stock solution, add 251 μL DEPC water.
   For example, if the nmoles of the primer = 32.8 nmoles
   To make a 100 μM stock solution, add 328 μL DEPC water.
7. Here, we use touchdown PCR (TD-PCR). The TD-PCR is another modification of conventional PCR that may result in a reduction of nonspecific amplification. It involves the use of an annealing temperature that is higher than the target optimum in early PCR cycles. The annealing temperature is decreased by 0.5 °C every cycle or every second cycle until a specified or "touchdown" annealing temperature is reached. The touchdown temperature is then used for the remaining cycles. This allows for the enrichment of the correct product over any nonspecific product [10].
8. The manager or designee should review the data and approve the acceptance criteria.
   (a) NTC PCR for each amplicon must be negative for amplification. If amplified bands are observed in the NTC, the PCR reaction may be set up using a new set of reagents.
   (b) Positive control actin PCR must show expected band size.
   (c) If a single band is observed in the sample, proceed to gel extraction; then proceed to StrataClone Blunt PCR cloning.
   (d) If multiple bands are observed in the sample, isolate the predominant band by gel extraction; then proceed to cloning.
   (e) If multiple bands are observed with no predominant band, the PCR may be repeated with a slightly higher annealing temperature.
9. To identify the lymphoma-associated V gene, 20 % above (4/20) clones sequence must be the same CDR3 V gene sequences.

Acknowledgement

This work was supported by the Cancer Prevention and Research Institute of Texas.

References

1. Schuster SJ et al (2011) Vaccination with patient-specific tumor-derived antigen in first remission improves disease-free survival in follicular lymphoma. J Clin Oncol 29:2787–2794
2. Biragyn A et al (1999) Genetic fusion of chemokines to a self tumor antigen induces protective, T-cell dependent antitumor immunity. Nat Biotechnol 17:253–258
3. Biragyn A et al (2004) Chemokine receptor-mediated delivery directs self-tumor antigen efficiently into the class II processing pathway in vitro and induces protective immunity in vivo. Blood 104:1961–1969
4. Dimopoulos MA et al (2005) Diagnosis and management of Waldenstrom's macroglobulinemia. J Clin Oncol 23:1564–1577
5. Dimopoulos MA et al (2009) Update on treatment recommendations from the Fourth International Workshop on Waldenstrom's macroglobulinemia. J Clin Oncol 27:120–126
6. Tiller T et al (2008) Efficient generation of monoclonal antibodies from single human B cells by single cell RT-PCR and expression vector cloning. J Immunol Methods 329:112–124
7. Kobrin CB, Kwak LW (1997) Development of vaccine strategies for the treatment of B-cell malignancies. Cancer Invest 15:577–587
8. Mahvi DM et al (2007) Intratumoral injection of IL-12 plasmid DNA—results of a phase I/IB clinical trial. Cancer Gene Ther 14:717–723
9. Lee SW et al (2000) Development of a polynucleotide vaccine from melanoma antigen recognized by T cells-1 and recombinant protein from melanoma antigen recognized by T cells-1 for melanoma vaccine clinical trials. J Immunother 23:379–386
10. Korbie DJ, Mattick JS (2008) Touchdown PCR for increased specificity and sensitivity in PCR amplification. Nat Protoc 3:1452–1456

Chapter 25

Heat Shock Proteins Purified from Autologous Tumors Using Antibody-Based Affinity Chromatography

Christian Kleist, Marco Randazzo, Janina Jiga, and Peter Terness

Abstract

Heat shock proteins (HSP) isolated from autologous tumors have become a promising tool for active-specific anticancer immunotherapy due to their properties as carriers of antigenic peptides on one hand and as immunostimulatory adjuvants on the other. Rapid and efficient isolation of HSP-peptide complexes from a patient's tumor is fundamental for their clinical application. Herein, we describe the purification of the HSP Gp96 and Hsc70/Hsp70 from human autologous tumor sources by one-step antibody-based affinity chromatography. Recombinant anti-Gp96 and anti-Hsp70 single-chain Fv antibodies are covalently coupled to a chromatographic bead resin to obtain highly specific affinity matrices. Chromatographic columns are assembled and then used to simultaneously isolate various HSP from the supernatant of lysates of human tumor samples of different origin in a single chromatographic step.

Key words Heat shock protein, Gp96, Hsc70/Hsp70, Active-specific cancer immunotherapy, Single-chain Fv antibody, Affinity chromatography, Native proteins, Autologous tumor antigens

1 Introduction

Within the plethora of cellular and humoral immunotherapeutical approaches comprehensively described in this volume, heat shock proteins (HSP) have been extensively studied for their potential use as cancer vaccines [1, 2]. In various animal models, members of different HSP families, including glycoprotein (Gp) 96, Hsp90, heat shock cognate protein (Hsc) 70, Hsp70, calreticulin, Hsp110, and glucose-regulated protein (Grp) 170, have been shown to specifically induce immune responses towards malignant tumors and infectious pathogens and, more importantly, elicit protective immunity [1, 3–7]. HSP are constitutively expressed in mammalian cells and act as intracellular molecular chaperones accounting for the maintenance of regular cellular functions. Upon conditions of stress challenging cellular integrity and survival, the expression

Michael J.P. Lawman and Patricia D. Lawman (eds.), *Cancer Vaccines: Methods and Protocols*, Methods in Molecular Biology, vol. 1139, DOI 10.1007/978-1-4939-0345-0_25, © Springer Science+Business Media New York 2014

of such proteins can be strongly upregulated. Therefore, HSP are also known as stress proteins [8]. As a result of their chaperone functions, HSP are associated with an array of various proteins and peptides, representing a molecular intracellular fingerprint of the specific cell in which they are being expressed. Regarding malignant tumor cells or tissues, HSP-peptide complexes would also harbor tumor-associated antigens [7]. A number of different peptides of viral, tumor, and mycobacterial origin bound to the chaperones have been identified [1, 7]. Most important for their potential use as cancer vaccines, exogenous HSP can be taken up by antigen-presenting cells (APC), such as macrophages and dendritic cells, via distinct receptors. The associated peptides are then cross-presented to T lymphocytes in a MHC-restricted manner resulting in antigen-specific immune activation [6, 9, 10]. As known for vaccine adjuvants, HSP per se have been shown to mediate the activation and maturation of APC by upregulating costimulatory molecules and inducing cytokine expression [1, 7].

As a consequence, the intriguing dual function of HSP as antigenic peptide carriers as well as immunostimulatory adjuvants makes them an ideal tool for active-specific immunotherapy in cancer patients. In several clinical trials, preparations of HSP from autologous tumor sources, especially Gp96 and Hsc70/Hsp70, were used to vaccinate tumor patients and specifically induce immune responses against the antigens distinctively expressed by the patients' own tumors [1]. Although so far a beneficial outcome could only be observed for limited cohorts of patients, the clinical results encourage further comprehensive investigations of HSP-based personalized tumor immunotherapy.

Due to the limited amount of autologous tumor tissue, the generation of such precious cancer vaccines requires fast and efficient isolation of pure HSP-peptide complexes. Established procedures mainly consist of serial purification steps including protein precipitation and several chromatographic preparations [11–16].

In contrast, we developed a one-step affinity-chromatography purification protocol for the isolation of HSP [17, 18]. Monoclonal antibodies (mAbs), recognizing their corresponding target molecules with remarkable specificity, represent the ideal tool to be used in purification procedures of distinct HSP entities. We had selected various antibody clones from human recombinant single-chain (sc) Fv antibody libraries binding to either Gp96 or Hsc70/Hsp70 [17, 19]. These recombinant antibody fragments can easily be produced in large amounts in *Escherichia coli* (*E. coli*) expression systems [20] and used in chromatographic affinity purification settings [17, 21]. Very importantly, our recombinant scFv antibodies (Abs) were shown to only bind to HSP Gp96 in its native conformation which would guarantee the isolation of functional HSP complexes still carrying the immunogenic peptides [17]. The chosen anti-HSP-mAbs (recombinant Abs in our case but also any other

Ab that is available) are covalently immobilized onto a solid matrix, e.g., activated sepharose bead resin, from which chromatography columns with different antigen binding capacities can be manufactured.

Cleared supernatants of tumor lysates, either derived from single tumor-cell suspensions or solid cancer tissue, are run through the affinity columns to capture distinct HSP on the corresponding Ab-matrices. When different affinity columns are combined in series by transferring the flow-through of one column directly onto a subsequent column, it allows the simultaneous preparation of various HSP entities from 1 single tumor sample (Fig. 1a).

After thoroughly washing the affinity resin, pure HSP-peptide complexes can be eluted from the columns in defined fractions of volume using a high salt buffered solution (Fig. 1b). HSP-containing fractions are detected and checked for purity via sodium dodecyl sulfate polyacrylamide-gel electrophoresis (SDS-PAGE) [23] and subsequent Coomassie or silver staining (Fig. 1c)—when establishing a purification procedure, Western blotting [24] should be performed to verify the identity of the purified HSP—pooled, concentrated, and stored in storage buffer at –70 °C until use.

Depending on the expression level and the storage and handling of the original primary tumor sources, up to several hundred micrograms purified HSP (Gp96 and Hsc70/Hsp70) per gram of tumor material can be obtained when following this affinity-based chromatography purification protocol we describe in this chapter.

2 Materials

General remarks: Labware and equipment routinely used and therefore commonly available in a research laboratory such as disposable tubes and standard centrifuges are not specifically mentioned in the Materials section, though they may appear in the Methods section when this information might help the researcher with experimental performance. Reagents (analytical grade), labware, and equipment suggested are related to our experiences and availability. Therefore, equivalent materials can be obtained from other sources provided that quality and application are comparable to those described herein. Additional information on general materials and methods can be found in the laboratory manual by Green and Sambrook [22], as well as in the references provided with the specific procedures.

All solutions are prepared with ultrapure water (conductivity 0.055 μS/cm and 18.2 MΩ·cm at 25 °C) using water purification systems such as TKA (Thermo Electron LED, Niederelbert, Germany), Milli-Q (EMD Millipore, Billerica, MA, USA), or ELGA PURELAB (VWS Deutschland, Celle, Germany).

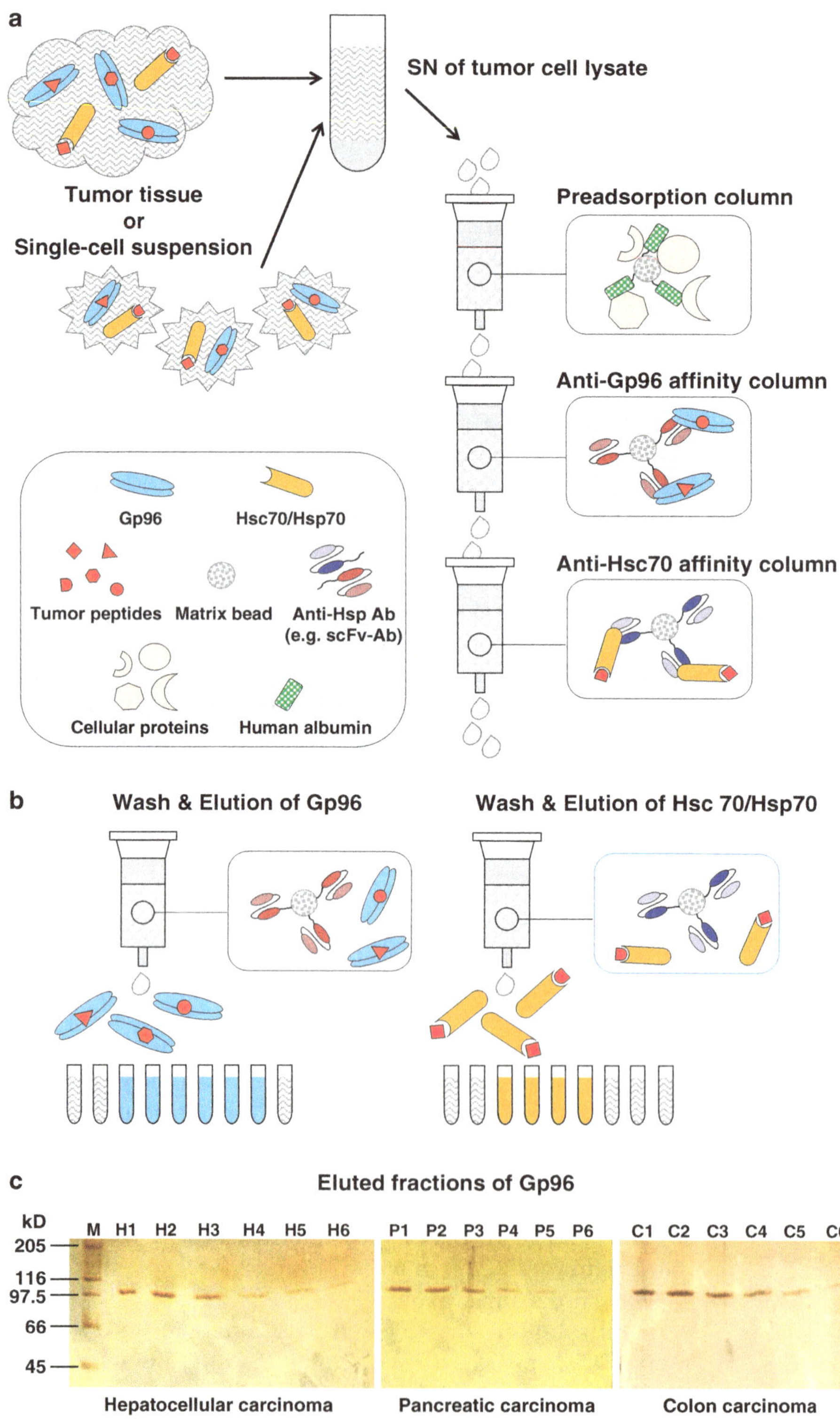

Fig. 1 Antibody-based affinity chromatographic purification of heat shock proteins (HSP) from autologous tumor samples for vaccine preparation. (**a**) Schematic representation of the isolation principles. Solid tumor tissues or tumor cell suspensions from cancer patients are lysed in hypotonic buffer solution by mechanical

2.1 HSP-Specific Affinity Columns

1. Multi-axle rotating mixer or rotating shaker (neoLab Migge GmbH, Heidelberg, Germany).
2. UV/Visible spectrophotometer, e.g., NanoDrop™ 2000 (Thermo Fisher Scientific, Waltham, MA, USA).
3. Empty chromatography columns in different sizes (2.5 mL, 5 mL, 10 mL) with lids, filters, and stopcocks (MoBiTec, Goettingen, Germany) (*see* **Note 1**).
4. PD-10 desalting columns (GE Healthcare Europe, Freiburg, Germany).
5. CNBr-activated Sepharose 4 Fast Flow or 4B (GE Healthcare Europe) (*see* **Note 2**).
6. Purified anti-HSP Abs, such as anti-Gp96 or anti-Hsc70/Hsp70 single-chain Fv (scFv)-Ab fragment specifically recognizing native HSP-peptide complexes (*see* **Note 3**).
7. Human serum albumin (HSA) (Sigma-Aldrich, St. Louis, MO, USA) or Human-Albumin Kabi 20 % (Octapharma, Langenfeld, Germany).
8. Matrix activation solution: 0.1 M hydrochloric acid (HCl).
9. Glycine buffer: 0.2 M glycine, pH 8.0–8.5.
10. Coupling buffer: 0.1 M $NaHCO_3$, 0.5 M NaCl, pH 8.3.
11. Bead washing buffer I: 0.1 M sodium acetate, 0.5 M NaCl, pH 4.0.
12. Bead washing buffer II: 0.1 M Tris–HCl, 0.5 M NaCl, pH 8.0.
13. Blocking buffer: 0.1 M Tris–HCl, pH 8.0.
14. Column storage solution: 20 % (v/v) ethanol in water or phosphate-buffered saline (PBS) containing 0.02 % (w/v) sodium azide (*see* **Note 4**).

2.2 Preparation of the Tumor Samples

1. Ultracentrifuge (Beckman Coulter, Indianapolis, IN, USA; Thermo Fisher Scientific, Waltham, MA, USA).
2. Polyallomer ultracentrifuge tubes (Herolab, Wiesloch, Germany).

douncing or homogenization. The ultracentrifuged cleared tumor cell lysate is then loaded onto a preadsorption column (coated with human albumin) to remove potential cellular molecules nonspecifically binding to the chromatographic matrix. The flow-through is then consecutively applied to the affinity columns coupled with the monoclonal antibodies (recombinant scFv-Ab fragments or complete Ab molecules) specifically recognizing their corresponding HSP (Gp96 and Hsc70/Hsp70). (**b**) After extensive washing of the columns to remove all unbound and nonspecifically adsorbed cellular material, Gp96 and Hsc70/Hsp70 are eluted with a high-salt buffer and collected in fractions. (**c**) The fractions are examined for the presence of the desired target HSP Gp96 by SDS-polyacrylamide gel electrophoresis (SDS-PAGE) and subsequent silver staining. Fractions containing purified protein are pooled, concentrated, and sterile filtered. The pure HSP is cryopreserved in aliquots in storage buffer at −70 °C until use for analysis or as vaccine for autologous active-specific anticancer immunotherapy. The images show pure fractions of Gp96 isolated from three human tumor samples of different origin: hepatocellular (fractions H1–H6), pancreatic (P1–P6), and colon (C1–C6) carcinoma. A molecular weight marker (M) was used for identification of purified Gp96 according to its molecular weight of around 96–99 kDa

3. Sterile glass or disposable plastic Petri dishes.
4. Disposable scalpels (Feather Safety Razor, Osaka, Japan; Aesculap, Tuttlingen, Germany).
5. Forceps (Aesculap; Fine Science Tools, Heidelberg, Germany).
6. Glass Dounce tissue grinder sets consisting of grinder tube or mortar and pestle for different working volumes (B. Braun Melsungen, Melsungen, Germany; neoLab Migge; Omni International, Kennesaw, GA, USA; Sigma-Aldrich; VWR International, Darmstadt, Germany).
7. Tissue sample homogenizer Polytron® PT 1200 (Kinematica, Luzern, Switzerland), IKA® Ultra-Turrax® disperser (IKA®-Werke, Staufen, Germany), Omni Tissue Master (Omni International), or TissueRuptor (Qiagen, Hilden, Germany) with various saw teeth or probes (5–12 mm) for efficient breakdown of tumor tissue of various sizes and volumes (*see* **Note 5**).
8. Tumor tissue surgically removed from cancer patients or collected single-cell suspensions from hematological malignancies (immediately stored in PBS or tissue culture medium, e.g., Roswell Park Memorial Institute (RPMI)-1640, and kept at about 4 °C on ice or frozen at −70 °C) (*see* **Note 6**).
9. Protease inhibitor stocks: 100 mM Pefabloc SC in water, 2 mg/mL of pepstatin in dimethyl sulfoxide (DMSO), 2 mg/mL of leupeptin in DMSO, and protease inhibitor cocktail ULTRA cOmplete tablets (mini and regular size) (all from Roche Diagnostics Deutschland, Mannheim, Germany). Make aliquots of inhibitor solutions and store at −20 °C. Add tablets to the buffer just before use.
10. Hypotonic lysis buffer: 30 mM $NaHCO_3$, pH 7.1. Directly before use, add protease inhibitors: Pefabloc (1:500), leupeptin, and pepstatin (each 1:1,000) and 1 inhibitor cocktail tablet (mini to 10 mL and regular to 50 mL of lysis buffer) (*see* **Note 7**).

2.3 Chromatographic Purification of HSP

1. System for protein gel electrophoresis and blotting, e.g., complete PhastSystem including separation-control and staining unit (GE Healthcare) or any other available equipment (e.g., Bio-Rad Laboratories, Munich, Germany; Life Technologies, Darmstadt, Germany) for quick analysis of small protein samples (*see* **Note 8**).
2. Thermomixer with thermoblock for small (1.5- and 2-mL) reaction tubes (e.g., Eppendorf, Hamburg, Germany).
3. Laboratory stands, clamp holder, and clamps.
4. Disposable sample concentrating devices: Vivaspin® 6 mL (Sartorius, Goettingen, Germany) or Amicon® Ultra 4 mL

(EMD Millipore, Billerica, MA, USA) with appropriate molecular weight cutoff, e.g., 30 kDa for HSP Gp96 and Hsc70/Hsp70) (*see* **Note 9**).

5. Chromatography columns containing CNBr-activated sepharose coated with anti-HSP antibodies generated in Subheading 2.1.
6. Disposable plastic Pasteur pipettes.
7. Column washing buffer I: PBS, pH 7.4.
8. Column washing buffer II: PBS containing 0.5 M NaCl.
9. Elution buffer: PBS, pH 7.4 containing 1.3 M NaCl.
10. Column regeneration buffer: PBS, pH 7.4 containing 2 M NaCl.
11. Column storage solution: 20 % (v/v) ethanol in water or PBS containing 0.02 % (w/v) sodium azide (*see* **Note 4**).
12. Dilution/Storage buffer for purified HSP antigens, e.g., Gp96: 10 mM sodium phosphate, 0.38 M NaCl, and pH 7.0 (*see* **Note 10**).
13. 2× SDS protein sample buffer: 100 mM Tris–HCl, pH 6.8, 4 % (w/v) sodium dodecyl sulfate (SDS), 0.2 % (w/v) bromophenol blue, and 20 % (v/v) glycerol. Add dithiothreitol (DTT) just before use to a final concentration of 200 mM.
14. PhastGel homogenous precast polyacrylamide gels, e.g., 12.5 % (GE Healthcare), other precast or self-made polyacrylamide gels according to the electrophoretic system used (*see* **Note 11**).
15. PhastGel SDS buffer strips (GE Healthcare) or electrophoresis running buffer: 25 mM Tris–HCl, pH 8.3, 192 mM glycine, and 0.1 % (w/v) SDS.
16. PhastGel sample applicators, 8× 1 μL and sample well stamp (GE Healthcare).
17. Parafilm® M sealing film.
18. Prestained molecular weight standards (e.g., Bio-Rad Laboratories; GE Healthcare; Sigma-Aldrich).
19. PlusOne Silver staining kit, protein or Coomassie R 350 staining solution (GE Healthcare). Use PlusOne Coomassie tablets Phast blue R-350 (GE Healthcare) to prepare a 0.2 % stock and 0.02 % final staining solution as described by the supplier.
20. Destaining solution for Coomassie-stained polyacrylamide gels: 30 % (v/v) methanol, 10 % (v/v) acetic acid in water.
21. Conservation solution for polyacrylamide gels: 5 % (v/v) glycerol, 10 % (v/v) acetic acid in water.

3 Methods

3.1 HSP-Specific Affinity Columns

1. Pretreat the CNBr-activated sepharose beads for 15 min with bead activation solution at room temperature in a 50-mL tube. Use 20 mL of the solution for 0.5 g of beads. The dry sepharose will swell immediately; whereas 0.5 g of dry beads correspond to 2 mL final volume of swollen beads. Spin down the beads at 700×*g* for 5 min and remove the supernatant. Alternatively, the activation solution can be applied in aliquots to the beads by adding 3–4 times the bead volume of activation solution, mixing gently by inverting the tube a few times and then spinning down the beads at 700×*g*. Discard the supernatant and repeat the wash procedure several times as per the instructions of the supplier (*see* **Notes 12** and **13**).
2. Equilibrate the beads: add coupling buffer (20 mL for 0.5 g beads), mix gently, and spin for 5 min at 700×*g*.
3. Change the buffer of the antibody solution to coupling buffer by using PD-10 desalting columns. Dilute the antibody solution with coupling buffer to a concentration of about 0.5–1 mg/mL. Use approximately 5–10 mg scFv-Ab to couple 0.5 g of beads (*see* **Notes 14** and **15**).
4. Add the Ab coupling solution to pre-swollen beads. The volume of the beads should represent approximately 20 % of the coupling solution.
5. Gently rotate the suspension overnight at 4 °C or for 1 h at room temperature (*see* **Note 16**).
6. To determine the efficiency of the coupling process, measure the optical density at 280 nm (OD_{280}) of the antibody coupling solution in a spectrophotometer before adding to the activated beads and after the incubation period. The coupling efficiency should be >50 %.
7. Wash the beads as in **step 2** by alternating bead washing buffer I with bead washing buffer II. Apply each buffer 3×.
8. Incubate the beads with 20 mL of the blocking buffer rotating for 1 h at room temperature.
9. Wash the beads 2× with PBS, pH 7.4, as in **step 2**.
10. Add fresh PBS, pH 7.4, to obtain a 20 % bead-suspension. Store the beads at 4 °C.
11. If the Ab-coupled bead matrix is not immediately used for the manufacturing of chromatography columns, equilibrate the gel matrix with 20 % ethanol and store at 4 °C until use. For preparation of columns, proceed with **step 13**.
12. In addition, prepare beads by coupling 10–15 mg HSA/0.5 g beads to the matrix instead of anti-HSP Abs (*see* **Note 17**).

When a purification protocol is to be established, also prepare control beads coupled with glycine. Use 0.2 M glycine, pH 8.0 (*see* **Note 18**). For preparation of columns, proceed with **step 13**.

13. Prepare an empty column by placing an appropriate filter inside at the base and fixing a stopcock at the outlet. Set the stopcock to the closed position.
14. Transfer the bead matrix to empty chromatography columns using a plastic Pasteur pipette (*see* **Note 19**). Let the solid chromatographic matrix settle. Carefully regulating the flow-through via the stopcock helps packing the matrix to a dense column. Cover the matrix with an appropriate filter while buffer is still present above the matrix. Soak the filter before use to ensure the removal of any air. Slowly push down the filter until touching the gel matrix lightly. Do not compress the matrix bed to prevent any impairment of subsequent chromatographic performance (*see* **Note 20**).
15. Equilibrate the column with the appropriate buffer with at least 5–10 times the volume of the matrix. For storage, use 20 % (v/v) ethanol. Make sure to leave some buffer above the filter.
16. Close the columns with appropriate lids and store them at 4 °C in an upright position.

3.2 Tumor Sample Preparation

1. Hematological single-cell suspension from tumor samples are prepared by resuspending the tumor cell pellet, previously washed with cold PBS, in ice-cold hypotonic lysis buffer supplemented with protease inhibitors, using a total of 10× the pellet volume.
2. Allow the cells to swell by incubating them with gentle rotation on a mixer or shaker for 1 h at 4 °C.
3. Transfer the cell suspension into the dounce tissue grinder mortar (placed on ice) and homogenize the cells with the pestle by dunking with approximately 15 long and 10 short strokes. Make sure the cell sample is cooled on ice during the entire duration of the homogenization procedure.
4. Solid tumor tissue samples are prepared by transferring the tumor tissue to a sterile Petri dish (placed on ice containing hypotonic lysis buffer) with the forceps and mincing it to pieces as small as possible with the scalpels. Use sterile hypotonic lysis buffer (containing protease inhibitors) during the cutting to wet the tissue and suspend the cut pieces. Small tumor samples (a few grams of weight only) can be homogenized with a dounce tissue grinder as described above. For larger samples, the minced tissue is transferred into a tube with hypotonic lysis buffer containing protease inhibitors and disrupted with

electric tissue sample homogenizers placed on ice. Make sure that the sample is suspended and covered in a sufficient volume of lysis buffer (*see* **Notes 21** and **22**).

5. Remove large cellular fragments and cell debris by spinning the homogenate at 2,100 × *g* at 4 °C for 20 min.
6. Transfer the supernatant to ultracentrifuge tubes and spin at 100,000 × *g* for 1 h.
7. Carefully retrieve the supernatant. It may be stored briefly on ice or in the fridge at 4 °C before loading onto the chromatographic columns.

3.3 Chromatographic Purification of HSP

1. During the ultracentrifugation step, equilibrate the antibody-coupled sepharose columns as well as the control HSA column with 5–10 column volumes of cold PBS, pH 7.4. The columns should be mounted via clamps on a laboratory stand.
2. Load the cold precleared supernatant several times onto the columns by starting with the HSA pre-column and allowing the supernatant to run directly onto the affinity column by gravity flow at 4 °C. Repeat this at least 3–5 times (Fig. 1a) (*see* **Note 23**).
3. Wash the columns separately with column washing buffer I followed by a wash with column washing buffer II and a final wash with buffer I again. Use 5 bed volumes of wash buffer for each step. The washing procedure is carried out at room temperature. Collect the buffers of the washing steps on ice for subsequent analysis (*see* **Note 24**).
4. Elute the proteins from both columns at room temperature with 5 bed volumes elution buffer into cooled tubes in consecutive fractions of a distinct volume, e.g., 1 mL aliquots (Fig. 1b) (*see* **Note 24**).
5. Heat a small aliquot of each fraction with an equal volume of 2× SDS protein sample buffer to 95 °C for 5 min. Immediately cool down samples very briefly on ice and centrifuge the samples at 14,000 × *g* for 1 min. Keep the samples at room temperature.
6. Check the fractions of the elution step for the presence of HSP by SDS-PAGE and Western blotting [23, 24]. Refer to appropriate detailed protocols elsewhere [22] (*see* **Note 8**). The stained gels can be kept in conservation solution for analysis and documentation.
7. Pool the fractions containing Gp96, Hsc70/Hsp70, or other purified HSP and determine the approximate protein concentration in a UV spectrophotometer by using the Warburg–Christian formula [25]. To get a quick but rough estimation, the absorption of the HSP at 280 nm can be measured and the

concentration calculated using an extinction coefficient ε_{280} of 1: protein concentration = $A_{280}/\varepsilon_{280} \times d$ [mg/mL] (*see* **Note 25**).

8. Concentrate the solution to approximately 0.5–1 mg/mL by centrifugation in a concentrating device at 4 °C (*see* **Note 26**).
9. Quantify the protein as described in **step 8** and/or by choosing a suitable protein assay [22, 26, 27].
10. Store the HSP in aliquots at −80 °C (*see* **Note 27**).

4 Notes

1. Any suitable columns from other suppliers, e.g., Bio-Rad Laboratories or GE Healthcare, can be chosen alternatively.
2. CNBr-activated Sepharose 4 Fast Flow resin, covalently attaching ligands via their amino groups, worked best in our hands for immobilization of recombinant scFv-Ab proteins and subsequent efficient purification of HSP. Alternatively, activated Sepharose matrices (GE Healthcare Europe) or other rigid polymers such as SEPABEADS®EC and ReliZyme™ (Resindion, Binasco, Italy) or Immobead-150 (ChiralVision, Leiden, The Netherlands) can be used according to the specific needs, ease, and efficiency of handling and application, especially regarding large-scale protocols and isolation procedures in compliance with the stringent requirements for good manufacturing practices (GMP). The carrier EUPERGIT® C 250L (Evonik Industries, Darmstadt, Germany) can only be obtained in large bulk quantities for industrial scale use.
3. Any mAbs specifically binding the HSP entities to be isolated can be used for affinity chromatographic isolation. Purification protocols have to be comprehensively established for each chosen antibody. Recombinant Abs have been found to be particularly suitable, since they can be easily produced in large scale by bacterial or yeast cultures. This constitutes an important advantage to mammalian hybridoma cultures regarding practicability and cost-effective production, especially under GMP conditions.
4. Be aware of the toxic properties of sodium azide. Wear gloves while handling it. Make sure there is no sodium azide present when purified HSP are used in functional cellular assays or in in vivo vaccination approaches.
5. Disposable probes or saw teeth are preferable in order to prevent cross-contamination between different tumor sample preparations, especially in preclinical and clinical settings.
6. Make sure to only use native fresh or cryopreserved tissue for HSP preparations. Do not take any samples prepared for pathological diagnostics, e.g., formaldehyde fixed tissue.

7. Inhibitor cocktail tablets should be sufficient to supplement the hypotonic lysis buffer in order to block enzymatic activity of cellular proteases.
8. The system chosen should give results within a few hours after purification of HSP with minimal consumption of the precious HSP samples. The semiautomated PhastSystem is the ideal equipment for fast analysis of very small samples (minimal gel loading volume of only 1 μL is sufficient for applications described herein).
9. The chosen cutoff should not measure less than 2–3 times the molecular weight of the target HSP to prevent loss of protein by passing through the filter membrane during the centrifugal concentration procedure. The capacity of the filtration device should be chosen by the total sample volume to be concentrated.
10. The appropriate storage solution and conditions must be specifically determined for each HSP selected. Usually, a phosphate-buffered low-concentrated salt solution with a physiological pH is chosen to start with and subsequently can be adjusted according to experience and/or published literature.
11. Currently available gels show good performance. Nevertheless, we still experience best results with freshly cast gels. These gels can be stored for 1–2 days up to 1 week at 4 °C. Make sure to adjust gels to room temperature before use.
12. Avoid applying high *g* forces to the beads in order to avoid breakage. When using larger volumes of resin, the beads can also be washed on a sintered glass filter (*see* supplier's protocol).
13. The coupling can be carried out in the chromatography columns themselves. Buffers can easily be drained out through the stopcock without the necessity of centrifugation.
14. Remember that the original sample will be diluted 1.4 times. The coupling buffer should not contain any reactive groups itself that may interfere with the covalent linkage of the proteins to the resin. The abundant buffer substance, Tris–HCl, must not be used in the coupling step.
15. The optimal concentration must be determined for each chosen mAb according to format (recombinant Ab fragments, e.g., scFv- or Fab-Ab, or native complete immunoglobulins) and performance with respect to efficiency and purity of HSP isolation.
16. In order to avoid damage to the sepharose beads, do not use a magnetic stirrer.
17. These beads are prepared to adsorb nonspecific binding proteins of the tumor cell lysates prior to applying the lysate onto the affinity column.

18. These beads will provide data concerning nonspecific binding of cellular molecules including your target HSP to the matrix.
19. Remaining beads in tubes and Pasteur pipettes can be flushed out with buffer, e.g., PBS, pH 7.4, and transferred to the columns.
20. If uneven packing of the matrix bed occurs, remix the beads to a homogenous suspension and let the beads settle again to pack the column bed. The filters to cover the matrix bed are tightly fitted and are not easily placed horizontally above the matrix without disturbing the packed bed. Take a plunger of a syringe and use the flat end to help push down the filter carefully. Choose the size of the plunger to be a few millimeters smaller than the diameter of the column. This will ensure that buffer can easily escape through the filter while pushing the filter towards the gel bed, but the plunger should still be wide enough to be able to horizontally move down the filter. In case of uneven position of the filter and compression or disturbance of the matrix bed, repack the column.
21. It is extremely important to avoid any heating of the sample during the homogenization process! Make sure to keep the container on ice at all times. Homogenization should be interrupted by short breaks to ensure not to heat the lysate.
22. Any other suitable tissue disruption devices can be used as long as they allow easy and fast performance.
23. If using different columns to purify multiple HSP proteins, make sure to repeatedly load the lysate supernatant onto each column before applying it to the subsequent one. It is also possible to serially load the lysate onto the columns as schematically depicted in Fig. 1.
24. When establishing a purification protocol, the washing and elution buffers must be determined empirically for each chosen antibody and corresponding HSP to be purified. Start with wash buffers gradually increasing the salt concentration and/or varying the pH. Choosing inappropriate conditions may result in impurity of the eluted fraction, lack of HSP elution, or even loss of antigenic peptides from the HSP-peptide complex. In consequence, the immunogenicity of the isolated HSP may not be retained [17]. Collect all washing and elution buffers in fractions to determine potential elution of the desired HSP. Check fractions by SDS-PAGE and Western blotting [23, 24].
25. The Warburg–Christian formula only provides an estimation of the protein concentration: $1.55 \times A_{280} - 0.757 \times A_{260} =$ protein concentration [mg/mL] [25]. If a more accurate determination is required, a protein assay such as the Bradford assay may be performed using bovine serum albumin (BSA) standards provided to create the calibration curve [26, 27].

26. Pretreat the concentrator with 0.2 M glycine to block nonspecific adsorption of HSP to the membrane.
27. Preparations of HSP might be quite unstable and should not be stored at 4 °C for longer than a few days. Therefore, prepare small aliquots that suit your experiments and store them at −70 °C. Avoid repeated freeze-thaw cycles.

Acknowledgments

We would like to thank Prof. Dr. Helmut Friess (Heidelberg University Hospital, Department of Surgery, Division of General, Visceral and Transplantation Surgery, Heidelberg, Germany) for generously providing tumor tissue samples. This work was partly supported by a grant (LR02/07) from the Deutsche José Carreras Leukämie-Stiftung e.V., Munich, Germany.

References

1. Randazzo M et al (2012) Active-specific immunotherapy of human cancers with the heat shock protein Gp96-revisited. Int J Cancer 130:2219–2231
2. Srivastava P (2002) Roles of heat-shock proteins in innate and adaptive immunity. Nat Rev Immunol 2:185–194
3. Tamura Y et al (1997) Immunotherapy of tumors with autologous tumor-derived heat shock protein preparations. Science 278:117–120
4. Navaratnam M et al (2001) Heat shock protein-peptide complexes elicit cytotoxic T-lymphocyte and antibody responses specific for bovine herpesvirus 1. Vaccine 19:1425–1434
5. Zugel U et al (2001) gp96-peptide vaccination of mice against intracellular bacteria. Infect Immun 69:4164–4167
6. Udono H et al (1994) Cellular requirements for tumor-specific immunity elicited by heat shock proteins: tumor rejection antigen gp96 primes $CD8^+$ T cells in vivo. Proc Natl Acad Sci USA 91:3077–3081
7. Srivastava P (2002) Interaction of heat shock proteins with peptides and antigen presenting cells: chaperoning of the innate and adaptive immune responses. Annu Rev Immunol 20:395–425
8. Lindquist S (1986) The heat-shock response. Annu Rev Biochem 55:1151–1191
9. Suto R, Srivastava PK (1995) A mechanism for the specific immunogenicity of heat shock protein-chaperoned peptides. Science 269: 1585–1588
10. Colaco CA (1999) Why are dendritic cells central to cancer immunotherapy? Mol Med Today 5:14–17
11. Peng P et al (1997) Purification of immunogenic heat shock protein 70-peptide complexes by ADP-affinity chromatography. J Immunol Methods 204:13–21
12. Srivastava PK (1997) Purification of heat shock protein-peptide complexes for use in vaccination against cancers and intracellular pathogens. Methods 12:165–171
13. Menoret A, Bell G (2000) Purification of multiple heat shock proteins from a single tumor sample. J Immunol Methods 237:119–130
14. Meng SD et al (2002) Three-step purification of gp96 from human liver tumor tissues suitable for isolation of gp96-bound peptides. J Immunol Methods 264:29–35
15. Menoret A (2004) Purification of recombinant and endogenous HSP70s. Methods 32:7–12
16. Srivastava PK, Jaikaria NS (2001) Methods of purification of heat shock protein-peptide complexes for use as vaccines against cancers and infectious diseases. Methods Mol Biol 156:175–186
17. Arnold-Schild D et al (2000) One-step single-chain Fv recombinant antibody-based purification of gp96 for vaccine development. Cancer Res 60:4175–4178
18. Kleist C et al (2003) Single-chain Fv-based affinity purification of the cellular stress protein gp96 for vaccine development. Methods Mol Biol 207:393–420

19. Little M et al (1999) Generation of a large complex antibody library from multiple donors. J Immunol Methods 231: 3–9
20. Kipriyanov SM et al (1997) High level production of soluble single chain antibodies in small-scale Escherichia coli cultures. J Immunol Methods 200:69–77
21. Kipriyanov SM, Little M (1997) Affinity purification of tagged recombinant proteins using immobilized single chain Fv fragments. Anal Biochem 244:189–191
22. Green MR, Sambrook J (2012) Molecular cloning: a laboratory manual. Cold Spring Harbor Laboratory Press, Woodbury, NY, USA
23. Laemmli UK (1970) Cleavage of structural proteins during the assembly of the head of bacteriophage T4. Nature 227:680–685
24. Towbin H et al (1979) Electrophoretic transfer of proteins from polyacrylamide gels to nitrocellulose sheets: procedure and some applications. Proc Natl Acad Sci USA 76:4350–4354
25. Warburg O, Christian W (1941) Isolierung und Kristallisation des Gärungsfermentes Enolase. Biochem Z 310:384–421
26. Stoscheck CM (1990) Quantitation of protein. Methods Enzymol 182:50–68
27. Bradford MM (1976) A rapid and sensitive method for the quantitation of microgram quantities of protein utilizing the principle of protein-dye binding. Anal Biochem 72:248–254

Chapter 26

Invariant Chain-Peptide Fusion Vaccine Using HER-2/neu

Sonia A. Perez, George E. Peoples, Michael Papamichail, and Constantin N. Baxevanis

Abstract

A novel method for amplifying the activity of major histocompatibility complex (MHC) class II helper epitopes entails linking a 4-amino-acid moiety (LRMK) from the invariant chain (Ii) of MHC (referred to as Ii-Key) to the N-terminal end of the epitope peptide either directly or using a simple polymethylene spacer (-ava-). Ii-Key catalyzes binding of the linked epitope to the MHC class II molecule, thereby enhancing the overall potency of presentation. HER-2(776–790) (or AE36), which is derived from the intracellular domain of HER-2/neu, has been intensively used as an Ii-key/HER-2(776–790) (or AE37) fusion (hybrid) vaccine in clinical trials. This chapter describes procedures for the synthesis, reconstitution, sterility testing, and storage of both AE36 and AE37 for their use in clinical trials. Also provided is a detailed information about their in vivo administration and analysis of in-depth protocols for monitoring of immune activation upon vaccination with AE37.

Key words Cancer immunotherapy, Peptide vaccine, HER-2/neu, Ii-key, Clinical trial

1 Introduction

During the last decade, a large number of tumor-associated antigens (TAA) have been identified, which can be recognized by T cells. This has led to the use of active immunization as a modality for the therapeutic or preventive and adjuvant treatment of cancer patients. TAAs have been classified into several categories including differentiation, tissue-specific, mutated, and overexpressed antigens. HER-2/neu, a member of the last category, is a transmembrane glycoprotein and member of the epidermal growth factor receptor family. HER-2/neu protein is overexpressed through gene amplification in various cancer types including breast, ovarian, colon, uterine, gastric, prostate, and adenocarcinoma of the lung [1]. In addition, HER-2/neu contains multiple immunogenic epitopes [1] and therefore represents an attractive target for cancer immunotherapy.

Michael J.P. Lawman and Patricia D. Lawman (eds.), *Cancer Vaccines: Methods and Protocols*, Methods in Molecular Biology, vol. 1139, DOI 10.1007/978-1-4939-0345-0_26,

Initially, vaccination-based therapies have focused on eliciting a cytotoxic T lymphocyte (CTL) response, primarily due to the fact that CTL can directly recognize and lyse tumor cells. However, in the past few years, accumulating evidence especially from preclinical studies has placed increasing importance on the stimulation of a $CD4^+$ T helper (Th) cell response in cancer immunotherapy [2]. The major contribution of Th cells for enhancing antitumor effects is thought to be by providing the required activating signals for generating and augmenting tumor-specific CTL responses. T cell help may be directly accessible to the CTL, for instance, by the secretion of interleukin-2 (IL-2), which can activate and also recruit CTLs at the tumor site [3]. Moreover, interferon-γ (IFN-γ) production by Th results in the upregulation of MHC molecules on tumor cells leading to enhanced CTL recognition [2]. However, Th cells may also indirectly activate CTLs through antigen-presenting cells (APC), i.e., "licensing" of dendritic cells (DC) for promoting CTL function and can markedly influence both primary and memory CTL responses.

1.1 Role of Th Cells in Potentiating Anti-HER-2/neu⁺ Tumor Responses

There are several studies reporting the existence of MHC class II-restricted T cell responses to HER-2/neu. $CD4^+$ Th cells from HER-2/neu^+ breast and ovarian cancer patients can proliferate and produce lymphokines in response to stimulation with HER-2/neu recombinant protein or synthetic peptides corresponding to immunodominant regions of HER-2/neu, such as HER-2(p369–384), HER-2(p776–788), and HER-2(p884–899) [4–6]. Some of these patients exhibited preexistent immunity to these peptides in that they responded moderately after a short-term stimulation period. We have reported [7] on the generation and characterization of $CD4^+$ T cell clones specifically recognizing HER-2(p776–788). Such clones yielded specific proliferative and cytokine responses after exposure to DC loaded with HER-2(p776–788).

Most importantly, studies reported by [8] and others [9] with BALB-neuT mice have made it clear that protection against the growth of autochthonous mammary tumors relied on the activation of $CD4^+$ T cells. This activation results in the release of IFN-γ and the reduction of T regulatory cells in the tumor microenvironment, both of which contribute to breaking tolerance against HER-2/neu CTL epitopes in these mice. In addition, activation of HER-2/neu-specific $CD4^+$ Th cells results in the induction of anti-HER-2/neu antibodies. $CD4^+$ Th cells that release IFN-γ have a central role in controlling the switch of antibody isotype to IgG2a [10]. Anti-HER-2/neu antibodies are both necessary and sufficient for protecting BALB-neuT mice, and the IgG2a isotype is the most effective [10, 11]. From the aforementioned points, it is reasonable to postulate that stimulating an effective Th cell response is a way to boost antigen-specific immunity as $CD4^+$ T cells generate the specific cytokine environment required to support an evolving immune response. Furthermore, as CTL and B cell immunity may have a significant effect on HER-2/neu-overexpressing tumor growth, targeting $CD4^+$ T cells in a vaccine strategy would result in the potential to augment these arms of the immune system.

1.2 The Ii-Key Modification of HER-2/neu Helper Peptides Increases Their Efficacy to Act as Tumor Vaccines

Th cells generally respond to long peptides (usually 15–20 aa long) presented to them by class II MHC molecules [3]. Efficient T cell activation is only triggered when the interaction of the specific T cell receptor with its cognate antigenic peptide and MHC reaches a specific half-life threshold. T cell receptor binding kinetics required for T cell activation depend on the density of cognate ligand on the antigen-presenting cell [12]. Thus, increased epitope density coupled with enhanced MHC class II exchange would result in a higher apparent affinity with reduced dissociation rate resulting in enhanced generation of Th cells. To achieve increased density of an epitope onto MHC class II alleles, helper peptides are modified at their COOH terminus with Ii-Key, a fragment of the Ii that is known to promote exchange of the peptides in the MHC class II molecules at the site of action of HLA-DM [13]. Such Ii-Key hybrid peptides catalyze direct charging of MHC class II epitopes to the peptide-binding groove, circumventing the need for intracellular epitope processing [14]. Covalent linkage of this Ii-Key segment to MHC class II epitopes significantly augments antigen presentation [14, 15]. Initially, a homologous series of Ii-Key/HER-2/*neu*(776–790) epitope hybrids were synthesized by systematically varying the structure and length of the spacer which connects the Ii-Key LRMK segment to the promiscuous HER-2/*neu*(776–790) MHC class II epitope (GVGSPYV SRLLGICL) through a flexible polymethylene, *ava*, (5-aminovaleric acid = 5-aminopentanoic acid) chain (Table 1). Full-length hybrids independent of the presence of a spacer were proven to be most immunogenic [16]. Moreover, the Ii-Key/HER-2(776–790) hybrid (AE37) was consistently found to induce more potent immunologic responses both in vitro and in vivo compared with the nonmodified HER-2(776–790) peptide (AE36) [15–19]. These studies fostered human clinical trials in which disease-free breast cancer patients (phase I and phase II) [20, 21] or prostate cancer patients at various stages of the disease (phase I) [22] were immunized with AE37. The vaccine did not induce toxic effects beyond grade 2, and the majority of the patients developed robust HER-2/neu-specific immunity.

In this chapter, we provide a detailed description of the methods and procedures applied for the use of AE37 and AE36 in clinical trials. We also refer to experiments we employed for accurately assessing the immunogenic efficacy of the AE37 vaccine.

Table 1
Ii-Key/HER-2/*neu* (776–790) MHC class II epitope hybrid design

Peptide	Position	Sequence
NP	776–790	Ac-GVGSPYVSRLLGICL-NH2
B	776–790	Ac-LRMK-ava-GVGSPYVSRLLGICL-NH2
C	777–790	Ac-LRMK-ava-VGSPYVSRLLGICL-NH2
E	779–790	Ac-LRMK-ava-SPYVSRLLGICL-NH2
F	776–790	Ac-LRMK-GVGSPYVSRLLGICL-NH2

NP is the native peptide HER-2/*neu*(776–790), whereas peptides B through F are the Ii-Key/HER-2/*neu*(776–790) hybrid peptides

The Ii-Key (LRMK) segment of the immunoregulatory Ii protein was linked through a simple polymethylene *ava* spacer to the promiscuous HER-2/*neu*(776–790) MHC class II epitope by systematically deleting amino acids N-terminal to the P1 (Y) site residue

2 Materials

2.1 Vaccine Preparation

1. Bacteriostatic normal saline for injection.
2. 2-mL Polypropylene freezer-safe cryovials.
3. Freezer-safe boxes.
4. 1-mL syringes.
5. Parafilm M®.
6. Freezer (−20 °C) with temperature recorder.
7. Refrigerator with temperature recorder.
8. Biological Safety Hood class II.

2.2 Immune Monitoring

2.2.1 Peripheral Blood Mononuclear Cell (PBMC) Isolation

1. Cell preparation tubes (CPT).
2. Bench refrigerated centrifuge.
3. Phosphate-buffered saline (PBS) sterile or CTL wash medium (CTL Cellular Technology Ltd, Shaker Heights, OH, USA).

2.2.2 ELISPOT and Proliferation Assays

1. RPMI-1640 with L-Glutamine.
2. Fetal bovine serum (FBS).
3. IFN-γ ELISPOT kit with pre-coated plates (or strips) (BD Biosciences, Franklin Lakes, NY, USA).
4. *Candida albicans* (C. alb) (Lofarma, Milano, Italy).
5. Pokeweed mitogen (PWM).
6. CTL test medium.
7. Tritiated-thymidine (^{3}H-TDR), specific activity 30–40 Ci/mmol, 1 mCi/mL. Prepare a 20 μCi/mL working solution in CTL medium.

8. CO_2 Incubator.
9. ELISPOT analyzer.
10. Cell harvester.
11. β-counter.

2.2.3 Regulatory T Cell (Treg) Determination

1. Red blood cell lysis buffer.
2. Labeled monoclonal antibodies: anti-CD45-PerCP (use 5 μl/50 μl sample), anti-CD4-APC (use 5 μL/50 μL sample), anti-CD25-FITC (use 5 μL/50 μL sample), and anti-CD127-PE (use 1 μL/50 μL sample).
3. Fluorescence-activated cell analyzer.
4. Complete blood count (CBC) tubes.

3 Methods

3.1 GMP Production of AE37 and AE36

AE37 (Ii-key modified HER2/*neu*, 776–790, LRMK-GVGSPYVSRLLGICL) and the native peptide AE36 (HER2/*neu*, 776–790, GVGSPYVSRLLGICL) are produced commercially by a good manufacturing practices production facility for patient use, approved by the competent authorities of each country, such as the Food and Drug Administration (FDA)-approved PolyPeptide Laboratories Group (PPL, http://www.polypeptide.com). The peptides are purified to >95 %, purified and verified by high-performance liquid chromatography and mass spectrometry. The amino acid content is determined by amino acid analysis. Sterility, endotoxin, limulus amebocyte lysate test, and general safety testing are carried out by the manufacturer. In addition, the manufacturer should perform purity/stability testing periodically. Lyophilized peptide is shipped to clinical centers in 100-mg sealed vials, each bearing a label noting the vial content, i.e., AE36 or AE37 peptide, the production lot number, and peptide sequence. The vials are stored in a −20 °C freezer.

3.2 AE37 and AE36 Peptide Reconstitution

Only a single 100-mg sealed vial of AE37 is removed and used at a given time; peptide mixing is carried out in a Clinical Laboratory by trained individuals and under the supervision of a research pharmacist. In a biological safety hood, the vial's seal is broken and the peptide is suspended in bacteriostatic saline for injection (*see* **Note 1**). After suspension and thorough mixing, the 100 mg of peptide will be divided into individual aliquots as described in the next section.

3.2.1 Aliquoting Peptides

1. 166 single-dose vials of 500 μg (0.5 mg) consuming 83 mg of peptide, for vaccines.
2. 170 vials of 100 μg (0.1 mg) consuming 17 mg of peptide, for delayed-type hypersensitivity (DTH) and sterility testing.

3.2.2 Resuspending Lyophilized Peptide

1. Using aseptic technique, 100 mL of bacteriostatic normal saline for injection is added to the 100-mg container of lyophilized peptide to make a solution of 1 mg peptide/1 mL normal saline.
2. After thorough mixing (*see* **Note 2**) and using aseptic technique, 83 mL are withdrawn from the 100 mL solution and 0.5 mL of the solution is injected into 166 sterile, single-dose polypropylene freezer-safe cryovials. The concentration injected into the vials is 0.5 mg peptide/0.5 mL normal saline, i.e., 500 μg peptide/0.5 mL of normal saline. Each vial is labeled with the content (AE37 peptide 500 μg plus saline) and the peptide lot number, then dated and sealed with Parafilm M®. There will be 17 mL of solution with a concentration of 1 mg/1 mL remaining in the vial.
3. To the remaining 17 mL of the original 1 mg/mL of solution is added 68 mL of normal saline to result in 85 mL of 0.2 mg peptide/1 mL normal saline.
4. Inject 0.5 mL of this solution into 170 sterile, single-dose polypropylene freezer-safe cryovials. The concentration injected into the vials is 0.1 mg peptide/0.5 mL of normal saline, i.e., 100 μg peptide/0.5 mL of normal saline. Each vial is labeled with the content (AE37 peptide 100 μg plus saline) and the peptide lot number, then dated and sealed with Parafilm M®.
5. At the conclusion of **steps 1–4**, the original 100 mg peptide will have been suspended and divided into the following individual dose amounts:

   83 mg peptide for 166 doses of 500 μg (**steps 1** and **2**)

   17 mg peptide for 170 doses of 100 μg (**steps 3** and **4**)
6. 100 μg single-dose vials of AE36 peptide (for DTH testing only) will be prepared similarly: part of an initial reconstitution of the AE36 lyophilized peptide to 1 mg/mL in normal saline will be subsequently diluted, with normal saline to 0.2 mg/mL, and aliquoted at 0.5 mL/cryovial, i.e., 100 μg/0.5 mL. The remaining 1 mg/mL preparation can be stored at −75 °C in aliquots for the next batch of AE36 single-dose preparation.

3.3 Peptide Storage and Sterility Testing

3.3.1 Peptide Storage

1. All sealed and labeled vials from steps a–f above are then placed in labeled freezer-safe boxes according to their peptide and dose amount, i.e., all AE36 or AE37 100 μg or AE37 500 μg amounts in separate boxes, and stored in a −20 °C freezer in the Clinical Laboratory.
2. Prior to the initiation of the trial and every 6 months after initiation of the trial, the stability of each peptide must be confirmed by purity testing by manufacturing facility, e.g., PPL,

utilizing RP-HPLC. The tested aliquots are then compared to the original test result to confirm stability.

3.3.2 Sterility Assurance Plan

1. In order to reduce the possibility of contamination and product decomposition, only 1× 100 mg bulk peptide container is opened, and the lyophilized peptide suspended as described above, at a single time.
2. After the lyophilized peptide is distributed in the appropriate number of aliquoted doses, there are 170 vials of 0.1 mg (100 μg) peptide/0.5 mL of normal saline created for DTH and sterility testing.
3. The last 100 μg sample from the bulk 100 mg container after aliquoting is completed should be sent to the Hospital Microbiology Laboratory to be tested for bacterial and fungal contaminants.
4. If the first test vial of the first bulk peptide container from which peptide was suspended, i.e., AE37 bulk #1, renders a positive result, a second 100 μg sample should be tested by the Microbiology Laboratory. This second sample should be the next to the last aliquoted sample from the bulk 100 mg container of peptide. If this second 100 μg/0.5 mL sample renders a positive test result, all of the remaining 500 μg and 100 μg single-dose vials previously aliquoted from that 100 mg bulk container must be destroyed.
5. After destruction of the contaminated samples from the first 100 mg container, the last 100 μg sample from the second 100 mg container from which peptide was suspended, i.e., AE37 bulk #2, should be sent to the Microbiology Laboratory to be tested for bacterial contaminants as described above. If this first vial renders a positive result, a second 100 μg/0.5 mL vial should be sent for sterility testing. If this second vial also renders a positive test result, all remaining vials of suspended peptide and all unopened 100 mg containers of peptide must be destroyed (*see* **Note 3**).

3.3.3 Fluid Thioglycollate Medium Sterility Test (See Note 4)

Sterility testing should be conducted by the Hospital Microbiology Laboratory and should consist of two separate tests: (1) fluid thioglycollate medium to test for bacterial contaminants and (2) soybean-casein digest medium to test for fungal contaminants. As noted above, the last 100 μg/0.5 mL vial from each bulk 100 mg vial should be sent to the Microbiology Laboratory to be tested according to 21CFR610.12. Also, representative samples of the final single-dose vials (1 test per vaccinated patient) should also be sent for sterility testing (approximately 10 % of the vials).

1. Inoculate the 100 μg/0.5 mL sample from the bulk container of peptide into test vials of fluid thioglycollate medium.

(a) Mix the inoculum and medium thoroughly and incubate at 30–35 °C for no less than 14 days and examine visually for evidence of growth on the third, fourth, or fifth day, and on the seventh or eighth day, and on the last day of the incubation period.

(b) If growth appears (a positive test result), then a second vial from the same dose cohort should be tested with fluid thioglycollate medium to rule out the possibility of the receipt of a false-positive test result.

(c) Only 1 repeat bulk test may be performed. If the second 100 μg/mL vial renders a positive test result, then all of the remaining vials bearing the same lot number should be destroyed.

3.3.4 Soybean-Casein Digest Test (See Note 4)

The soybean-casein digest test follows the same steps as outlined above for the fluid thioglycollate test, with the exception that the medium will be soybean-casein digest medium and the incubation will occur at a temperature of 20–25 °C.

3.4 Vaccine Administration and Monitoring

3.4.1 Vaccine Administration

Each enrolled and properly consented patient should receive a total of six vaccinations with AE37 plus granulocyte-monocyte colony stimulating factor (GM-CSF) or six inoculums of GM-CSF alone every 3–4 weeks plus 2 DTH injections (1 before delivery of the first vaccination and 1 after delivery of the sixth and final vaccination (*see* **Note 5**)). Patients receiving six inoculums of GM-CSF alone should also receive two DTH injections. For each vaccinated patient, the research nurse coordinator should send one test vial of 100 μg of peptide/0.5 mL normal saline to the Microbiology Laboratory for sterility testing 2 weeks before delivery of the first vaccine injection. Test vials are not required for patients receiving GM-CSF alone.

Upon written confirmation from the Microbiology Laboratory of product sterility, the contents of the first DTH vial for that patient's inoculation regimen should be administered in the following manner according to the protocol submitted with this formulation plan:

1. One frozen, sterile AE37 DTH vial containing 100 μg of peptide/0.5 mL normal saline is removed from the −20 °C freezer and thawed at room temperature. The thawed solution is withdrawn into a single-dose, sterile syringe and immediately administered intradermally (Fig. 1) on the left anterior thigh approximately 9 in. (~22 cm) superior to the knee.
2. One frozen, sterile AE36 DTH vial containing 100 μg of peptide/0.5 mL of normal saline is removed from the −20 °C freezer and thawed at room temperature. The thawed solution is withdrawn into a single-dose, sterile syringe and immediately

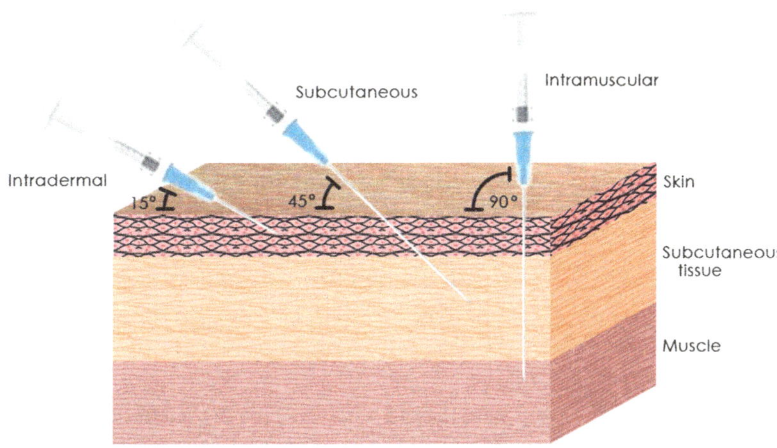

Fig. 1 Intradermal inoculation: comparison of the angles of insertion of intramuscular (IM, 90°), subcutaneous (SC, 45°) in thin and average-size individuals, and intradermal (ID, 15°) injections

administered intradermally on the left anterior thigh approximately 11 in. (~27 cm) superior to the knee, i.e., approximately 2 in. (5 cm) apart from the AE37 inoculation site.

3. After the above is accomplished, 0.5 mL of normal sterile saline is withdrawn into a single-dose, sterile syringe. The 0.5 mL inoculum is immediately administered intradermally approximately 6 in. (~15 cm) superior to the knee. This second inoculum of sterile saline is administered to serve as a negative control for the DTH test.
4. At the time of vaccine delivery, one frozen, sterile vial containing 500 μg of peptide/0.5 mL of saline is removed from the freezer and thawed at room temperature. To this individual container is added GM-CSF at 125 μg in 0.5 mL, withdrawn under a sterile hood using a large-bore single-dose needle from a 1 mL container obtained from the pharmacy. Mixing of the 1 mL solution is accomplished by repeatedly withdrawing the fluid into the syringe and gently injecting it back into the container without producing bubbles and using aseptic technique. The preparation of the inoculum is performed in a biological safety hood by a licensed, trained individual under the supervision of a research pharmacist. For GM-CSF-only patients, the appropriate corresponding amount of GM-CSF should be diluted to a final volume of 1 mL with sterile saline.
5. After mixing is accomplished, the vaccine or GM-CSF alone is immediately administered intradermally in 0.5 mL inoculums at two different sites within 5 cm of each other on the left anterior thigh by a licensed medical doctor or nurse. The lot number of the peptide and the GM-CSF is recorded for each inoculation throughout the trial.

3.4.2 Patient Monitoring

Patients should be monitored postinjection in the Clinical Laboratory for 1 h to note any local or systemic reactions to the vaccine or immunoadjuvant and are required to return to the Clinical Laboratory 48–72 h after inoculation for assessment of local and/or systemic reactions. Additionally, patients should be given the phone number to the vaccine research nurse, principal investigator, and emergency department in case of reaction/side effects and educated as to the local and systemic signs of infection. If any adverse events occur, these must be reported as per the protocol. If infection is detected, then vaccinations should be halted and the sterility of the remaining single-dose vials reconfirmed. The patient should be medically treated as appropriate.

3.5 Monitoring of AE37 Vaccine-Induced Immunity

3.5.1 DTH Reaction

The DTH reaction is performed before the vaccination regimen (baseline DTH) and at post and long term. The DTH reaction is assessed with 100 μg of AE36 and 100 μg of AE37 as described in Subheading 3.4. DTH reactions, as well as dermal reactions to the vaccine, are measured in 2 dimensions at 48–72 h using the sensitive ballpoint pen method [23] in two directions (including the longer and the shorter dimension) and results are reported as an orthogonal mean of the two measurements.

The basis of reading the skin test is the presence or absence of induration, which is a hard, dense, raised formation. This is the area that is measured. Sometimes the site has erythema, a reddening of the skin that can also have swelling. The erythema should NOT be measured. Patients must have an induration of >5 mm postvaccinations to be considered as having developed a positive DTH reaction.

1. Palpate the injection site.
2. Using a medium ballpoint pen held at right angles to the skin, move towards the induration while pressing lightly on the skin. The pen will stop when it reaches the raised area, indicating the edge of the induration (Fig. 2).
3. Mark this point.
4. Repeat from the opposite site of the reaction.
5. Measure the transverse diameter of the induration, perpendicular to the direction of the injection, disregarding any redness. The distance between the two points indicates the diameter of the induration.
6. Record the result in millimeter; if there is no induration, record the result as 0 mm.

Whatever induration is present at 48–72 h should be measured and recorded. Only the part of the reaction recorded by the ballpoint pen method, which is the induration, is measured, even if there is soft swelling or redness at the site. Keep in mind there might not be any induration.

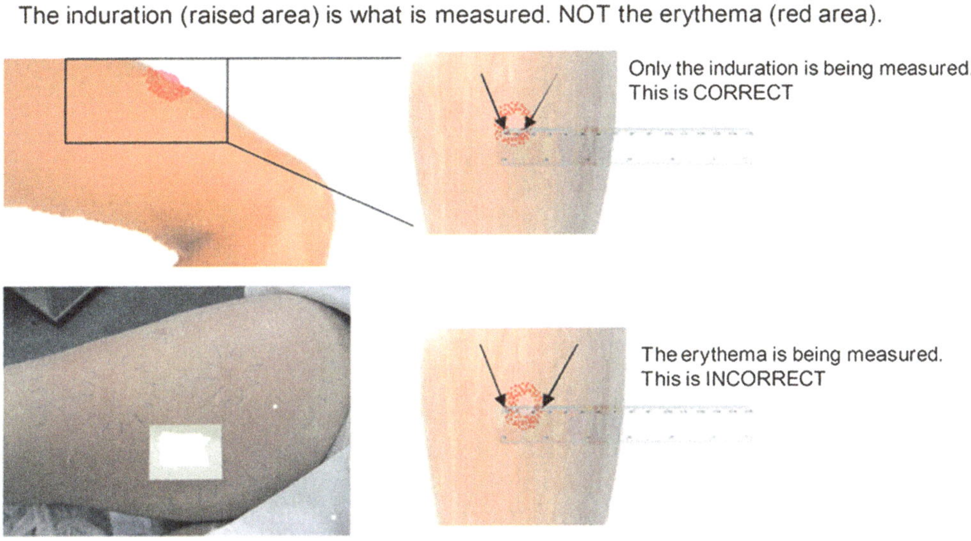

Fig. 2 DTH measurement: the induration (*raised area*) is what is measured, NOT the erythema (*red area*)

3.5.2 Peripheral Blood Collection and Processing

In order to determine in vivo induction of peptide-specific immune responses in the vaccinated patients and in the immunoadjuvant-only patients, 50 mL of blood should be drawn prior to the first inoculation in the series and before each successive inoculation for immunologic studies. In addition, 50 mL of blood should be drawn at 3–4 weeks after completion of the primary inoculation series for immunologic studies. Fifty milliliters of blood should also be drawn before administration of each booster inoculation and as well as at 3–4 weeks postinoculation to record the immunologic response to each of four booster inoculations.

The peripheral blood drawn in blue tiger cap CPTs is processed as described by the manufacturer. PBMC are collected either on the same day or next morning (kept overnight at 4–6 °C). After two washes with sterile PBS or CTL wash medium (prepared as described by the manufacturer), cells are counted and resuspended at 25×10^6 PBMC/mL in CTL medium used as recommended by the manufacturer (*see* **Note 5**).

3.5.3 ELISPOT Assay (See Note 6)

1. For ELISPOT and proliferation assays, 0.4 mL of cell suspension is transferred in 3.6 mL of complete medium (2.5×10^6 PBMC/mL). Remaining cells are frozen in aliquots of 10^7–1.5×10^7 in 1 mL of FBS and 10 % dimethyl sulfoxide.
2. Peptides are diluted in culture medium (CM) at 20 μg/mL (1/50 for AE37, AE36 from a stock of 1 mg/mL). C. alb is diluted 1/50 and PWM at 2 μg/mL in complete medium (working dilutions).
3. ELISPOT plates are washed and blocked as described by the manufacturer and 100 μL/well of complete medium and of working dilutions of peptides. C. alb and PWM are added in two columns for each patient as follows:

A	CM	CM
B	CM	CM
C	AE36	AE36
D	AE36	AE36
E	AE37	AE37
F	AE37	AE37
G	C. alb	C. alb
H	PWM	PWM

4. Then, 100 μL of PBMC suspension (2.5×10^5 cells) is added to each well. Plates are incubated for 40 h at 37 °C in a humidified incubator with 5 % CO_2 and then developed as described by the manufacturer. Spots are enumerated using an ELISPOT analyzer (Fig. 3). Data are presented as the number of spots/10^6 PBMC or as a calculated 1/frequency of IFN-γ-secreting cells in 10^6 PBMC and discussed as the ratio of responding cells to PBMC (*see* **Note 7**).

3.5.4 Proliferation Assay (See Note 6)

A series of 100 μL working dilutions and cell suspensions prepared as for the ELISPOT assay are plated in 1 row/patient in a flat 96-well plate as follows:

CM	CM	CM	AE36	AE36	AE36	AE37	AE37	AE37	C.Alb.	C.Alb.	PWM

Plates are incubated in a 5 % CO_2 humidified incubator for 4 days. Tritiated thymidine (^{3}H-TDR, 1 μCi/50 μL/well in complete medium) is added for the last 16–18 h of incubation. Cells are harvested and radioactivity is measured. Data are presented as mean counts per minute (cpm), Δcpm, i.e., corrected for background with CM alone, and stimulation index (SI: cpm with peptide/cpm with CM).

3.5.5 Phenotypic Characterization of Regulatory T Cells (Treg)

Peripheral blood is collected in complete blood count (CBC) tubes from patients at the same time points as for the ELISPOT and proliferation assays. Treg are detected in whole blood by a lyse-no-wash method (*see* **Note 8**). Fifty microliters of whole blood is stained for 15 min at room temperature with pre-titrated combinations of anti-CD45-PerCP, CD4-APC, CD25-FITC, and CD127-PE antibodies. Red blood cells are lysed with 450 μL of ammonium chloride lysing solution and analyzed within an hour on a cytometer. Treg are defined by gating on low SSC $CD45^+$ $CD4^+$ lymphocytes expressing high CD25 (higher than the non-$CD4^+$ lymphocytes) and negative/low for CD127 (Fig. 4) [18]. The percentage of Treg among $CD4^+$ T cells is recorded.

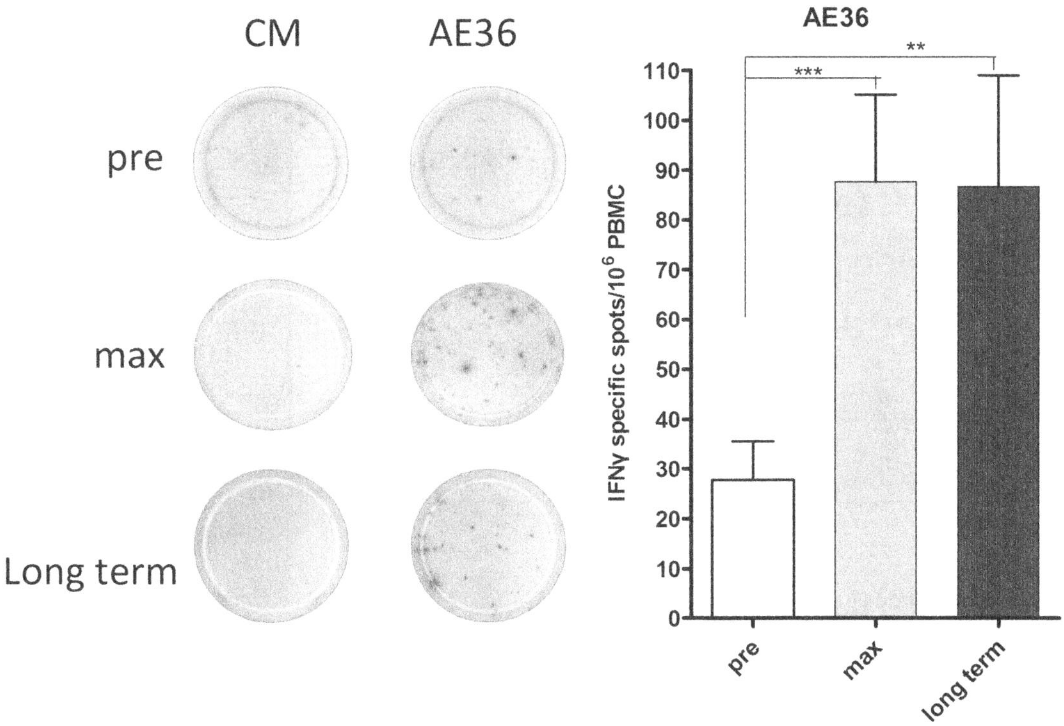

Fig. 3 Detection of the individual patients' PBMC producing IFN-γ in response to AE36 using the ELISPOT assay. ELISPOT plates showing IFN-γ spots in unstimulated cultures (CM) or in cultures stimulated with AE36 (AE36), before (pre), at any time point during vaccinations reaching maximal levels (max) and 6 months post-vaccinations (long term) (*left panel*). A graph from pooled data of vaccinated patients (means ± SD) (*right panel*)

4 Notes

1. If bacteriostatic normal saline is not available, use sterile normal saline for injection.
2. Peptide is not completely dissolved and should be periodically mixed by swirling of the container after dispensing 10 aliquots.
3. The microbiological tests are not described in detail because they are intended to be performed by the routine Hospital Microbiology Laboratory.
4. The final single-dose vials may also be tested for sterility in accordance with the regulatory guidelines of every country, e.g., FDA 21CFR610.12.
5. Initially, we used RPMI-1640 with 10 % FBS as complete medium for the functional assays. However, the background and the efficiency of the assay were greatly influenced by the different FBS batches. X-VIVO™-15 plus 2 % human serum gave less variation supplemented with different batches of human serum. Finally, when compared X-VIVO™-15 plus 2 %

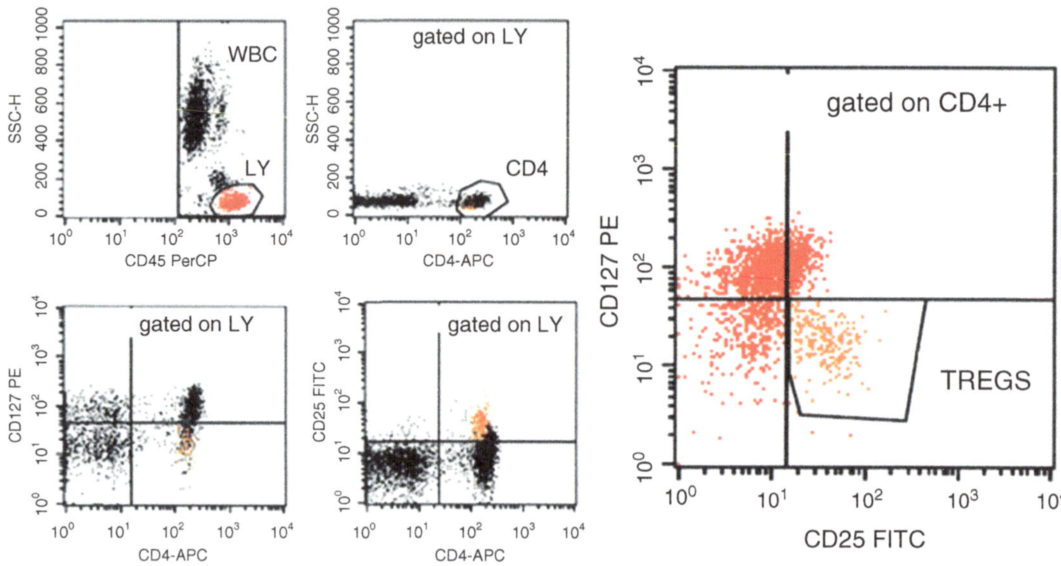

Fig. 4 Gating strategy used to identify the CD4$^+$CD25^{high}CD127^{low} Treg by flow cytometry. Red blood cells (CD45^{neg}) are excluded during acquisition. *WBC* white blood cells (CD45$^+$), *LY* lymphocytes, *CD4*$^+$ CD4$^+$ T lymphocytes, *TREGS* Tregs, and CD4$^+$CD25^{high} CD127^{low} lymphocytes are depicted in different color

human serum with the CTL medium, we found that for the same samples, the background was lower, but more importantly, the sensitivity of the assay was significantly improved. Thus, we decided to use CTL medium for all functional assays.

6. The setup of these assays is indicative for in vitro stimulating ex vivo-isolated patients' T cells. The number of cells/well is the lowest to give reliable results. Up to 0.5×10^6 cells/well can be used. Other protocols suggest a pre-stimulation of PBMC with the peptides, in the absence or presence of cytokines, e.g., IL-12 and IL-7, for a given time period and then testing them on an ELISPOT plate for a shorter time. The purpose of this approach is to increase the sensitivity of the assay. It is important to note that in any case, the response, either IFN-γ production or proliferation, obtained when using unsorted PBMC is not exclusively peptide specific: an effective anti-peptide immune response will initiate a cascade of events leading to activation of other immune cell populations induced to proliferate and/or to produce IFN-γ or other cytokines/chemokines. However, the magnitude of the final response recorded in each assay reflects the magnitude of the specific anti-peptide T cell response.

7. In several analyses, data can be presented as IFN-γ spots per well corrected for background or described as the number of spots per 10^6 PBMC postvaccination minus the number of spots prevaccination. Patients are considered to have preexisting immunity if, at baseline, the mean antigen-specific spots

per well are statistically different ($p < 0.05$) from background, i.e., PBMC in complete medium. Patients are considered to have increased response if the mean number of spots per well (MSPW) is greater than 2 standard deviations (SD) above the previous value, remained the same if the MSPW is within 2 SD of the previous value, and decreased if the MSPW is greater than 2 SD below the previous value [18].

8. We have compared the results obtained by determination of Treg in isolated PBMC using FOXP3 or CD127, along with CD25 and CD4, and we found that both methods give similar results. Furthermore, the lyse-no-wash method for whole blood described here is much easier (less steps, less time) and cost-effective (less consumables) when analyzing many samples, as in the case of clinical trials.

References

1. Baxevanis CN et al (2006) Immunogenic HER-2/neu peptides as tumor vaccines. Cancer Immunol Immunother 55(1):85–95
2. Baxevanis CN et al (2010) HER-2/neu as a target for cancer vaccines. Immunotherapy 2(2):213–226
3. Kennedy R, Celis E (2008) Multiple roles for CD4+ T cells in anti-tumor immune responses. Immunol Rev 222:129–144
4. Anderson BW et al (2000) Induction of determinant spreading and of Th1 responses by in vitro stimulation with HER-2 peptides. Cancer Immunol Immunother 49(9):459–468
5. Disis ML et al (2002) Flt3 ligand as a vaccine adjuvant in association with HER-2/neu peptide-based vaccines in patients with HER-2/neu-overexpressing cancers. Blood 99(8):2845–2850
6. Perez SA et al (2010) Results from a phase I clinical study of the novel Ii-Key/HER-2/neu(776-790) hybrid peptide vaccine in patients with prostate cancer. Clin Cancer Res 16(13):3495–3506
7. Sotiriadou R et al (2001) Peptide HER2(776-788) represents a naturally processed broad MHC class II-restricted T cell epitope. Br J Cancer 85(10):1527–1534
8. Gritzapis AD et al (2010) Peptide vaccination breaks tolerance to HER-2/neu by generating vaccine-specific FasL(+) CD4(+) T cells: first evidence for intratumor apoptotic regulatory T cells. Cancer Res 70(7):2686–2696
9. Lollini PL et al (2006) Vaccines for tumour prevention. Cancer 6(3):204–216
10. Quaglino E et al (2004) Electroporated DNA vaccine clears away multifocal mammary carcinomas in her-2/neu transgenic mice. Cancer Res 64(8):2858–2864
11. Nanni P et al (2004) Immunoprevention of mammary carcinoma in HER-2/neu transgenic mice is IFN-gamma and B cell dependent. J Immunol 173(4):2288–2296
12. Gonzalez PA et al (2005) T cell receptor binding kinetics required for T cell activation depend on the density of cognate ligand on the antigen-presenting cell. Proc Natl Acad Sci USA 102(13):4824–4829
13. Adams S, Humphreys RE (1995) Invariant chain peptides enhancing or inhibiting the presentation of antigenic peptides by major histocompatibility complex class II molecules. Eur J Immunol 25(6):1693–1702
14. Humphreys RE et al (2000) Increasing the potency of MHC class II-presented epitopes by linkage to Ii-Key peptide. Vaccine 18(24):2693–2697
15. Gillogly ME et al (2004) Ii-Key/HER-2/neu MHC class-II antigenic epitope vaccine peptide for breast cancer. Cancer Immunol Immunother 53(6):490–496
16. Sotiriadou NN et al (2007) Ii-Key/HER-2/neu(776-790) hybrid peptides induce more effective immunological responses over the native peptide in lymphocyte cultures from patients with HER-2/neu+ tumors. Cancer Immunol Immunother 56(5):601–613
17. Voutsas IF et al (2007) Induction of potent CD4+ T cell-mediated antitumor responses by a helper HER-2/neu peptide linked to the Ii-Key moiety of the invariant chain. Int J Cancer 121(9):2031–2041
18. Perez SA et al (2010) A new era in anticancer peptide vaccines. Cancer 116(9):2071–2080
19. Erskine CL et al (2011) MHC class II epitope nesting modulates dendritic cell function and improves generation of antigen-specific CD4 helper T cells. J Immunol 187(1):316–324
20. Holmes JP et al (2008) Results of the first phase I clinical trial of the novel II-key hybrid

preventive HER-2/neu peptide (AE37) vaccine. J Clin Oncol 26(20):3426–3433
21. Sears AK et al (2011) AE37: a novel T-cell-eliciting vaccine for breast cancer. Expert Opin Biol Ther 11(11):1543–1550
22. Perez SA et al (2002) HER-2/neu-derived peptide 884-899 is expressed by human breast, colorectal and pancreatic adenocarcinomas and is recognized by in-vitro-induced specific CD4(+) T cell clones. Cancer Immunol Immunother 50(11):615–624
23. Sokal JE (1975) Editorial: measurement of delayed skin-test responses. N Engl J Med 293(10):501–502

Chapter 27

TLR-9 Agonist Immunostimulatory Sequence Adjuvants Linked to Cancer Antigens

Hidekazu Shirota and Dennis M. Klinman

Abstract

The primary goal of cancer vaccines is to elicit tumor-specific cytotoxic T lymphocytes (CTL) capable of eradicating established tumors and preventing/eradicating their metastatic spread. CpG oligonucleotides (CpG ODN) activate and support the maturation of immune cells, including plasmacytoid dendritic cells and B lymphocytes, that express Toll-like receptor 9 (TLR9) and are capable of presenting tumor antigens to T cells. Thus, CpG ODN are effective vaccine adjuvants. The adjuvant activity of CpG ODN is improved by maintaining them in close physical and temporal proximity to the co-administered vaccine antigen. This work describes a method of chemically conjugating CpG ODN to antigens and/or cancer cells that improve the resulting CTL response.

Key words CpG oligonucleotide, Vaccine, Adjuvant, Tumor

1 Introduction

Improving the host's ability to recognize and reject tumor cells is a key goal of cancer immunotherapy. Animal studies and clinical trials utilizing tumor-associated antigens (TAA) and whole non-viable cancer cells as vaccines demonstrate the feasibility of inducing an adaptive immune response capable of eradicating established tumors and tumor metastasis [1–3]. Key to the success of such immunotherapy is the ability to magnify the immunogenicity of TAA by inclusion of adjuvants capable of inducing a strong CTL response [4, 5]. In this context, whole killed tumor cells represent an excellent source of diverse TAA and also eliminate the need to identify individual antigens on tumors from different individuals [6].

Non-methylated CpG motifs are present at high frequency in bacterial, but not vertebrate DNA [7]. These motifs are sensed by immune cells which express the Toll-like receptor 9 (TLR9). The resulting interaction triggers an innate immune response that facilitates the elimination of the infectious pathogen. Characteristic of

Michael J.P. Lawman and Patricia D. Lawman (eds.), *Cancer Vaccines: Methods and Protocols*, Methods in Molecular Biology, vol. 1139, DOI 10.1007/978-1-4939-0345-0_27, © Springer Science+Business Media New York 2014

CpG-mediated immune responses is the activation of antigen-presenting cells (APC), Th1-cytokine-producing cells, antibody-secreting B cells, and CTL, all of which support the development of adaptive immunity [8, 9]. From these reported studies, CpG ODN are findings used as adjuvants to enhance the adaptive immune response.

We and others previously documented that the efficacy of CpG-based adjuvants is critically dependent on maintaining close physical and temporal proximity between ODN and Ag, as free ODN diffuse from the site of Ag delivery [10–12]. Physically cross-linking ODN to the target can improve the resulting immune response by up to a 100-fold over that induced by simply mixing ODN with the immunogen [10, 13, 14]. We also have shown that chemically cross-linking CpG ODN to the surface of apoptotic tumor cells generates a highly immunogenic vaccine capable of accelerating tumor rejection in murine models [15]. CpG ODN conjugation improves the uptake of apoptotic tumor cells by host APC and promotes the functional maturation of dendritic cells thereby facilitating the induction of tumor-specific responses. These findings suggest that CpG-conjugated TAA or autologous cancer cells may be useful in cancer immunotherapy.

2 Materials

A number of different methods have been evaluated for their ability to induce antitumor immunity. Below is a description of how protein-based TAA and whole apoptotic tumor cell vaccines can be prepared in conjunction with CpG ODN.

2.1 Oligodeoxynucleotides (ODNs)

The following ODNs (MW 6,500) were used:

CpG ODN 1826 (TCCATGACGTTCCTGACGTT).
Control ODN 1745 (TCCATGAGCTTCCTGAGTCT).

Both of these ODNs can be purchased as thiolated or NH_2-modified phosphorothioate from multiple sources. The ODN should be free of detectable protein or endotoxin contamination.

2.2 Chemical Conjugation of ODN to TAA

1. Lyophilized thiolated phosphorothioate ODN.
2. Sterile endotoxin-free water.
3. Sulfo-SMCC (sulfosuccinimidyl 4-[N-maleimidomethyl] cyclohexane-1-carboxylate) (Thermo Scientific, Rockford, IL, USA) MW 436 (*see* **Notes 1** and **2**).
4. Conjugation Buffer, phosphate-buffered saline (PBS): 100 mM sodium phosphate, 150 mM sodium chloride, and pH 7.2 (*see* **Note 3**).
5. Amine-modified recombinant tumor antigen (Protein-NH_2).

6. Desalting column to separate modified protein from excess cross-linker.
7. Dialysis equipment, MW cut-off 10,000.
8. BCA protein assay reagent (Thermo Scientific).

2.3 Conjugation of ODN to Apoptotic Tumor Cells

1. Lyophilized NH_2 modified phosphorothioate ODN.
2. Sterile endotoxin-free water.
3. BS^3 (bis[sulfosuccinimidyl] suberate). Prepare this cross-linker immediately before use by dissolving BS^3 in water or 50 mM PBS. BS^3 may be added directly to cells to decrease the extent of hydrolysis (*see* **Notes 4** and **5**).
4. Conjugation Buffer: Use a non-amine-containing buffer at pH 8.0, such as NaOH-adjusted PBS.
5. Apoptotic tumor cells. Induce apoptosis by irradiation (15,000 rad) or chemical treatment, e.g., incubation with 10 μg/mL of mitomycin C for 8–12 h.

3 Methods

3.1 Chemical Conjugation of CpG ODN to TAA Protein (Reaction Scheme, Fig. 1)

1. Dissolve lyophilized thiolated phosphorothioate ODN in sterile endotoxin-free water at a concentration of 5 mg/mL. This material can be stored at −20 °C.
2. Dissolve amine-modified recombinant tumor antigen in conjugation buffer.
3. Add the appropriate amount of cross-linker to the protein solution. The concentration of the protein-NH_2 determines the amount of cross-linker to use. Suggested cross-linker molar excesses are shown in Table 1.
4. Incubate reaction mixture for 30 min at room temperature or 2 h at 4 °C.
5. Remove excess cross-linker by passing the mixture through a desalting column equilibrated with Conjugation Buffer.
6. Combine and mix CpG ODN-SH and desalted cross-linker-activated protein in a molar ratio corresponding to that desired for the final conjugate and consistent with the relative number of sulfhydryl and activated amines that exist on the protein and ODN (*see* **Note 6** and Table 2).
7. Incubate the reaction mixture overnight at 4 °C.
8. Remove unconjugated ODN by dialysis against 20 mL of PBS overnight at 4 °C.
9. Measure the unconjugated ODN in dialysis buffer by NanoDrop and calculate/estimate protein-bound CpG ODN (*see* **Note 7**).

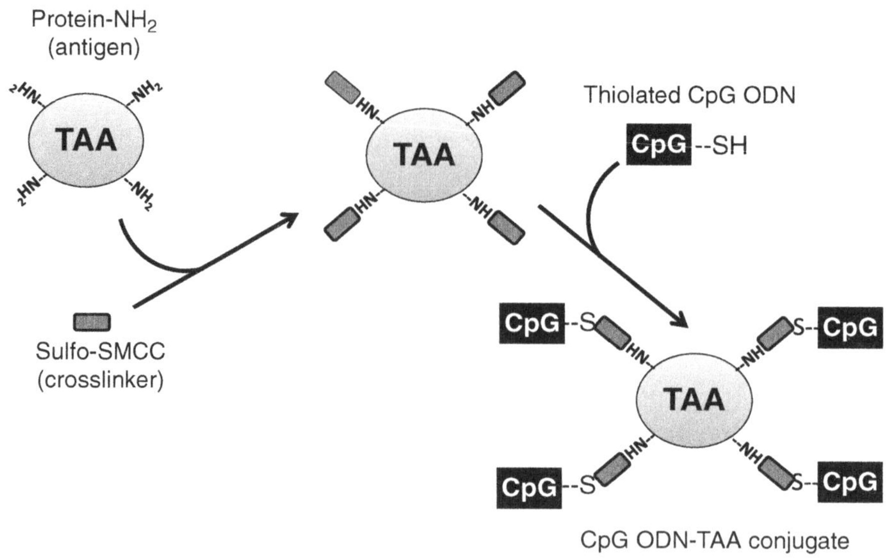

Fig. 1 Schema for conjugation of protein to CpG ODN

Table 1
Cross-linker preparation and molar excess to use for 1 mL of sample

NH_2 protein concentration (based on a 50 kDa protein)	10 mg/mL	1 mg/mL	0.5 mg/mL
Cross-linker molar excess	5×	20×	50×
Sulfo-SMCC (50 mM, 4.8 mg/mL)	100 μL	40 μL	50 μL

Table 2
Preparation of cross-linker-activated protein and ODN-SH for 1 mL of sample

Cross-linker-activated protein (based on a 50 kDa protein, 1 mg/mL)			
Molar ratio of protein:CpG ODN	20:1	5:1	2:1
ODN-SH			
(5 mg/mL)	520 μL	130 μL	52 μL

10. Change the dialysis buffer and dialyze two more times at 4 °C.
11. Measure protein concentration using a protein assay kit.

In the process of protein-ODN conjugation, the protein may aggregate. An example of this effect is seen in Fig. 2 where CpG ODN was conjugated to ovalbumin. We recommend separating the unconjugated material by gel filtration chromatography and visualizing the outcome using SDS-PAGE stained for protein (A) and ODN (B). In the example provided, the lane furthest on the right

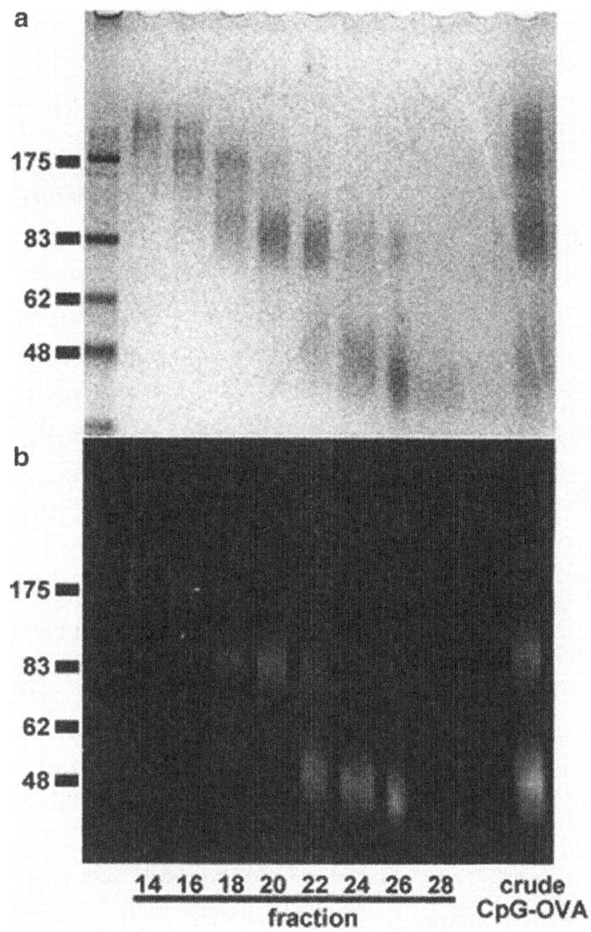

Fig. 2 Synthesis of protein—CpG ODN conjugate. The molar ratio of CpG ODN:protein in this conjugation was 5:1. CpG ODN was bound to ovalbumin protein. The lane on the far right shows the crude, unseparated conjugate. This was separated over a Sephacryl S-200 HR column and the fractions collected analyzed on SDS-PAGE gel stained for protein (*A*) or CpG (*B*). Note that fractions 24–26 were strongly stimulatory

represents crude freshly synthesized OVA-ODN. The output of the gel filtration shows that some fractions stain for protein, but not DNA. These are unconjugated protein and they lack immunostimulatory activity. Other fractions stain for both protein and DNA. These correspond to stimulatory CpG-OVA conjugates and strongly induce Th1 differentiation. In our experience, both aggregates and monomers containing CpG ODN and protein are immunostimulatory.

3.2 Chemical Conjugation of CpG ODN to Cells

1. Induce apoptosis by irradiation (15,000 rad) or chemical treatment of target cells using 10 μg/mL of mitomycin C for 8–12 h.

2. Wash cells extensively with ice-cold PBS, pH 8.0, to remove amine-containing culture medium and proteins released by apoptotic cells.
3. Suspend 5×10^7 cells in 1 mL of PBS, pH 8.0, and add NH_2-modified ODN at a final concentration of 500 μg/mL, i.e., 10 μg/1×10^6 cells. Incubate for 1 h at 4 °C.
4. Add BS^3 solution to a final concentration of 1–5 mM and incubate for 30 min at 4 °C.
5. Wash cells 1× by centrifugation to remove unbound ODN.
6. Measure the unconjugated ODN in the supernatant and use this to calculate the amount of ODN bound to the cells (*see* **Note 8**).
7. Count the cells (*see* **Note 9**).

4 Notes

1. Sulfo-SMCC is moisture-sensitive. Therefore, you should store the material frozen in an airtight container that includes a desiccant. Allow the vial containing the sulfo-SMCC to reach room temperature before opening it to avoid any water condensing inside the container. Dissolve only the amount of reagent needed for use and add it immediately (before hydrolysis occurs) to the protein. Discard any excess dissolved sulfo-SMCC as it will be inactive.
2. We recommend the use of "No-Weigh Microtubes" for sulfo-SMCC. Immediately before use, puncture the microtube foil with a pipette tip, add 200 μL of ultrapure water, and pipette up and down to mix. Store unused microtubes frozen in the presence of a desiccant.
3. Avoid buffers containing primary amines, e.g., Tris or glycine, or sulfhydryls during conjugation because they will compete with the intended reaction. If necessary, dialyze or desalt samples into an appropriate buffer such as PBS.
4. BS^3 is moisture-sensitive. To avoid moisture condensation in the storage vial, it must be equilibrated to room temperature before opening.
5. The NHS-ester moiety readily hydrolyzes and becomes nonreactive. Therefore, prepare the cross-linking reagent immediately prior to use. Discard any unused reconstituted cross-linker.
6. The typical molar ratio of CpG ODN to protein in the conjugate is 5–10:1.
7. Subtract total free CpG ODN (ODN concentration in dialysate × 20 mL) from total added-CpG ODN.
8. Subtract total free CpG ODN (ODN concentration in supernatant x volume) from total added-CpG ODN.

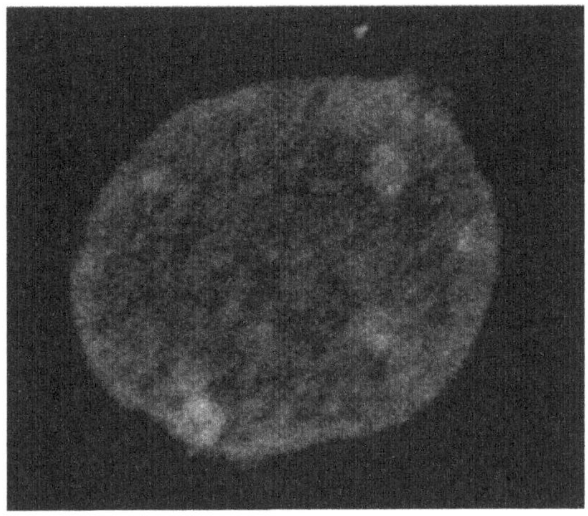

Fig. 3 Binding of CpG ODN to the surface of apoptotic tumor cells. E.G7 cells were treated with mitomycin C for 24 h to induce apoptosis. The cells were then conjugated to FITC-labeled CpG ODN and binding examined by confocal microscopy (*see* **Note 10**)

9. The typical number of CpG ODN-conjugated cells used as a vaccine in mice is 2×10^6.
10. We found that 80–90 % of ODN bind to cells using this technique. This can be visualized directly by using FITC-modified ODN and studying the cells using confocal microscopy (E.G7 cells) (Fig. 3).

Acknowledgement

This research was supported by the Intramural Research Program of the NIH, National Cancer Institute.

References

1. Greten TF, Jaffee EM (1999) Cancer vaccines. J Clin Oncol 17:1047–1060
2. Lollini PL et al (2006) Vaccines for tumour prevention. Nat Res Cancer 6:204–216
3. Gilboa E (2004) The promise of cancer vaccines. Nat Rev Cancer 4:401–411
4. Schijns VE, Lavelle EC (2011) Trends in vaccine adjuvants. Expert Rev Vaccines 10:539–550
5. Chiang CL et al (2011) Adjuvants for enhancing the immunogenicity of whole tumor cell vaccines. Int Rev Immunol 30:150–182
6. Klebanoff CA et al (2011) Therapeutic cancer vaccines: are we there yet? Immunol Rev 239:27–44
7. Krieg AM et al (1995) CpG motifs in bacterial DNA trigger direct B-cell activation. Nature 374:546–548
8. Hemmi H et al (2000) A Toll-like receptor recognizes bacterial DNA. Nature 408:740–745
9. Takeshita F et al (2001) Cutting Edge: role of toll-like receptor 9 in CpG DNA-induced activation of human cells. J Immunol 167: 3555–3558
10. Shirota H et al (2000) Regulation of murine airway eosinophilia and Th2 cells by antigen-conjugated CpG oligodeoxy-nucleotides as a novel antigen-specific immunomodulator. J Immunol 164:5575–5582

11. Tighe H et al (2000) Conjugation of protein to immunostimulatory DNA results in a rapid, long-lasting and potent induction of cell-mediated and humoral immunity. Eur J Immunol 30:1939–1947
12. Heit A et al (2005) Protective CD8 T cell immunity triggered by CpG-protein conjugates competes with the efficacy of live vaccines. J Immunol 174:4373–4380
13. Shirota H et al (2001) Novel roles of CpG oligodeoxynucleotides as a leader for the sampling and presentation of CpG-tagged antigen by dendritic cells. J Immunol 167:66–74
14. Sano K et al (2003) Oligodeoxy-nucleotides without CpG motifs work as adjuvant for the induction of Th2 differentiation in a sequence-independent manner. J Immunol 170: 2367–2373
15. Shirota H, Klinman DM (2011) CpG-conjugated apoptotic tumor cells elicit potent tumor-specific immunity. Cancer Immunol Immunother 60:659–669

Chapter 28

Production of Multiple CTL Epitopes from Multiple Tumor-Associated Antigens

Rena Morita, Yoshihiko Hirohashi, Munehide Nakatsugawa, Takayuki Kanaseki, Toshihiko Torigoe, and Noriyuki Sato

Abstract

Identification of antigenic peptides derived from tumor-associated antigens (TAA) enables cancer vaccine therapy using antigenic peptides. Here, we summarize the design of antigenic peptides and induction of cytotoxic T lymphocytes (CTL) using antigenic peptides and validation of CTL.

Key words Tumor-associated antigen, Cytotoxic T lymphocyte, Antigenic peptide, HLA

1 Introduction

In recent years, immunotherapies for malignant diseases have been regarded as the fourth strategy following surgery, chemotherapy, and radiotherapy. The molecular biological characteristics of immunotherapies have been analyzed and have been partially applied in clinical settings. Previous studies showed that antigen-specific immunotherapies such as peptide vaccine therapy were less effective and successful in vivo than in vitro [1, 2]. These results might be due to various escape mechanisms from the immune system, including antigen molecules targeted by immune cells, actions of immune suppression, e.g., regulatory T lymphocytes, or inhibiting cytokines and loss of human leukocyte-associated antigen (HLA) and β2-microglobulin. It is essential to design antigenic peptides to prevent escape from the immune system [3]. Loss of antigens is thought to be one of the main causes of escape from the immune system, therefore, functional antigens are thought to be suitable targets.

An antigen derived from the melanoma-associated antigen (MAGE) family that was recognized by cytotoxic T lymphocytes from a human melanoma patient was discovered in 1991 [4]. Since then, many tumor-associated antigens (TAA) have been identified and analyzed. Various methods have been used for identifying

Michael J.P. Lawman and Patricia D. Lawman (eds.), *Cancer Vaccines: Methods and Protocols*, Methods in Molecular Biology, vol. 1139, DOI 10.1007/978-1-4939-0345-0_28, © Springer Science+Business Media New York 2014

candidate TAA, including cDNA expression cloning, cDNA microarray, DNA subtraction methods, serological identification of antigens by recombinant expression cloning (SEREX methods), and a reverse-immunogenetical approach [4–7]. Although cancer cell-specific proteins are potential immunological targets, it is necessary to determine whether a peptide from a candidate protein can induce a CTL response. In this chapter, we summarize (1) prediction of antigenic peptides, (2) generation of CTL, and (3) validation of CTL and establishment of CTL clones.

2 Materials

2.1 Selection of HLA-Restricted Peptides Derived from Candidate Antigens

1. Putative antigenic peptides can be designed by several website programs (e.g., BIMAS, SYFPEITHI, CTLPred, ProPred1, MAPPP, nHLAPred, LPPEP, SVMHC, NetMHC, MHCPred, Epitope binding, MMPRED, and PREDEP) (Fig. 1) (*see* **Note 1**) [8, 9].
2. Synthetic peptides.
3. Dimethyl sulfoxide (DMSO).
4. T2 cells cultured in Roswell Park Memorial Institute (RPMI)-1640 supplemented with 10 % FBS (*see* **Note 2**).
5. Phosphate-buffered saline (PBS) without Ca^{2+} and Mg^{2+} on ice.
6. Opti-MEM® (Life Technologies, Inc., Carlsbad, CA, USA).
7. Anti-HLA-class I monoclonal antibody (mAb) (*see* **Notes 3** and **4**).
8. ITC-conjugated rabbit antimouse IgG + IgM (KPL, Gaithersburg, MD, USA).

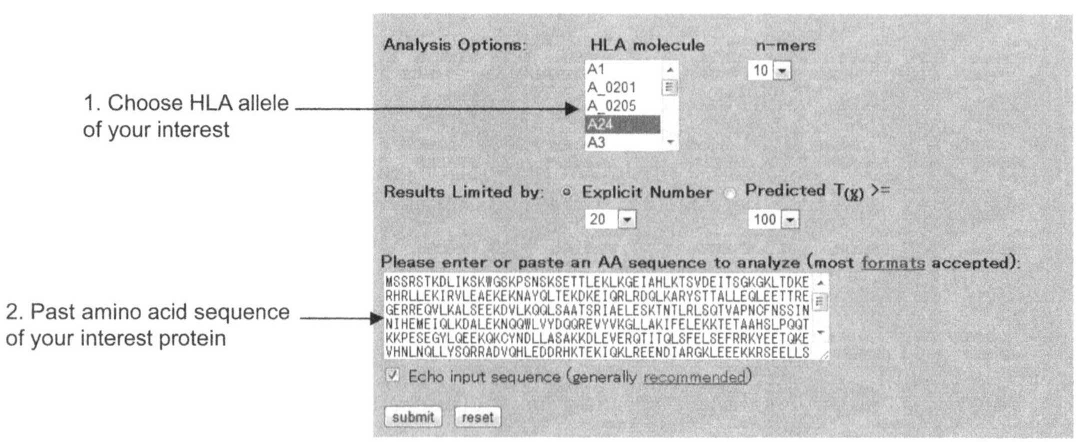

Fig. 1 Representative prediction of antigenic peptides by BIMAS website. BIMAS website: http://www-bimas.cit.nih.gov/molbio/hla_bind/

9. PBS containing 1 % formaldehyde.
10. Disposable pipettes and Pasteur pipettes (sterile).
11. Sterile tubes for flow cytometry.
12. Sterile micropipettors and tips.
13. Centrifuge (refrigerated) with swing-out rotor and appropriate carriers.
14. Hemocytometer and microscope for cell counting.
15. 5 % CO_2 incubator at 26 and 37 °C.
16. Flow cytometer.

2.2 Preparation of APC and CD8⁺ T Cells Isolated from Peripheral Blood Mononuclear Cells (PBMC)

1. Blood sample (*see* **Note 4**).
2. Lymphoprep (Nycomed, Oslo, Norway).
3. Anticoagulant agent, e.g., heparin sodium, EDTA, and sodium citrate.
4. PBS with 2 mM EDTA, at room temperature.
5. AIM-V medium.
6. 2-Mercaptoethanol.
7. 4-(2-Hydroxyethyl)-1-piperazineethanesulfonic acid buffer (HEPES).
8. Human recombinant interleukin-2 (IL-2) (R&D Systems, Minneapolis, MN, USA).
9. Human recombinant interleukin-4 (IL-4) (R&D Systems).
10. Human granulocyte/macrophage-colony stimulating factor (GM-CSF) (R&D Systems).
11. Tumor necrosis factor-α (TNFα) (R&D Systems).
12. Phytohaemagglutinin (PHA-P).
13. MACS separation system (Miltenyi Biotech, Bergisch Gladbach, Germany) using anti-CD8 mAb coupled with magnetic microbeads.
14. Sterile disposable pipettes and Pasteur pipettes.
15. Sterile 50-mL high-clarity polypropylene conical centrifuge tube.
16. Sterile micropipettors and tips.
17. Centrifuge (not refrigerated) with swing-out rotor and appropriate carriers.
18. Sterile 10-cm culture flasks (dish) and 24-well plates.

2.3 Induction of CTL

1. Synthesized peptides dissolved in 20 mg/mL of DMSO.
2. β2-Microglobulin.
3. AIM-V medium supplemented with 10 % human serum, 100 IU/mL of IL-2, 50 μM 2-mercaptoethanol, and HEPES buffer.

4. Human recombinant IL-2 (R&D Systems).
5. Human recombinant interleukin-7 (IL-7) (R&D Systems).
6. Human AB serum.
7. Complete RPMI-1640 medium, i.e., RPMI-1640 supplemented with 10 % fetal bovine serum (FBS).
8. Sterile disposable pipettes and Pasteur pipettes.
9. Sterile 24-well plates.
10. Enzyme-linked immunospot (ELISPOT) Human interferon-γ (IFN-γ) ELISPOT set (Becton Dickinson Biosciences, Franklin Lakes, NJ, USA).
11. Sterile micropipettors and tips.
12. KS ELISPOT assay system (Carl Zeiss, Oberkochen, Germany).
13. Gamma counter (PerkinElmer, Waltham, MA, USA).
14. X-ray irradiation device for cells (SOFTEX, Tokyo, Japan).

2.4 Establishment of CTL Clone

1. $CD8^+$ T cells (CTL).
2. PBMC from donors.
3. AIM-V medium supplemented with 10 % human serum, 100 IU/mL of IL-2, 50 μM 2-mercaptoethanol, and 10 mM HEPES.
4. Human recombinant IL-2 (R&D Systems).
5. PHA-P.
6. Human AB serum.
7. Sterile disposable pipettes and Pasteur pipettes.
8. Sterile 96-, 48-, and 24-well plates.
9. Sterile micropipettors and tips.
10. X-ray irradiation device for cells (SOFTEX, Tokyo, Japan).

3 Methods

3.1 Selection of HLA-Restricted Peptides Derived from Candidate Antigens

1. Predict putative antigenic peptides with protein sequence (*see* **Note 1**). The synthesized peptides should be dissolved in DMSO and stored at −80 °C before use (*see* **Note 2**).
2. After incubation of T2 cells in RPMI-1640 culture medium supplemented with 10 % FBS at 26 °C for 18 h, wash the cells with ice-cold PBS (*see* **Note 5**).
3. For flow cytometric analysis, divide the cells equally into two sterile tubes and suspend T2 cells with 1 mL of Opti-MEM® with or without 100 μg of peptide, followed by incubation at 26 °C for 3 h and then at 37 °C for 3 h.

4. After washing 1× with ice-cold PBS, incubate the cells with anti-HLA-class I mAb at 4 °C for 30 min (*see* **Notes 3** and **4**).
5. After washing with ice-cold PBS 1×, incubate the cells with FITC-conjugated rabbit antimouse IgG+IgM at 4 °C for 30 min.
6. Then suspend the cells with 1 mL of PBS containing 1 % formaldehyde and analyze the cells by flow cytometry.
7. Binding affinity is evaluated by comparing mean fluorescence intensity of HLA-class I expression in the presence of peptide with mean fluorescence intensity in the absence of the peptide (*see* **Note 4**).

3.2 Preparation of APC and CD8$^+$ T Cells from PBMC (Summarized in Fig. 3) [10–12]

1. Obtain 50 mL of a blood sample with an anticoagulant agent, e.g., heparin sodium, EDTA, and sodium citrate (*see* **Note 6**).
2. Add 15 mL of Lymphoprep to each of two 50-mL high-clarity polypropylene conical centrifuge tubes. Carefully add 25 mL of a blood sample onto the top of Lymphoprep and centrifuge at 780×g for 20 min at room temperature using a swing-out rotor (*see* **Note 7**).
3. After centrifugation, the PBMC form a white–light yellow band at the plasma/Lymphoprep interface as shown in Fig. 2. Obtain the PBMC layer from the interface using micropipettors without removing the upper plasma layer and transfer the PBMC to a fresh 50-mL conical centrifuge tube (*see* **Note 8**).
4. Add 1× or more volume of PBS with EDTA to the tube with the isolated PBMC cells. Pellet PBMC by centrifugation at 630×g for 7–10 min at room temperature using a swing-out rotor.
5. Following centrifugation, wash the pellet 2× with 10 mL of PBS with EDTA (centrifugation at 440×g for 5 min at room temperature).
6. Incubate PBMC in AIM-V medium supplemented with 50 μM 2-mercaptoethanol and 10 mM HEPES for 2–24 h at 37 °C in a culture flask to separate adherent cells and nonadherent cells (*see* **Note 9**).
7. To generate dendritic cells (DC) from adherent PBMC, incubate adherent cells in AIM-V medium supplemented with 1,000 U/mL of IL-4 and 1,000 U/mL of GM-CSF for 5 days and then add 10 ng/mL TNFα to facilitate maturation of monocyte-derived DC (*see* **Note 10**).
8. Isolation of CD8$^+$ T lymphocytes and CD8$^-$ lymphocytes from nonadherent cells: CD8$^+$ T lymphocytes are isolated from nonadherent cells utilizing the MACS separation system with anti-CD8 mAb coupled with magnetic microbeads according to the manufacturer's instructions.

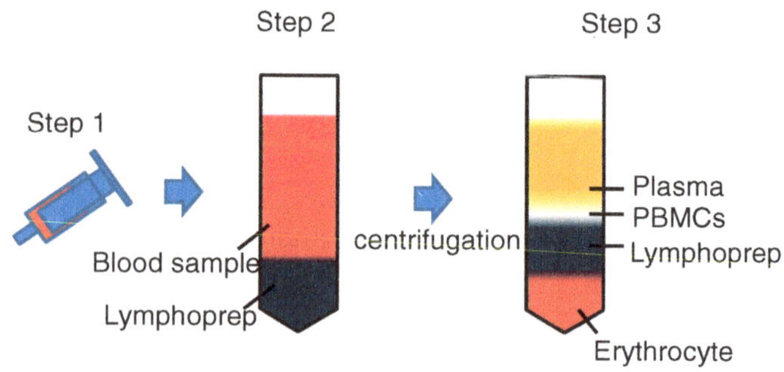

Fig. 2 Isolation of peripheral blood mononuclear cells (PBMC) from peripheral blood

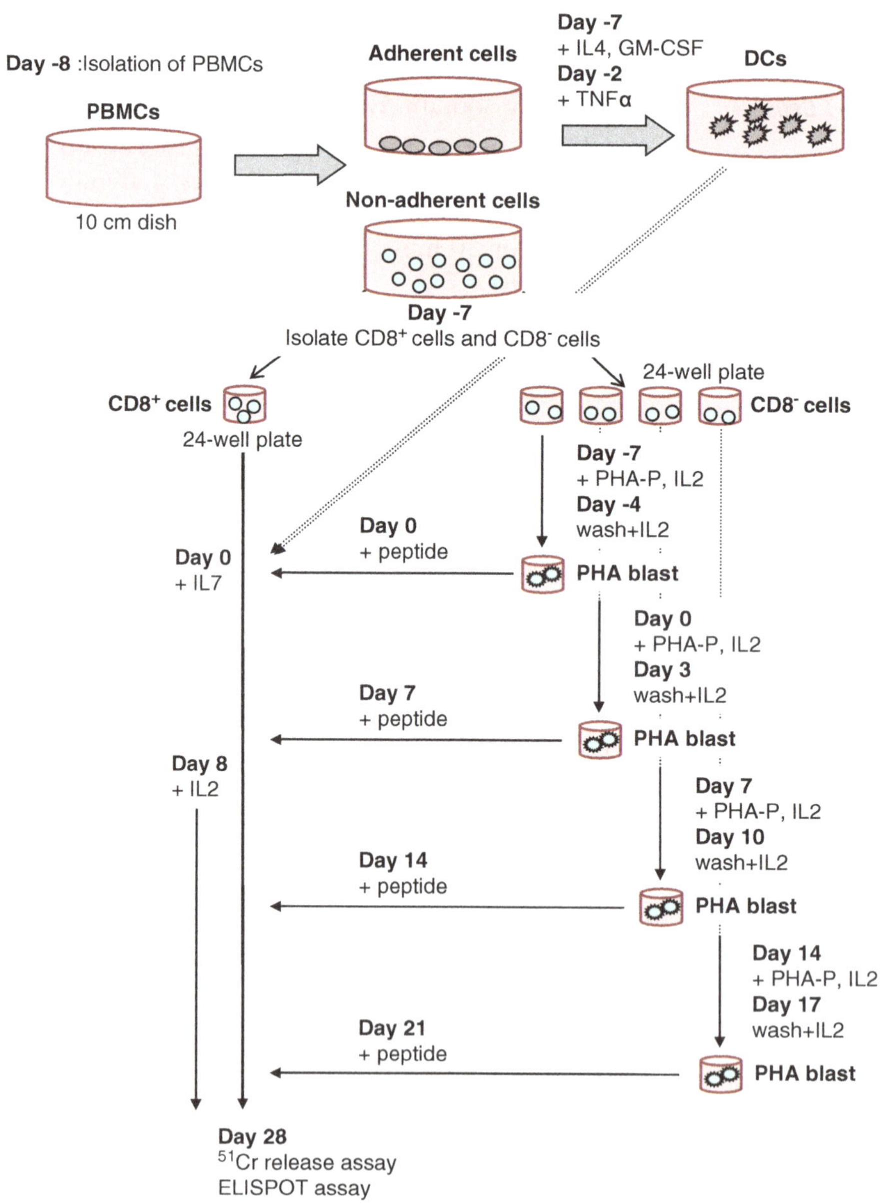

Fig. 3 Summary of CTL induction from PBMC

9. Generation of PHA-blasts from nonadherent PBMC: $CD8^-$ cells derived from nonadherent PBMC are seeded into four wells of a 24-well plate and cultured in AIM-V medium containing 1 μg/mL of PHA-P and 100 U/mL of IL-2 for 3 days, followed by washing with AIM-V medium and culture in AIM-V medium supplemented with 100 U/mL of IL-2 for 4 days (*see* **Note 11**).

3.3 Induction of CTL (Summarized in Fig. 3)

1. On day 0, autologous APC (DC or PHA-blasts) are incubated at room temperature for 2 h in AIM-V medium with 2.5 μg/mL of β2-microglobulin and 50 μg/mL of synthetic peptide. APC are then irradiated (100 Gy) using an X-ray irradiation device and washed with AIM-V medium. One hundred thousand peptide-pulsed-irradiated APC are incubated with 1×10^6 $CD8^+$ cells in 2 mL of AIM-V medium supplemented with 10 % human AB serum, recombinant 10 ng/mL of IL-7, 50 μM 2-mercaptoethanol, and 10 mM HEPES in 1 well of a 24-well plate (*see* **Note 11**).
2. On day 7, autologous PHA-blasts are incubated at room temperature for 2 h in AIM-V medium with 50 μg/mL peptide. PHA-blasts are then irradiated (100 Gy) and washed with AIM-V medium. One million $CD8^+$ T cells are stimulated with 2×10^5 peptide-pulsed PHA-blasts in 2 mL of AIM-V medium.
3. On day 8, add IL-2 to each well at a concentration of 50 U/mL.
4. The peptide stimulation procedure using PHA-blasts is repeated every 7 days. During CTL induction, cells are fed with fresh AIM-V medium supplemented with 10 % human serum, 50 U/mL of IL-2, 50 μM 2-mercaptoethanol, and 10 mM HEPES every 2–5 days (*see* **Note 12**).
5. On day 28, $CD8^+$ T cell reactivity is assessed by IFN-γ ELISPOT assay or conventional 6-h ^{51}Cr release assay (see below).

3.4 IFN-γ ELISPOT Assay

Multiscreen 96-well plates are coated with 100 μL/well of 5 μg/mL of anti-IFN-γ capture antibody in PBS at 4 °C overnight. Plates are washed once with 200 μL/well of complete RPMI-1640 and blocked with 200 μL/well of complete RPMI-1640 at room temperature for 2 h. Then, 2×10^5 $CD8^+$ T cells are incubated with 5×10^4/well T2 cells pulsed with each peptide at 50 μg/mL. After 40 h of incubation at 37 °C, IFN-γ spots are developed and counted as per the manufacturer's instructions (*see* **Note 13**).

3.5 ^{51}Cr Release Assay

Target cells are labeled with 100 μCi of ^{51}Cr for 1 h at 37 °C, washed 3×, and resuspended in AIM-V medium. ^{51}Cr-labeled target cells at 2×10^3 cells/well are incubated with various numbers of effector cells for 6 h at 37 °C in 96-well microtiter plates. Radioactivity of the culture supernatant is measured using a gamma counter. The percentage of cytotoxicity is calculated as follows:

% cytotoxicity = (experimental release − spontaneous release)/(maximum release − spontaneous release) × 100 (*see* **Note 14**).

3.6 Establishment of CTL Clone [13]

1. Seed CTL at 0.3–30/well by limiting dilution in a 96-well round-bottom plate. Fifty thousand irradiated PBMC derived from three healthy donors are placed in each well in 200 μL of AIM-V medium with 10 % normal human serum, 100 IU/mL of IL-2, 50 μM 2-mercaptoethanol, 10 mM HEPES, and 5 μg/mL of PHA-P (*see* **Note 15**).
2. The cells are fed with fresh AIM-V medium supplemented with 10 % human serum, 100 IU/mL of IL-2, 50 μM 2-mercaptoethanol, and 10 mM HEPES every 7 days.
3. Growing wells can be observed on days 14–20. Transfer the cells to a 48- or 24-well plate. $CD8^+$ cell reactivity is assessed by a cytotoxicity assay such as ^{51}Cr release or ELISPOT assays.

4 Notes

1. We usually use the BIMAS website: (http://www-bimas.cit.nih.gov/molbio/hla_bind/) (Fig. 1). A peptide with a score of more than 100 binds strongly to HLA molecules in the described HLA-binding assay.
2. Predicted peptides are often hydrophobic and are very difficult to dissolve in PBS or water. Therefore, DMSO is recommended to dissolve synthetic peptides.
3. Use an appropriate anti-HLA mAb, e.g., anti-HLA-A2 mAb clone BB7.2 is available for detection of HLA-A2.
4. The use of an appropriate positive control peptide (HLA-binding) and negative control peptide (HLA-nonbinding) is necessary. We use HLA-A2-restricted influenza peptide (GILGFVFTL), HLA-A24-restricted HIV peptide (RYLRDQQLLGI), and EBV peptide (TYGPVFMSL) as positive controls for HLA-A2 and -A24, respectively [14–16].
5. T2 cells lack the transporter associated with antigen transport, and thus endogenous peptide loading onto HLA molecules is extensively impeded and the expression level of HLA molecules on the cell surface is very low. Cell culture at a lower temperature (26 °C) facilitates the expression of antigenic peptide unbound to HLA molecules. After incubation with exogenous synthetic peptides, peptide-HLA complex is stabilized

even under a normal temperature condition (37 °C). The genotype of T2 cells is HLA-A*0201/ B*5101/ Cw*0102, and T2 cells can therefore be used for HLA-A*0201/ B*5101/ Cw*0102-binding peptides. Furthermore, since other HLA molecules are expressed on T2 cells, they are also available for detection of those HLA types, e.g., T2-A24 cells for detection of HLA-A24-binding peptides [12, 13, 17].

6. Before acquiring blood samples, it is necessary to obtain informed consent from all patients and volunteer donors according to the guidelines of the Declaration of Helsinki.
7. This is a very delicate procedure and care should be taken not to disturb the surface of separation between the blood sample and Lymphoprep. For centrifugation, minimum acceleration and deceleration are highly recommended to avoid disturbing the surface of separation.
8. Obtain monocyte layer carefully not to disturb the layer. Eliminate contamination of Plasma layer and Lymphoprep layer as possible.
9. Adherent cells can be washed gently 2× or 3× in PBS to eliminate contamination of nonadherent cells.
10. Dendritic cells are floating cells that have many dendrites. Some adherent cells can be observed after 7 days of culture. These adherent cells are macrophages. DO NOT use these adherent cells as APC. Macrophages inhibit CTL induction in the described CTL induction procedure.
11. DC are commonly used to induce CTL; however, we could induce CTL more efficiently by PHA-blasts as APC than by DC in our experiments. Thus, we strongly recommend the use of PHA-blasts rather than DC as APC.
12. Viability of $CD8^+$ cells is critical for generation of CTL. Highly viable $CD8^+$ are small with a round shape (Fig. 4). Activated $CD8^+$ cells form clusters (Fig. 4).
13. We usually stimulate $CD8^+$ cells with multiple peptides-pulsed PHA-blasts. Following stimulation, the reactivities to peptides are screened using the ELISPOT assay.
14. Both peptide-pulsed T2 cells and cancer cells are available as target cells. For peptide-pulsed T2 cells, add 10 μg/mL of peptide onto T2 cells for 1 h and wash with PBS before the assay. For cancer cells, it is recommended to add 100 units/ mL of IFN-γ in the culture for 48–72 h to increase the expression of HLA.
15. For feeder cells, we use a mixture of PBMC from three different donors. A mixture yields higher CTL clone establishment efficiency than that of feeder cells from a single donor. The reason for this is unknown.

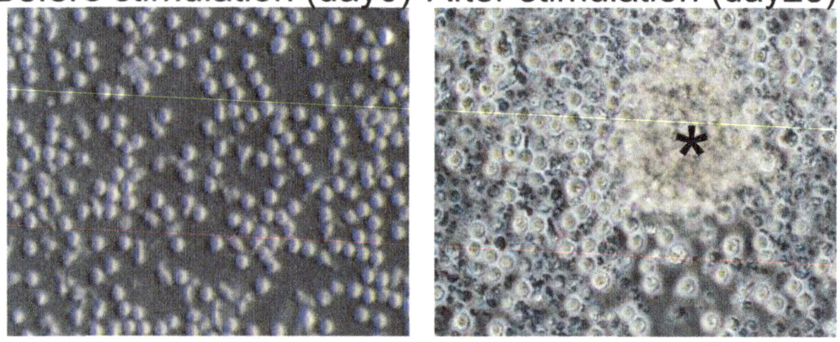

Fig. 4 Morphological change of CTL after stimulation by APC. Before and after stimulation. $CD8^+$ cells make clusters (*asterisk*) in a good culture conditions. Magnification, 400×

Acknowledgements

This study was supported by a Grant-in-Aid for Scientific Research from the Ministry of Education, Culture, Sports, Science and Technology of Japan (to N.S.) program for developing the supporting system for upgrading education and research from the Ministry of Education, Culture, Sports, Science and Technology of Japan (to N.S.) and Takeda Science Foundation (to Y.H.).

References

1. Rosenberg SA et al (2004) Cancer immunotherapy: moving beyond current vaccines. Nat Med 10:909–915
2. Perez SA et al (2010) A new era in anticancer peptide vaccines. Cancer 116:2071–2080
3. Hirohashi Y et al (2009) The functioning antigens: beyond just as the immunological targets. Cancer Sci 100:798–806
4. van der Bruggen P et al (1991) A gene encoding an antigen recognized by cytolytic T lymphocytes on a human melanoma. Science 254:1643–1647
5. Sahin U et al (1995) Human neoplasms elicit multiple specific immune responses in the autologous host. Proc Natl Acad Sci USA 92:11810–11813
6. Rosenberg SA (1999) A new era for cancer immunotherapy based on the genes that encode cancer antigens. Immunity 10:281–287
7. Polyak K, Riggins GJ (2001) Gene discovery using the serial analysis of gene expression technique: implications for cancer research. J Clin Oncol 19:2948–2958
8. Parker KC et al (1994) Scheme for ranking potential HLA-A2 binding peptides based on independent binding of individual peptide side-chains. J Immunol 152:163–175
9. Lin HH et al (2008) Evaluation of MHC class I peptide binding prediction servers: applications for vaccine research. BMC Immunol 9:8
10. Hirohashi Y et al (2002) An HLA-A24-restricted cytotoxic T lymphocyte epitope of a tumor-associated protein, survivin. Clin Cancer Res 8:1731–1739
11. Hariu H et al (2005) Aberrant expression and potency as a cancer immunotherapy target of inhibitor of apoptosis protein family: livin/ML-IAP in lung cancer. Clin Cancer Res 11:1000–1009
12. Inoda S et al (2009) Cep55/c10orf3, a tumor antigen derived from a centrosome residing protein in breast carcinoma. J Immunother 32:474–485
13. Maeda A et al (2001) Identification of human antitumor cytotoxic T lymphocytes epitopes of

recoverin, a cancer-associated retinopathy antigen, possibly related with a better prognosis in a paraneoplastic syndrome. Eur J Immunol 31:563–572

14. Morrison J et al (1992) Identification of the nonamer peptide from influenza A matrix protein and the role of pockets of HLA-A2 in its recognition by cytotoxic T lymphocytes. Eur J Immunol 22:903–907
15. Koup RA et al (1991) Limiting dilution analysis of cytotoxic T lymphocytes to human immunodeficiency virus gag antigens in infected persons: in vitro quantitation of effector cell populations with p17 and p24 specificities. J Exp Med 174:1593–1600
16. Lee SP et al (1997) Conserved CTL epitopes within EBV latent membrane protein 2: a potential target for CTL-based tumor therapy. J Immunol 158:3325–3334
17. Andersen MH et al (1999) An assay for peptide binding to HLA-Cw*0102. Tissue Antigens 54:185–190

Chapter 29

Preparation of Polypeptides Comprising Multiple TAA Peptides

Bing Ni, Zhengcai Jia, and Yuzhang Wu

Abstract

Polypeptides consisting of multiple tumor-associated antigen epitopes (multiepitope peptides) are commonly used as therapeutic peptide cancer vaccines in experimental studies and clinical trials. These methods include polypeptides composed of multiple major histocompatibility complex (MHC) class I-restricted cytotoxic T cell (CTL) epitopes and those containing multiple CTL epitopes and one T helper (Th) epitope. This chapter describes a complete set of methods for preparing multiepitope peptides and branched multiple antigen peptides (MAPs), including sequence design, peptide synthesis, purification, preservation, and the preparation of polypeptide solutions.

Key words Tumor-associated antigen (TAA), Peptide, Synthesis, Identification, Multiple antigenic peptide (MAP), Branched peptide

1 Introduction

Since van der Bruggen and colleagues cloned the first tumor-associated antigen (TAA) gene and identified the first TAA CTL epitope in 1991 [1], techniques including cDNA expression cloning and autoantibody screening have been applied to identify a variety of TAAs and their epitopes recognized by the immune system. Specifically, MAGE, GAGE, NY-ESO-1, and other TAAs, as well as their human leukocyte antigen (HLA) class I-restricted CTL epitopes and HLA class II Th epitopes, have been identified [2–7]. Identification of these TAAs and their epitope peptides provides a large number of antigens and epitopes for studies on therapeutic peptide cancer vaccines.

In 1996, Hu et al. published the first clinical trial on a therapeutic cancer vaccine based on the MAGE-A1 epitope [8]. Subsequently, various forms of therapeutic peptide cancer vaccines have been developed and tested in clinical trials for the treatment of cancer. These include single-epitope peptide vaccines made of one CTL epitope, long-chain polypeptides containing multiple

Michael J.P. Lawman and Patricia D. Lawman (eds.), *Cancer Vaccines: Methods and Protocols*, Methods in Molecular Biology, vol. 1139, DOI 10.1007/978-1-4939-0345-0_29,

sequences for different epitopes, multiepitope polypeptide vaccines containing multiple CTL epitopes or both CTL and Th epitopes, peptide cocktail vaccines containing multiple CTL epitopes, dendritic cell (DC) vaccines made after incubation with epitope peptides, and branched MAPs [9, 10].

The methods described in this chapter are for the preparation of multiepitope polypeptides containing multiple CTL epitopes or both CTL and Th epitopes and branched MAPs based on multiepitope polypeptides.

Distinct from natural long-chain polypeptides containing multiple epitope sequences, multiepitope polypeptides, whether they consist of multiple CTL epitopes or both CTL and Th epitopes, are artificial polypeptides in which different epitope sequences are connected artificially using linker sequences. In multiepitope polypeptides containing multiple CTL epitopes, the CTL epitopes may be derived from one or multiple antigens, which can be presented by the same or different MHC class I molecules. In multiepitope polypeptides containing both CTL and Th epitopes, the epitopes can also be derived from the same or different antigens. The linkers used to connect these epitope sequences are typically nonantigenic polyvalines or polyglycines, composed of three or more valine or glycine residues, respectively [11].

Branched MAPs commonly consist of a nonantigenic lysine core linked to multiple peptide chains of the same sequence. This increases the number of copies of the epitope on the antigen polypeptides, enhancing their ability to induce immune responses. The lysine cores are composed of different numbers of lysine residues. Those containing one lysine can be linked to two polypeptide chains, forming 2-branch MAPs; whereas those containing three lysines can be linked to four polypeptide chains, forming 4-branch MAPs. Similarly, those containing seven lysines can be linked to eight polypeptide chains, forming 8-branch MAPs. Currently, the most common branched MAPs are 8-branch MAPs [10].

2 Materials

2.1 Reagents and Supplies

1. Peptide synthesis reagents.
2. Amino acids: according to the chemical method applied during polypeptide synthesis, the amino groups of amino acids used for peptide synthesis may be protected by Fmoc or Boc groups, and the amino acid side chains are protected by corresponding protecting groups.
3. Resin, including HMP resin (Wang resin).
4. Reagents needed for the preparation of cleavage buffer: appropriate cleavage buffer formulations are selected according to the amino acid sequence of the multiepitope polypeptides and

the side-chain protecting groups chosen for polypeptide synthesis. Ingredients include trifluoroacetic acid (TFA), needed for hydrolyzing peptide-resins prepared using the Fmoc method, and crystalline phenol. Cleavage buffer should always be prepared fresh.

5. Anhydrous ether, preserved at 4 °C.
6. Solvents including dimethyl sulfoxide (DMSO).
7. Phosphate-buffered saline (PBS).
8. Acetic acid.
9. Round-bottom flasks.
10. G4 fritted funnel.
11. G6 fritted funnel.

2.2 Equipment

1. Peptide synthesizer.
2. Vacuum drying apparatus.
3. Electronic balance.
4. Magnetic stirrer.
5. Vacuum pump.
6. Fume hood.
7. High-performance liquid chromatography (HPLC) analyzer.
8. Spectrophotometer.
9. Freeze-drying apparatus.

3 Methods

3.1 Designing the Polypeptide Sequence

1. Based on the test object and experimental purpose, appropriate epitopes are selected from identified TAACTL epitopes, such as Th epitopes, and serve as a component of the multiepitope polypeptide. For example, the epitopes could be the HLA-A1-restricted CTL epitope MAGE-A1$_{161-169}$ (EADPTGHSY), HLA-A2-restricted CTL epitope MAGE-A3$_{271-279}$ (FLWGPRALV), HLA-DRB1*1301-restricted Th epitope MAGE-A1$_{121-134}$ (LLKYRAREPVTKAE), or HLA-DRB1*1101-restricted Th epitope MAGE-A3$_{281-295}$ (TSYVKVLHHMVKISG).
2. Linkers, polyvalines, or polyglycines are inserted between the selected epitope sequences to link the epitopes into a multiepitope polypeptide, e.g., a multi-CTL epitope polypeptide contains multiple HLA-A2-restricted epitopes of MAGE-A2 and HLA-TRAG-3 or a multiepitope polypeptide contains the CTL epitope of MAGE-A1 and Th epitope (Table 1).
3. If MAPs with branches of the same sequence based on the multiepitope polypeptide are desired, then a small lysine core

Table 1
Sequences of multiepitope peptides composed of different epitopes

Peptide sequence	CTL epitope	Linker	CTL epitope	Linker	Th epitope
1	KMVELVHFL	GGG	ILLRDAGLV		
2	EADPTGHSY	AAA	NYKHCFPEI	AAA	LLKYRAREPVTKAE

composed of the appropriate number of lysines (according to the number of branches) is added to the carboxy terminus of the peptide sequence. For example, Table 2 illustrates the sequences of 2-, 4-, and 8-branch MAPs composed of multiepitope peptides containing 2 CTL epitopes.

3.2 Polypeptide Synthesis (See Note 1)

1. A suitable resin is used as the carrier, and a multiepitope polypeptide is synthesized according to its amino acid sequence from the carboxyl to the amino terminus using a peptide synthesizer following the Fmoc or Boc method. This obtains the peptide-resin. At this point, the polypeptide chain is connected to the resin, and the amino acid side chains are still protected by the side-chain protecting groups.
2. During the synthesis of branched MAPs, the first polylysine core is synthesized on the resin. The multiepitope polypeptide is then synthesized according to its amino acid sequence from the carboxyl to the amino terminus (*see* **Note 2**).
3. The synthesized peptide-resin is vacuum dried and then further processed or stored at −20 °C (*see* **Note 3**).

3.3 Preparation of the Crude Polypeptide

After the polypeptide has been synthesized, the peptide chain is connected to the resin, and there are still side-chain protecting groups on the amino acid residues. Therefore, it is necessary to cleave the polypeptide from the resin using cleavage buffer. The following method describes the preparation of crude polypeptide from peptide-resin synthesized using the Fmoc method:

1. According to the amino acid sequence of multiepitope polypeptide and the side-chain protecting groups used, a suitable cleavage buffer such as 95 % TFA is prepared. The cleavage buffer is precooled on ice (*see* **Note 4**).
2. A specific amount of peptide-resin is weighed and placed in a round-bottom flask. A stir bar is added, and the flask is precooled on ice.
3. The precooled cleavage buffer is transferred to the round-bottom flask containing the peptide-resin, and the ice bath is removed. After the cleavage buffer warms to room temperature, it is stirred constantly for 1–2 h.

Table 2
MAPs with different numbers of branches

MAP	Peptide sequence	Lysine core		
	KMVELVHFLGGGILLRDAGLV			
2-branch		K		
	KMVELVHFLGGGILLRDAGLV			
	KMVELVHFLGGGILLRDAGLV			
		K		
	KMVELVHFLGGGILLRDAGLV			
4-branch			K	
	KMVELVHFLGGGILLRDAGLV			
		K		
	KMVELVHFLGGGILLRDAGLV			
	KMVELVHFLGGGILLRDAGLV			
		K		
	KMVELVHFLGGGILLRDAGLV			
			K	
	KMVELVHFLGGGILLRDAGLV			
		K		
	KMVELVHFLGGGILLRDAGLV			
8-branch				K
	KMVELVHFLGGGILLRDAGLV			
		K		
	KMVELVHFLGGGILLRDAGLV			
			K	
	KMVELVHFLGGGILLRDAGLV			
		K		
	KMVELVHFLGGGILLRDAGLV			

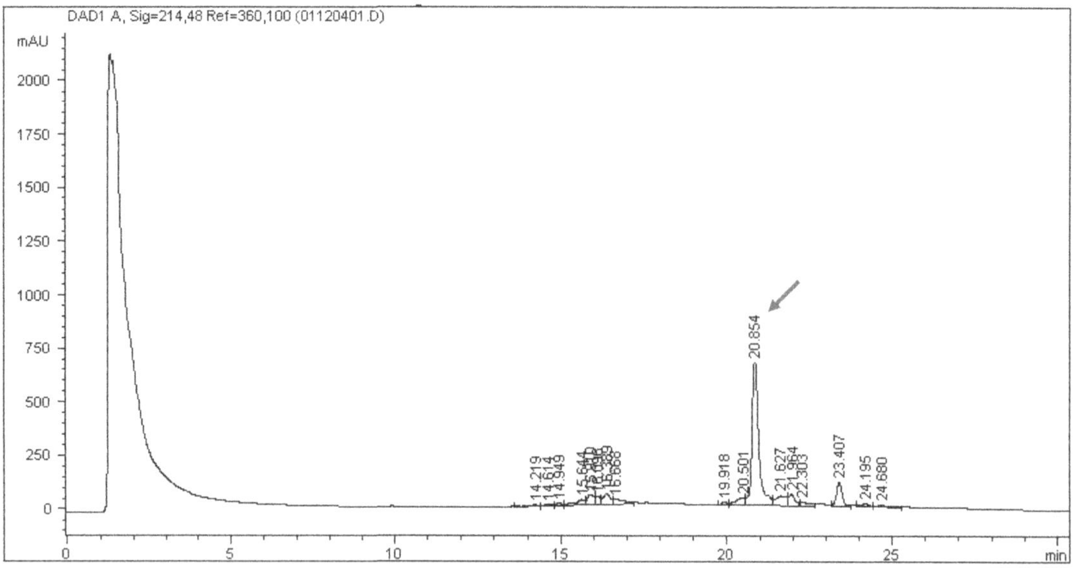

Fig. 1 HPLC purification of polypeptides. Here, the 2-branch peptide KMVELVHFLGGGILLRDAGLV-K-KMVELVHFLGGGILLRDAGLV is used as an example. The crude-synthesized peptide is purified by HPLC, and the main eluting peak (denoted by the *arrow*) is collected

4. A G4 fritted funnel is then used for filtering. The filtrate is collected and concentrated in a vacuum to 1–2 mL.
5. Anhydrous ether, precooled to 4 °C, of at least 25× the volume of the concentrated filtrate is then added to the filtrate under constant stirring to precipitate the polypeptide.
6. A G6 fritted funnel is then used for filtering, and the precipitate is collected.
7. The precipitate is vacuum-dried, and crude peptide is obtained.

3.4 Purification and Identification of the Polypeptide

1. In order to purify the synthesized polypeptide, an appropriate solvent, e.g., DMSO, is used to dissolve the crude polypeptide, e.g., the 2-branch peptide, as shown in Table 2. HPLC is used to purify the crude polypeptide, and the main eluting peak is collected (Fig. 1). The purity of the purified polypeptide is then assessed using HPLC (Fig. 2). In general, the purity can reach 95 % and above.
2. In order to confirm the identification of the synthesized polypeptide, mass spectrometry is used to determine the molecular mass of the synthesized and purified polypeptide as a means of identification. As shown in Fig. 3, mass spectrometry revealed that the molecular weight matched that of the 2-branch polypeptide.

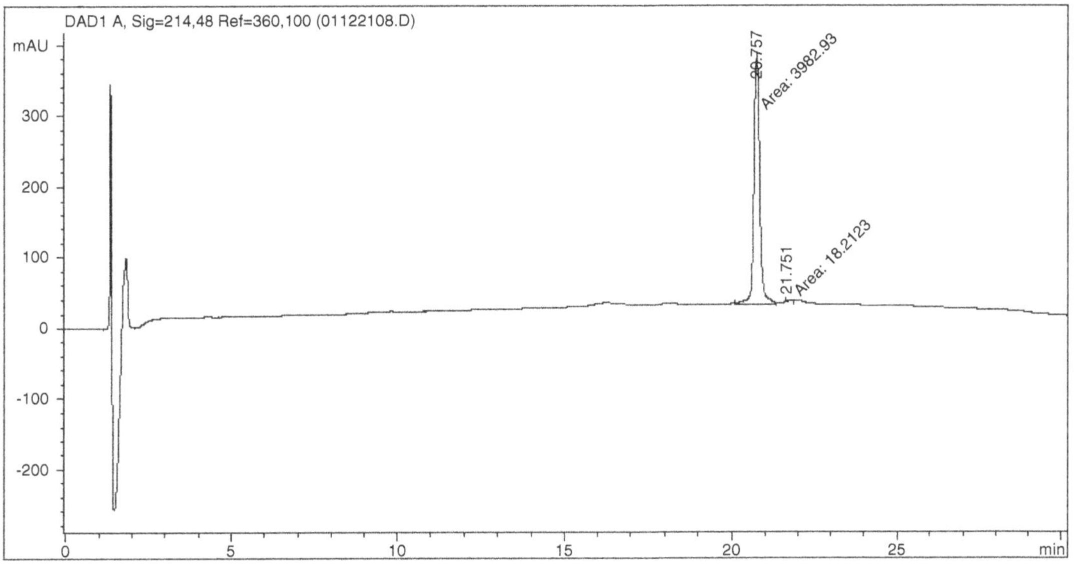

Fig. 2 Purity test for the purified polypeptide. The peptide purified by HPLC in the previous step is measured again using HPLC to determine its purity after purification

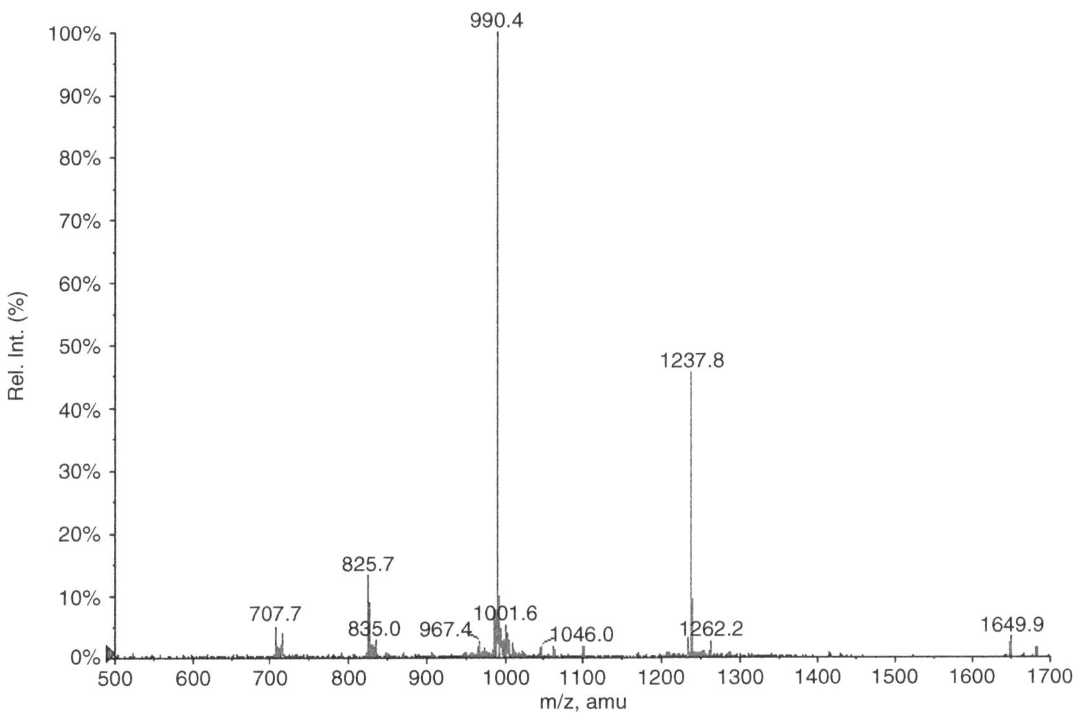

Fig. 3 Molecular mass of the polypeptide determined using mass spectrometry. The 2-branch purified peptide is analyzed by mass spectrometry and cleavage to determine its molecular weight

3.5 Preservation of the Polypeptide

The purified and identified polypeptide is freeze-dried and then stored at −20 °C for future use.

3.6 Preparation of Polypeptide Solution

1. A small amount of polypeptide powder is weighed, and the solubility is tested using PBS, DMSO, and other solvents to determine the solubility of the peptide in different solvents.
2. Polypeptides with good water solubility can be dissolved in PBS or other aqueous solvents. When conducting an experiment, the polypeptide is dissolved directly in PBS or aqueous solvents at the desired concentration (*see* **Note 5**).
3. Polypeptides with poor water solubility are dissolved in DMSO to make high-concentration polypeptide stock solutions of 10 or 20 mg/mL. Based on the needs of the experiment, a small amount of stock solution is used for dilution tests in PBS and other solvents to determine the suitable diluent and dilution factor. The polypeptide stock solution is then stored at −20 °C (*see* **Note 6**). The polypeptide is equilibrated at room temperature, and a specific volume of the stock solution is diluted with the diluent and dilution factor determined in the dilution test.

4 Notes

1. During polypeptide synthesis, the purity of the amino acids can affect the coupling efficiency, which ultimately affects the purity of the target polypeptide within the crude polypeptide. Therefore, peptides with increased purity are therefore preferred.
2. During the synthesis of branched MAPs, the materials used for synthesizing the polylysine core should be lysines where the two amino-protecting groups are Fmoc or Boc groups. To ensure a satisfactory coupling efficiency, the amount of amino acid used should be increased according to the number of branches in the MAPs to be synthesized, based on the amino acid/resin molar ratio of the non-branching peptide. For example, if the amino acid/resin molar ratio of the non-branching peptide is 4:1, then the amino acid/resin molar ratio of 8-branch MAPs is 32:1.
3. The stability of peptide-resin is good, and so it can be stored long term at −20 °C.
4. Before cleaving the polypeptide from the peptide-resin, a cleavage experiment should be performed using a small amount of peptide-resin to determine the appropriate ratio of peptide-resin/cleavage buffer and cleavage reaction time. The peptide-resin/cleavage buffer ratio is considered to be optimal when the cleavage buffer is clear, and there is no polypeptide precipitate after cleavage is complete. If there are polypeptide precipitates, the amount of cleavage buffer used should be

increased. Different cleavage outcomes are also achieved with different reaction times. A reaction time that is too short will result in polypeptides that are not fully cleaved from the resin or where the protecting groups are not fully removed; whereas a cleavage reaction time that is too long may cause the polypeptide chain to break. Both can cause decreases in the concentration of the target polypeptide in the crude polypeptide and reduce the yield of the target polypeptide. Therefore, after the optimal peptide-resin/cleavage buffer ratio has been determined, tests using different reaction times, e.g., 0.5, 1, 1.5, and 2 h, should be performed, using HPLC to measure the purity of the polypeptide to determine the optimal cleavage reaction time.

5. When cleaving a small amount of peptide-resin in a low volume of cleavage buffer, e.g., less than 2 mL, the filtrate does not need to be concentrated after cleavage is complete before precipitation using ether.
6. Freeze-dried polypeptide and polypeptide stock solutions stored in DMSO are both stable and thus can be stored long term at −20 °C. Because the stability of the prepared polypeptide solution is relatively low, polypeptide solutions should be prepared fresh.

Acknowledgment

This work was supported by grants from the Major State Basic Research Development Program of China (973 Program) (2013CB531503) and the Program for Changjiang Scholars and Innovative Research Team in University (PCSIRT 10521).

References

1. van der Bruggen P et al (1991) A gene encoding an antigen recognized by cytolytic T lymphocytes on a human melanoma. Science 254(5038):1643–1647
2. Gaugler B et al (1994) Human gene MAGE-3 codes for an antigen recognized on a melanoma by autologous cytolytic T lymphocytes. J Exp Med 179(3):921–930
3. Kawakami Y et al (1994) Cloning of the gene coding for a shared human melanoma antigen recognized by autologous T cells infiltrating into tumor. Proc Natl Acad Sci U S A 91(9):3515–3519
4. Huang LQ et al (1999) Cytolytic T lymphocytes recognize an antigen encoded by MAGE-A10 on a human melanoma. J Immunol 162(11):6849–6854
5. Parmigiani RB et al (2006) Characterization of a cancer/testis (CT) antigen gene family capable of eliciting humoral response in cancer patients. Proc Natl Acad Sci U S A 103(48):18066–18071
6. Jäger E et al (2000) Identification of NY-ESO-1 epitopes presented by human histocompatibility antigen (HLA)-DRB4*0101-0103 and recognized by CD4$^{(+)}$ T lymphocytes of patients with NY-ESO-1-expressing melanoma. J Exp Med 191(4):625–630
7. Novellino L et al (2005) A listing of human tumor antigens recognized by T cells: March

2004 update. Cancer Immunol Immunother 54(3):187–207
8. Hu X et al (1996) Enhancement of cytolytic T lymphocyte precursor frequency in melanoma patients following immunization with the MAGE-1 peptide loaded antigen presenting cell-based vaccine. Cancer Res 56(11):2479–2483
9. Yamada A et al (2013) Next-generation peptide vaccines for advanced cancer. Cancer Sci 104(1):15–21
10. Zhang J et al (2013) Peptide FLNPDVLDI of heparinase is a novel HLA-A2-restricted CTL epitope and elicits potent immunological antitumor effects in vitro with an 8-branched design. Oncol Rep 29(5):1955–1961
11. Takahashi N et al (2012) First clinical trial of cancer vaccine therapy with artificially synthesized helper/killer-hybrid epitope long peptide of MAGE-A4 cancer antigen. Cancer Sci 103(1):150–153

Chapter 30

Idiotype Vaccine Production Using Hybridoma Technology

Susana Inoges, Ascensión López Díaz de Cerio, Helena Villanueva, Fernando Pastor, and Maurizio Bendandi

Abstract

Non-Hodgkin's lymphoma (NHL) is the most common hematological malignancy both in Europe and in the United States. Follicular lymphoma (FL), a tumor comprised of mature B cells, represents one fourth of all NHL and, despite good response rates to standard treatments, tends to frequently relapse to such an extent that it is still considered incurable. Among several alternative therapeutic options actively being pursued, immunotherapy by idiotypic vaccination is in the forefront of clinical experimental medicine. The idiotype vaccine consists of the tumor-specific immunoglobulin conjugated with keyhole limpet hemocyanin (KLH) and administered together with an adjuvant. Over the last 20 years, researchers have proven that this vaccine can induce specific immune responses. Too, those patients with such responses experience a disease-free survival longer than normally achievable, although these latter results require further confirmation in large clinical trials. Traditionally, idiotype vaccines have been produced through hybridoma technology. In this chapter this technology is described.

Key words Idiotype vaccine, Follicular lymphoma, Hybridoma technology, Sequencing, Tumor immunoglobulin, Conjugation of tumor immunoglobulin to KLH

1 Introduction

An idiotype vaccine is a form of active immunotherapy which has demonstrated clinical benefit when associated with other treatments for patients with follicular lymphoma. This chapter describes the protocol for the production of idiotype vaccines using hybridoma technology. In particular, the aim of this effort is to reproduce, in vitro, an idiotype that closely resembles that which is displayed on the lymphoma cell membrane. Since the idiotype is contained within the tumor-specific immunoglobulin, the ultimate protein obtained from the selected hybridoma will be an immunoglobulin idiotype that also is virtually identical to that expressed on the lymphoma cell. This complex process includes the following steps: (1) the preparation of a single cell suspension from a lymph node biopsy; (2) the freezing of the single cell suspension until use;

Michael J.P. Lawman and Patricia D. Lawman (eds.), *Cancer Vaccines: Methods and Protocols*, Methods in Molecular Biology, vol. 1139, DOI 10.1007/978-1-4939-0345-0_30,

(3) sequencing of tumor immunoglobulin; (4) preparation of cells necessary for the hybridoma production; (5) fusing tumor cells with the K6H6/B5 cell line; (6) maintenance, selection, and expansion of hybridomas; (7) purification of the tumor immunoglobulin; and (8) conjugation of tumor immunoglobulin to KLH.

2 Materials

2.1 Preparation of the Single Cell Suspension from a Lymph Node Biopsy

1. Petri dishes.
2. Forceps.
3. Scalpels.
4. GentleMACS C Tubes (Miltenyi Biotec, Auburn, CA, USA).
5. GentleMACS Dissociator (Miltenyi Biotec).
6. Sterile 2.5-cc syringes.
7. 2-mL Pasteur pipettes.
8. Cell strainer (40-μm) (Becton Dickinson Biosciences, Franklin Lakes, NJ, USA).
9. 50-mL conical tubes.
10. Complete Roswell Park Memorial Institute (RPMI)-1640: "complete" medium is RPMI-1640 containing 10 % FBS, 2 mM glutamine, and 1 % penicillin–streptomycin. To prepare 100 mL of RPMI complete medium, mix 1 mL of 200 mM glutamine solution, 1 mL of penicillin–streptomycin (PenStrep) solution that contains 10,000 U of penicillin and 10,000 μg of streptomycin per mL, 10 mL of fetal bovine serum (FBS), and 88 mL RPMI-1640.
11. Neubauer hemocytometer.
12. Laminar-flow hood.

2.2 Freezing the Single Cell Suspension

1. Sterile 2-mL cryopreservation vials.
2. RPMI-1640 complete medium containing glutamine, PenStrep, and FBS, as described in Subheading 2.1.
3. CryoSure dimethyl sulfoxide (DMSO).
4. Freezing mixture: 40 % RPMI-1640 complete, 40 % FBS, 20 % DMSO.
5. Pipettes (range 100–1,000 μL).
6. Sterile pipette tips (range 100–1,000 μL).
7. 2.5-mL syringes with needles.
8. Cryo 1 °C Freezing Container: "Mr. Frosty."
9. Laminar-flow hood.
10. Freezer (–80 °C).
11. Liquid nitrogen tank (for long-term storage).

2.3 Sequencing the Tumor Immunoglobulin

1. 2-mL sterile tubes.
2. 0.2-mL sterile tubes.
3. Micropipettes.
4. RNA extraction kit (Qiagen, Life Science, Valencia, CA, USA).
5. PCR purification kit.
6. Gel band purification kit.
7. Purification and sequencing kit.
8. DNTPs and 10× buffer.
9. $MgCl_2$.
10. Taq polymerase.
11. Specific primers.
12. Ethidium bromide.
13. Agarose gel: Prepare the agarose gel at a 2 % concentration, mixing 3 mL 50× Tris–borate–EDTA (TBE), 3 g agarose, and up to 150 mL of deionized H_2O.
14. DNase.
15. β-Mercaptoethanol (BME).
16. Big Dye.
17. DMSO.
18. Ethanol 70 %.
19. Hexamers.
20. RNase Inhibitor.
21. Reverse transcriptase (RT) enzyme.
22. Deionized and sterile H_2O.
23. 50× TBE.
24. Loading buffer: 30 % Glycerol, 0.005 % w/v of Orange G.
25. Formamide.
26. Laminar-flow cabinet.
27. Thermocycler.
28. Vortex/mixer.
29. Micropipettes.
30. Electrophoresis system.
31. Transilluminator.
32. Nanodrop.
33. Speed-Vac.
34. Sequencer.
35. Computer, Chromas program.
36. GFX™ PCR DNA kit.

2.4 Preparation of Cells Necessary for Hybridoma Production

1. Mouse heteromyeloma tumor cells K6H6/B5 (ATCC CRL-1823).
2. Cryopreserved human lymphoma cells.
3. Sterile calcium-magnesium-free PBS.
4. 50-mL conical tubes.
5. Neubauer hemocytometer.
6. Trypan blue.
7. 5-mL conical tubes.
8. Complete RPMI-1640 medium.
9. CD10 MicroBead (Miltenyi Biotec).
10. Ficoll-Hypaque.

2.5 Fusion of Tumor Cells with K6H6/B5 Cell Line

1. Water bath at 37 °C.
2. 50-mL conical tubes.
3. Warm sterile calcium-magnesium-free phosphate buffered saline (PBS).
4. 40 % Polyethylene glycol (PEG). If it is necessary, dilute PEG in PBS.
5. BME.
6. Complete RMPI-1640 with BME: Dilute 18.5 μL of BME in 15 mL of complete medium. Then to prepare 500 mL of complete RMPI-1640 with BME, add 500 μL of the diluted BME to the bottle.
7. 96-well plates.
8. 50× Hypoxanthine–aminopterin–thymidine medium (HAT).
9. 50× Hypoxanthine–thymidine medium (HT).

2.6 Maintenance and Selection of the Hybridomas

1. 6-, 24-, and 48-well plates.
2. T-25-cm^2, T-75-cm^2 and T-150cm^2 tissue culture flasks.
3. Complete RPMI-1640.
4. 0.2-μm filtration system.
5. 25 % Sodium azide: 25 % sodium azide (25 g) in 100 mL of deionized and sterile H_2O.
6. Incubators at 37 °C and humidified 5 % CO_2 in air.
7. Inverted microscope.
8. Laminar-flow hood.
9. Vacuum pump.

2.7 Concentration of Culture Supernatant

1. Filtration module (100,000 MWCO PES) Vivascience Vivaflow 200 (Sartorius Stedim Biotech GmbH, Goettingen, Germany).
2. 5-mL sterile pipettes.

3. Deionized and sterile H_2O.
4. Ethanol 10 %.
5. NaOH.
6. Sodium hypochlorite.
7. PBS without calcium or magnesium.
8. pH indicator strips.
9. MasterFLex® L/STM (peristaltic pump-head).
10. Laminar-flow hood.

2.8 Purification of the Immunoglobulin

1. Glass columns.
2. HiTrap protein G columns.
3. Anti-human IgM–agarose.
4. Anti-human IgA–agarose.
5. PBS without calcium or magnesium.
6. Solution A (binding solution): 20 mM PBS, pH 7.0.
7. Solution B (elution solution): 0.1 M glycine, pH 2.5.
8. 1.5 M Tris–HCl, pH 8.8.
9. 0.05 % sodium azide: Dilute 0.05 g of sodium azide in 100 mL of deionized and sterile H_2O.
10. 20 % ethanol.
11. 70 % ethanol.
12. 5-mL polypropylene tubes.
13. 0.45-μm filters.
14. Vivaspin concentrators 100,000 molecular weight cut off (MWCO) PES (Sartorius Stedim Biotech GmbH, Goettingen, Germany).
15. Pipette (range 10–100 μL).
16. Pipettes range (100–1,000 μL).
17. pH indicator strips.
18. Dialysis cassette 10,000 MWCO.
19. Biologic-LP Chromatography System.
20. Spectrophotometer.

2.9 Conjugation

1. 50-mL conical tubes.
2. Specific tumor idiotype at 1 mg/mL.
3. KLH clinical grade at 1 mg/mL.
4. 25 % glutaraldehyde.
5. 2 M glycine.
6. Sterile calcium-magnesium-free PBS.

7. 0.9 % saline.
8. Dialysis cassette 10,000.
9. 1 L glass beaker.
10. Magnet.
11. Agitator.

3 Methods

3.1 Preparation of the Single Cell Suspension from a Lymph Node Biopsy

1. Place the sample into a Petri dish with enough complete medium to prevent the tissue from dehydrating.
2. Using a scalpel, trim away any fatty, necrotic, vascular, or connective tissue not directly part of the tumor.
3. Transfer the sample to a clean Petri dish with 5–10 mL of complete medium.
4. Cut the lymph node into 2–4 mm pieces.
5. Transfer several pieces of tissue to the GentleMACS "C" tube and add 5–10 mL of complete medium. Secure the lid and, after the lid is tight, twist the lid one more time to click it into place.
6. Place the tube in the slot on the GentleMACS dissociator and run the appropriate program (h_tumor_03.01 program).
7. After the first cycle, open the lid carefully, collect the cells suspension, and transfer it through a 40-μm nylon filter into a 50-mL conical tube.
8. Repeat the **steps 5–7** until all the tissue is well dissociated into a single cell suspension. Use more than one GentleMACS "C" tube and more than 1 50-mL conical tube if necessary.
9. Centrifuge all 50-mL conical tubes at 750 × *g* for 8 min.
10. Following centrifugation, discard the supernatant and resuspend the pellet in complete medium.
11. Collect all cells in a 50-mL conical tube and fill with complete medium up to 50 mL: Remove a 100 μL aliquot to perform a cell count and viability determination. Remove an aliquot of 5×10^7 cells for phenotypic studies especially if it is necessary to characterize the tumor immunoglobulin. Remove an aliquot of 5×10^7 cells to sequence the tumor immunoglobulin.
12. Adjust to 1.5×10^8 cells/mL for freezing as described in the following section. The final concentration of freezing will be 7.5×10^7cells/mL.
13. Freeze in liquid nitrogen until needed; *see* Subheading 3.2 (*see* **Note 1**).

3.2 Freezing the Cell Suspension

1. Prepare the cryotubes and properly mark them with the identification of the sample. Then, put them in the Freezing Container at 4 °C until needed.
2. Retrieve the cryopreservation vials from their container that had been kept at 4 °C and place them in the laminar-flow hood. Add 500 μL of the prepared single cell suspension to each of the vials.
3. Under continuous agitation using a 2.5-mL syringe, add slowly (drop by drop) 500 μL of the freezing solution to each of the vials, ensuring that each drop slides down the side of the vials without falling directly onto the cells.
4. Close the tubes straight away and place the Freezing Container containing the vials into the −80 °C freezer immediately.
5. Twenty-four hours later, frozen vials should be transferred into liquid nitrogen where they should remain until needed.

3.3 Sequencing of Tumor Immunoglobulin

The aim of this protocol is to obtain the complementarity-determining region (CDR) sequences of the tumor immunoglobulin. It is expected to obtain clean electropherograms corresponding to the sequences of the samples studied [1–3].

3.3.1 RNA Extraction

Once the sample is received, RNA extraction is initiated and requires approximately $1–2 \times 10^7$ cells. The extraction takes place following the Qiagen RNA extraction kit protocol:

1. Centrifuge the sample for 10 min at 8,000 × *g*.
2. Remove the supernatant and break the cells through the addition of 500 μL of RLT buffer, to which BME had been previously added.
3. Homogenize the mixture by thorough pipetting and vortexing.
4. Add 500 μL of 70 % ethanol and mix by pipetting.
5. Pass the sample to a column, close, and centrifuge for 15 s at 8,000 × *g*, removing the obtained liquid.
6. Add 350 μL of RW1 buffer to the column and centrifuge for 15 s at 8,000 × *g*. Remove the obtained liquid.
7. Add 10 μL of DNase to 70 μL of RDD buffer. Mix by inverting the tube.
8. Place in the column and incubate at room temperature for 15 min.
9. Add 350 μL of RW1 buffer and centrifuge for 15 s at 8,000 × *g*.
10. Add 500 μL of RPE buffer and centrifuge for 2 min at 8,000 × *g*.
11. Elute in 30 μL of RNase-free water and centrifuge for 1 min at 8,000 × *g*. (Make 2 elutions.)
12. Quantify RNA using Nanodrop.

3.3.2 cDNA Aquisition (RT-PCR)

1. Once the RNA is extracted, it is converted into DNA. To a 1-mL Eppendorf vial, the following reagents are added:
   (a) 10 μL of 10× buffer.
   (b) 22 μL of $MgCl_2$ Solution.
   (c) 20 μL of DNTPs.
   (d) 5 μL of Hexamers.
   (e) 2 μL of RNase Inhibitor.
   (f) 2 μL of RT enzyme.
   (g) 2 μg of RNA.
   (h) H_2O until total volume = 100 μL.
2. Next, the samples are placed into the thermocycler with the following program:
   (a) 25 °C for 10 min.
   (b) 48 °C for 30 min.
   (c) 95 °C for 5 min.
   (d) 4 °C ∞.

3.3.3 Polymerase Chain Reaction (PCR)

Once the cDNA is obtained, PCR will be performed using the specific primers for each isotype of immunoglobulin (A, M, G):

1. In each 0.2-mL tube, place the following mixture:
   (a) 4 μL of DNTPs.
   (b) 5 μL of 10× PCR buffer.
   (c) 4 μL of MgCl2 solution.
   (d) 0.5 μL of Taq polymerase.
   (e) 19.5 μL of H2O.
   (f) 4 μL of forward primer.
   (g) 4 μL of reverse primer.
   (h) 10 μL of cDNA.
2. Tubes containing the mixture above are placed into the thermocycler with the following program:

(a) 95 °C for 10 min.	
(b) 95 °C for 30 s.	35 cycles
(c) 53 °C for 30 s.	
(d) 72 °C for 1 min.	
(e) 72 °C for 7 min.	
(f) 4 °C ∞.	

3.3.4 Electrophoresis

When the thermocycler program is completed, the resultant PCR products are then loaded into an agarose gel for DNA electrophoresis.

1. Place the 2 % agar in the microwave until it is melted and transparent.
2. Add 10 μL of ethidium bromide into the molten agar and place the mixture in the gel plate with the combs that create the slots for the samples. Let the agar solidify.
3. Once the gel has solidified, the combs are removed. Place the gel in the electrophoresis chamber.
4. Add the electrophoresis buffer (1× TBE), and then load into the slots 5 μL of sample plus 5 μL of loading buffer.
5. Finally, the electrophoresis chamber is connected to the current supply and a 140 V current is applied for approximately 40 min. Once the electrophoresis time is completed, the gel is removed and visualized under *uv* light using a transilluminator.

3.3.5 Purification of PCR Products

When the gel is visualized, the bands corresponding to amplified products using the specific primers can be observed. Those products that are to be purified can be sequenced. The purification is performed following the GFX™ PCR DNA kit protocol and gel band purification kit protocol:

1. Add 500 μL of capture buffer to each column.
2. Take the entire sample that is to be purified and pour it onto the column, pipetting for a good mixture.
3. Centrifuge at 8,000 × *g* for 1 min.
4. Remove the liquid and add 500 μL of washing buffer.
5. Centrifuge at 8,000 × *g* for 1 min.
6. Place the column in a clean 2-mL tube and elute the sample in 30 μL of H_2O.

3.3.6 Sequencing Reaction

1. Prepare two tubes for each PCR product to be sequenced. In one of the tubes, add 0.3 μM final concentration of forward primer; in the other tube, add 0.3 μM final concentration of reverse primer.
2. Add to both tubes:
   (a) 1 μL of DMSO.
   (b) 9 μL of H2O.
   (c) 4 μL of Big Dye.
   (d) 4 μL of PCR purified product.
3. Place the tubes into the thermocycler with the following program:

(a) 96 °C for 10 min.	25 cycles
(b) 50 °C for 5 s.	
(c) 60 °C for 4 min.	
(d) 4 °C ∞.	

3.3.7 Purification of the Sequencing Reaction

The purification of the sequencing reaction is started following the CentriSep purification kit protocol:

1. Remove as many columns as samples to be purified and add 800 μL of H_2O.
2. Shake the column so that the resin is well hydrated.
3. Let the column rest at room temperature for at least 30 min.
4. Reduce the volume of the column by opening and closing the lid 10×.
5. Centrifuge columns at 750×*g* for 1 min.
6. Place the columns in clean 2-mL tubes and add the resulting product from the sequencing reaction to the columns.
7. Centrifuge columns at 750×*g* for 1 min.
8. Discard the columns and place the 2-mL tubes in the Speed-Vac at 37 °C for approximately 40 min.
9. Resuspend samples in 10 μL of formamide.
10. Once samples are purified and reconstituted in formamide, the samples are loaded into the DNA sequencer.

3.3.8 Sequence Analysis

After loading samples into the DNA sequencer, the electropherograms corresponding to the sequences of the samples under study are obtained. These electropherograms can be analyzed using the Chromas program and the ORF Finder from the website: http://www.ncbi.nlm.nih.gov.

3.4 Preparation of Cells Necessary for the Hybridoma Production

To obtain hybridomas that produce the tumor immunoglobulin, two cell types are fused: the patient lymphoma cells and mouse heteromyeloma tumor cells (K6H6/B5) [4, 5]. The first step is to prepare both cell types.

3.4.1 Preparation of K6H6/B5

The K6H6/B5 cells are used when they are growing in log phase (*see* **Note 2**).

1. Harvest K6H6/B5 from flasks in 50-mL conical tubes.
2. Spin down at 750×*g* for 5 min.
3. Decant the supernatant and resuspend the pellet gently.

4. Add 20 mL of PBS and count the cells in a Neubauer hemocytometer. Add 90 μL of Trypan blue in a 5-mL conical tube. Add 10 μL of cell suspension to the same conical tube. Mix and put 10 μL in the Neubauer hemocytometer.
5. Count the cells and determine viability. If the viability of the cells is less than 60 %, a density gradient centrifugation (Ficoll-Hypaque) is performed to remove dead cells and increase the concentration of viable cells as described below.
   (a) Prepare 50-mL conical tubes with 15 mL of Ficoll-Hypaque, carefully underlay the cells.
   (b) Spin at 1,125 × g for 22 min. Allow the centrifuge to stop without operating the brake mode.
   (c) Collect cells at interface and dilute in PBS up to 50 mL.
   (d) Spin at 750 × g for 8 min.
   (e) Decant the supernatant and resuspend the pellet gently.
   (f) Add 20 mL of PBS and take an aliquot to count in a Neubauer hemocytometer as previously described.

3.4.2 Preparation of Lymphoma Tumor Cells

A patient tumor cell suspension obtained from a lymph node must be thawed immediately before the fusion (*see* **Note 3**) and processed as stated below:

1. Prepare 50-mL conical tubes with 49 mL of complete RPMI-1640 (as many as the number of vials that are being thawed).
2. Remove cryotube from liquid N_2 and immerse in a water bath at 37 °C until the ice comes off the walls.
3. Decant the vial contents in 50-mL conical tube with complete medium (from **step 1**).
4. Centrifuge at 750 × *g* for 8 min.
5. Decant the supernatant and resuspend the pellet gently.
6. Add 50 mL of complete RPMI-1640.
7. Centrifuge at 750 × *g* for 8 min.
8. Decant the supernatant and resuspend the pellet gently.
9. Add 20 mL of PBS and count in a Neubauer hemocytometer as described above.
10. Count the cells and determine viability (*see* **Note 4**).

3.5 Fusion of Tumor Cells with K6H6/B5 Cell Line

Cell fusion is accomplished using PEG. This entire procedure should be performed in a 37 °C water bath with continuous agitation of the tubes.

1. Mix tumor cells and K6H6/B5 cells at a ratio of 4:1 (tumor cells to K6H6/B5 cells) in 50-mL conical tubes.
2. Bring up the volume to 50 mL with PBS.

3. Centrifuge the cells at 525 × *g* for 5 min at 37 °C.
4. Decant the supernatant and resuspend the pellet gently.
5. Place the tube in a water bath at 37 °C and add 1 mL of 40 % PEG over a 1-min period with gentle stirring (*see* **Note 5**).
6. Maintain the tube in the water bath for 1 min under continuous stirring.
7. Add 4 mL warm PBS over a 4-min period while stirring continuously.
8. Add 14 mL warm PBS over 2 min while stirring continuously.
9. Adjust the volume to 50 mL using warm PBS.
10. Centrifuge the cells at 230 × *g* for 5 min at 37 °C.
11. Decant the supernatant and resuspend the cells gently in complete RMPI-1640 with BME at a cell concentration of 0.5×10^6 cell/mL.
12. Plate at 50,000 cells/well (100 μL/well) in a 96-well plate.
13. As a control, use eight wells containing K6H6/B5 only.
14. The next day, add 100 μL of 2× HAT (HAT 50× diluted in complete medium with BME) to each well.
15. One week later, replace 100 μL of supernatant from each well with 100 μL/well of 1× HAT (HAT 50× diluted in complete medium).
16. One week later, replace 100 μL of supernatant from each well with 100 μL/well of 1× HT (HT 50× diluted in complete medium).

3.6 Maintenance and Selection of the Hybridomas

The aim of this portion of the protocol is to obtain as many hybridomas as possible that both proliferate in culture and secrete a clonal immunoglobulin (*see* **Note 6**).

3.6.1 Assessment of Hybridoma Viability and Growth Characteristics

1. If the degree of confluence in the 96-well plates is greater than 75 %, the cells are resuspended and transferred into a 48-well plate. Then, 200 μL/well of fresh complete medium is added to 96-well plates and 1 mL/well of fresh complete medium to the 48-well plates.
2. If the degree of confluence in the 96-well plates is less than 75 %, 100 μL of supernatant are removed and 100 μL of complete medium is added.

3.6.2 Reassessment of Hybridoma Growth Characteristics

1. If the hybridoma has grown to a confluence level of 75 % in the 48-well plates, the cells are passed to a 6-well plate.
   a) The contents of the 48-well plate are stirred and the cells are passed onto a 6-well plate.
   b) 500 μL/well of complete medium are added in 48-well plate.

c) 3 mL/well of complete medium are added to 6-well plate and 1 mL/well of medium is added to the 48-well plate.

2. If the degree of confluence is less than 75 % in the 48-well plates and cell viability is not good, leave the hybridoma in 48-well plates. The medium is removed and replaced by 1.5 mL/well of fresh medium.
3. Growth also needs to be assessed in the 96-well plates and dealt with as described in the previous section.
4. One week later, if the hybridoma has grown in a 6-well plate to a confluency of 75 %, it will be transferred into a 25-cm^2 culture flask.
   a) The contents of the wells of the 6-well plate are stirred and passed to the 25-cm^2 culture flask.
   b) 4 mL/well of complete medium is added in the 6-well plate and 12 mL of medium is added to the 25-cm^2 culture flask.
5. If the degree of confluence is less than 75 % and/or the cell viability is poor, the hybridomas should remain in the 6-well plate. The medium is removed and replaced with 4 mL/well of fresh medium.
6. Growth in 96- and 48-well plates will be evaluated and the same procedure described in the previous section will be carried out but eliminating the 96-well plates after harvesting the cells.

3.6.3 Evaluation of Hybridoma Growth in 25-cm^2 Flasks (see Notes 7 and 8)

1. If the degree of confluence is greater than 75 %, the cells are taken off smoothly and half of the flask content is transferred to another 25-cm^2 flask. Fresh medium is added to the two flasks to give a total volume of 15 mL each.
2. If the degree of confluence in the 25-cm^2 flasks is less than 75 %, the supernatant is removed and 15 mL of fresh medium are added to the flask.
3. The handling of all 48- and 6-well plates will be carried out as described above, but eliminating the plates after harvesting the cells.

3.6.4 Harvesting the Hybridomas

1. Gently remove the cells from two 25-cm^2 flasks and transfer 8 mL of cells from each flask to a 50-mL conical tube.
2. Add 8 mL of fresh medium to each of the flasks.
3. Bring up the volume in the conical tube to 50 mL with complete medium and centrifuge at $750 \times g$ for 7 min.
4. Decant the supernatant and resuspend the pellet in 1 mL of PBS.
5. Count and adjust the cells to 5×10^6 cells/mL prior to their use in sequencing the CDR3 region. As soon as there are three hybridomas with the CD3 region sequence identical to the tumor's, the rest of the hybridomas that remain positive in the ELISA are frozen.

3.6.5 Weekly Evaluation of Hybridoma Growth

1. If the degree of confluence is greater than 75 %, double the volume of medium and transfer the cells to 75-cm^2 culture flasks.
2. If the degree of confluence is less than 75 %, the supernatant is removed and fresh medium is added (15 mL while the hybridomas are in 25-cm^2 flasks and 75 mL when the hybridomas are in 75 cm^2 flasks).
3. Every 2 weeks, the ELISA is repeated to confirm that the hybridomas still produce the immunoglobulin.

   Depending on the growth, the cell cultures are expanded and then transferred to other 75-cm^2 or to 150-cm^2 culture flasks. When there are four 150-cm^2 culture flasks, the culture supernatant is finally collected to purify the tumor immunoglobulin. Importantly, from the moment the hybridomas are identified as "Identical sequence" ("IS"), if the tumor immunoglobulin belongs to the IgG class, the culture is continued with RPMI-1640 + FBS without IgG in order to avoid possible contamination with bovine IgG from the FBS.
4. If the degree of confluence is greater than 75 %, harvest the cells and double the volume of medium.
   a) Remove the cells by gently shaking the flask.
   b) Double the volume with fresh medium and move to a new 75-cm^2 culture flask.
   c) When there are 2× 75-cm^2 flasks, proceed in the same way, but transferring the contents of the flasks to a 150-cm^2 flask.
   d) When the cells are growing in T150-cm^2 flasks, gently harvest the cells by shaking the flask, double the volume with fresh complete medium and move to new 150-cm^2 culture flasks, and repeat the procedure each week.
5. If the degree of confluence is less than 75 %, the supernatant is collected and fresh medium is added (75 mL to the 75-cm^2 flasks or 150 mL to the 150-cm^2 culture flasks):
   a) Collect the supernatant in 50-mL conical tubes.
   b) Centrifuge at 1,125 × g for 8 min.
   c) Filter the supernatant through a 0.2-μm filter and store at −20 °C in properly labeled flasks until needed.
6. When there are 4× T150-cm^2 flasks, collect the supernatant produced by the cells as follows:
   a) Place the contents of the 150-cm^2 flask into 50-mL conical tubes.
   b) Centrifuge at 1,125 × g for 10 min.

c) Collect the supernatant and filter it through a 0.2-μm filter.
d) Add 200 μL sodium azide per 100 mL of supernatant collected.
e) Store the supernatant in properly labeled flasks at 4 °C until needed.
f) Add new medium to the 150-cm2 culture flasks.
g) Repeat the last step weekly.

7. Cultures are maintained until there is enough purified immunoglobulin. While the cultures are being maintained, ELISA assays are repeated every other week in order to confirm that the hybridomas keep producing the immunoglobulin:
   a) If the ELISA is positive, proceed as described in the previous sections.
   b) If the ELISA is negative, the test should be repeated 1 week later and, if confirmed, the culture will be terminated.

3.7 Concentration of Culture Supernatant

The aim of this method is to concentrate the culture supernatants to obtain an adequate volume to pass through the chromatography columns to purify the immunoglobulin (*see* **Note 9**).

1. Flush the system with 1 L of deionized water with the filtrate going to waste.
2. Prepare cleaning solutions suitable for the membrane (500 mL of 0.5 mM NaOCl in 0.5 M NaOH) and pass through the circuit with the filtrate going to waste.
3. Drain the system with air and pass 1 L of deionized water through the system over 5–10 min.
4. Pass 500 mL of PBS through the system with the filtrate going to waste. The system is now ready for use.
5. Pass the sample (a maximum of 2.5 L) through the concentrator, recirculating as many times as necessary to obtain a final volume of 50 mL:
   (a) Fill the feed reservoir with sample solution.
   (b) Pump liquid through the system. The recirculation rate should be 200–400 mL/min and suitable flow should exit the filtrate line.
   (c) Concentrate the sample.
   (d) When nearing the desired volume, reduce the recirculation rate to 20–40 mL/min and recirculate the concentrated sample for 1–2 min to increase sample recovery.
6. Store the concentrated sample at 4 °C until needed.
7. Clean the concentrator as described in points 1, 2 and 3 and store at 4 °C.

3.8 Purification of the Immunoglobulin

The goal is to purify the tumor immunoglobulin from the supernatant of the hybridoma cultures selected for vaccine production [6–12] (*see* **Note 10**).

3.8.1 Thawing of Samples

1. Remove the samples from the freezer and place them at 4 °C, where the samples are thawed.
2. Immediately before immunoglobulin purification, pass the sample through a 0.45-μm filter.

3.8.2 Purification of IgG Immunoglobulin

1. Use a commercial HiTrap protein G column (*see* **Note 11**).
2. Once the chromatograph is properly prepared and programmed as described above, place the column in the chromatograph and proceed to the purification of immunoglobulin.
3. When the sample eluted into the tube containing 1.5-M Tris–HCl buffer, check that the pH is 7.
4. If the pH is below 7.0, add 200 mL of Tris–HCl, mix well, and measure the pH again.
5. Repeat the previous step until the pH is 7.0.

3.8.3 Purification of IgM

1. Use a glass column in which anti-human IgM–agarose has been added.
2. Shut the lockable bottom of the column and add 5 mL of PBS.
3. Open the lockable bottom, drain, and return to close position.
4. Add 4 mL of the anti-human IgM–agarose to the glass column and hold at room temperature for 30 min to sediment the gel.
5. Add PBS to complete the volume of the column.
6. Place the column into the chromatograph system and proceed in the same manner as described in paragraph above.

3.8.4 Purification of IgA Immunoglobulin

1. Use a glass column containing an anti-human IgA-linked-agarose.
2. Shut the lockable bottom of the column and add 5 mL of PBS.
3. Open the lockable bottom, drain, and return to the closed position.
4. Add 4 mL of the anti-human IgA-linked-agarose to the glass column and hold at room temperature for 30 min to sediment the gel.
5. Add PBS to complete the volume of the column.
6. Place the column into the chromatograph system and proceed in the same manner as described above.

3.8.5 Storage of the Columns

Following the purification procedures above, the columns should be stored at 4 °C as follows:

1. Storage of a protein G column:
   (a) Remove the column from the system.
   (b) With a 5-mL syringe, slowly add 5 mL of 20 % ethanol.
   (c) Place the cap on the bottom of the column, fill the column with 20 % ethanol, and replace the top plug.
   (d) Store at 4 °C until needed.
2. Storage of either an anti-IgM or anti-IgA column:
   (a) Remove the column from the system.
   (b) With a 5-mL syringe, slowly add 5 mL of 0.05 % sodium azide.
   (c) Place the bottom cap on the column, fill the column with 0.05 % azide, and replace the top plug on the column.
   (d) Store at 4 °C until needed.

3.8.6 Processing the Sample After Purification

This step is common to all purified samples:

1. Collect the sample eluted and neutralized with 1.5 M Tris–HCl buffer, pH 8.8.
2. Transfer the sample to a Vivaspin with a 100,000 MWCO and centrifuge at 1,125 × g for 15 min.
3. Repeat the previous step until the sample is concentrated to a final volume of 5 mL.
4. Quantify the purified protein concentration using the Nanodrop.
5. Adjust the concentration to 1 mg/mL protein:
   (a) If the concentration is lower, repeat the centrifugation as in the previous paragraph.
   (b) If the concentration is higher, add PBS accordingly.

3.9 Conjugation of the Idiotype and KLH

The last step to produce the complete idiotype vaccine consists of conjugating the specific tumor idiotype with KLH [13].

1. Mix the same amount of immunoglobulin and KLH (depending on the number of vaccine doses needed) and place in a dialysis cassette (*see* **Note 12**).
2. Dialyze for 24 h against PBS. Change the PBS twice during that period.
3. Remove the contents from the dialysis cassette.
4. Add 4 μL of 25 % glutaraldehyde per mL of reaction and maintain gentle stirring for 2 h (*see* **Note 13**).

5. Add 10 μL of 2 M glycine/mL and maintain gentle stirring for 30 min.
6. Place the material into a dialysis cassette.
7. Dialyze for 48 h against saline. Change the saline 4×.
8. Extract the content of the dialysis cassette and aliquot into vials for storage.
9. Take a sample to run on an acrylamide gel and check that all the idiotype is conjugated to KLH.
10. Store the vials at −80 °C until needed.

4 Notes

1. If the sample cannot be processed immediately after receiving it, it is possible to keep the biopsy completely covered in RPMI supplemented with antibiotics for 24 h at 4 °C without significant loss of cell viability.
2. The K6H6/B5 cells are obtained when they are in log phase of growth, so these cells must be duplicated the day before.
3. Tumor cells proceed from a cell suspension obtained from a lymph node. This cell suspension must be thawed immediately before the fusion. Once thawed, both cell number and viability will be assessed. Also, if the infiltration of tumor cells in the cell suspension is less than 30 %, it is necessary a selection of tumor cells by magnetic separation in order to increase the chance of selecting hybridomas that produce the tumor immunoglobulin. When the viability of the cells is less than 60 %, after thawing or after selecting, a density gradient centrifugation (Ficoll-Hypaque) is performed to remove dead cells and thereby increase cellular viability.
4. If the number of tumor cells in the cell suspension is less than 30 %, it is necessary to perform a selection of tumor cells by magnetic separation in order to increase the likelihood of selecting hybridomas producing the tumor immunoglobulin. In this process, $CD10^+$ cells are selected using CD10 microbeads.
5. It is important to note that PEG is very dense, and therefore the most appropriate method to remove it from the vial is to use a 1-mL syringe without needle.
6. The hybridomas obtained after fusion are tested by enzyme-linked immunosorbent assay (ELISA) to select those clones that produce the same immunoglobulin isotype as that of the tumor immunoglobulin. Such selected hybridomas are expanded from the 96-well to a 48-well culture plate. The growth of hybridomas is assessed weekly, and complete

medium is added or the hybridomas will be transferred to a 24-well plate or to a 25-, 75-, or 150-cm^2 culture flask depending on the proliferation of each. Every 15 days, an ELISA is repeated to confirm that the selected hybridomas continue producing the immunoglobulin. When some hybridomas are in 2× 25-cm^2 culture flasks, a small aliquot is used to sequence the CDR3 region of the immunoglobulin produced by the hybridomas, the aim being to select those hybridoma clones whose CDR3 region is identical to the CDR3 region of the tumor immunoglobulin. Once the sequence data confirms that these clones are correct, then those hybridomas will be expanded to produce the tumor immunoglobulin.

7. Once we have the hybridomas in 25-cm^2 culture flasks, the ELISA is repeated to confirm that the growing hybridomas keep producing the same immunoglobulin isotype expressed by the tumors. ELISA is done on samples from 25-cm^2 flasks as well as from all plates. If it is confirmed that the hybridomas in flasks and in the plates are positive for immunoglobulin production, the expansion of the hybridomas will be continued. If the ELISA is negative, the test will be repeated 1 week later, and if it is confirmed that the hybridomas have stopped to produce the immunoglobulin, these cultures will be terminated.
8. The growth of hybridomas is assessed weekly. When there are 2 25-cm^2 flasks, an aliquot of these cells will be used to sequence the immunoglobulin CDR3 region in order to confirm that it is identical to the tumor's CDR3 region. This is completed with various hybridomas (selecting the best both in terms of growth and immunoglobulin secretion), when there are three hybridomas with identical immunoglobulin sequence to the tumor's. These hybridomas will be called "identical sequence" (IS) hybridomas and will be used for vaccine production.
9. The volume should not exceed 50 mL. In order to concentrate the culture supernatant, a maximum volume of 2.5 L of supernatant is passed, making it recirculate through the system as many times as necessary to obtain a maximum volume of 50 mL.
10. The day prior to the immunoglobulin purification, culture supernatants containing the tumor immunoglobulin are thawed. On the day of purification, the chromatograph system is prepared and the sample is purified.

    Preparation of chromatograph system: Before passing the sample, the chromatograph system should be prepared properly. Briefly, all circuits should be washed with sterile, deionized water, then with 70 % ethanol, and finally with sterile deionized water once again. After that, PBS should be passed around the circuit, to make it ready for the passage of the sample. Then, the program for the purification of the sample is completed using the following steps:

(a) Pass 25 mL of Solution A at a flow rate of 1 mL/min.

(b) Pass the sample (the volume will be different depending on how many samples we have, but should not be more than 50 mL) at a flow rate of 0.5 mL/min.

(c) Wash with 25 mL of Solution A at a flow rate of 1 mL/min.

(d) Elute with 20 mL of Solution B at a flow rate of 1 mL/min.

(e) Wash with 25 mL of Solution A at a flow rate of 1 mL/min.

(f) Collect the elution fraction into a tube containing the neutralization buffer (1 mL of 1.5 M Tris–HCl, pH 8.8).
To prevent the column from becoming saturated and therefore not retaining the immunoglobulin adequately, repeat the cycle as many times as necessary to pass the entire sample. The types of column differ depending on the type of immunoglobulin being purified.

11. The column to be used is different if the immunoglobulin being purified is of the IgG or IgA or IgM class: If the immunoglobulin is IgG, a HiTrap protein G column is used. If the immunoglobulin is IgM, a glass column with agarose containing anti-human IgM is used. If the immunoglobulin is IgA, a glass column with agarose containing anti-human IgA is used.

12. A vaccine contains 0.5 mg of idiotype and 0.5 mg of KLH.

13. The glutaraldehyde must be added slowly in order to prevent the protein from precipitating.

References

1. Kobrin CB, Kwak LW (1997) Development of vaccine strategies for the treatment of B-cell malignancies. Cancer Invest 15:577–587
2. Hawkins RE et al (1994) Idiotypic vaccination against human B-cell lymphoma. Rescue of variable region gene sequences from biopsy material for assembly as single-chain Fv personal vaccines. Blood 83(11):3279–3288
3. Bendandi M et al (2001) Identification of the B-cell tumor-specific molecular fingerprint using non-radiolabelled PCR consensus primers. Ann Oncol 12(10):1479–1484
4. Carroll WL et al (1986) Mouse × human heterohybridomas as fusion partners with human B-cell tumors. J Immunol Methods 89:61–72
5. Rodríguez-Calvillo M et al (2004) Variations in "rescuability" of immunoglobulin molecules from different forms of human lymphoma: implications for anti-idiotype vaccine development. Crit Rev Oncol Hematol 52:1–7
6. Grodzki AC, Berenstein E (2010) Antibody purification: ammonium sulfate fractionation or gel filtration. In: Oliver C, Jamur MC (eds) Immunocytochemical methods and protocols, vol 588, Methods in molecular biology. Humana, Totowa, pp 15–26
7. Harlow E, Lane D (1988) Antibodies: a laboratory manual. Cold Spring Harbor Laboratory Press, Cold Spring Harbor, NY
8. Gagnon PS (1996) Purification tools for monoclonal antibodies. Validated Biosystems. In: Rathore Gail Sofer AS (ed) Process validation in manufacturing of biopharmaceuticals, 3rd edn. CRC, Tuscon, AZ
9. Nethery A et al (1990) Single-step purification of immunoglobulin M on C1q-Sepharose.

J Immunol Methods 126(1):57–60, Erratum in: J Immunol Methods 130(2), 287
10. Nevens JR et al (1992) Affinity chromatographic purification of immunoglobulin M antibodies utilizing immobilized mannan binding protein. J Chromatogr 597(1–2):247–256, April 24
11. Roque-Barreira MC, Campos-Neto A (1985) Jacalin, an IgA-binding lectin. J Immunol 134(3):1740–1743
12. Aucouturier P et al (1987) Characterization of jacalin, the human IgA and IgD binding lectin from jackfruit. Mol Immunol 24(5):503–511
13. Kwak LW et al (1992) Induction of immune responses in patients with B-cell lymphoma against the surface-immunoglobulin idiotype expressed by their tumors. N Eng J Med 327:1209–1215

Chapter 31

Preparation of Cancer-Related Peptide Cocktails that Target Heterogeneously Expressed Antigens

Reshu Gupta and Pradip P. Sachdeva

Abstract

A number of outstanding descriptions of the techniques linked to peptide chain assembly have already been published (Atherton and Sheppard, Solid phase peptide synthesis: a practical approach, pp 55–150, 1989; Stewart and Young, Solid phase peptide synthesis, pp 91–120, 1984; Wellings and Atherton, Methods in enzymology, p 44, 1997). These processes are also described in the operator manuals supplied by the manufacturers of peptide synthesis instrumentation. Accordingly the protocols presented in this chapter are to provide further information on those topics not covered in those publications.

Key words Synthetic peptides, Fmoc, Dimethylformamide, Resins, Linkers

1 Introduction

There has been an increasing need for synthetic peptides, and many techniques for their assembly have been published [1–3]. Synthetic peptides are being used in a wide variety of applications, including, but not limited to, the development of synthetic peptide vaccines [4–8], the study of antigen–antibody interactions [9–14], the preparation of biologically active analog peptides [15–17], the optimization of peptide antigens of clinical diagnostic value [18–20], the mapping of protein products of brain-specific genes [21, 22], and the study of parameters related to protein conformation [23].

Recently, Bae's [24] investigations concluded that targeting multiple myeloma-associated antigens using a cocktail of specific peptides may provide an effective therapeutic application in patients with the blood cancer and related diseases. In the majority of these studies, the restrictive factor has been the availability and expenditure of the desired peptides. Clearly, these studies would be significantly facilitated if synthetic methods were available that would permit the synthesis of larger numbers of peptides in a more cost-efficient manner and in a shorter time period. For the generation of cancer-related peptide cocktails, solid phase

Michael J.P. Lawman and Patricia D. Lawman (eds.), *Cancer Vaccines: Methods and Protocols*, Methods in Molecular Biology, vol. 1139, DOI 10.1007/978-1-4939-0345-0_31, © Springer Science+Business Media New York 2014

peptide synthesis (SPPS) has been utilized as an effective method. SPPS is a technique by which a number of diverse compounds can be synthesized simultaneously and screened rapidly for a useful compound. In particular, the SSPS method described by Merrifield [25] has become an important advancement in the field of combinatorial chemistry. Additionally, as the use of solid phase synthesis and screening methods increase, a variety of research-related fields such as solid supports, linkers and peptide coupling chemistry, automated synthesis systems, and screening methods have been developed. One of the most popular approaches for SPPS is Fmoc/tBu. Unlike the Merrifield approach [25] which utilizes a regime of graduated acidolysis to remove temporary and permanent protection group to get selectivity, the Fmoc/tBu method [26] is based on an orthogonal protecting group strategy. This method utilizes the base-labile *N*-Fmoc group for protection of the alpha-amino group and acid-labile side-chain protecting groups and resin linkage agents. Since removal of temporary and permanent protection is effected by completely different chemical mechanisms, linkage agents and side-chain protecting groups can be employed which can be removed under considerably milder setting than those used in the Merrifield method. In practice, t-butyl- and trityl-based side-chain protection and alkoxybenzyl-based linkers are used as they can be removed with trifluoroacetic acid (TFA). There are two primary types of deprotection reagents used in solid phase peptide synthesis. N-deprotection reagents remove only the N-terminal protection group of the peptide attached to the resin. These are TFA in Boc chemistry and piperidine in Fmoc chemistry. 1,8-diazabicyclo[5.4.0]undec-7-ene (DBU) may also be used to selectively remove Fmoc groups when deprotection with piperidine is sluggish. Cleavage reagents are the second type of deprotection reagents utilized in solid phase peptide synthesis. Cleavage reagents typically cleave the peptide product from the resin and, at the same time, remove all of the side-chain protecting groups producing the free peptide. The volatile nature of TFA makes it an excellent solvent that can be used in standard glass laboratory glassware; and it is readily removed by evaporation. Indeed, it is this convenience of the cleavage reaction and the ease with which the method can be adapted to multiple peptide synthesis that have increased the use of the Fmoc/tBu approach. In this method, the C-terminal residue is anchored to a TFA-labile linkage agent. The side-chain functionalities are protected with TFA-labile protecting groups. The temporary *N*-Fmoc protecting group is removed with 20 % piperidine in *N*,*N*-dimethylformamide (DMF). Coupling is typically carried out in DMF or *N*-methylpyrrolidone (NMP) with preformed active esters or activation reagents that generate in situ benzotriazolyl esters. Cleavage of the peptide from the resin and global side-chain deprotection is affected with 95 % TFA. The background and development of the Fmoc approach to SPPS has been the subject of a number of exceptional reviews [27, 28]. The protocols so far reported utilize a manual peptide synthesis vessel. While it is appreciated that the majority of scientists preparing synthetic peptides will be using automated peptide synthesizers, these protocols are not well described. In this chapter, particular emphasis has been given to those procedures which are typically carried out off-instrument, such as first residue attachment and peptide-resin cleavage.

2 Materials

2.1 Basic Resin Handling (See Notes 1–4)

1. Polyethylene glycol polyacrylamide copolymer (PEGA) or polyethylene glycol-polystyrene (PEG-PS) Resins.
2. Dichloromethane (DCM) or dimethylformamide (DMF) or isopropanol or methanol.

2.2 Symmetrical Anhydride Method

1. Fmoc-amino acid derivatives.
2. Dry, acid-free DCM.
3. 1,3-Diisopropylcarbodiimide (DIC).
4. DMF.
5. Hydroxyl-functionalized peptide synthesis resin.
6. 4-(*N*,*N*-dimethylamino)pyridine (DMAP).

2.3 Dichlorobenzoyl Chloride Method

1. Fmoc-amino acid derivatives.
2. DMF.
3. 1,4 Dichlorobenzene (DCB).
4. Pyridine.
5. Hydroxyl-functionalized peptide synthesis resin.

2.4 MSNT/MeIm Method

1. Fmoc-amino acid derivatives.
2. Dry, acid-free DCM.
3. 1-(Mesitylene-2-sulphonyl)-3-nitro-1*H*-1,2,4-triazole (MSNT).
4. 1-Methylimidazole (MeIm).
5. Dry tetrahydrofuran (THF).
6. DMF.
7. Hydroxyl-functionalized peptide synthesis resin.

2.5 Chlorination of Trityl Alcohol Resins

1. Dry toluene.
2. Freshly distilled acetyl chloride (AcCl).
3. 4-(Hydroxy (diphenyl) methyl) benzoyl.
4. Dry DCM aminomethyl resin.

2.6 Manual Removal of Fmoc Groups

1. 20 % Piperidine in DMF (v/v) or DBU/piperidine/DMF (1:1:48 v/v).

2.7 Hydroxy-benzotriazole Method

1. Fmoc-amino acid derivatives.
2. 1-Hydroxy-7-azabenzotriazole(HOAt)or1-hydroxybenzotriazole (HOBt).
3. 1,3-Diisopropylcarbodiimide (DIC).
4. DMF.

2.8 Pentafluorophenyl Ester Method

1. Fmoc-amino acid pentafluorophenyl ester (OPfp).
2. HOBt.
3. DMF.

2.9 Symmetrical Anhydrides Method

1. Fmoc-amino acid derivatives.
2. Dry, acid-free dichloromethane (DCM).
3. DIC.
4. DMF.

2.10 TBTU/PyBOP Method

1. Fmoc-amino acid derivatives.
2. *O*-(Benzotriazol-1-yl)-*N*,*N*,*N*′,*N*′-tetramethyluronium tetrafluoroborate (TBTU) or benzotriazol-1-yloxytris(pyrrolidino) phosphonium.
3. Hexafluorophosphate (PyBOP).
4. HOBt.
5. VV-Diisopropylethylamine (DIPEA).
6. DMF.

2.11 HATU Method

1. Fmoc-amino acid derivatives.
2. DIPEA.
3. *N*-[(Dimethylamino)-1*H*-1,2,3-triazolo[4,5-6]pyridin-lylmethylene]-*N*-methylmethanaminium (HATU).
4. DMF.

2.12 TFFH Method

1. Fmoc-amino acid.
2. DIPEA.
3. Tetramethyl fluoro formamidinium hexafluorophosphate (TFFH).
4. DMF.

2.13 Analytical Methods

1. 5 % Ninhydrin in ethanol (w/v).
2. KCN in pyridine: 2 mL 0.001 M KCN in 98 mL, 80 % Phenol in ethanol (w/v) pyridine.

3. 5 % DIPEA in DMF (v/v).
4. 1 % 2,4,6-Trinitrobenzenesulphonic acid (TNBS) in water (w/v).
5. 2 % *p*-Chloranil in DMF (w/v).
6. 2 % Acetaldehyde in DMF (v/v).
7. 20 % Piperidine in DMF.

2.14 Cleavage

1. TFA.
2. *m*-Cresol.
3. 1,2-Ethanedithiol (EDT).
4. Thioanisole.
5. Trimethylsilyl bromide (TMSBr).
6. Peptidyl resin.

2.15 Peptide Isolation

1. Rotary evaporator equipped with CO_2.
2. Peroxide-free diethyl ether or t-butyl acetone cold finger.
3. Oil pump protected methyl ether by a soda-lime trap.
4. 1 % TFA in DCM.
5. 10 % Pyridine in MeOH.

3 Methods

The protocols set out below would be carried out using a manual peptide synthesis vessel or in a sintered glass funnel fitted with a three-way stopcock.

3.1 Basic Resin Handling

3.1.1 Swelling of Polystyrene-Based Resin

1. Place the dry desired resin in a peptide synthesis reactor.
2. Add adequate DCM to cover up resin with three-time bed volume.
3. To remove air bubbles, shake reaction vessel softly and form a suspension of resin (*see* **Note 1**).
4. Let stand for 30 min.
5. Apply vacuum to remove DCM.

3.1.2 Washing

1. Washing can be performed by adding an appropriate amount (three bed volumes) of solvent.
2. Agitate for 1 min, followed by applying vacuum to drain resin.
3. Repeat **steps 1** and **2** 4×.

3.1.3 Drying the Resin

1. Wash resin sequentially as described in Subheading 3.1.2 with either DMF, DCM, MeOH, and/or hexane (polystyrene-based resins); DMF, isopropanol, and/or hexane (loaded 2-chlorotrityl resins); or DMF, DCM, and/or ether (PEG-PS resins).

2. Apply vacuum to air-dry the resin for 10 min.
3. The resin can now be transferred to a sample tube.

3.2 Symmetrical Anhydride Method

Appropriate procedures can be applied for the attachment of first residue to the resins based on their functional group. Resins can be easily divided into three categories on the basis of their reactive functional groups (hydroxymethyl-, trityl chloride-, and aminomethyl-based resins).

The protocols described in this section are applicable to all hydroxyl methyl-based resins which involve esterification of the first amino acid to a linker hydroxyl group. There are three methods which are used for the attachment of Fmoc-protected amino acids to the resins: (1) the symmetrical anhydride method, (2) the dichlorobenzoyl chloride method, and (3) the MSNT/Melm method. To ensure acceptable results when using these protocols, it is essential that several precautions are observed (*see* **Notes 5–9**):

1. Attachment of the first amino acid residue to alcohol-based resins can be performed by using the symmetrical anhydrides method.
2. Place resin in a dry reaction vessel.
3. Swell and wash with DMF as described in Subheading 2.1.
4. Prepare the appropriate Fmoc-amino acid anhydride (5 eq) according to Subheading 3.9. Dissolve in least amount volume of DMF followed by addition of the resin. If needed, add additional DMF to ensure complete coverage of the resin bed.
5. Dissolve DMAP (0.1 eq) in DMF and add this solution to the resin/amino acid mixture. Close the vessel and allow the mixture to agitate at room temperature for 1 h (*see* **Notes 10** and **11**).
6. The resin can now be washed 5× with DMF.
7. Transfer 10 mg of resin with a wide-mouth Pasteur pipette to a small, sintered glass funnel. Wash and dry-down as described in Subheading 3.1. Find out the extent of loading using Subheading 3.14.4. If the loading is below 70 %, repeat **steps 2–5**.
8. Add benzoic anhydride (5 eq) and pyridine (1 eq) in DMF and agitate for 30 min.
9. Wash and shrink-down the resin as described in Subheading 3.1.

3.3 Dichlorobenzoyl Chloride Method

1. Put dry resin in a reaction vessel.
2. Swell and wash with DMF as described in Subheading 3.1. If needed, add extra DMF to ensure complete coverage of the resin.
3. Add the suitable Fmoc-amino acid (5 eq) followed by pyridine (8.25 eq). Gently agitate to dissolve amino acid completely.

4. Add DCB (5 eq) and agitate the mixture softly for 18 h.
5. Wash and shrink-down the resin as described in Subheading 3.1.

3.4 MSNT/MeIm Method (See Note 12)

1. Place resin in a dry reaction vessel.
2. Swell and wash with DCM as described in Subheading 3.1. Add sufficient DCM to cover resin and flush vessel with nitrogen followed by its sealing.
3. Weigh the desired Fmoc-amino acid (5 eq) and place into a dry round-bottom flask equipped with a magnetic stirrer. Then, add approximately 3 mL/mmol of dry DCM to dissolve the amino acid derivative. To aid complete dissolution, one or two drops of THF can be added.
4. Now add MeIm (3.75 eq) followed by MSNT (5 eq). Flush flask with nitrogen and seal with a septum and then stir the mixture until the MSNT has dissolved.
5. Using a syringe, transfer the amino acid solution to the resin containing vessel.
6. Allow the mixture to stand at room temperature for 1 h, with mild agitation.
7. Wash with DCM and DMF, 5× each.
8. Transfer 10 mg of resin with a wide-mouthed Pasteur pipette to a small, sintered glass funnel. Wash and dry-down as described in Subheading 3.1. Determine the degree of loading using Subheading 3.14.4. If the loading is under 70 %, repeat **steps 2–7**.
9. Add benzoic anhydride (5 eq) and pyridine (1 eq) in DMF and agitate softly for 30 min.
10. Wash and dry the resin as described in Subheading 3.1.
11. Two trityl-based supports (*see* **Note 13**) are presently in frequent use for the production of peptide acids by Fmoc SPPS: 2-chlorotrityl chloride resin [29] and 4-(chloro (diphenyl) methyl) benzoyl resin [30]. These resins are extremely moisture sensitive, and so it is essential that all reagents and glassware should be dried completely before use. 2-Chlorotrityl chloride resin can be stored desiccated at room temperature; 4-(chloro-(diphenyl) methyl)benzoyl resins should be generated from the precursor trityl alcohol immediately before use as described elsewhere.

3.5 Chlorination of Trityl Alcohol Resins

1. Place the resin in a sintered glass funnel.
2. Swell and wash with DCM as described in Subheading 3.1.
3. Wash with toluene 5×.
4. Transfer resin to a round-bottom flask. Add adequate toluene to cover resin bed.

5. Add 1 mL AcCl/g resin and fit flask with reflux condenser and $CaCl_2$ guard tube to absorb moisture.
6. Heat mixture at 60 °C for 3 h.
7. Allow to cool to room temperature.
8. Slurry resin with toluene into a dry reaction vessel and wash with DCM.
9. Load immediately.
10. For the addition of the first amino acid to supports derivatized with peptide amide-forming linkers, such as trialkoxybenzhydrylamine, trialkoxybenzylamine, and aminoxanthenyl resins, any of the standard peptide coupling methods described in this chapter can be used.

3.6 Removal of Fmoc Groups

Removal of the Fmoc group from the N-terminus of the resin-bound peptide chain is usually achieved by treating the resin with 20–50 % piperidine in DMF. In the case of aggregated sequences, treatment with piperidine in DMF will not always be successful. In such cases, the use of the non-nucleophilic base 1,8-diazabicyclo[5.4.0]undec-7-ene (DBU) is recommended [31].

1. Place the peptidyl resin in a sintered glass funnel or reaction vessel.
2. Dry and swell the resin as described in Subheading 3.1.
3. Then, wash resin with DMF 5× followed by addition of deprotection reagent to cover resin.
4. Agitate gently for 2 min and drain off reagent.
5. Repeat **steps 3** and **4**, 2–3×.
6. Again, wash resin with DMF 5×.

3.7 Hydroxybenzotriazole Method

For the addition of amino acids in the sequential manner, in situ carboxyl activation of the incoming amino acid or the use of preformed derivatives of activated amino acid is required. The coupling time depends on the nature of the active species, on the peptide sequence, and on the concentration/functionality of the reagents and resin. For highly reactive species, reagents like TFFH [32], PyBOP [33], TBTU [34], and HATU [35], 30 min of coupling time is usually sufficient.

1. Place the appropriate Fmoc-amino acid (5 eq) and HOXt (5 eq) in a dry round-bottom flask or sample vial equipped with a magnetic stirrer.
2. To dissolve the amino acid, add a minimum amount of DMF.
3. Add DIC in a dropwise manner (5 eq).
4. Stir the mixture for 20 min and add the solution to the N-deblocked peptidyl resin.

5. Agitate resin softly for 1 h.
6. Transfer 10 mg of resin to a sintered glass funnel. Wash and dry the resin as described in Subheading 3.1. Perform Kaiser or 2,4,6-trinitrobenzenesulphonic acid (TNBS) test (Subheading 3.14). If positive, repeat **steps 5** and **6**.
7. If resin still gives a positive color test after 4 h, wash resin with DMF 5× and repeat coupling reaction with fresh reagents.
8. Collect the derivatized resin.

3.8 Pentafluorophenyl Ester Method

1. Weigh the desired Fmoc-amino acid pentafluorophenyl ester (5 eq) and HOBt (5 eq) in a sample vial which should be completely dry.
2. Add the least amount volume of DMF to dissolve amino acid.
3. Add the solution to the N-protected peptidyl resin.
4. Agitate resin gently for 1 h and transfer 10 mg of resin to sintered glass funnel. Wash and dry-down as described in Subheading 3.1. Perform Kaiser or TNBS test (Subheading 3.14). If positive, repeat **steps 4** and **5**.
5. Follow **step 7** of Subheading 3.7 and collect the resin.

3.9 Symmetrical Anhydrides Method

1. Put the appropriate Fmoc-amino acid (10 eq) in a dry round-bottom flask, connected with a magnetic stirrer.
2. Add dry DCM to dissolve the amino acid derivative.
3. Add a solution of DIC (5 eq) in the mixture.
4. Mix the mixture for 10 min at 0 °C and keep the reaction mixture free of moisture. If a symmetrical anhydride precipitates, add dry DMF dropwise to redissolve and mix again for a further 10 min.
5. Remove the DCM by evaporation using a rotary evaporator.
6. Redissolve the residue in the lowest volume of DMF and add the solution to the N-deprotected peptidyl resin.
7. Agitate resin gently for 1 h and follow **steps 7** and **8** of Subheading 3.7.

3.10 TBTU/PyBOP Method

1. Weigh out Fmoc-amino acid (5 eq) (*see* **Note 14**), HOBt (5 eq), and PyBOP (5 eq) or TBTU (4.9 eq) and place in a dry glass vial.
2. Add a lowest amount of DMF to dissolve completely.
3. Add DIPEA (10 eq) and mix completely.
4. Add the solution right away to the N-deblocked peptidyl resin.
5. Follow **steps 6–8** of Subheading 3.7.

3.11 HATU Method

1. Weigh out into a dry glass vial Fmoc-amino acid (5 eq) and HATU (4.9 eq).
2. Follow **steps 2–5** of Subheading 3.10.

3.12 TFFH Method

1. Weigh out into a dry glass vial Fmoc-amino acid (5 eq) and TFFH (4.9 eq).
2. Follow **steps 2–5** of Subheading 3.10.

3.13 Assembly of the Peptide Residue

1. Add 20 % piperidine, agitate for 2 min, drain, and wash appropriately
2. Wash resin with DMF 5× (*see* **Note 15**).
3. Add activated and dissolved amino acid derivative to resin.
4. Agitate gently for 30 min and perform color test.
5. Continue agitations if necessary.
6. Wash resin with DMF.

3.14 Analytical Procedures

3.14.1 Kaiser Test

The ninhydrin test, devised by Kaiser [35], is the most broadly used qualitative test for the presence or absence of free amino groups. Other methods such as picric acid monitoring [36] or the TNBS test [37] are also available. For proline, the chloranil test [38] is recommended.

1. Sample a few resin beads and wash a number of times with ethanol.
2. Transfer to a small glass tube and add two drops of each of the solutions above.
3. Mix well and heat to 120 °C for 4–6 min.

The presence of resin-bound free amine is indicated by blue coloration of resin beads.

3.14.2 TNBS Test

1. Sample a few resin beads and wash several times with ethanol.
2. Put the sample on a microscope slide followed by addition of one drop of each solution.
3. Watch the sample under the microscope and look for changes in color (*see* **Note 16**).
4. The test is positive when the resin beads turn yellow or red within 10 min and negative when the beads show no color.

3.14.3 Chloranil Test

1. Add one drop of acetaldehyde solution and *p*-chloranil solution to a few mg of resin beads placed on a microscope slide.
2. Keep the slide at room temperature for 10 min.
3. Blue-stained resin beads indicate the presence of amines.

3.14.4 Fmoc Determination

The theoretical substitution of a peptidyl resin can be calculated from the substitution of the base resin using below mentioned equation:

$$A = B \times 1{,}000 / [1{,}000 + (B \times (M - X)]$$

A = theoretical substitution (mmol/g).

B = substitution of starting resin (mmol/g).

M = molecular weight of target peptide, plus all protecting groups.

X = 18 for hydroxymethyl, 36 for trityl chloride, 17 for aminomethyl-based resins, but 239 if resin is initially protected with Fmoc.

Estimation of level of first residue attachment can be performed by this method.

1. Take three 10 mm matched silica UV cells.
2. Weigh dry Fmoc-amino acid resin (approx. 1 μmol with respect to Fmoc) into two of the cells.
3. Distribute freshly prepared 20 % piperidine in DMF into each of *uv* cells.
4. Agitate the resin suspension for the duration of 5–10 min (*see* **Note 17**).
5. Place the reference cell (which contains only 20 % piperidine solution) into a spectrophotometer and set the absorbance zero at 290 nm.
6. Then, place cells containing the settled resin into the spectrophotometer and read the absorbance at 290 nm. Take an average of two values.
7. Calculate the loading using the below mentioned equation:

$$\textit{Loading}\ (\textit{mmol} / \textit{g}) = (\textit{Abs sample}) / (\textit{mg of sample} \times 1.75)$$

3.15 TFA-Mediated Cleavage

This section describes the procedures used for cleavage of peptides from acid-sensitive linkages. Before performing the cleavage reaction, it is essential that DMF should be completely removed from the peptidyl resin as described in Subheading 3.1. Because of the different behavior of the peptidyl resins, it is recommended that a small-scale cleavage of peptide resin by using 20–30 mg sample should be carried out to conclude the optimum cleavage conditions.

1. Place dry resin in a flask and add desired cleavage reagent.
2. Wash out flask with nitrogen and seal it by stopper. Let stand at room temperature with occasional swirling for 1.5–18 h, depending on sequence.
3. Remove the resin by filtration and wash it 2× with clean TFA.
4. Combine filtrates and isolate the peptide as described in Subheading 3.17.

3.16 TMSBr Cleavage

1. Place dry resin in a flask followed by addition of 0.25 mL *m*-cresol/g resin, 1.25 mL EDT/g resin, 2.35 mL thioanisole, and 18 mL TFA/g resin.
2. Add peptide resin and cool to 0 °C.
3. Wash flask with N_2 and quickly add 3.3 mL of TMSBr/g resin.
4. Wash out flask again with N_2 and seal it by stopper. Leave it to stand at room temperature with occasional swirling for 15 min.
5. Follow **steps 3** and **4** of Subheading 3.15.

3.17 Peptide Isolation

The peptide is commonly precipitated by adding cold diethyl or t-butyl methyl ether. A rotary evaporator equipped with CO_2, a peroxide-free diethyl ether or t-butyl acetone cold finger, and oil pump protected methyl ether by a soda-lime trap are used for this procedure.

3.17.1 Quick Method

1. Move the cleavage mixture to an appropriate-sized round-bottom flask.
2. Evaporate the TFA and scavenger mixture to a glassy film.
3. Add cold ether slowly.
4. Wash the peptide film mildly by using ether.
5. Pour out the ether and repeat the washing step minimum of 4×.
6. Now air-dry the peptide.
7. Dissolve in appropriate aqueous buffer and lyophilize.

3.17.2 Filtration

1. Perform **steps 1–3** of Subheading 3.17.1.
2. Suspend the peptide in the ether solution.
3. Filter the precipitated peptide in a Hirsch funnel under light vacuum.
4. Wash it further with cold ether.
5. Dissolve and lyophilize the buffer.

3.17.3 Centrifugation

1. Carry out **steps 1–4** of Subheading 3.17.1.
2. Transfer the suspension to a centrifuge tube and seal.
3. Centrifuge at 1,500 × *g* for 10 min followed by removal of the ether (supernatant) from the tube.
4. Add fresh ether, seal, and shake the tube to resuspend the peptide and centrifuge as above.
5. Repeat **steps 3–4** 4×.
6. Dissolve the pellet in a suitable aqueous buffer and lyophilize. The peptide can then be analyzed by LC-MS equipped with diode array detection.

3.18 Release of Fully Protected Peptides

Peptides attached to resins can be free under conditions that leave most of their side-chain protecting groups intact. Peptide release is normally affected by repetitive treatment with 1 % TFA in DCM or by using TFE in DCM (*see* **Note 18**).

1. Swell 1 mmol peptidyl-resin in DCM in a manual peptide synthesis vessel followed by washing 3× with DCM.
2. Drain off extra DCM.
3. Add 10 mL TFA solution, seal the funnel by stopper, and agitate it gently for 2–3 min.
4. Replace stopper with adaptor connected to a nitrogen supply.
5. Filter solution by nitrogen into a flask that contains 2 mL pyridine solution.
6. Repeat **steps 3–5** up to 10×.
7. Wash the residual protected peptide with DCM and MeOH.
8. Check out filtrates by TLC or HPLC.
9. Evaporate product-containing filtrates under low pressure.
10. Add 40 mL of water and cool mixture with ice.
11. Filter the precipitated peptide through in a Hirsch funnel under light vacuum.
12. Wash product consecutively with water 3×, with 5 % $NaHCO_3$ aq. 2×, with water 3×, with 0.05 M $KHSO_4$ 2×, and with water 6×.
13. Dry the peptide sample in desiccators.

4 Notes

1. Agitation of any resin with a magnetic stirrer is not suggested as the action results in slow destruction of the resin particles.
2. All resins must be swollen with an appropriate solvent before use, with the exception of PEGA resins which are supplied as a slurry in methanol or water.
3. Underivatized polystyrene resins do not swell well in DMF; hence the resin must be first swollen in DCM.
4. In contrast, packaging of dry PEG-PS resins can be performed directly in the reaction vessel and then can be swollen directly with DMF.
5. All reagents and glassware must be dried completely before use as the presence of moisture can affect loading efficiencies.
6. Amino acids containing water should be dried either by dissolving in ethyl acetate or by drying the solution over anhydrous magnesium sulfate and isolating by evaporation or by repeated evaporation from dioxane.

7. Reactions should be conducted using the least amount of solvent to ensure highest reagent concentration.
8. For the synthesis of peptide acids which contain C-terminal cysteine, histidine, proline, methionine, and tryptophan residues, it is recommended to use trityl-based resins.
9. After each reaction, the loading efficiency should be checked using the method described in Subheading 3.14.4 and, if necessary, the reaction repeated using fresh reagents.
10. With arginine to be the first residue, this reaction may need to be repeated 3× to achieve acceptable loading owing to rapid conversion of the symmetrical anhydride to the unreactive δ-lactam.
11. While using DMAP, some enantiomerization and dipeptide formation can be expected. Enantiomerization is particularly challenging with cysteine and histidine. For the majority of other amino acids, the levels of enantiomerization can be usually controlled to within acceptable limits by using minimum amount of DMAP.
12. It has proved mainly effective in loading Fmoc-amino acids to the relatively unreactive hydroxyl group of 4-hydroxymethylbenzoyl-derivatized resins [39] and in situations where enantiomerization is a problem.
13. This method is free from enantiomerization and dipeptide formation [40], making these techniques ideal tools for the preparation of peptides containing C-terminal histidine or cysteine residues. Their use is also recommended for the synthesis of peptides containing C-terminal proline [41], methionine, or tryptophan residues [40].
14. Cysteine is best introduced using the appropriate symmetrical anhydride or OPfp ester.
15. DMF is usually employed as the wash solvent, although *N*-methylpyrrolidone (NMP) or *N*,*N*-dimethylacetamide (DMA) can also be used.
16. It may be more suitable to perform this procedure by placing the resin beads in an ignition tube, followed by addition of three drops of each reagents, and by leaving the suspension for 10 min. Decant off the supernatant, resuspend the resin beads in DMF, and look for color formation of the beads.
17. For polystyrene-based resins that have high substitution levels, leave the suspension with occasional agitation for 2–3 h.
18. The cleavage should be performed in a sealed manual peptide synthesis reaction vessel, and the filtration should be performed by applying nitrogen pressure rather using vacuum.

References

1. Atherton E, Sheppard RC (1989) Solid phase peptide synthesis: a practical approach. IRL Press, Oxford, pp 55–150
2. Stewart JM, Young JD (1984) Solid phase peptide synthesis, 2nd edn. Pierce Chemical Company, Rockford, pp 91–120
3. Wellings DA, Atherton E (1997) Methods in enzymology, vol 289. Academic, New York, p 44
4. Lerner RA (1982) Tapping the immunological repertoire to produce antibodies of predetermined specificity. Nature 299:592–596
5. Sutcliffe JG et al (1980) Chemical synthesis of a polypeptide predicted from nucleotide sequence allows detection of a new retroviral gene product. Nature 287:801–805
6. Green N et al (1982) Immunogenic structure of the influenza virus hemagglutinin. Cell 23: 477–487
7. Bittle JL et al (1982) Protection against foot-and-mouth disease by immunization with a chemically synthesized peptide predicted from the viral nucleotide sequence. Nature 298: 30–33
8. Houghten et al (1985) In: Lerner RA et al (eds) Vaccines '85: molecular and chemical basis of resistance to parasitic, bacterial, and viral diseases. Cold Spring Harbor Laboratory Press, Cold Spring Harbor, NY, pp 91–94
9. East IJ et al (1980) On topographic antigenic determinants in myoglobins. Mol Immunol 17:519–525
10. Wilson IA et al (1984) The structure of an antigenic determinant in a protein. Cell 37: 767–778
11. McMillan S et al (1983) Synthetic idiotypes: the third hypervariable region of murine anti-dextran antibodies. Cell 35:859–863
12. Geysen HM et al (1984) Use of peptide synthesis to probe viral antigens for epitopes to a resolution of a single amino acid. Proc Natl Acad Sci U S A 81:3998–4002
13. Geysen HM et al (1985) Small peptides induce antibodies with a sequence and structural requirement for binding antigen comparable to antibodies raised against the native protein. Proc Natl Acad Sci U S A 82:178–182
14. Niman HL et al (1983) Generation of protein-reactive antibodies by short peptides is an event of high frequency: implications for the structural basis of immune recognition. Proc Natl Acad Sci U S A 80:4949–4953
15. Yamashiro D, Li CH (1984). In: Meienhofer H (ed) The peptides, vol 6. Academic, New York, pp 191–217
16. Hruby V (1984). In: Vida JA, Gordon M (eds) Conformationally directed drug design. American Chemical Society, Washington, DC, pp 9–27
17. Veber DF et al (1978) Conformationally restricted bicyclic analogs of somatostatin. Proc Natl Acad Sci U S A 75:2636–2640
18. Chen PP et al (1984) Anti-hypervariable region antibody induced by a defined peptide: an approach for studying the structural correlates of idiotypes. Proc Natl Acad Sci U S A 81: 1784–1788
19. Klipstein FA et al (1984) Enzyme-linked immunosorbent assay for Escherichia coli heat-stable enterotoxin. J Clin Microbiol 19: 798–803
20. Chen PP et al (1985) Characterization of an epibody. An antiidiotype that reacts with both the idiotype of rheumatoid factors (RF) and the antigen recognized by RF. J Exp Med 161: 323–331
21. Bloom FE et al (1985) Immunocytochemical mapping of 1B236, a brain-specific neuronal polypeptide deduced from the sequence of a cloned mRNA. J Neurosci 5:1781–1802
22. Sutcliffe JG et al (1983) Identifying the protein products of brain-specific genes with antibodies to chemically synthesized peptides. Cell 33: 671–682
23. Freidinger RM et al (1980) Bioactive conformation of luteinizing hormone-releasing hormone: evidence from a conformationally constrained analog. Science 210:656–658
24. Bae J et al (2012) Myeloma-specific multiple peptides able to generate cytotoxic T lymphocytes: a potential therapeutic application in multiple myeloma and other plasma cell disorders. Clin Cancer Res 18(17):4850–4860
25. Merrifield RB (1963) Solid phase peptide synthesis. I. The synthesis of a tetrapeptide. J Am Chem Soc 85:2149–2154
26. Atherton E et al (1978) A mild procedure for solid phase peptide synthesis: use of fluorenylmethoxycarbonylamino-acids. J Chem Soc Chem Commun 13:537–539
27. Fields GB, Noble RL (1990) Solid phase peptide synthesis utilizing 9-fluorenylmethoxycarbonyl amino acids. Int J Pept Protein Res 35:161–214
28. Grant G (ed) (1992) Synthetic peptides. W. H. Freeman & Co., New York, pp 77–183
29. Barlos K et al (1989) Darstellung geschutzter peptid-fragmente unter einsatz substituierter triphenylmethyl-harze. Tetrahedron Lett 30: 3943–3946

30. Bayer E et al (1994). In: Hodges RS, Smith JA (ed) Peptides: chemistry, structure and biology, Proc 13th American Peptide Symposium. ESCOM, Lieden, p 156
31. Carpino LA, El-Faham A (1995) Tetramethylfluoroformamidinium hexafluorophosphate: a rapid acting peptide coupling reagent for solution and solid phase peptide synthesis. J Am Chem Soc 117:5401–5402
32. Coste J et al (1990) PyBOP a new peptide coupling reagent devoid of toxic by product. Tetrahedron Lett 31:205–208
33. Knorr R et al (1989) New coupling reagents in peptide chemistry. Tetrahedron Lett 30: 1927–1930
34. Carpino LA (1993) 1-hydroxy-7-azabenzotriazole. An efficient peptide coupling additive. J Am Chem Soc 115:4397–4398
35. Kaiser E et al (1970) Color test for detection of free terminal amino groups in the solid-phase synthesis of peptides. Anal Biochem 34:595–598
36. Arad O, Houghten RA (1990) An evaluation of the advantages and effectiveness of picric acid monitoring during solid phase peptide synthesis. Pept Res 3:42–50
37. Hancock WS, Battersby JE (1976) A new micro-test for the detection of incomplete coupling reactions in solid-phase peptide synthesis using 2,4,6-trinitrobenzenesulphonic acid. Anal Biochem 71:260–264
38. Vojkovsky T (1995) Detection of secondary amines on solid phase. Pept Res 8:236–237
39. Meldal M et al (1998) Inhibition of cruzipain visualized in a fluorescence quenched solid-phase inhibitor library assay. D-amino acid inhibitors for cruzipain, cathepsin B and cathepsin L. J Pept Sci 4:83–91
40. Barlos K et al (1991) 2-Chlorotrityl chloride resin. Studies on anchoring of Fmoc-amino acids and peptide cleavage. Int J Pept Protein Res 37:513–520
41. Steinauer R, White P (1994). In: Epton R (ed) Innovations and perspectives in solid phase synthesis. 3rd international symposium, Mayflower Worldwide Ltd., Birmingham, UK, p 689

Part V

Delivery Mechanisms

Chapter 32

Making an Avipoxvirus Encoding a Tumor-Associated Antigen and a Costimulatory Molecule

Paul M. Howley, Kerrilyn R. Diener, and John D. Hayball

Abstract

Fowlpox virus (FPV) is a double-stranded DNA virus with a history of use as a live attenuated vaccine in commercial poultry production systems. FPV is also highly amenable to genetic engineering, with a large cloning capacity and many nonessential sites available for integration, meaning that in recombinant form, several transgenes can be expressed simultaneously. Recombinant FPV has proven an effective prophylactic vaccine vector for other diseases of birds, as well as other animal species (Brun et al., Vaccine 26:6508–6528, 2008). These vectors do not integrate into the host genome nor do they undergo productive replication in mammalian cells; thus they have a proven and impeccable safety profile and have been progressed as prophylactic and therapeutic vaccine vectors for use in humans (Beukema et al., Expert Rev Vaccines 5:565–577, 2006; Lousberg et al., Expert Rev Vaccines 10:1435–1449, 2011). Furthermore, repeated immunization with FPV does not blunt subsequent vaccine responses, presumably because it is replication-defective, and thus larger doses can be routinely administered (Brun et al., Vaccine 26:6508–6528, 2008). This strengthens the case for FPV as a viable platform vaccine vector, as it means it can be used repeatedly in an individual to achieve different immunological outcomes. Here we describe in detail the construction of a recombinant variant of FPV expressing the prostate tumor-associated antigen prostatic acid phosphatase (PAP) in conjunction with the immunostimulatory cytokine, interleukin-2 (IL-2), which, if undertaken under the appropriate regulatory conditions and with approvals in place, would theoretically be amenable to clinical trial applications.

Key words Fowlpox virus, Viral vaccine vectors, Co-expression, Tumor-associated antigens, Cytokines

1 Introduction

Fowlpox virus (FPV) and canarypox virus (CNPV) both belong to the *Avipoxvirus* genus, the only genus of the *Chordopoxviridae* to infect non-mammalian hosts [4]. Recombinant CNPV has been licensed for commercial use in a number of veterinary vaccines including for CNPV itself, equine influenza, and West Nile virus [5, 6], with a single dose of a CNPV vaccine sufficient to elicit long-lasting protection [7, 8]. In addition to its veterinary applications, CNPV is currently in clinical trials for human diseases

Michael J.P. Lawman and Patricia D. Lawman (eds.), *Cancer Vaccines: Methods and Protocols*, Methods in Molecular Biology, vol. 1139, DOI 10.1007/978-1-4939-0345-0_32, © Springer Science+Business Media New York 2014

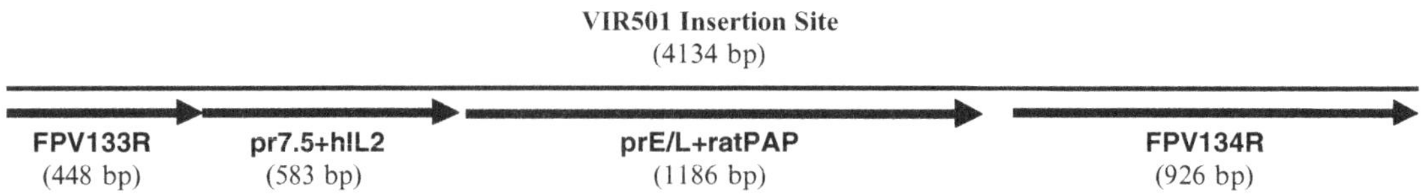

Feature	Description
FPVM3	Parental virus of VIR501: FPVm3 is a tissue culture adapted (chicken embryo cells) plaque purified clone of Websters vaccine strain M
FPV133R	Fowlpox virus protein coding sequence of ORF 133R
Pr7.5+human IL2	Human interleukin 2 (hIL2) expression cassette consisting of a vaccinia virus p7.5 promoter and the protein coding sequence of IL2. The protein coding sequence was obtained by RT-PCR amplification from total RNA extracted from human white blood cells.
prE/L+rat PAP	Rat prostatic acid phosphatase (PAP) expression cassette consisting of an early/late fowlpox virus promoter and the protein coding sequence of PAP of rat species. DNA of the protein coding sequence was obtained from Professor Michael Brown, Royal Adelaide Hospital, Adelaide, Australia. He obtained the DNA by RT-PCR amplification of total RNA extracted from prostate cells extracted from rats.
FPV134R	Fowlpox virus protein coding sequence of ORF 134R

Fig. 1 Details of VIR501 insertion site highlighting the FPV M3 flanking regions targeted for homologous recombination (FPV133R and FPV 134R) and the vaccinia virus p7.5 promoter to drive IL-2 expression as compared to the early/late FPV promoter which controls expression of rat-PAP

including human immunodeficiency virus (HIV), cytomegalovirus prevention, and cancer, where it has shown an excellent safety profile but limited efficacy [9–12]. Fowlpox virus, which naturally infects poultry, has been used successfully to prevent FPV itself in chickens and turkeys since the 1920s. With the advent of recombinant DNA techniques in the 1980s, FPV has subsequently been employed in the construction of recombinant vaccine vectors [2, 3] targeting other poultry diseases [13–15], as well as for the development of vectored vaccines for various mammalian and human diseases, most notably HIV and cancer [16–21]. Here we describe the stepwise processes by which a recombinant variant of FPV (rFPV) can be prepared (VIR501, Virax Holdings, Melbourne, Victoria, Australia), expressing the rat prostate tumor-associated antigen prostatic acid phosphatase (rPAP) in conjunction with the human immunostimulatory cytokine, interleukin-2 (hIL-2) which if undertaken under the appropriate regulatory conditions and with approvals in place would be theoretically amenable to clinical trial applications.

VIR501 (Fig. 1) is a recombinant fowlpox virus (M3 strain) that expresses rPAP and hIL-2 upon infection. The rPAP protein-coding sequence is under the control of an early/late fowlpox promoter. The hIL-2 protein-coding sequence is under the control of the vaccinia p7.5 promoter. The rPAP and hIL-2 expression cassettes where cloned into pKG10a (FPV transdominant shuttle vector, provided by Dr David Boyle, Australian National University,

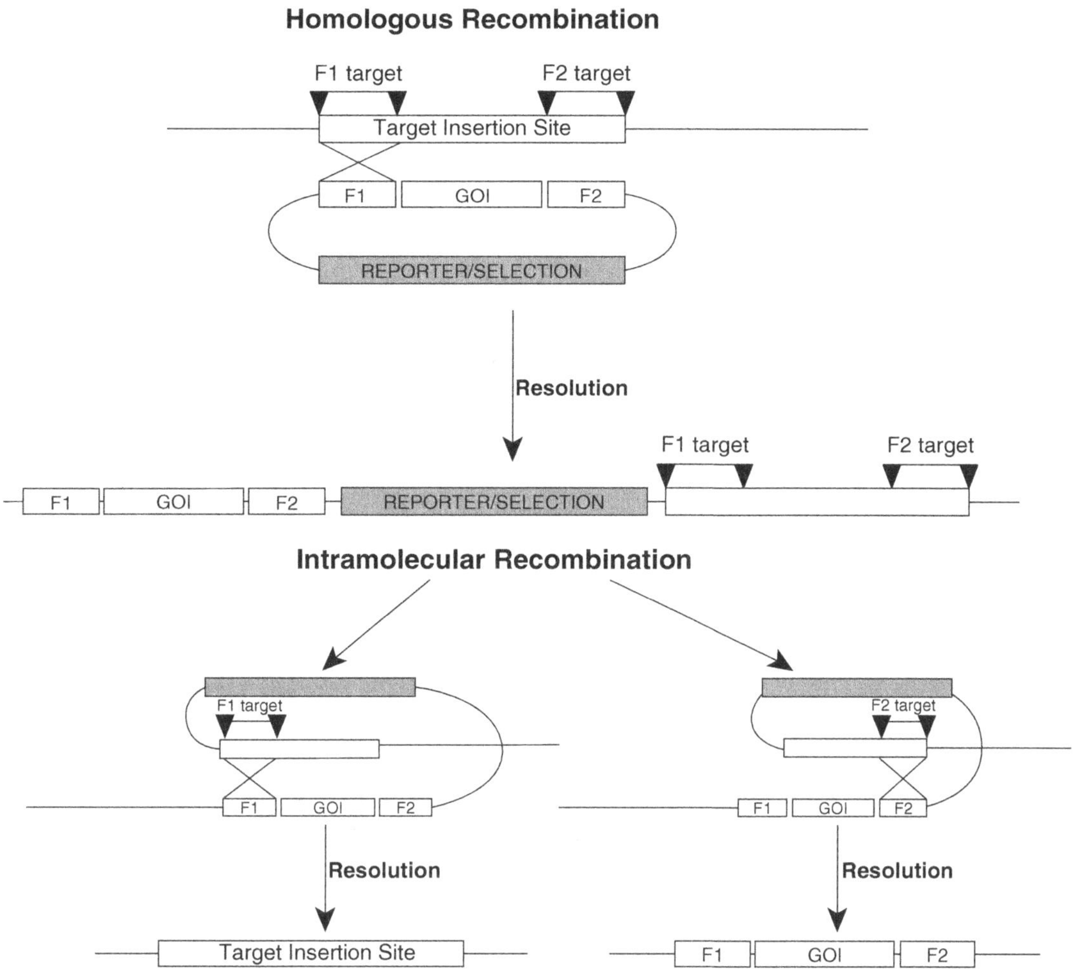

Fig. 2 Diagrammatic presentation of the homologous recombination event involving two crossover events. First crossover event will insert the gene of interest (GOI) by recombining the whole plasmid shuttle vector into the FPV genome at the target site. The second crossover event, intramolecular recombination, will result in the removal of all sequences outside of F1 and F2 arms. The first crossover event has to be positively selected for and maintained by using drug resistance strategies. Removing the positive selection will encourage the second crossover event to occur

Canberra, Australia) and used to insert the two cassettes into the FPV M3 genome by homologous recombination between ORFs FPV133R and FPV134R (reference to FPV genome Genbank AF198100). Recombinant virus VIR501 was amplified and blue plaque-purified using drug selection and Xgal agarose overlays. The reporter cassette was eliminated by further plaque purification (white plaque purification using Xgal agarose overlays) in the absence of drug selection. This process of homologous recombination to insert the expression cassettes into the FPV genome followed by reporter cassette elimination is shown diagrammatically in Fig. 2.

The pKG10a shuttle vector was designed so that the gene of interest (GOI) to be stably inserted into the FPV genome is cloned-in in between FPV133R homologous recombination arm (Flank 1 arm, F1 in Fig. 2) and FPV134R homologous arm (Flank 2 arm, F2 in Fig. 2). These homologous recombination arms are short sequences identical to the target sequences within the FPV genome for insert. The reporter/drug selection cassette must be located outside of the F1 and F2 configuration. PKG10a report/drug selection cassette consists of the beta-galactosidase poxvirus-expression cassette and the *Escherichia coli* (*E. coli*) guanine phosphoribosyltransferase (Ecogpt) poxvirus-expression cassette. Recombinant viruses expressing Ecogpt are able to replicate in the presence of mycophenolic acid (MPA) which can arrest DNA synthesis by blocking purine synthesis [22]. Recombinant viruses expressing beta-galactosidase can be visualized as blue plaques in the presence of Xgal in the culture medium. Because of the configuration of the pKG10a shuttle vector, insertion of the GOI together with the beta-galactosidase/Ecogpt cassettes, a single crossover event must take place thereby inserting the whole shuttle vector into the FPV gene. A double crossover event between F1 and F2 will insert the GIO only into the genome of FPV; however, there will be no mechanism to visualize and positively select recombinants over nonrecombinant virus. Without such a visual and/or positive selection capability, finding a recombinant virus will be as hard as looking for a needle in a haystack.

After homologous recombination, amplification in the presence of MPA plus required supplements (MXHAT media) and blue plaque purification in the presence of Xgal will enrich and isolate recombinant viruses containing the whole shuttle vector as shown in Fig. 2. Once insertion has been confirmed and nonrecombinant virus has been eliminated, the second crossover event can be encouraged to take place by amplifying the virus in the absence of MPA and plaque purifying white plaques. This second crossover event will result in two possibilities as shown in Fig. 2, 50 % no insertion, i.e., complete deletion of the pKG10a vector from the genome, or 50 % with GOI present but deletion of the shuttle vector backbone plus reporter/selection cassette. Now, finding the recombinant virus (Fig. 3) among nonrecombinant viruses becomes manageable by screening a hand full of white plaques for gene insertion (Fig. 4). In this chapter, we describe the construction of a recombinant variant of FPV expressing the PAP in conjunction with IL-2.

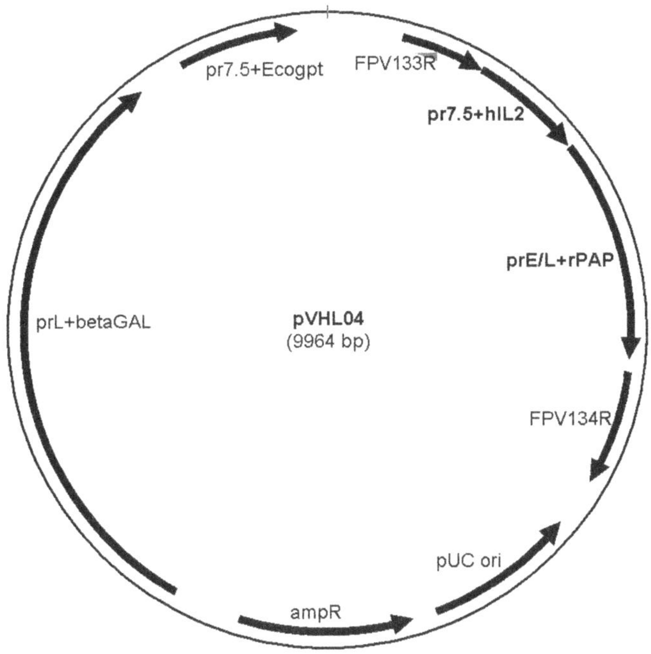

Fig. 3 The configuration of the shuttle vector used to insert the rPAP and hIL-2 expression cassettes into the FPV133R–FPV134R target site of FPV M3. pVHL04 plasmid is a pKG10a shuttle vector clone for recombining the rat-PAP (rPAP) and human-IL2 (hIL-2) expression cassettes into FPV M3 between ORFs PFV133 and FPV134R. In relation to Fig. 2, the F1 arm is FPV133R sequence and the F2 arm is FPV134R sequence. The rPAP and hIL-2 expression cassettes are flanked by both F1 and F2 arms. The reporter cassettes beta-galactosidase (betaGAL) and the *E. coli* guanine phosphoribosyltransferase (Ecogpt) are located outside of F1 and F2 arms. *Pr7.5* vaccinia virus p7.5 promoter, *prE/L* FPV early late promoter, *prL* FPV late promoter, *ampR* ampicillin resistance gene, *pUC ori* plasmid origin of replication

2 Materials

2.1 Stock Solutions and Materials

1. TrypLE Select (Gibco-Invitrogen, Mulgrave, Victoria, Australia) (*see* **Notes 1** and **2**).
2. Minimal Essential Media (MEM).
3. Fetal bovine serum (FBS).
4. Glutamax.
5. (4-(2-Hydroxyethyl)-1-piperazineethanesulfonic acid) (HEPES).
6. Gentamicin.
7. Mycophenolic acid (MPA) powder: 10 mg/mL stock in 0.1 M NaOH, filter sterilized, stored at −20 °C (Sigma-Aldrich, St. Louis, MO, USA).

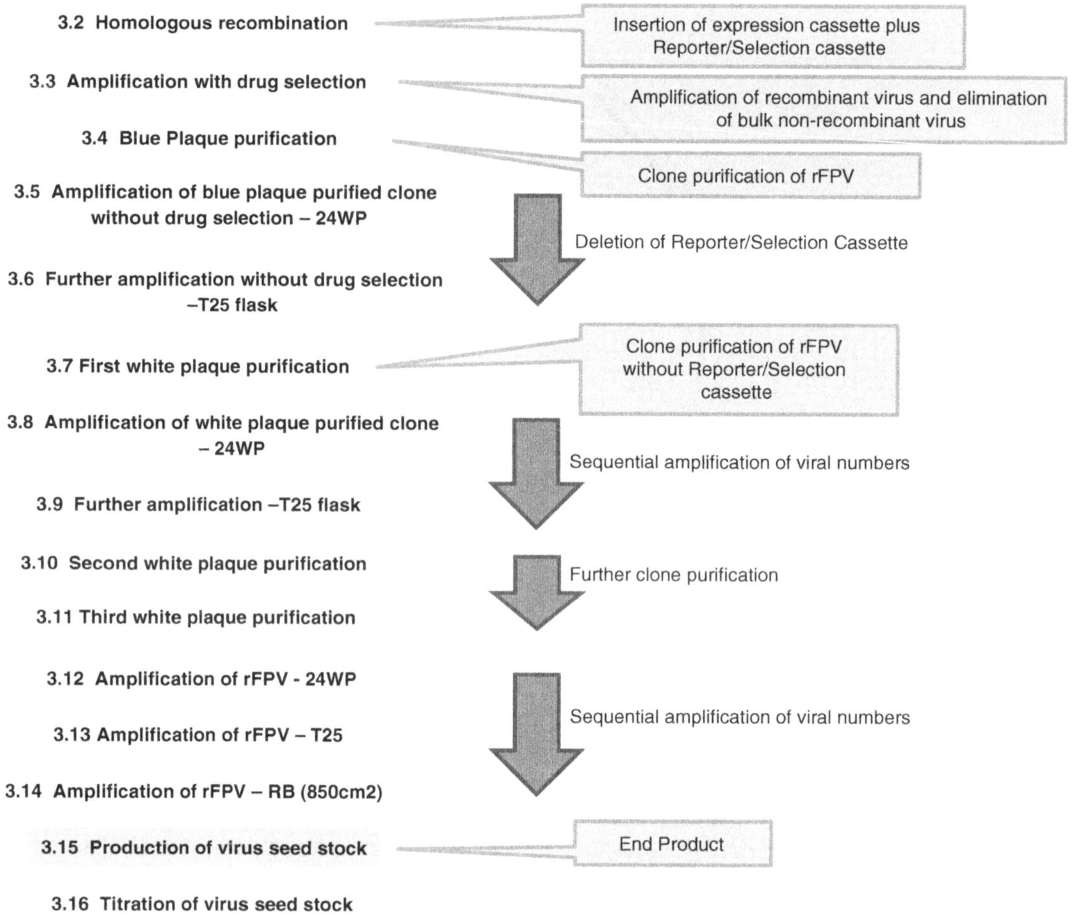

Fig. 4 Summary of the protocol steps used in our lab to construct recombinant FPVs employing the pKG10a shuttle vector as was the case for constructing VIR501

8. Xanthine powder: 10 mg/mL stock in 0.1 M NaOH, filter sterilized, stored at −20 °C.
9. HAT 50×, stored at −20 °C.
10. Stock Xgal: 50 mg/mL Xgal in sterile dimethyl sulfoxide (DMSO), stored at −20 °C.
11. Stock Neutral red (NR) 0.33 % solution.
12. Autoclaved stock 5 % low-temperature gelling agarose or low-melting point agarose in water.
13. Sterile 1 M stock Tris–HCl, pH.
14. Methanol.
15. Effectene kit (Qiagen, Valencia, CA, USA) (*see* **Note 3**).
16. Qiagen DNA extraction spin column kit (Qiagen) (*see* **Note 4**).
17. Autoclaved glass plugged Pasteur pipettes.

18. Autoclaved rubber teats for Pasteur pipettes.
19. 850-cm^2 tissue culture grade roller bottles.
20. Tissue culture grade T25-flasks (T25).
21. Tissue culture grade T150-flasks (T150).
22. Tissue culture grade 24-well plates (24-WP).
23. Tissue culture grade 60-mm dishes.
24. MantaRay single use cell culture vessels (LabSource, Romeoville, IL, USA) (*see* **Note 5**).
25. Sterile dissecting scissors and forceps.
26. Sterile disposable bottle for embryo digestion.
27. Sterile magnetic stir bar.
28. Sterile stainless-steel sieves 40-μm mesh (*see* **Note 6**).

2.2 Working Solutions for the Preparation of Chicken Embryo Fibroblast (CEF) Cells

1. Ten-day-old embryonated eggs (*see* **Note 7**).
2. 70 % Ethanol (EtOH).
3. Phosphate buffered saline (PBS) without calcium and magnesium.
4. TrypLE Select (Gibco-Invitrogen) Minimal Essential Media (MEM) plus 5 % FBS, 2-mM glutamax, 1-mM HEPES, 50 μg/mL of gentamicin.
5. Sterile dissecting scissors and forceps.
6. Sterile disposable bottle for embryo digestion.
7. Sterile magnetic stir bar.
8. Sterile stainless-steel sieves 40-μm mesh × 2.

2.3 Construction of VIR501

1. Primary extracted CEF cells and secondary cultured CEF cells.
2. Growth medium (GM): MEM, 5 % FBS, 10-mM HEPES, 2-mM glutamax, 0.05 mg/mL of gentamicin.
3. Maintenance medium (MM): MEM, 2 % FBS, 10-mM HEPES, 2-mM glutamax, 0.05 mg/mL of gentamicin.
4. MM plus MXHAT: MM plus 25 μg/mL of MPA, 250 μg/mL of Xanthine, 1× HAT.
5. PBS without calcium and magnesium.
6. 0.1-M Tris–HCl, pH 8, sterilized by autoclaving.
7. 10-mM Tris–HCl, pH 8, sterilized by autoclaving.

2.4 Titration Assay

1. Secondary cultured CEF cells.
2. GM (growth medium): MEM, 5 % FBS, 10-mM HEPES, 2-mM glutamax, 0.05 mg/mL gentamicin.
3. MM (maintenance medium): MEM, 2 % FBS, 10-mM HEPES, 2-mM glutamax, 0.05-mg/mL gentamicin.

3 Methods

3.1 Chicken Embryo Fibroblast Cells

1. Position the 10-day-old embryonated eggs with air space up and spray with 70 % EtOH or disinfectant effective against bacteria and fungi.
2. Crack the top of an egg with sterile dissecting scissors and cut off the shell to just above the membrane while keeping the latter intact. Remove membrane with sterile forceps. Repeat with remaining eggs (*see* **Note 8**).
3. Remove the embryo from each egg and combine in a sterile container containing 5 mL of PBS per embryo (*see* **Note 9**).
4. Rinse embryos 1× with PBS.
5. Remove head and feet from the embryos and place the rest of the body (trunk) into another sterile container containing 5 mL of PBS per embryo.
6. Put ten trunks into a 20-mL syringe and mince by squeezing through the syringe into a sterile digestion flask.
7. Add 5 mL of TrypLE Select per embryo prewarmed to room temperature (*see* **Notes 9** and **10**).
8. Incubate for 30 min at room temperature with stirring.
9. Decant fluid from the digestion bottle into a sterile stainless-steel 40 mesh sieve (*see* **Note 6**).
10. Pass the filtrate through another sterile stainless-steel 40 mesh sieve.
11. Centrifuge the filtrate for 10 min at $1,000 \times g$ at 20 °C.
12. Discard the supernatant and resuspend the cells in 10 mL PBS per original starting embryo (*see* **Note 9**).
13. Centrifuge the cells again for 10 min at $1,000 \times g$ at 20 °C.
14. Resuspend the cells in MEM plus 5 % FBS, 2-mM glutamax, 1-mM HEPES, and 50 μg/mL of gentamicin, and adjust the volume to 3 mL per original starting embryo (*see* **Note 9**).
15. The cells are ready for cell counting and can be stored for a week at 4 °C.
16. Seed 1×10^8 cells per roller bottle in 200 mL of MEM plus 5 % FBS, 2-mM glutamax, 1-mM HEPES, and 50 μg/mL of gentamicin, and incubate rolling at 35 °C (*see* **Note 11**).

3.2 Homologous Recombination (See Note 12)

3.2.1 CEF Cell Setup

Seed three T25-flasks each containing 5 mL of GM with 5×10^6 CEF cells and incubate at 35 °C/5 % CO_2 overnight.

3.2.2 Infection

When cells are subconfluent, i.e., 70–90 % confluent:

1. Dilute FPV M3 starting virus in GM to give a final concentration of 1×10^5 pfu/mL (minimum volume of 2 mL).
2. Remove medium from each flask and add 500 μL of diluted virus per flask. Ensure the liquid evenly coats the cell layer. This will give a multiplicity of infection of 0.01 pfu per cell.
3. Adsorb for 1 h at 35 °C/5 % CO_2.
4. Remove inoculum and add 4 mL of GM to each flask.

Flasks are now ready for transfection immediately; see next section below.

3.2.3 Transfection

This transfection method utilizes the Effectene Transfection kit (*see* **Note 3**).

Set up three transfection reactions and follow the method below based on one transfection per flask.

Warning: do not linearize the shuttle vector for transdominant plaque purification procedures.

1. Dilute 2 μg of shuttle vector DNA to a total volume of 150 μL with buffer EC and vortex to mix.
2. Add 8 μL of Enhancer to the diluted DNA and vortex.
3. Incubate at room temperature for 5 min standing.
4. Add 25 μL of Effectene Transfection Reagent to the DNA mix and vortex for 10 s.
5. Incubate at room temperature for 10 min.
6. Add 1 mL of GM to the DNA mix and *mix gently* by inversion.
7. Add the transfection mix to a flask already containing 4 mL of GM and gently rock to mix before incubating the flask overnight at 35 °C/5 % CO_2.

3.2.4 Medium Change

1. Day 1 post infection, remove transfection medium from each flask and wash cells with PBS.
2. Add 5 mL of MM per flask and incubate at 35 °C/5 % CO_2 until cytopathic effects can be seen in the cell monolayer.

3.2.5 Harvesting

Once substantial cytopathic effects or plaquing within monolayer can be seen (day 6 or 7 post infection):

1. Scrape cells into medium and pellet cells $1,000 \times g$ for 10 min.
2. Resuspend the cell pellets from all three flasks in 1-mL PBS and sonicate (*see* **Note 13**) until an even homogenate can be seen (sterilize sonication probe using 70 % ethanol flame before and after sonication) and store at −20 °C.

3.3 Amplification with Drug Selective Pressure (See Note 14)

3.3.1 Cell Setup

1. Seed five T150-flasks containing 50 mL of GM with 30×10^6 CEF cells and incubate at 35 °C/5 % CO_2 until cell monolayer has reached 100 % confluency.
2. At 100 % confluency, remove medium and replace with 50 mL per flask MM plus MXHAT and incubate at 35 °C/5 % CO_2 overnight.

3.3.2 Infection

1. Thaw homologous recombination virus from the section above.
2. For infection per flask, mix 200 μL of viral stock with 200 μL of TrypLE Select (*see* **Note 2**) and incubate at 37 °C for 30 min.
3. Add digested virus to 5 mL of MM plus MXHAT to quench the digestion.
4. Remove medium from T150-flask and add the 5 mL of diluted TrypLE digested virus to each flask. Rock the flask gently to ensure monolayer is evenly covered and incubate at 35 °C/5 % CO_2 for 1 h.
5. To each flask, add 50 mL of MM plus MXHAT and incubate at 35 °C/5 % CO_2 for 5–7 days.
6. Check the monolayer for the appearance of plaques after day 4 post infection.

3.3.3 Harvesting

Harvest when plaquing or substantial cytopathic effects within monolayer can be seen (day 4–6 post infection). If not, harvest at day 6 post infection.

1. Scrape cells into medium and pellet cells at $1{,}000 \times g$ for 10 min.
2. Resuspend cells in 2-mL PBS and sonicate until an even homogenate can be seen (sterilize sonication probe using 70 % ethanol flame before and after sonication) (*see* **Note 13**).
3. Store viral extract at −20 °C.

3.3.4 Analysis for the Presence of rFPV

1. Extract total DNA from 200 μL of virus using a Qiagen DNA extraction spin column kit—follow protocol for extracting DNA from whole blood given in the instruction kit manual (*see* **Note 4**).
2. Using 5–10 μL of template DNA from above and PCR primers specific for targeting the foreign sequence inserted into the FPV, carry out a PCR reaction for 10–15 cycles of amplification.
3. Electrophoreses 5–10 μL of the PCR reaction in an agarose gel.

If the amplification of recombinant virus has worked well, PCR amplification of target sequence should be clearly detected by agarose gel electrophoresis after 10 or 15 PCR cycles. If not, carry out further round of viral amplification with drug selection until PCR product can be detected after 10 or 15 PCR cycles—another two rounds of amplification maybe required.

3.4 First Clone Purification: Blue Plaque Selection Without Drug Selection (See Note 15)

3.4.1 Cell Setup

Seed 21 60-mm dishes with 5 mL per dish of secondary CEFs (*see* **Note 16**) at 8.4×10^5 cells/mL and incubate plates at 35 °C/5 % CO_2 until cells reach 100 % confluency.

3.4.2 Infection

1. Add 100 μL of amplified virus to 900 μL of TrypLE Select and incubate at 37 °C for 30 min (*see* **Note 2**).
2. Add the 1-mL digested virus to 9 mL of MM to quench the digestion—this equals approximately a 10^{-2} dilution.
3. From this prepare serial dilutions, i.e., 0.5 mL of virus plus 4.5 mL of MM down to a 10^{-7} dilution.
4. For each dilution, starting at 10^{-3}, infect four dishes by adding 1 mL of serially diluted virus to each dish after removing GM and incubate at 35 °C/5 % CO_2 for 1 h. With the remaining plate, dummy infect with PBS and process as with the others. This will be your cell control (*see* **Note 17**).
5. Add 4 mL of MM to each dish and incubate at 35 °C/5 % CO_2 until plaques start to develop.

3.4.3 Addition of Xgal Agarose Overlay

1. Set up 3×50-mL tubes containing the following: 40 mL of MM, 750 μL of NR stock solution, 300 μL of Xgal stock solution.
2. Warm and maintain tubes at 37 °C in a water bath.
3. Melt the 5 % low-temperature gelling agarose in a microwave and leave to stand until ready for use (*see* **Note 18**).
4. Remove seven dishes from incubator and aspirate off the culture medium.
5. Take one tube from water bath and spray down with 70 % ethanol and top up the tube with molten agarose to the 50 mL mark. Be careful agarose bottle will still be very hot.
6. Gently mix by inverting the tube several times, and when the tube feels warm to the touch, carefully add 5 mL of agarose solution to each plate. Do not rush. There is plenty of time before the agarose begins to set.
7. Leave the dishes to set undisturbed before transferring them back to the incubator.

8. Repeat these steps for the next seven dishes.
9. Incubate plates at 35 °C/5 % CO_2 for 1 day until blue plaques can be clearly seen.

3.4.4 Harvesting Blue Plaques

1. Identify the highest dilution plate that has the smallest number of blue plaques well separated from each other, and using a marker pen, circle approximately ten blue plaques.
2. Using a sterile glass plugged Pasteur pipette and a sterile rubber suction teat, pick all the circled plaques and dispense into 1.5-mL microfuge tubes containing 500 μL of PBS. Use a fresh Pasteur pipette for each plaque pick.
3. Briefly sonicate each tube (approximately 3–5 s burst) remembering to sterilize the sonication probe using 70 % ethanol flame before sonication and after last sonication (*see* **Note 13**).
4. Store each tube (clone) at −20 °C.

3.5 Amplification of Blue Plaque Clones in 24-WP (See Note 20)

3.5.1 Cell Setup

Seed one 24-WP with 1 mL per well of CEF at 4×10^5 cells/mL and incubate plates at 35 °C/5 % CO_2 until cells have reached 100 % confluency.

3.5.2 Infection

1. For each blue plaque clone, take 100 μL and add 100 μL of TrypLE Select and incubate at 37 °C for 30 min (*see* **Note 2**).
2. Add 800 μL of MM to each clone to quench the digestion.
3. Remove medium from each well and add 1 mL of each digested clone to separates wells.
4. Incubate plate at 35 °C/5 % CO_2 until signs of infection can be seen.

3.5.3 Harvesting

1. Using a 1-mL pipette with a 1-mL plugged tip (use a fresh tip for each well), dispense medium up and down to detach the cells from the well.
2. Transfer the cell suspension to a sterile 1.5-mL tube and pellet the cells by centrifugation at $1,000 \times g$ for 5 min.
3. Discard liquid and resuspend the cell pellet in 500 μL of PBS. Briefly sonicate each tube (approximately 3 s burst) remembering to sterilize the sonication probe using 70 % ethanol flame before sonication and after last sonication (*see* **Note 13**).
4. Store each tube (clone) at −20 °C.

3.6 Amplification of 24-WP Clones in T25-flasks (See Note 19)

3.6.1 Cell Setup

1. Seed one T25-flask per clone with 5 mL of CEF at 1×10^6 cells/mL and incubate at 35 °C/5 % CO_2 until cells reach confluency.

3.6.2 Infection

1. For each clone add 500 μL of virus clone to 500 μL of TrypLE Select and incubate at 37 °C for 30 min (*see* **Note 2**).
2. Add 4 mL of MM to quench the digestion.
3. Remove the medium from each flask and add the digested virus, one clone per flask, and incubate at 35 °C/5 % CO_2 for 4–6 days.

3.6.3 Harvesting

1. Scrape the cells into the medium and recover all by sucking up and dispensing into a sterile 15-mL centrifuge tube, and pellet the cells by centrifuging at 1,000 × *g* for 5 min in a centrifuge.
2. Discard the supernatant and resuspend the cell pellet in 1-mL PBS and briefly sonicate each tube (3–4 s burst) remembering to sterilize the sonication probe using 70 % ethanol flame before sonication and after last sonication (*see* **Note 13**).
3. Store each tube at −20 °C.

3.6.4 Analysis for the Presence of rFPV

1. Extract total DNA from 200 μL of virus using a Qiagen DNA extraction spin column kit. Follow protocol for extracting DNA from whole blood (*see* **Note 4**).
2. Using 5–10 μL of template DNA from above and PCR primers specific for targeting the foreign sequence inserted into the FPV, carry out a PCR reaction for 25 cycles of amplification.
3. Electrophorese 5–10 μL of the PCR reaction in an agarose gel and identify the clones that give best amplification of targeted sequence.

3.7 First White Plaque Purification (See Note 20)

Use the best clone from above for the first plaque purification. Repeat Subheading 3.4, except this time you are looking for white plaques to pick. Pick about 10–20 white plaques.

3.8 Amplification of White Plaque Clones in 24-WP (See Note 21)

Repeat Subheading 3.5.

3.9 Amplification of 24-WP Clones in T25-flasks (See Note 21)

Repeat Subheading 3.6.

3.9.1 Amplification

3.9.2 Analysis for the Presence of Contaminating Parental Vector

1. Extract total DNA from 200 μL of virus using a Qiagen DNA extraction spin column kit—follow protocol given in the kit instruction manual for extracting DNA from whole blood (*see* **Note 4**).

2. Using 5–10 μL of template DNA from above and PCR primers specific for targeting the foreign sequence inserted into the FPV and primers to detect parental virus, i.e., priming the genomic sequences flanking the insertion site, carry out a PCR reaction for 35 cycles of amplification.
3. Electrophorese 5–10 μL of the PCR reaction in an agarose gel and identify clones that give best amplification of target sequence and no contaminating original parental virus.

3.10 Second White Plaque Purification (See Note 22)

Use the five clones from above for third plaque purification.

3.10.1 Cell Setup

1. Seed 25 × 60-mm dishes with 5-mL per dish of secondary CEFs at 8.4×10^5 cells/mL and incubate plates at 35 °C/5 % CO_2 until cells have reach 100 % confluency.

3.10.2 Infection

1. For each clone, add 100 μL of amplified virus to 100 μL of TrypLE Select and incubate at 37 °C for 30 min.
2. Add 800 μL of MM to digestion. This is equal to a 10^{-1} dilution.
3. From this prepare serial dilution, i.e., 0.1 mL of virus plus 0.9 mL of MM down to 10^{-5} dilution.
4. For each dilution starting at 10^{-1}, infect one dish per serial dilution with the entire serial dilution volume, i.e., 0.9 mL, after removing GM and then incubate at 35 °C/5 % CO_2 for 1 h.
5. Add 4 mL of MM to each dish and incubate at 35 °C/5 % CO_2 until plaques start to develop.

3.10.3 Addition of Xgal Agarose Overlay

Repeat Subheading 3.4.3.

3.10.4 Harvesting White Plaques

Repeat Subheading 3.7.

3.11 Third White Plaque Purification (See Note 22)

Use the five clones from above for third plaque purification.

Repeat Subheading 3.10.

3.12 Amplification of White Plaque Clones in 24-WP (See Note 21)

Repeat Subheading 3.5.

3.13 Amplification of 24-WP clones in T25-flasks dishes (See Note 21)

Repeat Subheading 3.6.

3.13.1 Amplification of Clones

3.13.2 Analysis for the Presence of Contaminating Parental Vector

1. Extract total DNA from 200 μL of virus using a Qiagen DNA extraction spin column kit. Follow protocol given in the kit instruction manual for extracting DNA from whole blood (*see* **Note 4**).
2. Using 5–10 μL of template DNA from above and PCR primers specific for targeting the foreign sequence inserted into the FPV and primers to detect parental virus, i.e., priming the genomic sequences flanking the insertion site, carry out a PCR reaction for 35 cycles of amplification.
3. Electrophorese 5–10 μL of the PCR reaction in an agarose gel and identify clones that give best amplification of target sequence and no contaminating original parental virus.

3.14 Amplification of Best Clones in Roller Bottles (See Note 21)

Amplify all clones that are positive for insertion and negative parental virus by amplification of one clone per roller bottle.

3.14.1 Cell Setup

Seed one roller bottle per clone containing 200 mL with 1×10^8 cells/mL of CEF and incubate at 35 °C until cells reach confluency.

3.14.2 Infection

1. For each clone, add 500 μL of virus clone to 500 μL of TrypLE Select and incubate at 37 °C for 30 min (*see* **Note 2**).
2. Add 25 mL of MM to quench the digestion.
3. Remove the medium from each roller bottle and add the digested virus, one clone per roller bottle, and incubate at 35 °C for 4–6 days.

3.14.3 Harvesting

1. Recover the infected cell and medium into a 250-mL centrifuge tube and pellet the cells by centrifuging at $1{,}000 \times g$ for 10 min.
2. Discard the supernatant and resuspend the cell pellet in 5-mL PBS and sonicate resuspended cells until an even homogenate can be seen. Remember to sterilize the sonication probe using 70 % ethanol flame before sonication and after last sonication (*see* **Note 13**).
3. Store each tube at −20 °C.

3.14.4 Analysis for the Presence of Contaminating Parental Vector

1. Extract total DNA from 200 μL of virus using a Qiagen DNA extraction spin column kit—follow protocol for extracting DNA from whole blood (*see* **Note 4**).
2. Using 5–10 μL of template DNA from above and PCR primers specific for targeting the foreign sequence inserted into the FPV and primers to detect parental virus, i.e., primers targeting genomic sequences flanking the insertion site, carry out a PCR reaction for 35 cycles of amplification for testing for original parental virus contamination and 10–15 cycle to detect target sequence.
3. Electrophorese 5–10 μL of the PCR reaction in an agarose gel and identify the clone that gives best amplification of target sequence after 10–15 PCR cycles and show no signs of contaminating original parental virus after 35 PCR cycles.

3.15 Amplification and Processing of Best Clone to Produce Virus Seed Stock (VSS) in 4 × 1 L MantaRays (See Note 23)

3.15.1 Preparation of Virus for Infection

To 1 mL of best virus clone, add 1 mL of TrypLE Select and incubate at 37 °C for 30 min (*see* **Note 2**).

3.15.2 MantaRay Seeding and Infection (See Note 23)

1. To the four MantaRays, add 1 L of MEM with glutamax, HEPES, and gentamicin to each.
2. To each MantaRay, add 1×10^9 CEF cells freshly prepared from embryos and gently mix into the medium. The final cell density will be 1×10^6 cells/mL.
3. Add 500 μL of viral digest to each MantaRay and gently mix into cell suspension.
4. Incubate the four MantaRay with gentle stirring at 37 °C/5 % CO_2 for 5 days and then harvest.

3.15.3 Harvesting and Purification (See Note 24)

1. Recover the infected cells and medium into 500-mL centrifuge tubes and pellet the cells by centrifuging at $2,000 \times g$ for 5 min.
2. Discard the supernatants and resuspend all the cell pellets in 50 mL of TrypLE Select and sonicate using a probe appropriate to the volume being sonicated. Sonicate until an even homogenate can be seen remembering to sterilize the sonication probe using 70 % ethanol flame before start of sonication and after last sonication (*see* **Note 13**).
3. Top up the homogenate to 140 mL by adding an extra 100 mL of TrypLE Select to the centrifuge tube and gently mix and incubate at 37 °C for 45 min (*see* **Note 2**).

4. Centrifuge at 1,000 × *g* for 10 min at 4 °C to pellet insoluble debris and recentrifuge the supernatant to pellet any carryover of insolubles.
5. Add 45 mL of digest to a high-speed 50-mL centrifuge tubes (sterilized by autoclaving) and seal tube with its screw on cap or push on cap and centrifuge at 15,000 × *g* for 1 h at 6 °C to pellet the virus out of solution.
6. Carefully remove liquid from the tube without disturbing the viral pellet and resuspend each viral pellet in 10 mL (*see* **Note 9**) of 10-mM Tris–HCl, pH 8. The pellet will be tightly compacted and may require a brief sonication pulse to loosen it up.
7. Pool the resuspended viral pellets into sterile 50-mL tube and store each tube at −80 °C until ready for titration and PCR analysis.
8. After titration (*see* Subheading 3.16), dilute the virus to a desired titer, e.g., 1×10^8 or 1×10^9 pfu/mL with more than 10-mM Tris–HCl, pH 8, and aliquot into 1-mL lots for storage at −80 °C.

3.15.4 Analysis for the Presence of Contaminating Parental Vector

1. Extract total DNA from 200 μL of virus using a Qiagen DNA extraction spin column kit—follow protocol for extracting DNA from whole blood (*see* **Note 4**).
2. Using 5–10 μL of template DNA from above and PCR primers specific for targeting the foreign sequence inserted into the FPV and primers to detect parental virus, i.e., PCR primer targeting genomic flanking the insertion site, carry out a PCR reaction for 35 cycles of amplification for testing for original parental virus contamination and 10–15 cycle to detect target sequence.
3. Electrophorese 5–10 μL of the PCR reaction in an agarose gel.
4. The VSS should still have target sequence and still be free of original parental virus.

3.16 Titration of Recombinant FPV

Titration of FPV or rFPV is best done using secondary CEF cells cultured in 60-mm dishes (*see* **Note 16**). Plaque formation occurs between day 4 and day 5 post infection. Plaques are visibly seen as translucent/opaque foci of infection within the monolayer.

3.16.1 Cell Setup

Titration done in triplicates plates for each serial dilution.

1. For each virus to be titered, seed 18 × 60-mm dishes with 2×10^6 secondary cultured CEF cells per dish in 4 mL of growth medium and incubate at 37 °C/5 % CO_2 until the secondary CEF cell cultures reaches 100 % confluency.
2. Serially dilute the virus in tenfold dilution by adding 500 μL of virus or previous dilution to 4.5 mL of MM down to 10^{-10} dilution.

3. Remove the growth medium from each dish, and starting from the 10^{-10} dilution and ending with 10^{-5} dilution, add 1 mL of each serial dilution to each dish (three dishes per dilution).
4. Adsorb virus for 45 min at 35 °C/5 % CO_2.
5. Add 4 mL of MM to each plate and incubate dishes at 35 °C/5 % CO_2 for 4–6 days until plaques can be seen.
6. Remove medium from each plate and add 2–5 mL of methanol, and then leave plates in methanol for 10 min to fix the cells.
7. Remove the methanol and let the dishes air-dry.
8. Count only the dishes that have around 15–50 plaques (around 30 plaques/dish being preferred for titration calculation).

3.16.2 Calculation of Titration in pfu/mL

1. For the dilution that results in around 30 plaques per plate or at least in the 15–50 plaque count range, calculate the average from replicate plates.
2. Multiply this figure with the reciprocal of the dilution used.
3. Multiply resultant figure (above) with volume in the number of milliliters of inoculating virus, in the above case multiply by 1 as the inoculating volume was 1 mL.
4. The resulting figure is the titer expressed as pfu/mL.
5. Calculating the standard deviation or standard error will tell you to which decimal point the titration can reliably be cited.

Example:

1. The following counts were found on the 10^{-6} dilution plates: 29, 35, 37.
2. The average being, 33.667.
3. The titration is calculated as follows: $33.667 \times 1 \times 10^6 = 33.667 \times 10^6 = 3.3667 \times 10^7$ pfu/mL.
4. Standard deviation calculated to be 3.4×10^6. Therefore, the titration can be estimated to be no more than 34×10^6 or 3.4×10^7 pfu/mL.

4 Notes

1. TrypLE Select is a recombinant protease of nonanimal origin and can be used as a substitute for trypsin. It comes as a ready to use solution, more stable than trypsin, and we find it less aggressive to tissue culture cells than trypsin but just as active as trypsin. In these sets of protocols, TrypLE is used for dissociating single cells from macerated chicken embryos, digestion of crude viral extracts, and to help increase infectivity and to dissociate cell monolayers.

2. TrypLE Select digestion is employed to increase the infectivity of FPV viral preps made from whole cell extracts.
3. Alternative methods of transfecting DNA into tissue culture cells can be used. Qiagen's Effectene reagent was employed in the protocol as this works well with primary cell cultures and difficult to transfect cell lines.
4. Alternative genomic DNA extraction kits can be used from other manufacturers or supplies. Always follow the manufacturer's protocol for extracting DNA from liquid starting samples.
5. Alternative liquid culturing systems for culturing mammalian and avian cell line as suspension cultures can be used, e.g., spinner flasks.
6. Alternative cell sieving devices or apparatuses can be used as an alternative or just use multiple layers of sterile muslin or cheese cloths lining a glass sterile funnel.
7. Various region-specific chicken hatcheries can be used as suppliers of embryonated chicken eggs to produce recombinant FPV M3 for experimental laboratory use. It is however preferred to access eggs from brood stock which have not been vaccinated against FPV infection. Of course, specific pathogen-free eggs from authorized and certified producers must be used where resultant viruses are destined for clinical applications.
8. Healthy eggs have well-formed blood vessels.
9. General rule of thumb—approximately 10 mL of Tris–HCl, pH 8, is a convenient volume for manipulation purposes.
10. Trypsin/EDTA can be used as an alternative, use at a final concentration of 0.25 % w/v trypsin/0.02 % w/v EDTA.
11. Chicken embryonic cells grow better at 35 °C than 37 °C.
12. Homologous recombination is an in vivo process of recombining in a site-specific manner foreign DNA sequences into the genome of FPV. Refer to Fig. 2 for the mechanism of gene insertion into FPV M3 using the shuttle vector pKG10a harboring the gene of interest.
13. If a sonicator is not available, several rounds of freeze-thawing can be employed with vigorous vortexing during the thawing cycle. Three cycles of freeze-thawing is normally adopted to release poxviruses from infected cells.
14. This step is designed to amplify the number of newly created recombinant virus and to eliminate bulk nonrecombinant virus.
15. This step is designed to clone purify several recombinant viral clones.
16. Plaques occur as translucent to opaque foci of infection within the cell monolayer. These become difficult to see in heterogeneous monolayers and contain many different types as in the case

of primary CEF cell monolayers. However, secondary CEF cell monolayers are more homogenous and preferential to primary CEFs when visual identification of plaques is important.

17. Comparing the uninfected cell monolayer to the infected monolayer will help train the eye to recognize translucent plaques and subtle cytopathic effects occurring in the monolayer caused by a productive infection.
18. Molten 5 % low-temperature gelling agarose is "superheated" and therefore extremely hot and slow to cool down. Be careful when handling molten agarose as it can cause severe burns.
19. This step is designed to sequentially amplify the viral numbers of each plaque-purified clone to enable further manipulation and to encourage the second intramolecular crossover event to take place (as outlined in Fig. 2) in order to delete the reporter/selection cassette from the recombinant virus.
20. This step is designed to isolate recombinant virus clones that have deleted their reporter/selection cassette via the second crossover event. Bear in mind at this stage there is a 50 % chance that the clone giving rise to a white plaque maybe a nonrecombinant virus as demonstrated in Fig. 2.
21. Sequential amplification of viral numbers.
22. This step is designed to ensure the elimination of trace contamination of nonrecombinant virus.
23. Freshly prepared CEF cells seeded into a suspension culture do not require FBS in the growth medium to maintain growth and viability of the cells during culturing. In the absence of a viral infection, the cells aggregate to form uniform spheres of cell mass which progressively get larger with time. However, when cells are coinfected upon seeding, these cell spheres are absent or retarded in their growth and eventually disappear. This observation has been used as a "marker" of a productive infection taking place.
24. This step involves the partial purification of the recombinant virus by pelleting the virus from the clarified whole cell extract and resuspending in 10-mM Tris–HCl, pH 8. In this purified form in Tris buffer, we have found the recombinant virus to be extremely stable upon multiple freeze-thaw cycles when stored as −70 to 80 °C.

Acknowledgment

J.D.H. is in receipt of research funding support from Sementis Ltd. P.M.H. is the Chief Scientific Officer, co-founder, and a major shareholder of Sementis Ltd. K.R.D. is supported by a training fellowship and grant from the National Health and Medical Research Council of Australia.

References

1. Brun A et al (2008) Antigen delivery systems for veterinary vaccine development. Viral-vector based delivery systems. Vaccine 26: 6508–6528
2. Beukema EL et al (2006) The potential role of fowlpox virus in rational vaccine design. Expert Rev Vaccines 5:565–577
3. Lousberg EL et al (2011) Innate immune recognition of poxviral vaccine vectors. Expert Rev Vaccines 10:1435–1449
4. Tulman ER et al (2004) The genome of canarypox virus. J Virol 78:353–366
5. Soboll G et al (2010) Onset and duration of immunity to equine influenza virus resulting from canarypox-vectored (ALVAC®) vaccination. Vet Immunol Immunopathol 135:100–107
6. Seino KK et al (2007) Comparative efficacies of three commercially available vaccines against West Nile Virus (WNV) in a short-duration challenge trial involving an equine WNV encephalitis model. Clin Vaccine Immunol 14:1465–1471
7. Larson LJ, Schultz RD (2007) Three-year duration of immunity in dogs vaccinated with a canarypox-vectored recombinant canine distemper virus vaccine. Vet Ther 8:101–106
8. Taylor J et al (1994) Applications of canarypox (ALVAC) vectors in human and veterinary vaccination. Dev Biol Stand 82:131–135
9. Gilbert PB et al (2003) Long-term safety analysis of preventive HIV-1 vaccines evaluated in AIDS vaccine evaluation group NIAID-sponsored phase I and II clinical trials. Vaccine 21:2933–2947
10. Rerks-Ngarm S et al (2009) Vaccination with ALVAC and AIDSVAX to prevent HIV-1 infection in Thailand. N Engl J Med 361:2209–2220
11. Gonczol E, Plotkin S (2001) Development of a cytomegalovirus vaccine: lessons from recent clinical trials. Expert Opin Biol Ther 1: 401–412
12. Tartaglia J et al (2001) Therapeutic vaccines against melanoma and colorectal cancer. Vaccine 19:2571–2575
13. Boyle DB, Coupar BE (1988) Construction of recombinant fowlpox viruses as vectors for poultry vaccines. Virus Res 10:343–356
14. Taylor J et al (1988) Protective immunity against avian influenza induced by a fowlpox virus recombinant. Vaccine 6:504–508
15. Taylor J et al (1990) Newcastle disease virus fusion protein expressed in a fowlpox virus recombinant confers protection in chickens. J Virol 64:1441–1450
16. French MA et al (2010) Vaccine-induced IgG2 anti-HIV p24 is associated with control of HIV in patients with a 'high affinity' FcγRIIa genotype. AIDS 24:1983–1990
17. Baxby D, Paoletti E (1992) Potential use of non-replicating vectors as recombinant vaccines. Vaccine 10:8–9
18. Taylor J, Paoletti E (1988) Fowlpox virus as a vector in non-avian species. Vaccine 6: 466–467
19. Beard CW et al (1991) Protection of chickens against highly pathogenic avian influenza virus (H5N2) by recombinant fowlpox viruses. Avian Dis 35:356–359
20. Emery S et al (2007) Influence of IFNgamma co-expression on the safety and antiviral efficacy of recombinant fowlpox virus HIV therapeutic vaccines following interruption of antiretroviral therapy. Hum Vaccin 3:260–267
21. Emery S et al (2005) Randomized, placebo-controlled, phase I/IIa evaluation of the safety and immunogenicity of fowlpox virus expressing HIV gag-pol and interferon-gamma in HIV-1 infected subjects. Hum Vaccin 1: 232–238
22. Falkner FG, Moss B (1990) Transient dominant selection of recombinant vaccinia viruses. J Virol 64:3108–3111

Chapter 33

Bacterial Vectors for the Delivery of Tumor Antigens

Yan Wang, Bertrand Toussaint, and Audrey Le Gouëllec

Abstract

The use of bacterial vectors, which offer ease of production and efficiency, has become an important mechanism for the delivery of protein antigens to antigen-presenting cells (APCs) in vivo. Proof of concept studies has been carried out utilizing different bacteria in various cancer models with some in clinical trials. Here we described the way to prepare *Pseudomonas aeruginosa* (*P. aeruginosa*) vaccines based on a virulence-attenuated strain to test the efficacy of different fragments of a well-known tumor antigen. This protocol could be applied to efficacy studies in murine models of human cancers.

Key words *P. aeruginosa*, Antigen cloning, Secretion, Vaccination

1 Introduction

In the last decade, the use of bacterial vectors, such as *Salmonella* spp., *Listeria monocytogenes*, and *P. aeruginosa*, has attracted more and more attention for their potential use in cancer vaccine development [1–4]. Indeed, in order to generate and maintain a potent adaptive cellular immune response, stimulation of the innate immune system and adequate antigen delivery are both crucial. Recent advances in bacterial engineering, molecular biology, and our understanding of pathogenic bacterial biology have significantly accelerated the rational design of bacterial vectors. As a delivery system, they offer multiple advantages: (1) there are several well-characterized virulence-attenuating mutations; (2) the number, the amount, and the in vivo location of antigen expression can be regulated; (3) multiple vaccine delivery routes are possible; and (4) they potently stimulate the innate and adaptive immune systems.

Naturally, *P. aeruginosa* possesses a type III secretion system (T3SS), a critical virulence factor used by a broad range of gram negative pathogens, e.g., *Salmonella*, *Shigella*, *Yersinia*, and *Pseudomonas*. T3SS is a finely regulated system dedicated to the delivery of toxic proteins (exotoxins) into the cytoplasm of

Michael J.P. Lawman and Patricia D. Lawman (eds.), *Cancer Vaccines: Methods and Protocols*, Methods in Molecular Biology, vol. 1139, DOI 10.1007/978-1-4939-0345-0_33,

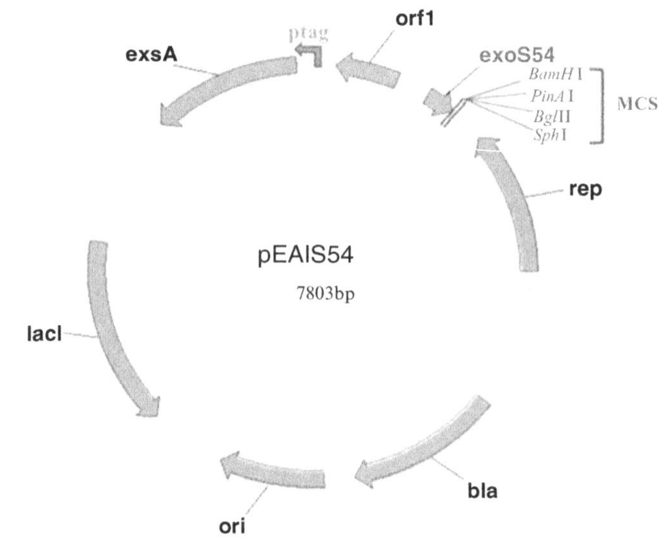

Fig. 1 The construction of pEAIS54. The plasmid pEAIS54 (JQ733380) contains the following: (1) the sequence of *exsA* gene which encode the transcriptional activator of total genes of T3SS. Here, the expression of *exsA* gene is under the control of one IPTG inducible promoter (ptac). (2) Multiple cloning sites (MCS) to clone the insert. The *ExoS54* sequence encodes the secretion tag. TRP2, TRP2L, and TRP2S fragments are cloned at *Bam*HI/*Sph*I sites. (3) The sequence of *lacI* gene which encodes the repressor of ptac. In non-induced situation, ptac is coupled with LacI and the transcription of ExsA is inhibited. With the presence of the ligand, IPTG, the quiescent effect imparted by LacI to ptac can be eliminated, consequently *ExsA* gene will be transcribed and T3SS genes will be expressed. (4) The sequence of *bla* gene encoding b-lactamase which allow specific antibiotic resistance for plasmid selection

host cells [5]. *P. aeruginosa* uses its T3SS to target immune cells such as polymorphonuclear neutrophils or antigen-presenting cells (APCs). We use a toxicity-attenuated *P. aeruginosa* strain in which all of the major secreted exotoxins are absent (ExoU), or deleted (ExoS, ExoT), and are unable to disseminate in vivo due to an *aroA* gene deletion which is responsible for aromatic amino acids synthesis [6]. We constructed a plasmid, pEAIS54 (Fig. 1), to easily clone antigen in fusion with 54 first amino acid of the exotoxin S (S54) which could further address the whole protein to the T3SS. Besides, this plasmid also contains an episomal copy of the ExsA activator of T3SS which is under the control of the anisopropylβ-D-1-thiogalactopyranoside (IPTG)-inducible promoter [7].

This system is also a useful tool for other applications that require high throughput screening of antigen(s) for use in immunotherapy protocols [8]. It is also useful for monitoring the effect of immunomodulators molecules in a well-established murine tumor model. The protocol described here was designed for efficacy screening of three different fragment of the tyrosinase-related protein 2 (TRP2), a well-known tumor-associated antigen (TAA) in glioma and melanoma. The protocol comprises the following steps: (1) polymerase chain reaction (PCR) amplification of the different inserts, (2) cloning in the pEAI54 plasmid and preparation for *E. coli* and transformation of plasmids in *P. aeruginosa*, (3) control of expression and secretion through T3SS of the different inserts, (4) storing of strains and culturing of strains before vaccination experiments, and (5) an example of a vaccination experiments in mice.

2 Materials

Prepare all solutions using ultrapure water (prepared by purifying deionized water).

2.1 Cloning Components

1. PCR: For example, the TRP2 encoding gene has been amplified by RT-PCR from the GL26 cells line and was used as template DNA. All primers used for antigen amplifications were commercially synthesized by (Metabion, Martinsried, Germany) and listed in Table 1: *PfuUltra*™ HF DNA polymerase (Stratagene, Massy, France), *PfuUltra*™ HF reaction buffer (Stratagene), dNTPs (Invitrogen, Saint Aubin, France), and Thermal cycler Mastercycler® Gradient (Eppendorf, NY, NY, USA).
2. Antigen cloning vector: In this work, pEAIS54 (JQ733380) was used as the antigen cloning vector for TAA expression. This plasmid has been constructed in our laboratory (Fig. 1).
3. Restriction enzymes, i.e., *Bam*HI and *Sph*I, and relative digestion buffers.
4. Rapid DNA Ligation Kit (Roche, Meylan, France).
5. QIAprep Spin Miniprep Kit and QIAquick Gel Extraction Kit (Qiagen, Courtaboeuf, France).

2.2 Agarose Gel Electrophoresis Components

1. Electrophoresis buffer: 40 mM Tris-Amino, 20 mM Acetate, 1 mM EDTA, pH 8. Dilute the 10× stock solution with H_2O to generate a 1× working solution immediately before use.
2. Agarose gel (1–2 %) (*see* **Note 1**): Dissolve 1–2 g ultrapure agarose powder (Invitrogen) in 100 mL electrophoresis buffer by heating the slurry in a microwave oven. Add 0.5 μg/mL ethidium bromide to the mixture. Shape gel at room temperature in a mold containing an appropriate comb for forming the sample slots.
3. 6× gel-loading buffer.
4. Molecular weight DNA ladder marker.
5. RunOne™ Electrophoresis apparatus with power supply device (EmbiTec, San Diego, CA, USA).
6. UV device (Bioblock Scientific, Illkirch, France).

Table 1
Primers used in PCR for antigens amplification

Name	Forward primer	Reverse primer
TRP2	AAGGATCCAGACGGAATATCCATTCCCTGACT	AAGCATGCTTACAACGCAAAGGACTCATTGCCA G
TRP2L	AAGGATCCA GACGGAATATCCATTCCCTGACT	AAGCA TGCTTACTTGCGGAAGGAGTGAGCCAAGTTATGAAG
TRP2S	AAGGATCCGACTACAACCGCCGGGTCACA	AAGCA TGCTTACTTGCGGAAGGAGTGAGCCAAGTTATGAAG
Sequencing	GCCAATCCTGATAGGCGATG	CGACTAACCCAGATGCCGCTG

2.3 Bacteria Strains

1. Competent Library efficient *Escherichia coli* DH5α strain (*E. coli*, DH5α) (Invitrogen).
2. *Pseudomonas aeruginosa* CHA-OAL strain is a mutant of the CHA strain (a mucoid strain isolated from the lungs of a cystic fibrosis patient) with the deletion of *exoS*, *exoT*, *aroA*, and *lasI* genes. This mutant line has been constructed in our laboratory and is recognized as non-virulent by the French Committee "Haut Conseil des Biotechnologies" rendering its manipulation as easy as *E. coli* laboratory strains [6].

2.4 Bacteria Manipulation Components

For bacteria culture, all media should be sterilized by autoclaving at 121 °C, 1.05 kg/cm^2 for 20 min.

1. Luria broth (LB) medium: Add 25 g LB Base powder into 0.5 L water. Mix well and make up to 1 L with water.
2. LB plates: Add 25 g LB Base powder and 15 g agar powder into 0.5 L water. Mix well and make up to 1 L with water. After sterilization, cool down medium to 45 °C, supplement with antibiotic as needed, and pour about 30 mL per 100 mm Petri dish. Allow to solidify overnight at room temperature.
3. Pseudomonas Isolation Agar (PIA) plates: Add 45 g Pseudomonas isolation agar and add 20 mL glycerol into 0.5 L water. Mix well and make up to 1 L with water. Following sterilization, cool down the medium, supplement with antibiotic as needed, and shape PIA plate at room temperature.
4. Super optimal broth with catabolite repression (SOC) medium: 2 % tryptone, 0.5 % yeast extract, 10 mM sodium chloride, 2.5 mM potassium chloride, 10 mM magnesium chloride, 10 mM magnesium sulfate, 20 mM glucose. Alternatively, this medium can be commercially purchased (Invitrogen).
5. LB medium-based T3SS activation culture medium: LB medium containing 300 μg/mL carbenicillin, 0.5 mM IPTG, 5 mM EGTA, and 20 mM $MgCl_2$ (*see* **Note 2**).
6. Antibiotics: 100 μg/mL ampicillin was added at the same concentration to all liquid and solid media; 300 μg/mL carbenicillin was added at in liquid medium and at 600 μg/mL in solid medium.
7. *P. aeruginosa* bacteria transformation: 300 mM sucrose, electroporation cuvette (VWR, Fontenay-sous-Bois, France), ElectroCell Manipulator ECM399 BTX system (Genetronic Inc., San Diego, CA, USA).
8. Cryo beads system (Dutscher, Brumath, France).
9. Perchloric acid, acetone.

2.5 SDS Polyacrylamide Gel Components

1. Acrylamide (Purity 99.9 %)/Bis-Acrylamide 40 % Solution.
2. Stacking gel buffer: 0.5 M Tris–HCl, pH 6.8.
3. Resolving gel buffer: 1.5 M Tris–HCl, pH 8.8.
4. Sodium dodecyl sulfate (SDS): 10 % (w/v) solution in water (*see* **Note 3**).
5. Ammonium persulfate 10 % (w/v) solution in water (*see* **Note 4**).
6. *N*,*N*,*N*′,*N*′-tetramethyl-ethylenediamine (TEMED). Store at 4 °C.
7. 5× SDS lysis buffer: 0.5 M Tris–HCl, 0.6 M DTT, 10 % SDS, 0.12 % bromophenol blue, 30 % glycerol.
8. SDS-PAGE running buffer: 25 mM Tris–HCl, pH 8, 200 mM glycin, 0.1 % SDS.
9. Protein molecular weight marker.
10. SDS polymerase gel staining solution: Coomassie Brilliant Blue R 250 solution.
11. SDS polymerase gel destaining solution: 5:1:4 methanol/glacial acetic acid/H_2O (v/v/v).

2.6 Mice

Female C57BL/6J mice (Janvier SA, Le Genest-Saint-Isle, France) are placed on experimental protocol at 6–8 weeks of age. They should be kept under pathogen-free conditions. All animal experiments should be approved by the Animal Experiment Committee of the Region and performed in accordance with institutional and national guidelines.

3 Methods

3.1 Antigen Cloning

1. PCR

   In a sterile 0.5 mL thin-wall microfuge tube, mix in the following order:

Template DNA	1–10 ng
10× *Pfu Ultra*™ HF reaction buffer	5 μL
5 mM solution of four dNTPs	2.5 μL
30 μM forward primer	0.5 μL
30 μM reverse primer	0.5 μL
2.5 U/μL *Pfu Ultra*™ HF DNA polymerase	0.5 μL
H_2O to final volume of	50 μL

The standard PCR program is as follows:

Step 1. Initial denaturation	95 °C	5 min
Step 2. Denaturation	95 °C	1 min
Step 3. Annealing	The melting temperature (T_m)	1 min
Step 4. Elongation	72 °C	1 min/kb
Repeat steps 2–4 for another 34 cycles		
Step 5. Final elongation	72 °C	10 min
Step 6.		Hold to 4 °C

2. Purification of amplified antigen fragments via agarose gel electrophoresis
Mount an agarose gel in an electrophoresis tank and add electrophoresis buffer to cover the gel. Mix individually PCR samples (TRP2, TRP2L, TRP2S) with 6× gel-loading buffer. Load the DNA marker and the sample mixtures into the slots of the submerged gel. Carry out the migration under constant voltage (50–100 V). Verify and recover antigen containing gel with the help of the UV device (*see* **Note 5**).
3. Recovery of antigen fragments from agarose gel
The different antigen fragments within agarose gel can be recovered from gel by using the QIAquick Gel Extraction Kit. All procedures were performed according to the manufacturer instructions.
4. Digestion of antigen fragments and plasmid vector
The standard recipe for the restriction enzyme digestion contains 0.1–0.5 μg DNA, 0.5 mL of each restriction enzymes (10 U/mL), and 1 μL 10× buffer for restriction enzymes, and make up to 10 μL with water. Incubate the reaction mixture at 37 °C for 1–3 h.
5. Purification of digested DNA fragments
Purify and recover digested antigen fragments and plasmid vector via agarose gel electrophoresis followed by gel extraction as described above.
6. Cloning of antigen fragments into the plasmid vector
The ligation between digested plasmid vector and insert antigen fragments can be achieved by using the Rapid DNA Ligation Kit. All procedures should be performed according to the instructions contained in the manual for the ligation kit.
7. Transformation of *E. coli* DH5α cells with ligation product for plasmids selection
Thaw competent *E. coli* DH5α cells on ice. Add individually 1–5 ng of ligation products to 25 μL of competent cells and mix well (*see* **Note 6**). Incubate the mixture on ice for 30 min,

and then, heat-shock the bacteria cells for 45 s at 42 °C and place back on ice for 2 min. Add 200 μL of pre-warmed SOC medium and shake at 250 rpm at 37 °C for 1 h to express the antibiotic resistance gene. Spread transformed cells onto the pre-warmed ampicillin containing LB plates. Incubate plates overnight at 37 °C. The next day, bacteria cells transformed by antigen containing plasmids should form colonies on the plate.

8. Plasmid amplification and extraction
   Pick bacteria colonies from ampicillin containing LB plate. Cultivate bacteria cells overnight in ampicillin containing LB medium at 250 rpm at 37 °C. The next day, amplified plasmids can be extracted by using QIAprep Spin Miniprep Kit from bacteria cells. All procedures should be performed according to the instructions contained in the manual for the Miniprep Kit. Accuracy of cloning can be confirmed by DNA sequencing.

3.2 Preparation of Electrocompetent *P. aeruginosa* Strain and DNA Transformation

1. Grow *P. aeruginosa* CHA-OAL strain in LB medium overnight at 37 °C with shaking at 250 rpm in a sterile culture tube.
2. Distribute the whole culture of *P. aeruginosa* CHA-OAL strain evenly into four sterile microcentrifuge tubes and centrifuge at 11,000 × *g* and room temperature for 3 min.
3. Use a sterile 1 mL disposable pipette tip, remove supernatant, and discard into a biological waste container. Resuspend each cell pellet in 1 mL of 300 mM sucrose (kept at room temperature) and centrifuge as in previous step (*see* **Note 7**).
4. Repeat **step 3** 2×.
5. Discard supernatant and suspend each cell pellet in a combined volume of 200 μL of 300 mM sucrose. At this step, competent cells can be frozen at −80 °C. However, it is advisable to use freshly prepared competent cells.
6. Transfer 100 μL of electrocompetent *P. aeruginosa* to a sterile microcentrifuge tubes. Add individually 1–3 μL (10–30 ng) pEAIS54-TRP2, pEAIS54-TRP2L, and pEAIS54-TRP2S plasmids and mix by gentle stirring with the gel-loading pipette tip. Incubate on ice for 20 min.
7. Add the mixtures in a cold electroporation cuvette (−20 °C for 30 min) (*see* **Note 8**) and electroporate using the following settings: 1,800 V, <5 min.
8. Immediately add 900 μL of pre-warmed SOC medium and shake at 37 °C for 1 h (*see* **Note 9**).
9. Plate 100 μL of transformed cells onto the pre-warmed PIA Cb_{600} plates. Centrifuge the remaining culture at 11,000 × *g* and room temperature for 3 min. Discard the supernatant but leave about 50 μL of medium to resuspend pellet and plate on PIA Cb_{600}. Incubate at 37 °C overnight.
10. The next day, the plasmid transformed bacteria cells should form colonies on the plates.

3.3 T3SS Activation Assay

This assay is for the verification of antigen expression and delivery by the *P. aeruginosa* CHA-OAL strain using an in vitro T3SS activation assay.

1. Cultivate CHA-OAL-TRP2, CHA-OAL-TRP2L, CHA-OAL-TRP2S strains in carbenicillin-containing LB medium overnight at 250 rpm at 37 °C.
2. The next day, wash pre-cultivated bacteria cells in fresh LB medium and resuspend cells to obtain an OD_{600} reading of 0.2 in pre-warmed LB medium-based T3SS activation culture medium until the OD_{600} reaches a value between 1.5 and 2 (*see* **Note 10**).
3. Centrifuge bacterial cultures at 13,000 × *g* for 10 min and recover the supernatants.
4. Precipitate bacteria-produced proteins by adding perchloric acid to the culture supernatants to obtain a final concentration of 15 % and incubate the mixture at 4 °C, overnight.
5. The next day, centrifuge the precipitated proteins at 17,000 × *g* at 4 °C for 30 min. Wash the proteins 2× with acetone, pelleting the proteins by centrifuging at 17,000 × *g* for 15 min (*see* **Note 11**).
6. Dry the precipitated proteins at room temperature (*see* **Note 12**).
7. Resuspend the dried protein samples in 50 μL SDS lysis buffer and heat at 95 °C for 5 min for SDS polyacrylamide electrophoresis (*see* **Note 13**).
8. Prepare a SDS polyacrylamide gel using the recipe in Table 2.
9. SDS polyacrylamide electrophoresis: Load the denatured protein samples and protein marker onto the SDS polyacrylamide gel. Apply a voltage of 8 V/cm to the stacking gel and then increase the voltage to 15 V/cm to the resolving gel. Run out

Table 2
SDS polyacrylamide gel preparation recipe

	Stocking gel	Resolving gel
Acrylamide/bis solution	5 %	15 %
10 % SDS solution	10 %	
Tris–HCl 0.5 M pH 6.8	25 %	
Tris–HCl 1.5 M pH 8.8		25 %
10 % (w/v) Ammonium persulfate	1 %	
TEMED	1 ‰	
H_2O	QSP	

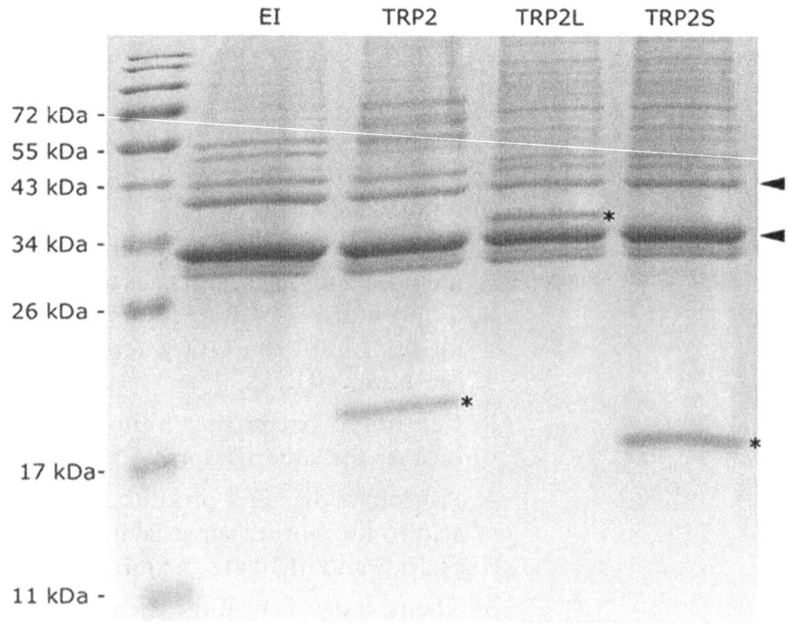

Fig. 2 Evaluation of T3SS-mediated protein secretion by SDS-PAGE. The positions of PopB (*bottom arrow*) and PopD (*top arrow*) are marked with *arrows* on the *right*. The positions of the ExoS54 fusion proteins are marked with *asterisks* within the gel

the proteins until the bromophenol blue in the sample buffer reaches the bottom of the gel.

10. Standard Coomassie Brilliant Blue staining: Following electrophoresis, immerse the gel in the 0.25 % Coomassie Brilliant Blue R 250 solution. Rotate slowly for a minimum of 1 h at room temperature. Remove the staining solution and destain the gel by soaking it in the destaining solution several times. Verify antigen secretion by CHA-OAL-fusion protein strains with an illumination device (Fig. 2).
11. Store indefinitely the fixed gel in H_2O containing 20 % glycerol before drying.

3.4 Storage of *P. aeruginosa* Strains

1. Grow 1 mL of each CHA-OAL-TRP2, CHA-OAL-TRP2L, CHA-OAL-TRP2S strains overnight in LB at 250 rpm at 37 °C.
2. Wash cultured bacterial cells 2× with fresh LB medium and resuspend cells in 100 μL LB medium.
3. Spread bacterial cells onto the pre-warmed carbenicillin-containing PIA plates. Incubate at 37 °C overnight.
4. The next day, recover bacteria layer from plates and store strains individually using the Cryo beads system. All procedures were performed according to the manufacturer's instructions.

5. Store at −80 °C. Functionally stored bacterial cultures are best for about 4–6 months but will probably work well up to 1 year.

3.5 Preparation of Bacteria-Based Vaccines

1. Cultivate 1 mL of CHA-OAL-TRP2, CHA-OAL-TRP2L, CHA-OAL-TRP2S strains overnight in carbenicillin-containing LB medium at 250 rpm at 37 °C.
2. The next day, wash pre-cultivated bacteria cells 2× with fresh LB medium and resuspend cells at 0.2 OD_{600} in 2 mL prewarmed LB medium containing 300 μg/mL carbenicillin and 0.5 mM IPTG until the OD_{600} reaches a value between 1.5 and 2.
3. Wash bacteria cells with sterile PBS, pH 7.2, and resuspend the cells in PBS at a concentration of 1×10^9/mL for animal injections.

3.6 Animal Vaccination

For all CHA-OAL-fusion protein strains, mice are injected 2× at the dose of 1×10^8 bacteria in 100 μL/time/mouse in right flank on 14 days and 7 days before tumor challenge experiment or immune response monitoring experiment. Mice are administered with bacteria vaccines through subcutaneous injection using insulin syringes. The quantity of bacteria is calculated with the measure of absorbance of the culture at 600 nm in a conventional spectrophotometer using the formula: 1 OD (600 nm) = 5×10^8 bacteria per mL (*see* **Note 14**).

4 Notes

1. Practically, 1 % gel will show good resolution of large DNA fragments (5–10 kb) and a 2 % gel will show good resolution for small fragments (0.2–1 kb).
2. The T3SS of *P. aeruginosa* can be induced in vitro utilizing calcium depletion methods. We believe that this condition can artificially open the secretory channel of the T3SS, leading to (1) a transcriptional activation of all T3SS genes in dependence of ExsA and (2) the secretion of toxins or toxin-protein fusion fragments. This calcium depletion can be achieved by incorporating 5 mM ethylene glycol tetraacetic acid, a calcium chelator, into culture medium. Moreover, we also added 20 mM $MgCl_2$ to the culture medium so that the bacteria have enough divalent cations. Carbenicillin allows the amplification of plasmid-containing bacteria cells. IPTG leads to the expression of ExsA and consequently the expression of exogenous antigen.
3. The SDS solution has a reduced respiratory toxicity and can be stored at room temperature.

4. We find that this solution is not stable at room temperature. Therefore, leave one aliquot at 4 °C for current use and store remaining aliquots at −20 °C.
5. The exposure of DNA fragments to UV can lead to mutations. To avoid this problem, divide one DNA sample into two aliquots that were simultaneously migrated in two agarose gel. At the end of the electrophoresis, divide the agarose gel, one part to be used to verify the migration by UV device and the other part to be used for later DNA extraction/purification.
6. *Do not* add more than 2.5 μL of ligation mixture to 25 μL of competent bacteria.
7. The sucrose solution must be stored at room temperature since cold sucrose results in a significant reduction in transformation competency. Sucrose should be sterilized by filtration only and manipulated under sterile condition. The washing steps with 300 mM sucrose are critical to avoid arching during the electroporation.
8. Pre-cooling of electroporation cuvettes is crucial to the outcome of transformation. Electrophoresis with cuvette conserved at room temperature might lead to the low efficiency of transformation.
9. Add medium to electroporation cuvettes as fast as possible to facilitate immediate recovery from the electroporation.
10. The concentration of bacteria cells can affect the efficiency of *P. aeruginosa*-based vaccine development. In our laboratory, we have demonstrated that when the bacteria concentration was over 2.0 OD_{600}, *P. aeruginosa* could produce several toxins to inhibit T3SS and thereby reduce the efficiency of the *P. aeruginosa* vaccine.
11. To discard the supernatant, do not overturn microcentrifuge tube several times. One inversion is sufficient to prevent the loss of the protein sample.
12. Complete drying of the protein samples is very important since the pellet can retain acetone which could affect sample loss during SDS polyacrylamide gel electrophoresis.
13. Residual samples can be stored at −20 °C for at least several months. Before the next SDS polyacrylamide gel electrophoresis, it is better to heat the samples one more time at 9 °C for 5 min.
14. The estimation of the quantity of bacteria could be verified by plating serial dilutions of the culture on Petri dishes containing LB agar and counting the colonies following overnight culturing. The number of colony forming units can then be calculated.

References

1. Carleton HA (2010) Pathogenic bacteria as vaccine vectors: teaching old bugs new tricks. Yale J Biol Med 83(4):217–222
2. Shahabi V et al (2010) Live, attenuated strains of Listeria and Salmonella as vaccine vectors in cancer treatment. Bioeng Bugs 1(4): 235–239
3. Singh R, Wallecha A (2011) Cancer immunotherapy using recombinant *Listeria monocytogenes*: transition from bench to clinic. Hum Vaccin 7(5):497–505
4. Le Gouellec A et al (2012) Bacterial vectors for active immunotherapy reach clinical and industrial stages. Hum Vaccin Immunother 8(10): 1454–1458
5. Deane JE et al (2010) Timing is everything: the regulation of type III secretion. Cell Mol Life Sci 67(7):1065–1075
6. Epaulard O et al (2008) Optimization of a type III secretion system-based Pseudomonas aeruginosa live vector for antigen delivery. Clin Vaccine Immunol 15(2):308–313
7. Derouazi M et al (2008) High-yield production of secreted active proteins by the Pseudomonas aeruginosa type III secretion system. Appl Environ Microbiol 74(11):3601–3604
8. Derouazi M et al (2010) Optimal epitope composition after antigen screening using a live bacterial delivery vector application to TRP-2. Bioeng Bugs 1(1):51–60

Chapter 34

Preparation of Peptide Microspheres Using Tumor Antigen-Derived Peptides

Santwana Bhatnagar, Raza Ali Naqvi, Riyasat Ali, and D.N. Rao

Abstract

Due to its distinct biological attributes, poly(D,L lactide-*co* glycolide) (PLGA) is one of the most preferred methods for DNA/protein/peptide encapsulation for therapeutics. Importantly, PLGA acts as an adjuvant for weakly immunogenic antigens and mimics booster responses after a single dose of administration, thereby serving as a single-shot vaccine delivery vehicle. Efficient delivery of antigens to antigen-presenting cells (APC) has been made possible by the use of a PLGA particle-based vaccine delivery system. Also, the plasma half-life of the PLGA-encapsulated vaccine increases as it is protected from degradation, prior to its further release. PLGAs are reported to be catabolized into individual nontoxic units once inside the host and further degraded via normal metabolic pathways. In this chapter, we have described the preparation and characterization of tumor peptide encapsulated PLGA microparticles as a model for controlled-release peptide delivery system.

Key words PLGA, Microspheres, Peptides, Vaccine delivery vehicles

1 Introduction

Biodegradable polymers such as gelatin, poly(D,L lactide-*co* glycolide) (PLGA), polymethyl methacrylate, polycaprolactone, and poly(lactide) have now been used for the preparation of microparticles for drug and vaccine delivery [1–5]. Distinctive properties of PLGA, e.g., higher stability, improved drug-loading capability, sustained biodegradability and release, and nontoxicity to the host, make it one of the best delivery vehicles to have been approved for certain human clinical trials by the Federal Drug Administration [6, 7]. There are many reported methods for the preparation of PLGA microspheres, e.g., phase separation or coacervation, spray drying, emulsification-solvent evaporation, emulsification-solvent diffusion, salting out, and the nanoprecipitation method, also known as solvent displacement. The choice of method depends on the hydrophilicity or the hydrophobicity of the

Michael J.P. Lawman and Patricia D. Lawman (eds.), *Cancer Vaccines: Methods and Protocols*, Methods in Molecular Biology, vol. 1139, DOI 10.1007/978-1-4939-0345-0_34,

protein or peptide to be entrapped in the microparticles. Double emulsion-solvent evaporation is the most preferred and widely used technique for encapsulation of the hydrophilic peptides. On the other hand, single emulsification-solvent evaporation, emulsification-solvent diffusion, salting out, and nanoprecipitation methods are preferred for insoluble or poorly water-soluble drugs.

PLGA is a copolymer consisting of lactic and glycolic acids. Because lactic acid is more hydrophobic than glycolic acid, polymers rich in lactic acid degrade more slowly [8]. The molecular weight of the polymer has also been shown to affect the size of PLGA. Important features of PLGA microspheres such as size, morphology, encapsulation efficiency, and in vitro release kinetics are governed by polymer concentration and molecular weight, nature and concentration of emulsion stabilizer in the external aqueous phase, speed and time of homogenization, temperature, and ratio of organic and aqueous phase [9, 10]. Also, Budhian et al. [9] substantiated that net shear stress for droplet breakdown can be reduced by increasing the molecular weight of the delivery vehicles. In this study, the remarkable increase in the viscosity of the organic phase by increasing the molecular weight of PLGA was considered as the most plausible explanation. The percentage of stabilizer, e.g., polyvinyl alcohol (PVA), as well as the speed of homogenization used during the entrapment also influences the size of the particle. Interestingly, particle size first decreases and then increases progressively with the increase in PVA concentration [9, 11]. The major advantages of microparticles are (1) elevated immunogenicity and plasma half-life as compared to soluble antigens; (2) history of biological safety [12]; (3) easy accessibility and deep penetration in various tissues due to their smaller size; (4) decrease in toxicity of various pharmacological agents due to slow and targeted release; (5) efficient ingestion, injection, or inhalation through various routes; (6) competent vaccination with no further booster administration, i.e., single-shot immunization [13]; and (7) capacity to encapsulate multiple peptides simultaneously within the same PLGA particle [14]. Importantly, during oral administration, microparticles protect encapsulated peptides from gastric pH and proteolytic enzymes. Furthermore, due to their smaller size, i.e., <10 μm, PLGA could come in close proximity to M cells of the *lamina propria* and *Peyer's patches* and trigger a strong immune response in the small intestine. This virtue enables PLGA to induce high antibody titer with high affinity antibodies, i.e., secretary IgA response, as compared to conventional modes of immunization [15]. Since the mucosal route of immunization elicits both systemic as well as mucosal antibodies, this approach is highly preferred over systemic immunization methods. Notably, one can also exploit this approach even if pathogens enter in the circulation through mucosal route. Contemplating the above advantages, we describe here the preparation and characterization of tumor peptide-targeted PLGA microparticles which are expected to improve the existing mode of tumor-targeted therapy.

2 Materials

2.1 Microsphere Preparation

1. PLGA lactide:glycolide (50:50), mol. wt. 30,000–60,000, is stored at −20 °C (Sigma, St Louis, MO, USA).
2. PVA, 87–90 % hydrolyzed, avg. MW 30,000–70,000 (Sigma).
3. Dichloromethane (DCM) >99 % in purity (AR grade).
4. Distilled and deionized Milli-Q water produced by Milli-Q purification system (Millipore, Billerica, MA, USA) and Homogenizer (Fisher Scientific, Mumbai, India).
5. Sigma 3-30K centrifuge (Newport Pagnell, Buckinghamshire, England).
6. Any tumor antigen-derived peptide.

2.2 Determination of Entrapment Efficiency

1. Acetonitrile >99 % in purity (AR grade), Milli-Q water.
2. 0.01 M phosphate-buffered saline (PBS) 1×, pH 7.4: Make a 10× stock solution by dissolving 12 g of anhydrous Na_2HPO_4, 2.2 g of $NaH_2PO_4.H_2O$, and 85 g of NaCl in 1 L of Milli-Q water. Dilute it to 1× immediately prior to use (*see* **Note 1**).
3. 1 N NaOH: Weigh 0.4 g of NaOH and add it carefully to 9 mL of Milli-Q water while stirring. Once the NaOH dissolves, add more water to make it up to 10 mL (*see* **Note 2**).
4. Bicinchoninic acids (BCA) assay (Sigma).
5. Sigma 1-15K centrifuge (Newport Pagnell).

2.3 Determination of Particle Size and Zeta Potential

1. Delsa™ Nano C (Beckman Coulter, Brea, CA, USA).
2. Diffraction spectrophotometer (Perkin Elmer, Waltham, Massachusetts, USA).
3. TEM CM-10 transmission electron microscope equipped with Mega view 3CCD camera (Philips, Beaverton, OR, USA).
4. Sonicator (Thomas Scientific, Swedesboro, NJ, USA).
5. Copper grids (Polysciences Inc., Warrington, PA, USA) (*see* **Note 3**).
6. Negative stain-saturated uranyl acetate (*see* **Note 4**) solution stored at 4 °C in the dark.

2.4 Morphological Studies

1. SEM Leo 435 VP scanning electron microscope.
2. Sputter gold coater (Denton Vacuum Inc., Cherry Hill, NJ, USA).
3. Microsphere sample.

2.5 In Vitro Release Kinetics

1. PBS, pH 7.4: Dissolve 1.44 g of Na_2HPO_4, 0.24 g of KH_2PO_4, 8.0 g of NaCl, and 0.2 g of KCl in 800 mL of Milli-Q water. Mix well and adjust pH if required with 0.1 N HCl or 0.1 N NaOH and make it to 1 L.
2. Sodium azide (AR grade).

2.6 Cell Culture and Cytotoxicity Studies

1. Ficoll-Hypaque Density Media (Histopaque).
2. RPMI-1640, fetal bovine serum (FBS), antibiotics, and trypan blue.
3. [3-(4,5 dimethylthiazol-2-yl)-2,5-(diphenyl tetrazolium bromide)] (MTT).
4. Dimethylsulfoxide (DMSO).
5. 96-well plate (Nunc), microplate reader (BioTek Instruments, Winooski, VT, USA).

3 Methods

3.1 PLGA Microsphere Preparation

Among the methods available for PLGA microsphere preparation, we explain here the double emulsion (w/o/w)-solvent evaporation method to entrap hydrophilic peptide and single emulsion (o/w)-solvent evaporation method for hydrophobic peptides.

3.1.1 Double Emulsion Method

1. Dissolve 1.5 g of PVA in 15 mL of pre-chilled Milli-Q water (*see* **Note 5**) and keep it over night at 4 °C.
2. Prepare the oil phase by slow mixing of 190 mg of PLGA in ~5 mL of DCM (*see* **Notes 6** and 7).
3. To this oil phase, add 100 μL of Milli-Q water containing 5 mg of dissolved peptide alone or peptide with adjuvant in a ratio of 1:2.5 (5 mg peptide:12.5 mg adjuvant) and homogenize it (*see* **Note 8**) at 20,000 rpm for 3 min in order to prepare primary emulsion (w1/o) (*see* **Note 9**).
4. Next, add 15 mL of aqueous solution of 10 % PVA (w2) in the above primary emulsion slowly and homogenize at 20,000 rpm for 4–5 min to form a stable "water-in-oil-in-water" emulsion (w1/o/w2).
5. Stir the above emulsion (w1/o/w2) overnight for 18 h on a magnetic plate at room temperature to allow solvent evaporation.
6. Centrifuge the emulsion at 11,068 ×g for 20 min at 4 °C to collect microspheres in the form of a pellet.
7. Wash the pellet 3× with Milli-Q water (*see* **Note 10**) and finally resuspend in 1 mL of Milli-Q water.

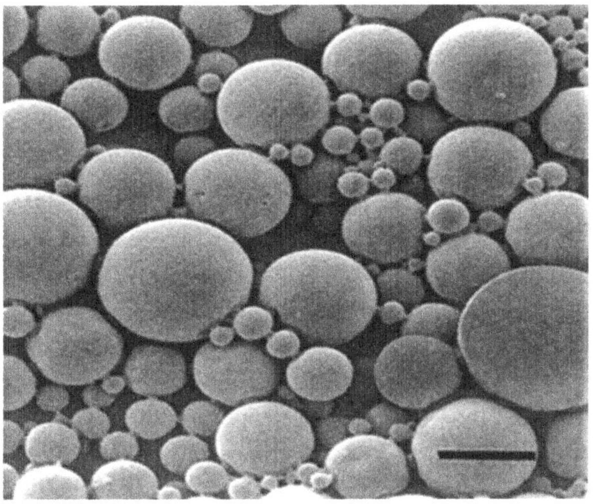

Fig. 1 Scanning electron micrograph of PLGA microspheres entrapping peptide produced by the standard double emulsion-solvent evaporation method (scale bar = 1 μm)

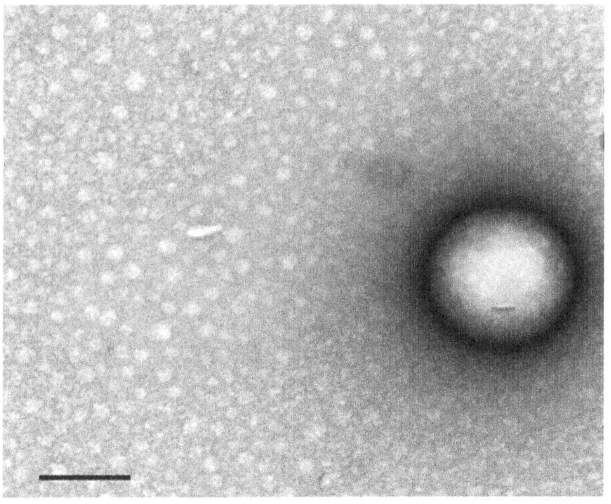

Fig. 2 Transmission electron micrograph of PLGA microspheres entrapping peptide produced by the standard double emulsion-solvent evaporation method (scale bar = 1 μm)

8. Keep the microsphere suspension at −70 °C for 4–5 h and then lyophilize it to obtain a fine powder.
9. Store the lyophilize powder at −20 °C until required. Figure 1 is a scanning electron micrograph of PLGA microspheres entrapping peptide produced by the standard double emulsion-solvent evaporation method, and Fig. 2 is a transmission electron micrograph of the same.

3.1.2 Single Emulsion Method

1. Dissolve 240 mg of PLGA and 60 mg of peptide in 3 mL of DCM in a water bath and sonicate the mixture for 10 min.

2. Add the above organic phase drop by drop using a Pasteur pipette to 20 mL of 10 % aqueous PVA solution and then homogenize it at 25,000 rpm for 4–5 min in order to form an emulsion.
3. Keep the above emulsion stirring overnight at room temperature to evaporate the organic solvent.
4. Harvest the microspheres by repeating **steps 6** and **7** of Subheading 3.1.1.

3.2 Calculation of Entrapment Efficiency of Peptide in Microspheres

The efficiency of the preparative method depends on the amount of peptide entrapped in the carrier system and can be determined by calculating the entrapment efficiency. The other term "loading efficiency" refers here to the incorporation of peptide into a carrier system. The entrapment efficiency can be improved when high peptide loading is achieved with minimum amount of peptide. The percentage loading for different peptide antigens can be ascertained by using the double solvent extraction method using the BCA assay.

1. Dissolve 10 mg of the peptide-encapsulated microspheres by adding 1 mL acetonitrile and centrifuge at 9,167 × *g* for 10 min at room temperature.
2. Discard the supernatant and keep the Eppendorf open to air dry the pellet.
3. Add 200 μL of PBS and incubate for 1 h.
4. Then centrifuge at 9,167 × *g* for 10 min at room temperature and preserve the supernatant for peptide content estimation.
5. Resuspend the pellet in 200 μL of 1 N NaOH to extract the remaining antigen and incubate it for 1 h.
6. Centrifuge it at 9,167 × *g* for 10 min and again remove the supernatant for peptide content estimation.
7. Assay the peptide concentration in both the PBS and NaOH fractions, separately, using the previously described BCA method as per the manufacturer's instructions.
8. Calculate the amount of peptide in both the supernatants using a standard curve generated with 200–1,000 μg of the same peptide.
9. The percentage entrapment efficiency and percentage loading efficiency can be determined by the following formula:

$$\text{Loading efficiency }(\%) = \frac{\text{amount of peptide in microspheres}}{\text{amount of microspheres formed}} \times 100$$

$$\text{Entrapment efficiency }(\%) = \frac{\text{total amount of peptide in supernatants}}{\text{original amount of peptide taken}} \times 100$$

3.3 Particle Size and Zeta Potential

The surface charges (zeta potential) of the microspheres are analyzed using a Delsa™ Nano C and the size distribution by diffraction spectrophotometry. 1 mg/mL samples are suspended in PBS, pH 7.4, and sonicated for 1 min to obtain a homogenous solution. The suspension is dispensed into a cuvette and the size is determined by diffraction spectrophotometry. A transmission electron microscope (TEM) is used to further confirm the size and structure of the microspheres (*see* **Note 11**).

1. Suspend the peptide-containing microspheres in deionized water and sonicate for 2 min to get a homogenous solution.
2. Take a drop of the suspension on a piece of plastic film or on a Petri dish with the help of tweezers.
3. Float the grid over the suspension droplet and leave it for 1–2 min, and remove excess solvent with the filter paper.
4. Add the negatively stained particles with uranyl acetate (saturated) solution for 20 s (*see* **Note 12**) and prepare approximately five to six grids per sample.
5. Dry the grids for 8–10 min and visualize the microparticles using TEM operated at 40–100 kV.

3.4 Scanning Electron Microscopy (SEM) of Microspheres

To study the morphology of the microspheres, place several drops of microsphere suspension on a double-stick tape over aluminum stubs and completely dry them at ambient temperature, thereby leaving only a thin layer of particles on the stub. All microspheres should be sputter-coated with gold at 300 Å using a sputter gold coater and be observed under scanning electron microscopy (*see* **Note 13**) (*see* Fig. 3).

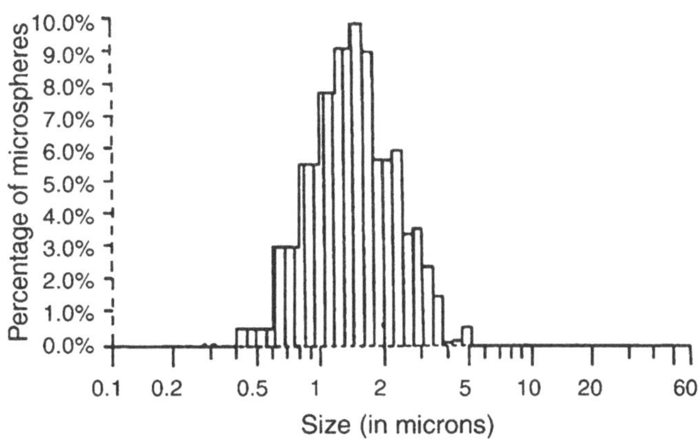

Fig. 3 Size distribution of typical microspheres preparation as determined by diffraction spectrophotometer

3.5 In Vitro Release Study of Microspheres [16]

1. Dispense 60 mg peptide-loaded microspheres in a tube containing 500 μL of PBS, pH-7.4, and 0.02 % (w/v) sodium azide.
2. Place the tube in water bath maintained at 37 °C under continuous shaking at 100 rpm.
3. After predetermined time intervals (such as 1, 2, 4, 8, 16, 32, 64 h), centrifuge the tube at 9,167 × *g* for 10 min and collect 400 μL of sample. Substitute it with an equal volume of fresh PBS at the same temperature as above.
4. Determine the peptide concentration in the collected samples by HPLC.

3.6 Cell Culture and Evaluation of Cell Cytotoxicity

1. Separate peripheral blood mononuclear cells (PBMC) from healthy donors using Ficoll-Hypaque density gradient centrifugation (*see* **Note 14**).
2. Carefully separate the buffy coat (the PBMC layer) from the middle layer.
3. Wash the isolated PBMC 3× in RPMI-1640 and resuspend the cells in 200 μL of RPMI (with 10 % FBS).
4. To examine cell viability and cell count, mix small volumes of PBMC with trypan blue (1:1) and observe under light microscopy.
5. Introduce 1×10^5 cells/100 μL/well into flat bottom 96-well culture plates.
6. Determine the effect of microspheres on the viability of the PBMC using the MTT assay.
7. Add peptide-loaded microspheres, blank microspheres, and peptide solutions in PBS (in different concentrations starting from 0 to 1 mg/100 μL) in each well and incubate at 37 °C in a CO_2 incubator under 5 % CO_2 in humidified air for 48 h.
8. Wash the cells with fresh PBS and then add 20 μL of MTT solution (1 mg/mL in PBS) (*see* **Note 15**) to each well and incubate for 2 h.
9. Decant the media and dry the plate to remove residue if necessary and add 200 μL of DMSO per well.
10. Place the plate on a shaker at 150 rpm for 5 min to mix the formazan crystals thoroughly in the solvent and take an OD at 570 nm.
11. Determined cell viability by the following formula:

$$\text{Cell viability percentage} = \frac{\text{O.D of test well}}{\text{O.D of reference well}} \times 100$$

4 Notes

1. To make 1× PBS, dilute one part of 0.1 M PBS stock solution with nine parts of Milli-Q water. To make 100 mL, take 10 mL of the stock solution and add 90 mL of distilled water. Mix well and adjust pH with 0.1 N HCl or 0.1 N NaOH if necessary.
2. 10 mL is sufficient for this method.
3. The copper grids used were self-coated with 2 % collodion in amyl acetate and dried before use. Use commercially available carbon-coated grids for better results.
4. Uranyl acetate is very toxic if it enters the body through skin cuts or ingestion or inhalation.
5. For preparing the 10 % (w/v) PVA solution, add 15 mL of chilled double-distilled water to a glass beaker. Weigh 1.5 g of PVA and transfer it to the glass beaker (kept on ice bath). Mix slowly on a magnetic stirrer so that the PVA mixes properly.
6. DCM is toxic and carcinogenic. While working with it, avoid skin and eye contact. Because of its volatile nature, chances of inhalation exposure are high with DCM. Thus, it is recommended to work under exhaust ventilation and wear a mask.
7. As DCM is volatile, perform this step in screw-capped tubes.
8. Before using a homogenizer, it is suggested to wash it 3× with Milli-Q water and then with DCM.
9. When preparing the blank microspheres, add HPLC-grade water to the oil phase without any dissolved peptide in it. All other steps are the same.
10. This step washes away the excess of PVA and peptide that escaped encapsulation.
11. For imaging by TEM, it is recommended to use freshly prepared microparticles. Also avoid waiting longer between negative staining and time of imaging.
12. Avoid staining for more than 20 s as it will increase the contrast and will lead to positive staining.
13. Before SEM observation, cool gold-coated particle samples over dry ice to avoid their melting under high magnification due to the electron beam exposure.
14. Maintain strict aseptic conditions during cell culture and cell cytotoxic studies.
15. Always use freshly prepared MTT solution as it is not stable.

References

1. Owusu-Ababio G, Rogers JA (1996) Formulation and release kinetics of cephalexin monohydrate from biodegradable polymeric microspheres. J Microencapsul 13(2):195–205
2. Dinarvand R et al (2006) Preparation, characterization and in vitro drug release properties of polytrimethylene carbonate/polyadipic anhydride blend microspheres. J Appl Polym Sci 101(4):2377–2383
3. Shokri N et al (2011) Preparation and evaluation of poly (caprolactone fumarate) nanoparticles containing doxorubicin HC1. Daru 19(1):12–22
4. Yousefpour P et al (2011) Targeted delivery of doxorubicin-utilizing chitosan nanoparticles surface-functionalized with anti-Her2 trastuzumab. Int J Nanomedicine 6:1977–1990
5. Dinarvand R et al (2011) Polylactide-co-glycolide nanoparticles for controlled delivery of anticancer agents. Int J Nanomedicine 6:877–895
6. Edlund U, Albertsson AC (2002) Degradable polymer microspheres for controlled drug delivery. Adv Polymer Sci 157:67–112
7. Muthu MS (2009) Nanoparticles based on PLGA and its copolymer: an overview. Asian J Pharm 3:266–273
8. Par T (1994) Degradation of poly (D, L-lactic acid) microspheres: effect of molecular weight. J Control Release 30(2):161–173
9. Budhian A et al (2007) Haloperidol-loaded PLGA nanoparticles: systemic study of particle size and drug content. Int J Pharm 336: 367–375
10. Benoit MA et al (1999) Preparation and characterization of protein-loaded poly (ε-caprolactone) microparticle for oral vaccine delivery. Int J Pharm 184:73–84
11. Cryan SA (2005) Carrier based strategies for targeting protein and peptide drugs to the lungs. AAPS J 7(1):E20–E41
12. Jiang W et al (2005) Biodegradable poly (lactic-co-glycolic acid) microparticles for injectable delivery of vaccine antigens. Adv Drug Deliv Rev 57:391–410
13. Khan AA et al (2008) Identifying B and T epitopes and studying humoral, mucosal and cellular immune response of V antigen of Y. pestis. Vaccine 26:316–332
14. Jayaprakash Babu US et al (2011) Enhanced humoral and mucosal immune responses after intranasal immunization with chimeric multiple antigen peptide comprising of defined epitopes of LcrV antigen of Yersinia pestis coupled to palmitate in mice. Vaccine 29: 9352–9360
15. Desai MP et al (1996) Gastrointestinal uptake of biodegradable microparticles: effect of particle size. Pharm Res 13:1838–1845
16. Diaz RV et al (1999) One month sustained release microspheres of ^{125}-I-bovine calcitonin: *in vitro–in vivo* studies. J Control Release 59: 55–62

Chapter 35

Production of Antigen-Loaded Biodegradable Nanoparticles and Uptake by Dendritic Cells

Vijaya Bharti Joshi, Sean M. Geary, and Aliasger K. Salem

Abstract

Particle-based cancer vaccines prepared from biodegradable polymers are a potentially attractive way of delivering antigen alone, or in combination with adjuvant molecules, to dendritic cells (DC). Non-viral modes of vaccination must ensure the activation of cellular immune responses in addition to humoral responses if an effective antitumor immune response is to be initiated. Here we describe in detail a method for manufacturing poly(D,L-lactide-*co*-glycolide) (PLGA) particles loaded with purified protein/antigen. We also describe a method for generating bone marrow-derived DC in vitro. These DC can be subsequently used to measure the adjuvant properties of the particle formulations.

Key words Biodegradable polymers, Dendritic cells, Antigen delivery systems, Antitumor immune response, Adjuvant molecules, Poly(D,L-lactide-*co*-glycolide)

1 Introduction

Recent studies have highlighted the potential for poly(D,L-LACTIDE-CO-glycolide) (PLGA)-based particles as cancer vaccines [1]. These particles are biodegradable, biocompatible, nontoxic vectors capable of delivering antigen to dendritic cells (DC) and promoting cross presentation of antigen in association with MHC class 1 [2]. The use of biodegradable particles in tumor immunotherapy has mainly involved PLGA particles primarily due to their capacity to protect their cargo from degradation along with their ability to prolong the release of that cargo. The relatively low toxicity and high safety profile of such particles are advantages that potentiate their utilization over viral-based cancer vaccines. PLGA-based particles have been extensively studied as antigen delivery systems and have been approved by the FDA for human use. Early animal studies with PLGA microparticle vaccinations showed that a single subcutaneous injection of the antigen ovalbumin (OVA) entrapped in PLGA particles was a superior immunogen to soluble OVA alone

Michael J.P. Lawman and Patricia D. Lawman (eds.), *Cancer Vaccines: Methods and Protocols*, Methods in Molecular Biology, vol. 1139, DOI 10.1007/978-1-4939-0345-0_35, © Springer Science+Business Media New York 2014

as well as soluble OVA combined with complete Freund's adjuvant (CFA) [3, 4]. PLGA particles have modest intrinsic adjuvant properties that can be substantially enhanced by co-encapsulating antigen with adjuvants such as CpG oligonucleotide (CpG ODN) [5]. Preclinical studies demonstrate the potential for PLGA particles, encapsulating adjuvants and tumor antigen, to act as cancer vaccines [6]. It has been demonstrated that PLGA-based particles are readily taken up by DC [7]. Coculture of particles with DC in vitro can yield informative data as to the potential immunogenicity of the particles in vivo as well as providing valuable mechanistic insights into particle uptake and DC maturation.

2 Materials

For PLGA particles, the solutions mentioned below should be prepared in ultrapure water (deionized, sterile, particle-free, bacteria-free, and pyrogen-free) and HPLC grade reagents. Reagents should be stored at room temperature unless otherwise indicated. For the generation of bone marrow-derived DC, all cell culture reagents are sterile, endotoxin-free, and stored at 4 °C unless otherwise stated.

2.1 Preparation and Characterization of PLGA Nanoparticles

1. Resomer® PLGA polymers (Boehringer Ingelheim KG, Ingelheim am Rhein, Germany) (*see* **Note 1**).
2. Polyvinyl alcohol (PVA): 1 % w/v solution of PVA in water (*see* **Note 2**).
3. Dichloromethane (DCM) (Sigma, Milwaukee, WI, USA).
4. NANOpure Diamond™ ultrapure water (Barnstead International, Dubuque, IA, USA).
5. 150-mL glass Pyrex® beaker, stir bar, magnetic stirrer, and sonic dismembrator Model 100 equipped with an ultrasonic converter probe (Fisher Scientific, Pittsburgh, PA, USA).
6. Purified protein/antigen.
7. FreeZone 4.5 (Labconco Corporation, Kansas City, MO, USA).

2.2 Characterization of PLGA Nanoparticles

1. Standard solution of antigen: Dissolve 20 mg of protein in 10 mL of 0.9 % saline to make a concentration of a 2 mg/mL (*see* **Note 3**).
2. 0.2 N NaOH and 0.5 N HCl solutions.
3. 0.01 M phosphate buffer saline, pH 7.4.
4. Argon beam K550 sputter coater (Emitech Ltd, Kent, England).

5. Hitachi S-4800 SEM (Hitachi High-Technologies, Ontario, Canada).
6. Micro BCA™ protein assay kit (Thermo Fisher Scientific, Wilmington, DE, USA).

2.3 Generation of Dendritic Cells from Mouse Bone Marrow

1. 8–12-week-old wild-type mice (*see* **Note 4**).
2. Dissection board.
3. Bacteriological Petri dishes (sterile, polystyrene, 100-mm diameter × 15-mm height).
4. 70 % ethanol in spray bottle.
5. Phosphate buffered saline (PBS), pH 7.4. For 1 L, weigh 8 g of NaCl, 0.2 g of KCl, 1.44 g of Na_2HPO_4, 0.24 g of KH_2PO_4. Adjust pH to 7.4 in final volume of 1 L of deionized H_2O, then autoclave (120 °C for 15 min).
6. Surgical equipment: scalpel holder/blade, small dissecting scissors, forceps.
7. Growth medium (500-mL final volume): To 430-mL RPMI-1640 medium, add 50 mL heat-inactivated fetal bovine serum (FBS) (*see* **Note 5**), 5 mL 200 mM GlutaMAX (Invitrogen, Grand Island, NY, USA) (*see* **Note 6**), 5 mL 10 mM Minimal Essential Medium nonessential amino acids, 0.5 mL of a stock solution 50 mM 2-mercaptoethanol (2-ME) (*see* **Note 7**), 5 mL 100 mM sodium pyruvate (Invitrogen), 5 mL 1 M HEPES buffer solution, and 0.5 mL 50 mg/mL gentamicin sulfate (Cellgro, Manassas, VA, USA).
8. Murine granulocyte-monocyte colony-stimulating factor (GM-CSF) 100 μg/mL stock solution (PeproTech, Rocky Hill, NJ, USA) (*see* **Note 8**).
9. 30-gauge needles and 3-mL syringes.
10. Class 2 biological safety cabinet.
11. Trypan blue: Add 0.4 g trypan blue to 100 mL PBS, mix well, and centrifuge at $400 \times g$ for 10 min. Filter supernatant through a 0.8-μm syringe-driven filter unit.
12. Hemocytometer.
13. Centrifuge.
14. Humidified 37 °C incubator (5 % CO_2 in air).

2.4 Nanoparticle Uptake Assays: Confocal Microscopy and Flow Cytometric Analyses

For confocal microscopy with chamber slides:

1. Lab-Tek™ Chamber Slides (Thermo Fisher Scientific, Rochester, NY, USA).
2. Growth medium (see above).
3. DC (prepared as per Subheading 3.2).

4. Nanoparticles (prepared as per Subheading 3.1).
5. Mounting medium Vectashield (Vector Laboratories, Burlingame, CA, USA).
6. Propidium iodide (PI) (Invitrogen).

2.5 Direct Immunofluorescence Assay

1. 96-well, V-bottomed, or U-bottomed plates.
2. Immunofluorescence (IF) buffer (500 mL): To 470 mL of PBS, add 25 mL of heat-inactivated FBS and 5 mL of a 10 % stock solution of sodium azide (*see* **Note 9**). Store and use at 4 °C.
3. Stock solution of 10 % sodium azide (100 mL): Add 10 g of sodium azide to 100 mL final volume of water. Filter through 0.4-μm syringe-driven filter unit to remove particulates. Store at room temperature indefinitely.
4. Fluorescently tagged lineage-specific antibodies. Details of each antibody used here are described in Subheading 3.
5. Fc receptor-blocking antibody: e.g., anti-mouse CD16/CD32 antibody, clone 93.
6. Fixative solution (100 mL): To 97 mL PBS, add 2 g of D-glucose, 2.7 mL of formalin, and 0.2 mL of 10 % sodium azide solution. Store at 4 °C (*see* **Note 10**).
7. Refrigerated centrifuge.
8. SealPlate™ adhesive sealing film for microplates (Research Products International Corp., Mount Prospect, IL, USA).
9. Flow cytometer.

3 Methods

Antigen-loaded PLGA particles are most commonly prepared by double emulsion-solvent evaporation process.

3.1 Preparation of Protein-Loaded PLGA Particles

1. Dissolve 200 mg of PLGA in 1.5 mL of DCM (oil phase). Dissolve 2 mg of protein antigen in 100 μL of 1 % PVA (water1 phase) (*see* **Note 11**). Prepare 8 mL of 1 % PVA in a 25-mL beaker (water2 phase). Prepare 24 mL of 1 % PVA in a 150-mL beaker.
2. Prepare primary emulsion (water1-*in*-oil) by sonication of the water1 phase into the oil phase for 30 s using the sonic dismembrator at an output power of 10 W.
3. Prepare secondary emulsion (water1-*in*-oil-*in*-water2) by sonication of primary emulsion into $water_2$ phase using sonic dismembrator for 30 s at 10 W (*see* **Note 12**).
4. Add secondary emulsion in 24 mL of 1 % PVA and keep it stirring on a magnetic stirrer in a fume hood for 150–180 min for complete evaporation of DCM.

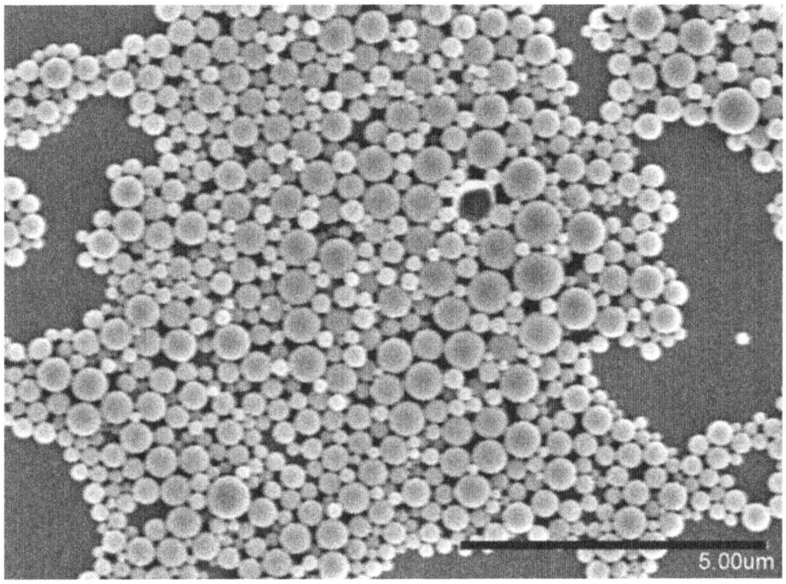

Fig. 1 SEM micrographs showing smooth morphology of PLGA nanoparticles

5. Transfer contents of beaker to a 50-mL conical tube and centrifuge at 6,800 × g for 5 min (*see* **Note 13**). Wash the pellet of particles 2× with water (*see* **Note 14**).
6. Resuspend the pellet in 5 mL of water and freeze it at −20 °C. Lyophilize the particles overnight in FreeZone 4.5.

3.2 Characterization of Morphology, Protein Loading, and Release Kinetics

1. Surface morphology and shape are examined using scanning electron microscopy (SEM):
   Suspend approximately 2 mg of particles in 1 mL of water and transfer a drop on a silicon wafer. Attach the silicon wafer to an SEM stub followed by a gold-palladium coating by an argon beam K550 sputter coater. Capture images with Hitachi S-4800 SEM at 5 kV accelerating voltage (Fig. 1).
2. Antigen loading is determined using a standard micro BCA™ protein assay kit:
   Incubate 20 mg of particles with 1 mL of 0.2 N NaOH for 12 h. Once clear solution is obtained, neutralize the solution to pH 7 using 0.5 N HCl. Perform standard micro BCA assay with 2 mg/mL protein solution as standard. Calculate loading of antigen using Eq. 1 and percentage entrapment efficiency (% EE) using Eq. 2:

$$Loading = (conc. \times volume) / weight\ of\ PLGA\ particles\ (mg) \quad (1)$$

(Loading = μg antigen encapsulated per mg of PLGA particles; conc. = concentration of antigen in the solution of degraded particles as calculated from standard curve (μg/mL); volume = volume of neutralized solution of degraded particles (mL))

$$\% EE = \left[weight\ of\ particles\,(mg) \times loading\,(\mu g / mg) \times 100 \right] / Initial\ weight\ of\ antigen\,(\mu g) \tag{2}$$

3. Take 50 mg of particles in a sealed glass vial and add 5 mL of PBS.
4. Keep the glass vial in a 37 °C incubator shaker at a speed of 200 rpm or higher to make sure the particles are not caking during the release study.
5. Take a 500 μL sample, centrifuge at 6,800 × *g*, and collect the supernatant to estimate antigen release using a micro BCA assay. Resuspend the particles in 500 μL of fresh PBS and add to the glass vial. Collect release study samples at regular intervals (*see* **Note 15**).

3.3 Preparation and Culture of Murine Dendritic Cells from Bone Marrow

This method for generating DC is derived from one published in 1999 by Lutz et al. [8]. Subsequently (2008) a very helpful visual aid (video) was published displaying the procedure in a step-by-step fashion [9]. By day 10 of culture, one can reliably generate at least 1×10^8 DC (immature and mature) from the marrow harvested from the hind limb of one mouse. The percentage of DC present in the floating cell population increases from approximately 75 % on day 9 of culture to approximately 90 % by day 13. These DC (days 9–13) can be used in subsequent in vitro experiments investigating the adjuvant properties of particle-based formulations:

1. Sacrifice mouse humanely and spray with 70 % ethanol to sterilize and dampen fur.
2. Remove skin surrounding hind leg using scissors and forceps.
3. Remove the leg using scissors high up in the pelvic region keeping femur and tibia intact.
4. Place the leg in approximately 10 mL of PBS in a Petri dish and remove the flesh and muscle surrounding the bone using scissors and scalpel blade (*see* **Note 16**).
5. Place the leg in approximately 10 mL 70 % ethanol for 1 min and complete the rest of the procedure in a class 2 biological safety cabinet to ensure sterile conditions.
6. Transfer the sterilized leg to a fresh Petri dish containing approximately 10 mL of PBS and further remove as much remaining soft tissue as possible using scissors and scalpel blade.

7. Transfer the leg to a fresh Petri dish containing approx. 10 mL of PBS to wash away debris, and then place the leg in a sterile dry Petri dish. Cut the leg using sterilized scissors at the extremities of the tibia and femur, i.e., above the ankle and below the knee and above knee and top of femur, creating two bone segments that have openings into bone marrow at either end.
8. Using a 30-gauge needle attached to a 3-mL syringe, flush 3–5 mL of growth medium through the marrow of each bone segment into a Petri dish (*see* **Note 17**).
9. Collect the cells in a centrifuge tube and centrifuge for 10 min at $230 \times g$.
10. Resuspend cells in 10 mL of growth medium and then count by mixing a 50-μL aliquot of cells 1:1 with 0.4 % trypan blue solution. Avoid counting red blood cells (*see* **Note 18**).
11. Using bacteriological grade Petri dishes, seed 2×10^6 white blood cells (WBC) per dish in 10 mL of growth medium containing 20 ng/mL of GM-CSF and incubate at 37 °C and 5 % CO_2 in a humidified incubator.
12. On day 3 of culture, i.e., 72 h after seeding, add 10 mL of growth medium containing 20 ng/mL GM-CSF. Do not remove the medium that is already there.
13. On days 6 and 8, transfer 10 mL of culture to a centrifuge tube, and centrifuge at $230 \times g$ for 5 min. Aspirate the supernatant and resuspend the cells in 10 mL of fresh growth medium containing 20 ng/mL of GM-CSF and place back into the original culture dish.
14. If cultures are extended beyond day 9, i.e., days 10 and 12, then maintain as per days 6 and 8 except that the amount of GM-CSF added to the fresh growth medium is halved (10 ng/mL in 10 mL of fresh growth medium).
15. On days 9–13, the DC can be harvested for experiments. To harvest the DC, flush off nonadherent and semi-adherent cells from the Petri dish by pipetting up and down and retain these cells (*see* **Note 19**). For maximum yield, rinse once with another 10 mL of growth medium and pool this with the initial harvest. The adherent cells, still attached to the Petri dish, can be discarded. Count a 50-μL aliquot of the harvested cells as described earlier using trypan blue and a hemocytometer. To ascertain the effect of PLGA formulations on uptake efficiency by these DC, refer to Subheading 3.3. For cell surface marker expression either before or after treatment with particles, direct immunofluorescence can be performed (*see* Subheading 3.5).

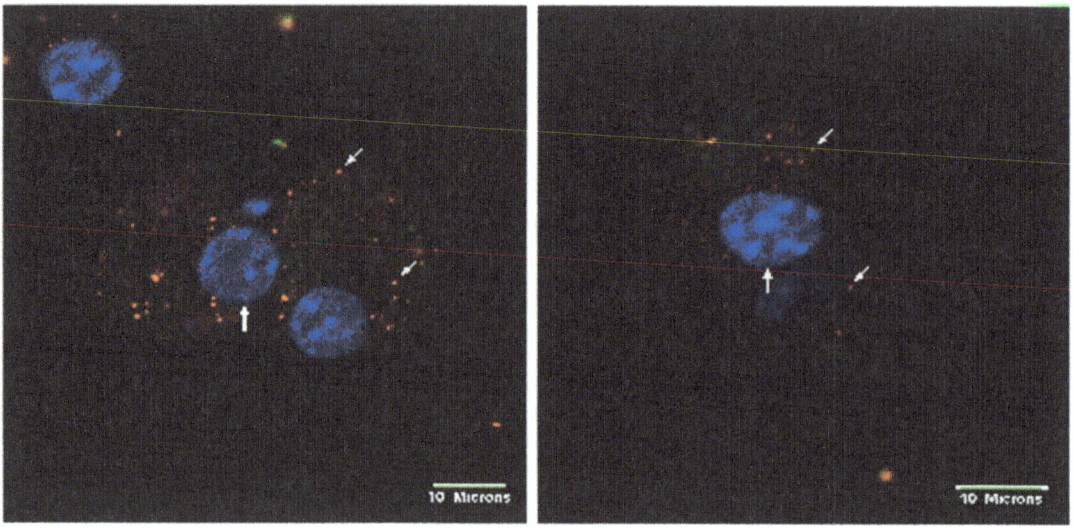

Fig. 2 Confocal micrographs representing internalization of fluorescently tagged PLGA nanoparticles in bone marrow-derived DC after 24 h of treatment. *Arrows* pointing *diagonally* depict particles and *arrows* pointing *upward* depict nuclei. Scale bar is 10 μm

3.4 Uptake of Nanoparticles by Antigen-Presenting Cells

Particles encapsulating a fluorescent protein, e.g., rhodamine or fluorescein isothiocyanate (FITC), can be used to study the uptake of particles by dendritic cells. These particles can be prepared by the method described in Subheading 3.1. The measurement of particle uptake by DC can be either qualitative, using confocal microscopy (**steps 1–7**) (Fig. 2), or quantitative, using flow cytometry (**steps 8–11**) (Fig. 3):

1. Coat chamber slide with poly-L-lysine solution (0.01 % w/v) for 6–8 h.
2. Aspirate the solution and allow the slides to dry.
3. Seed 10^4 cells/well in 200 μL of fresh growth medium and incubate overnight at 37 °C and 5 % CO_2.
4. Add 1-μg dose of loaded antigen in each well (*see* **Note 20**) and incubate for 24 h at 37 °C and 5 % CO_2.
5. Wash cells 3× with PBS (*see* **Note 21**).
6. Fix cells using 4 % paraformaldehyde for 30 min at room temperature followed by three washes with PBS.
7. Mount the cells with DAPI containing mounting medium and cover with a coverslip.

   The extent of antigen delivery can be quantified using flow cytometry. Prepare samples for flow cytometry using the following **steps 8–11**.
8. Seed 10^4 cells/well in a 12-well plate with 2 mL of fresh medium. Leave the cells overnight at 37 °C to settle and recover.

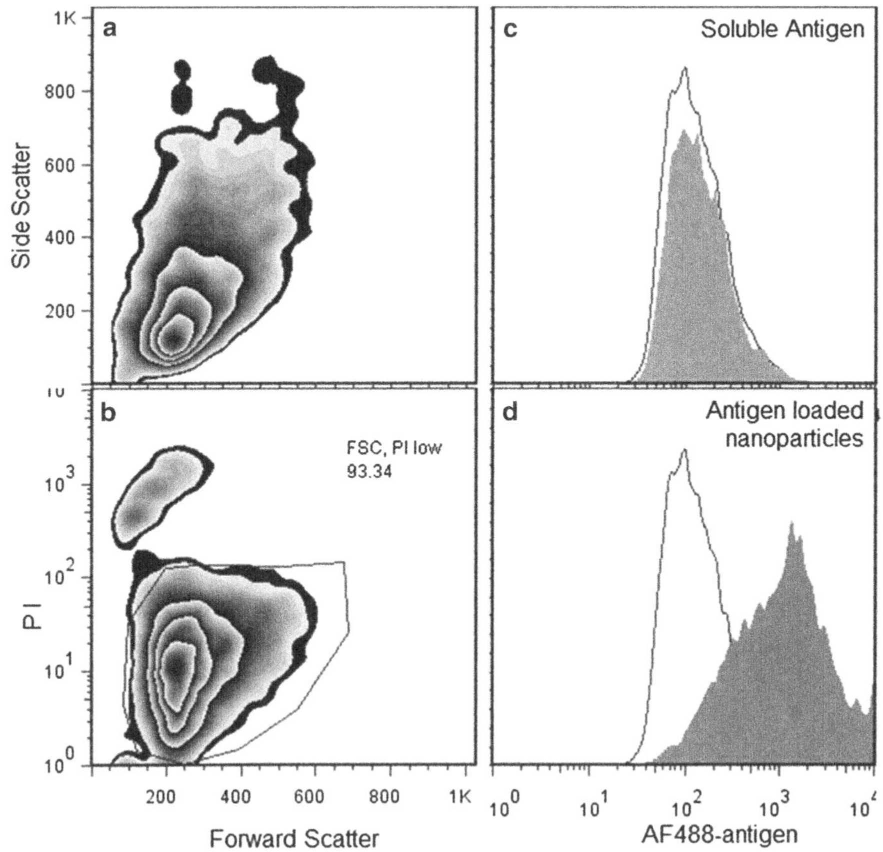

Fig. 3 Flow cytometry analysis of cells incubated with AF488-tagged antigen in solution and PLGA nanoparticles. (**a**) Forward vs. side scatter plot showing increase in side scatter due to particle uptake. (**b**) Forward scatter vs. PI stain to gate live cells for quantification of antigen uptake. (**c**, **d**) Histograms of antigen treatment in solution and nanoparticles, respectively. *Open histograms* represent untreated cells overlay with *closed histograms* of treatment group

9. Add 1 μg dose of loaded antigen in each well (*see* **Note 20**) and incubate for 24 h at 37 °C.
10. Harvest cells from wells by vigorously pipetting, collect cells into a centrifuge tube, centrifuge at 230 × *g* for 5 min, and wash cells 3× with PBS and incubate with PI to stain dead cells.
11. Acquire samples on a flow cytometer.

3.5 Direct Immunofluorescence on Harvested Dendritic Cells

Direct immunofluorescence can be performed to determine the phenotype of the harvested DC on days 9–13 of culture. Figure 4 shows the results of staining a day 9 culture with various lineage-specific antibodies to establish the percentage of DC in the population. In addition, one can determine the effect of PLGA particle formulations on the maturation of DC by staining for maturation markers such as CD86 and MHC class 2 antigen.

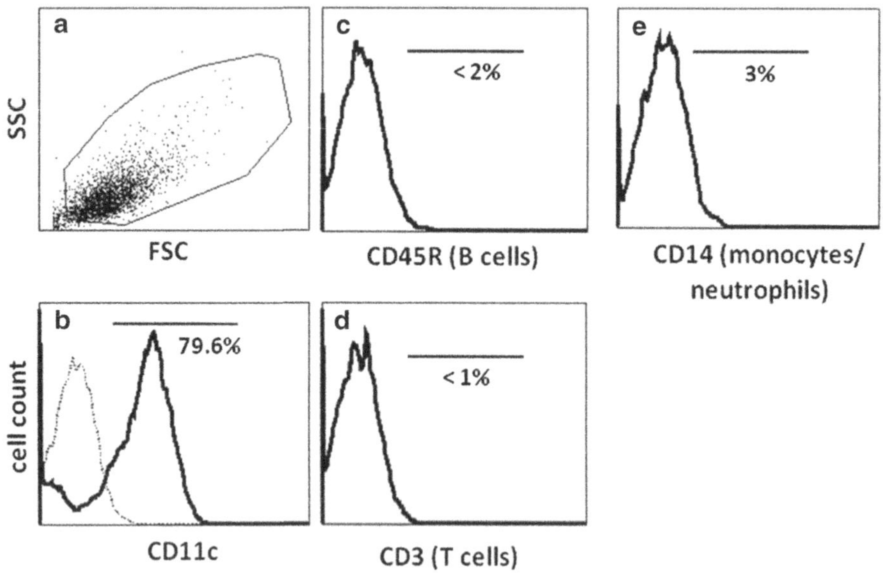

Fig. 4 Determining percent CD11c-positive bone marrow-derived cells after 9 days of culture. Floating and semi-adherent cells were harvested from a day 9 culture of bone marrow-derived cells (prepared as described in Subheading 3.3) and stained for the indicated cell surface markers using direct immunofluorescence (Subheading 3.5). Cells were fixed and run through a flow cytometer (FacScan, BD). (**a**) Forward scatter (FSC) (relative size) vs. side scatter (SSC) (relative granularity) plot where each *dot* represents a cell or event. Events within the drawn region were used to analyze for percentage of CD11c-positive cells. (**b**) Percentage of cells positive for CD11c was calculated by setting a gate (*horizontal black line*) based on excluding cells stained by a negative isotype control antibody (*dotted line*). Cells stained with FITC-labeled anti-CD11c antibody (*solid line*). (**c**) CD45R, a B cell marker. (**d**) CD3, a T cell marker. (**e**) CD14, a monocyte (and neutrophil) marker. The majority (>90 %) of the CD11c+ cells should be immature and mature dendritic cells based on the finding that <5 % of the cells in this culture contain cells of other lineages, as indicated by (**c**)–(**e**)

The following is a generalized method for staining DC with a single fluorescently tagged antibody:

1. Harvest the required DC populations, centrifuge for 5 min at 230 × *g*, and then wash 1× in 10 mL ice-cold IF buffer using a refrigerated (4 °C) centrifuge.
2. Resuspend cells at $<2 \times 10^7$ cells/mL in ice-cold IF buffer containing Fc block (1/100) and dispense 50 μL of cells to V-bottomed wells of a 96-well plate and incubate on ice for 15 min.
3. Add 50 μL of fluorescently tagged antibody diluted in IF buffer (10 μg/mL) to 50 μL of cells (*see* **Note 22**). Therefore final concentration of antibody is 5 μg/mL. Mix well without generating bubbles. Also, to a separate well(s), add a fluorescently tagged isotype control antibody to 50 μL of cells. Incubate on ice in a light-deprived environment for 30 min.
4. Add 100 μL/well of ice-cold IF buffer to each well, mix well, and then centrifuge for 5 min at 230 × *g* in a refrigerated centri-

fuge. Flick out supernatant (*see* **Note 23**) and then wash two more times using 200 μL/well/wash of ice-cold IF buffer.

5. After flicking out the final wash, resuspend the cells in 200 μL/well of ice-cold fixative solution. Mix well and store, and seal (*see* **Note 24**) in a light-deprived environment, at 4 °C.
6. Cells are now ready to be analyzed using flow cytometry.

4 Notes

1. The ratio of lactic acid and glycolic acid determines the release and degradation kinetics of PLGA particles. PLGA 50:50 is the fastest degrading polymer in the PLGA family. In contrast, poly(D,L-lactide) has the slowest degradation rate. The choice of PLGA polymer will depend on the desired release kinetics of the encapsulated antigen [10]. Inherent viscosity of the polymer can also influence the degradation kinetics of PLGA. Polymer chain length increases with increasing viscosity which leads to a slower degradation rate.
2. PVA is the most commonly used surfactant for the preparation of PLGA particles. Other surfactants that can prepare stable secondary emulsions are poly(ethylene oxide), cetrimonium bromide, dioctyl sodium sulfosuccinate, and poloxamer [11, 12].
3. A standard solution of bovine serum albumin can be used for the normalized quantification of cell lysate or mixed tumor antigen.
4. One should be able to harvest $1–2 \times 10^7$ leukocytes from the bone marrow of one hind limb. By day 10–12 of culture, at least 1×10^8 DC should be present.
5. To heat-inactivate serum, place thawed serum in a water bath at 56 °C for 30 min. This procedure will destroy complement.
6. There is no need to add GlutaMAX if the medium already contains L-glutamine. However, if the medium is more than 1 month old, it is advisable to then supplement the medium with GlutaMAX. GlutaMAX is a more stable and less toxic form of L-glutamine. However, L-glutamine (1/100 of 2-mM stock) can be used as an alternative to GlutaMAX if desired.
7. The stock solution of 50 mM 2-ME is made by adding 52 μL of 14.3 M 2-ME to 15 mL of deionized H_2O and then sterile filtered through a 0.2-μm syringe filter. This solution is labile and must be stored at 4 °C in a light-deprived environment and should be replaced every 3 months.
8. GM-CSF is very labile and should be stored long term at <–20 °C and only added to growth medium that is to be used immediately in culture. Avoid repeated freeze/thaw cycles of

stock solution of GM-CSF. Once thawed, the stock solution will retain full activity for no more than 2 weeks when stored at 4 °C.

9. Warning: Sodium azide is highly toxic. When weighing out the powder, follow safety instructions.

10. Fixative solution must be stored at 4 °C at all times. Extended periods of storage at room temperature will reduce its efficiency significantly.

11. Adjuvants like Toll-like receptor (TLR) agonists and lipopolysaccharides (LPS) can be added to $water_1$ phase for the preparation of antigen and adjuvant co-loaded particles. The volume of $water_1$ phase can be increased to 150 μL to increase the loading of the antigen. Further increase in volume can lead to porous particles with decreased loading.

12. Increase in the duration of sonication leads to a decrease in particle size. It is advisable to prepare the emulsion in an ice bath to prevent high-shear thermal damage of the emulsion.

13. Change in preparation parameters like sonication power, surfactant, and time of sonication can change the size of particles. Thus, large-size particles would fall out of suspension at lower centrifugation speed. After centrifugation at 6,800 × *g*, the supernatant should appear fairly clear. A cloudy supernatant is the indication of suspension of smaller particles. Centrifugation of cloudy supernatant at higher speeds, e.g., 10,000 × *g*, can collect this fraction of smaller-sized particles.

14. Resuspend the particles by pipetting in 5 mL of water. This helps in complete dispersion of aggregates. Once the particles are dispersed, make up the volume to 30 mL and centrifuge. Repeat the procedure for a second wash.

15. Particles usually show an early burst release followed by sustained release. Thus, it is important to collect early samples at intervals of 2–3 h. During the sustained release phase, samples can be collected at 24 h intervals. It is important that sink conditions are maintained at all times. However, adding an excess of PBS can dilute released protein. Samples that are too dilute could have a concentration below the detection limit of the micro BCA assay which, for all practical purposes, is 5 μg/mL in a 96-well plate. Thus, after estimation of the concentration of every sample, it is made sure that the concentration of PBS in glass vial is not more than 20 μg/mL of protein.

16. When removing tissue surrounding the leg bone, care must be taken not to cut into or break the bone, thus minimizing loss and contamination of marrow cells.

17. The 30-gauge needle should be inserted into the marrow, which should be apparent as a red circle in the center of the cross section of bone. The medium should squirt through the

marrow and come out the other side, being collected in the Petri dish. The solution in the Petri dish should appear cloudy. If this does not occur, reinsert the needle and try flushing the medium through again.

18. Red blood cells (RBC) can be distinguished from WBC, albeit sometimes with difficulty, when using a light microscope and a hemocytometer. RBC will often have a pink tinge combined with a slightly thicker dark perimeter compared to WBC. If your cultures fail to yield the predicted numbers by days 8–12 of culture, it is possible that you have underestimated the number of RBC present in your seeding culture.
19. The nonadherent and semi-adherent cells include the DC, while the unwanted adherent cells are mostly comprised of macrophages.
20. Dose can be varied depending on the degree of fluorescent conjugation of the antigenic protein and the duration of incubation. It is advisable to add soluble fluorescent antigen as a negative, or background, control.
21. Wash gently to avoid removal of loosely adherent cells. Place the plate at an angle of approximately 45° and slowly add PBS along the wall of each well. Gently aspirate the medium. The plate can be inverted on a Kimwipe to further absorb PBS.
22. Ensure that the fluorescent tag is compatible with the flow cytometer that you plan to use. Use an isotype or species-specific control antibody tagged with the same fluorescent tag.
23. When performing washes in 96-well plates, after centrifugation of the cells, the supernatant can be removed by quickly turning the tray upside down and firmly wrist-flicking (just once) into a sink. The cells should stay in the wells but may appear partially resuspended.
24. If cells are not going to be analyzed immediately, it is advisable to seal the tray using adhesive sealing film (*see* Subheading 2.4) to prevent desiccation of samples.

References

1. Krishnamachari Y et al (2011) Nanoparticle delivery systems in cancer vaccines. Pharm Res 28(2):215–236
2. Shen H et al (2006) Enhanced and prolonged cross-presentation following endosomal escape of exogenous antigens encapsulated in biodegradable nanoparticles. Immunology 117(1):78–88
3. O'Hagan DT et al (1993) Long-term antibody responses in mice following subcutaneous immunization with ovalbumin entrapped in biodegradable microparticles. Vaccine 11(9):965–969
4. Uchida T et al (1994) Dose and load studies for subcutaneous and oral delivery of poly(lactide-co-glycolide) microspheres containing ovalbumin. Pharm Res 11(7):1009–1015
5. Zhang XQ et al (2007) Potent antigen-specific immune responses stimulated by codelivery of CpG ODN and antigens in degradable microparticles. J Immunother 30(5): 469–478
6. Goforth R et al (2009) Immune stimulatory antigen loaded particles combined with depletion of regulatory T-cells induce potent tumor specific immunity in a mouse model of melanoma. Cancer Immunol Immunother 58(4): 517–530

7. Elamanchili P et al (2007) “Pathogen-mimicking” nanoparticles for vaccine delivery to dendritic cells. J Immunother 30(4): 378–395
8. Lutz MB et al (1999) An advanced culture method for generating large quantities of highly pure dendritic cells from mouse bone marrow. J Immunol Methods 223(1): 77–92
9. Boudreau JKS et al (2008) Culture of myeloid dendritic cells from bone marrow precursors. J Vis Exp 17:e769. doi:10.3791/769
10. Shive MS, Anderson JM (1997) Biodegradation and biocompatibility of PLA and PLGA microspheres. Adv Drug Deliv Rev 28(1):5–24
11. Sjostrom B et al (1993) A method for the preparation of submicron particles of sparingly water-soluble drugs by precipitation in oil-in-water emulsions. II: Influence of the emulsifier, the solvent, and the drug substance. J Pharm Sci 82(6):584–589
12. Sjostrom B et al (1995) Structures of nanoparticles prepared from oil-in-water emulsions. Pharm Res 12(1):39–48

Chapter 36

Development of Plasmid–Lipid Complexes for Direct Intratumoral Injection

Rama P. Kotipatruni and Ganji Purnachandra Nagaraju

Abstract

Gene therapy holds great promise as novel therapeutics for several major disorders, such as metabolic abnormalities and cancer. However, its use is limited by the lack of efficient, safe, and specific delivery strategies. Successful development of such strategies requires interdisciplinary collaborations involving expertise in lipid chemistry, cell biology, molecular biology, nanotechnology, systems biology, medical imaging methods, and clinical medicine. This methodological chapter summarizes cationic lipid-mediated gene transfer, which could be a safe and effective means of delivering potent therapeutic genes for transgene expression or gene suppression directly into tumors and gives references to studies on plasmid DNA delivery. These observations apply to gene therapy and DNA-based macromolecular drug synthesis, as well as in vitro and in vivo drug delivery studies.

Key words Intratumoral injection, Lipid complexes, DNA delivery

1 Introduction

In vivo gene delivery methods are widely used, including direct injection of naked DNA [1] and liposome–DNA complexes [2]. The direct injection procedure is a methodology that provides efficient transfection in skin and muscle [3]. The short gun or gene gun method is also very useful in introducing DNA into the cell by particle bombardment, which forces microscopic tungsten or gold particles coated with DNA into the tissues [4]. Over the past couple of decades, the significant progress in naked gene delivery has been unsuccessful in translation to gene therapy procedures in the clinic. DNA-based delivery vehicles thus require further improvement in development in order to successfully introduce therapeutic genetic material into its target site, e.g., tumor, in vivo. Most preclinical development projects in the nucleic acid-based drug delivery field focus on tumor targeting. DNA vector-based short hairpin RNA as a means of effecting RNA interference is a promising strat-

Michael J.P. Lawman and Patricia D. Lawman (eds.), *Cancer Vaccines: Methods and Protocols*, Methods in Molecular Biology, vol. 1139, DOI 10.1007/978-1-4939-0345-0_36, © Springer Science+Business Media New York 2014

egy for silencing the mRNA expression and will hopefully translate into therapeutic effects in the treatment of cancer.

The most common nucleic acid–liposome-based delivery systems for in vitro or in vivo applications are plasmid DNA–liposome complexes. The first cationic lipid to be introduced is *N*-[1-(2,3-dioleyloxy)propyl]-*N,N,N*-trimethylammonium chloride (DOTMA) [5]. Many different types of liposomes have been developed, and liposomes composed of cationic lipids are found to be most active in gene delivery. Since their introduction, more cationic lipids have been developed including 3-β-[*N*-*N*′,*N*′-(dimethylaminoethyl)carbamoyl] cholesterol (DC-CHOL) [6], *N*-[(2,3-dimyristyloxy)prolyl]-*N,N*-dimethyl-*N-hydroxyethylammonium* bromide (DMRIE) [7], and *N,N-dioleoyl-N,N*-dimethylammonium chloride (DODAC) [8]. These cationic lipids can form complexes with plasmid DNA with a fusogenic lipid and are capable of gene delivery into tumor cells with high efficiency [7]. The cationic region of the molecule associates with the negative charges of nucleic acid. An overall positive or neutral charge of the lipid–DNA complexes is generally correlated with higher transfection efficacy for cultured cells in vitro. It is hypothesized that the net neutral or positive charge effectively reduces electrostatic repulsion between the nucleic acid and the negatively charged cellular membrane. The lipid–DNA complexes appear to be endocytosed into cells. Nucleic acid entrapment in endosomal vesicles can be relieved by the presence of other lipids, such as dioleoylphosphatidylethanolamine (DOPE), in the liposome formulation [9]. It is thought that DNA encapsulated within the lipid complexes is protected from serum nucleases and small, long (~100 nm) circulating DNA–lipid complexes accumulate at solid tumor sites. Once at the disease site, an ideal delivery system would mediate efficient gene transfection. The large-size and positively charged character of these plasmid DNA–lipid aggregates also results in rapid clearance, and the highest expression levels are again observed in first-pass organs, particularly the lungs [10–13]. In in vivo gene transfer via intravenous administration by tail vein injection into mice of cationic lipid–protamine DNA complexes containing the luciferase reporter gene [14], luciferase gene expression was observed in all tissues including lung, heart, spleen, liver, and kidney, with the highest expression in the lung.

Various methods have been described for non-viral gene therapy, ranging from the direct intramuscular injection of purified DNA to the systemic administration of formulations comprising DNA and lipids, proteins, peptides, or polymers. The use of lipids as carriers of genetic material is well established in drug delivery methods [15]. For intratumoral therapy, plasmid DNA (pDNA) may be complexed with the cationic lipid *N*-(2-hydroxyethyl)-*N,N*-dimethyl 2,3-bis(tetradecyloxy)-1-propanaminium bromide and the neutral lipid dioleoylphosphatidylethanolamine at a 1:1 mol:mol ratio (DMRIE–DOPE) [7]. The use of pDNA–DMRIE–DOPE complexes has been shown to be effective for in vivo transfection of established tumors [16, 17].

Another cationic polymer, polyethylenimine (PEI), and its derivatives have been widely explored in gene delivery research. PEI has the distinct advantage of possessing the highest positive charge density among synthetic polycations, which enables effective condensation of pDNA by electrostatic interactions. Low-molecular-weight PEI has been shown to be well tolerated by eukaryotic cells with low toxicity. Several approaches have been proposed to provide DNA complexes with a higher level of in vivo stability. Phospholipid-grafted PEI conjugates (PLPEI), such as acetylated PEI and cholesteryl PEI, have been used to prepare polycationic liposomes (PCL) loaded with DNA. For example, a water-soluble lipopolymer consisting of a low-molecular-weight PEI and cholesterol was employed for in vivo gene therapy for cancer treatment and for gene delivery to ischemic myocardium [18].

Advantages of using cationic liposomes include the following: (1) the protocol for using cationic liposomes is relatively easy; often the reagents are mixed in a single tube prior to transfection; (2) many different cationic lipids are commercially available for gene transfer applications; (3) cationic liposome-mediated transfection can be used to generate transient and stable transfectants; (4) the method is versatile for the delivery of nucleic acids. RNA is effectively transferred to cells [19]; (5) these cationic lipid complexes can be used for in vivo gene transfer. Clinical trials have employed liposomes for gene delivery [20].

The use of nucleic acid-based drugs in the clinic has been hindered by a limited understanding of the basic mechanisms of plasma membrane transport. Advanced cell biological studies as well as in vivo experimental studies are required to provide a better understanding of how plasmid DNA–lipid complexes are processed by mammalian cells and tissues. Screening programs for novel synthetic vehicles of macromolecular DNA–lipid carriers in various biological systems are another obvious focus of future studies. The excitement over "nanobiotechnology" has served an important role in stimulating lipid chemists, molecular biologists, and clinicians to join interdisciplinary collaborations on the design of the ideal gene delivery vehicle. Once available, nucleic acid gene delivery drugs will revolutionize the treatment of various diseases as well as provide novel diagnostic tools for the benefit of cancer patients.

The focus of this chapter is to describe the techniques in the preparation of plasmid DNA–lipid complexes for intratumoral injections. The illustration below describes this technique:

Preparation of plasmid DNA and lipids

↓

Complexation of plasmid DNA and lipids

↓

Intratumoral injection of plasmid DNA–lipid complexes into tumors

The gene therapy procedure by plasmid DNA administration has several important advantages over traditional tumor treatments. Unlike recombinant protein therapies, serum levels of a therapeutic protein after intramuscular or intravenous or intracranial injection of a plasmid DNA encoding the protein-specific gene or the downregulation of specific gene expression by shRNA-encoding plasmid administration may reduce side effects while still maintaining a therapeutic effect. In current in vivo cancer gene therapy protocols, plasmid DNAs against specific target genes facilitate the treatment of small lesions in internal organs. Using plasmid DNA and lipid complexes may also be useful in treating primary tumors as well as minimizing or preventing the development of metastases in advanced cancer patients.

2 Materials

2.1 Lipid Conjugation to Plasmid DNA and Delivery

1. 1-Palmitoyl-2-azelaoyl-*sn*-glycero-3-phosphocholine (azPC ester), stored at −80 °C.
2. Branched polyethylene amine (bPEI) (1.8 kDa) (Polysciences, Inc., Warrington, PA, USA).
3. *N,N'*-Carbonyldiimidazole (CDI) (Fluka Chemie GmbH, Berlin, Germany).
4. 1 mg/mL plasmid DNA (pGFP or pLUC) encoding green fluorescent protein (GFP) or luciferase (Elim Biopharmaceuticals, Hayward, CA, USA).
5. Octylglucopyranoside (OGP), 4-(2-hydroxyethyl)-1-piperazineethanesulfonic acid (HEPES)-buffered glucose (HBS): 10 mM HEPES, 5 % (w/v) D-glucose, pH 7.4, sodium chloride (NaCl).
6. Dioleoylphosphatidylethanolamine (DOPE) (Northern Lipids, Vancouver, BC, Canada).
7. DNase I (Life Technologies, Mississauga, ON, Canada) and the luciferase assay kit (Promega, Madison, WI, USA).
8. Dioleoyl dimethylammonium chloride (DODAC) (Inex Pharmaceuticals, Burnaby, B.C. Canada).

9. Nuclease-free water.
10. Cell culture media and penicillin/streptomycin stock solutions.
11. Heat-inactivated fetal bovine serum (FBS).
12. DEAE-Sepharose CL-6B column.
13. Alzet miniosmotic pumps (Durect Corporation, Cupertino, CA, USA).
14. 6–10-week-old SCID mice, CD-1 nude mice.
15. Cancer cell lines (ATCC, Manassas, VA, USA).
16. Cell culture medium.
17. Dimethylsulfoxide (DMSO).
18. 1,2-dioleoyl-*sn*-glycero-3-phosphatidylcholine (DOPC) (Avanti Polar Lipids, Alabaster, AL, USA).
19. Phosphate buffered saline (PBS).

2.2 Oligofectamine and Plasmid DNA Complexes

1. Oligofectamine.
2. Plasmid DNA (shRNA) and scrambled shRNA (Origene, Rockville, MD).
3. Opti-MEM medium.
4. 1.5-mL Eppendorf tubes and pipette tips.

3 Methods

3.1 Intracranial Injection of Plasmid DNA–Lipid Complexes

3.1.1 Plasmid DNA

Plasmid DNA (pDNA) is produced by bacterial fermentation [21] and can be purified by standard double CsCl-ethidium bromide gradient ultracentrifugation followed by ethanol precipitation and dialysis. All plasmid preparations should be free of detectable RNA, and endotoxin levels should be less than 0.06 EU/μg of plasmid DNA. The spectrophotometric A_{260}/A_{280} ratios should be between 1.7 and 2.0 (*see* **Note 1**).

3.1.2 Complexation of Plasmid DNA with PLPEI

Tumors may be transfected in vivo with pDNA using cationic lipid-based delivery. Initial studies must determine the optimal in vivo pDNA–lipid ratio (*see* **Note 2**):

1. Take a fixed amount of plasmid DNA (100–200 μg) encoding GFP or luciferase tag and mix with varying amounts of PLPEI.
2. Dilute PLPEI separately in HBS solution to a final volume of 250 μL. The PLPEI solution is then transferred to the DNA solution by rapid addition and vortexing. The resulting PLPEI–DNA polyplexes are ready to use in vivo.

3.1.3 Complexation of Plasmid DNA with DOPE–DODAC–PEG-Cer

1. Incubate 60–400 μg of plasmid DNA with DODAC in 500 μL of 0.2 M octylglucoside, 150 mM NaCl, and 5 mM HEPES, pH 7.4 for 30 min at room temperature.
2. Add the plasmid–DODAC mixture to DOPE and PEG-$CerC_{14}$ or PEG-$CerC_{20}$ dissolved in 500 μL of 0.2 M OGP; 150 mM NaCl, 5 mM HEPES, pH 7.4. The final lipid concentration should be either 5 or 10 mg/mL with DOPE–DODAC–PEG-Cer at molar ratios of 84:6:10, unless otherwise indicated.
3. Dialyze the plasmid–lipid mixture against 5 mM HEPES in 150 mM NaCl, pH 7.4 (HBS), for 36–48 h with two buffer changes. Remove the non-encapsulated plasmid by anion exchange chromatography on a 1–4 cm DEAE-Sepharose CL-6B column.
4. To determine the encapsulation efficiency, take a 50 μL aliquot of each sample, load it onto a 1 mL DEAE-Sepharose CL-6B column, and equilibrate with HBS.
5. Elute the column with HBS and assess the collected fractions using ^{3}H-plasmid and ^{14}C-lipid by scintillation counting.

3.1.4 Preparation of Plasmid DNA Expressing shRNA–DOPC Complexes

1. Briefly, mix the plasmid DNA encoding a shRNA or scrambled control plasmid DNA with DOPC at a ratio of 10:1 (w/w) DOPC–pDNA and lyophilize.
2. Immediately before in vivo administration, hydrate the lyophilized preparations in 0.9 % saline at a concentration of 5 μg of pDNA per 200 μL and purify pDNA–DOPC complexes by using filter units with a size exclusion limit of 30,000 Da to separate free pDNA from the liposomes [22].

3.1.5 Complexation of Plasmid DNA with DMRIE–DOPE

1. For intratumoral injection, 100 μg of pDNA is diluted in 50 μL of 0.9 % saline.
2. In a second vial, add 100 μg of DMRIE (DMRIE–DOPE 1:1 mol:mol) and dilute in 50 μL of 0.9 % saline.
3. Combine the pDNA and DMRIE–DOPE and the 100 μL pDNA–lipid complex. The complex is then ready for intratumoral injection.

3.1.6 Stabilized Plasmid–Lipid Particle Protection of DNA from DNase and Serum Nucleases

DNase and serum nuclease from the external environment have an effect on encapsulated plasmid in the particles. By treating the plasmid DNA-PLP (plasmid–lipid particles) with DNase I, stability can be determined. Protection of PLP plasmid is compared to protection of free plasmid and plasmid in plasmid cationic lipid complexes prepared with DODAC–DOPE (1:1):

1. Samples containing 1 pg of plasmid are treated with 0, 1, 100, and 1,000 units of DNase I in a total volume of 1.0 mL of HBS for 30 min at 37 °C.

2. After incubation, the plasmid is isolated and analyzed by agarose gel electrophoresis.

3.1.7 Intracranial Injection of Plasmid DNA–Lipid Complexes

There is evidence of successful demonstration of non-viral cationic lipid-mediated gene therapy and expression of heat shock protein Hsp70 and reporter gene enzymes in the central nervous system of rats after injection into the lateral ventricle. Gene delivery is accomplished using optimized formulations of pDNA which have been complexed with the cationic lipid [23]. Luciferase-expressing pDNA carrying antisense or sense gene transcripts or shRNA molecules against targeted genes was used to test the ability to cause regression of human tumor xenografts transplanted into the intracranial region of female CD-1 nude mice [24]. All instruments should be sterilized and sterile surgical procedures followed for experiments involving animals:

1. Anesthetize the mice with an intraperitoneal injection consisting of 80–100 mg/kg of ketamine and 5–10 mg/kg of xylazine and place the mice in a Kopf stereotactic head frame that has been modified for use with small rodents or on a surgical flat form.
2. The area for the incision should be shaved and then treated with three alternating circular applications of betadine and ethanol.
3. Stereotactically inject 1×10^6 cells into the site which has been chosen relative to the bregma. The intracerebral site is located in the frontal white matter of the right hemisphere at the x, y, and z stereotactic coordinates of 3, 2, and 2, respectively. Place the sterile guide screw into the hole. A stylet could be used to close the 1-mm hole in the guide screw. The stylet that fits within the screw prevents tissue from growing into the screw hole when injections are not being performed.
4. Twenty days later determine the degree of tumor growth by bioluminescence imaging.
5. Although the animals may be asymptomatic, a single intraperitoneal or direct administration of pDNA–lipid complex of either control pDNA or experimental DNA in 10 μL of sterile PBS should be administered intracranially through the 1-mm burr hole into the right frontal parietal lobe at stereotaxic coordinates 3 mm lateral and 2 mm caudal to bregma using a 10-μL micro syringe or 27-gauge needle.
6. The plasmid DNA–lipid complex should be injected steadily over a period of 20 s, and the needle should be left in place for 1 min before it is withdrawn slowly. The injection site can be plugged with wax after completion of the intracranial injection.
7. Close the incision with skin clips and evaluate their tumor inhibitory effects.

3.2 Plasmid-Based shRNA Gene Delivery into Subcutaneous Tumors

3.2.1 Preparation of Oligofectamine and Plasmid DNA Complexes

1. Label two sterile 1.5-mL Eppendorf tubes A and B.
2. Add 250 μL of Opti-MEM solution to both the tubes.
3. Dissolve 140 μL of shRNA containing 20 pM/μL of pDNA in tube A and 60 μL of Oligofectamine in tube B and mix thoroughly.
4. Incubate the tubes for 5–10 min at room temperature in a tissue culture hood or in a sterilized chamber.
5. After incubation, mix the solutions from both the tubes and incubate for another 20–30 min at room temperature in a sterile hood.

3.2.2 Injection of Plasmid-Based shRNA and Lipid Complexes into Subcutaneous Tumors

1. Develop the subcutaneous tumors in 6-week-old female immune-deficient nude BALB/c-n mice by injecting subcutaneously with 200 μL of a 5×10^7/mL tumor cell suspension and monitor the mice daily. All the mice should form subcutaneous tumors.
2. When the tumor size has reached approximately 5 mm in length, remove the tumors surgically, cut them into 1–2 mm^3 pieces, and reseed them into another prespecified number of mice.
3. Again, when the tumor size reaches approximately 5 mm in length, randomly group the mice as shRNA, shRNA-N (nonsense shRNA), and controls ($n = 10$ each group).
4. Inject a total of 25–30 μL of shRNA or shRNA-N–lipid complexes, which have been mixed with Oligofectamine, into subcutaneous tumors using a multi-site-injection manner.
5. Mice in the control group should receive 25 μL of PBS, pH 7.4, only.
6. Administer the shRNA or shRNA-N–Oligofectamine complexes every day for 4 days in the same way.
7. Measure the tumor volume with a caliper, using the following formula [25]:
   $$\text{tumor volume } (\text{mm})^3 = (\text{length} \times \text{width} \times \text{height}) \times 0.52$$

3.3 Intravenous Injection of Plasmid DNA–Lipid Complexes

1. For intravenous injection of DNA–lipid complexes through the tail vein of the animal, 0.5 mL syringes with 27–29-gauge needles can be used.
2. The DNA–lipid complex suspension should be in no more than 200 μL of PBS. Inject the DNA–lipid complexes by immobilizing the animals, if necessary, in an open-ended tube such as a 50-mL Falcon tube with the conical end cut to insert the tail. Place the animals inside the tube with the tail inserted out of the other end.
3. This procedure will not induce pain in the animal except for the initial prick of the needle. This procedure may be done to minimize the trauma the animal might experience during tail vein

administration of DNA–lipid complexes [14]. The total time for the intravenous administration could be 10 min or more. Avoid quick injections in order to minimize blood vessel rupturing.

3.4 Statistical Analysis

The experimental animal data should be analyzed using a nonparametric test such as the Mann–Whitney U statistical test. Mouse survival may be analyzed using a Kaplan–Meier survival plot followed by a Logrank (Mantel–Cox) test. Differences are considered statistically significant when p value ≤ 0.05.

4 Notes

1. Plasmid DNA should be free of protein, RNA, and chemical contamination (A_{260}/A_{280} ratio of 1.7–1.9). The Pure Yield™ Plasmid Purification Systems will provide DNA of sufficient quality for most cell systems. Prepare purified DNA in sterile water or TE buffer at a final concentration of 0.2–1 mg/mL. The optimal amount of DNA to use in the tumor injection will vary widely depending upon the type of DNA and target tumor volume used.
2. Since different tumor types vary in the optimal in vivo pDNA–lipid ratio as well as the optimal plasmid DNA injection regimen, pilot studies to determine these must be conducted for each tumor model.

References

1. Choate KA, Khavari PA (1997) Direct cutaneous gene delivery in a human genetic skin disease. Hum Gene Ther 8(14):1659–1665
2. Zhu N et al (1993) Systemic gene expression after intravenous DNA delivery into adult mice. Science 261(5118):209–211
3. Ghazizadeh S et al (1999) *In vivo* transduction of mouse epidermis with recombinant retroviral vectors: implications for cutaneous gene therapy. Gene Ther 6(7):1267–1275
4. Nanney LB et al (2000) Boosting epidermal growth factor receptor expression by gene gun transfection stimulates epidermal growth *in vivo*. Wound Repair Regen 8(2):117–127
5. Felgner PL et al (1987) Lipofection: a highly efficient, lipid-mediated DNA-transfection procedure. Proc Natl Acad Sci USA 84(21):7413–7417
6. Gao X, Huang L (1991) A novel cationic liposome reagent for efficient transfection of mammalian cells. Biochem Biophys Res Commun 179(1):280–285
7. Felgner JH et al (1994) Enhanced gene delivery and mechanism studies with a novel series of cationic lipid formulations. J Biol Chem 269(4):2550–2561
8. Wong FM et al (1996) Cationic lipid binding to DNA: characterization of complex formation. Biochemistry 35(18):5756–5763
9. Farhood H et al (1995) The role of dioleoyl phosphatidylethanolamine in cationic liposome mediated gene transfer. Biochim Biophys Acta 1235(2):289–295
10. Huang L, Li S (1997) Liposomal gene delivery: a complex package. Nat Biotechnol 15(7):620–621
11. Templeton NS et al (1997) Improved DNA: liposome complexes for increased systemic delivery and gene expression. Nat Biotechnol 15(7):647–652
12. Hofland HE et al (1997) *In vivo* gene transfer by intravenous administration of stable cationic lipid/DNA complex. Pharm Res 14(6):742–749
13. Thierry AR et al (1995) Systemic gene therapy: biodistribution and long-term expression of a

transgene in mice. Proc Natl Acad Sci USA 92(21):9742–9746
14. Li S, Huang L (1997) *In vivo* gene transfer via intravenous administration of cationic lipid-protamine-DNA (LPD) complexes. Gene Ther 4(9):891–900
15. Ledley FD (1994) Non-viral gene therapy. Curr Opin Biotechnol 5(6):626–636
16. Saffran DC et al (1998) Immunotherapy of established tumors in mice by intratumoral injection of interleukin-2 plasmid DNA: induction of $CD8^+$ T-cell immunity. Cancer Gene Ther 5(5):321–330
17. Rubin J et al (1997) Phase I study of immunotherapy of hepatic metastases of colorectal carcinoma by direct gene transfer of an allogeneic histocompatibility antigen, HLA-B7. Gene Ther 4(5):419–425
18. Yockman JW et al (2008) Novel polymer carriers and gene constructs for treatment of myocardial ischemia and infarction. J Control Release 132(3):260–266
19. Muller SR et al (1990) Efficient transfection and expression of heterologous genes in PC12 cells. DNA Cell Biol 9(3):221–229
20. Felgner PL et al (1995) Improved cationic lipid formulations for *in vivo* gene therapy. Ann N Y Acad Sci 772:126–139
21. Horn NA et al (1995) Cancer gene therapy using plasmid DNA: purification of DNA for human clinical trials. Hum Gene Ther 6(5):565–573
22. Landen CN Jr et al (2005) Therapeutic EphA2 gene targeting *in vivo* using neutral liposomal small interfering RNA delivery. Cancer Res 65(15):6910–6918
23. Hecker JG et al (2001) Nonviral gene delivery to the lateral ventricles in rat brain: initial evidence for widespread distribution and expression in the central nervous system. Mol Ther 3(3):375–384
24. Ragel BT et al (2008) A novel model of intracranial meningioma in mice using luciferase-expressing meningioma cells. Laboratory investigation. J Neurosurg 108(2):304–310
25. Tomayko MM, Reynolds CP (1989) Determination of subcutaneous tumor size in athymic (nude) mice. Cancer Chemother Pharmacol 24(3):148–154

Part VI

The Advances, Challenges, and Future of Cancer Vaccines

Chapter 37

The Use of Dendritic Cells for Peptide-Based Vaccination in Cancer Immunotherapy

Mohamed L. Salem

Abstract

Effective antitumor immunity requires the generation and persistence of functional tumor-specific T-cell responses. Among the critical factors that often control these responses is how the antigen is delivered and presented to T cells. The use of peptide-based vaccination has been found to be a promising means to induce antitumor T-cell responses but with limited effects even if the peptide is co-delivered with a potent adjuvant. This limited response could be due to cancer-induced dysfunction in dendritic cells (DC), which play a central role in shaping the quantity and quality of antitumor immunity. Therefore, DC-based peptide delivery of tumor antigen is becoming a potential approach in cancer immunotherapy. In this approach, autologous DC are generated from their precursors in bone marrow or peripheral blood mononuclear cells, loaded with tumor antigen(s) and then infused back to the tumor-bearing host in about 7 days. This DC-based vaccination can act as an antigen delivery vehicle as well as a potent adjuvant, resulting in measurable antitumor immunity in several cancer settings in preclinical and clinical studies. This chapter focuses on DC-based vaccination and how this approach can be more efficacious in cancer immunotherapy.

Key words Cancer, Dendritic cells, Immunotherapy, Peptide, T cells, Tumor, Vaccination

1 Introduction

Generation of immune response is governed by the capability of immune cells to discriminate between self and non-self. To the immune system, however, a cancer cell is different in very small ways from a normal cell. As a result, the immune system largely tolerates cancer cells rather than attacking them. Therefore, antitumor immunotherapeutic regimens must not only provoke an immune response but stimulate the immune system strongly enough to overcome this tolerance [1]. In contrast to antitumor chemotherapy and radiation therapies, which kill tumor cells as well as hurt healthy cells, cancer immunotherapy harnesses the exquisite power and specificity of the immune system to specifically mediate tumor regression [2].

Michael J.P. Lawman and Patricia D. Lawman (eds.), *Cancer Vaccines: Methods and Protocols*, Methods in Molecular Biology, vol. 1139, DOI 10.1007/978-1-4939-0345-0_37, © Springer Science+Business Media New York 2014

2 Cancer Immunotherapy

The concept of modulating the immune system to achieve an antitumor response is not new, with numerous attempts documented throughout history. The first successful efforts at achieving an anticancer response via immunotherapy, however, were not achieved until the turn of the nineteenth to twentieth century when a surgeon, William Coley, noted the regression of an unresectable sarcoma subsequent to a postoperative wound infection. Building on this observation, he was able to show the objective regression of a variety of tumors using bacterial (*Streptococcus*) extracts (Coley's toxins), presumably through a mechanism of nonspecific immune stimulation. Despite treatment with Coley's toxins, resulting in the encouraging results of shrinking sarcoma, it came under criticism because many doctors did not believe his results. Even though this criticism caused Coley's toxins to gradually disappear from use, the modern science of cancer immunology revealed that Coley's principles were correct and that some cancers are sensitive to an enhanced immune system [3].

Cancer immunotherapy strategies aim to bridge innate and adaptive components of the immune system to augment the antitumor effects of T cells. There have been important advances in immunotherapy over recent years [2, 4, 5]. These immunotherapies can be broadly divided into two categories: adoptive cell transfer or antibodies (passive immunotherapy) and vaccination (active immunotherapy) [6]. Adoptive transfer involves the direct transfer of the actual components of the immune system already capable of producing a specific immune response. These components could be in a form of cell-based or antibody-based therapies. Antigenic elements could be in different forms, including killed tumor cells, whole tumor cell lysate, antigenic tumor protein, defined antigenic peptide of the tumor protein antigen, or naked DNA encoding the antigen of interest.

3 Active Anticancer Immunotherapy

Multiple phase I and II trials of cancer vaccines with tumor peptide antigens have involved patients with advanced disease and even impaired immune function [2, 4]. The goal of vaccination is to educate the immune system against antigens expressed by tumor cells in order to augment preexisting antitumor immunity and create a new repertoire against tumor epitopes that escaped recognition [7]. There are sufficient data from recent preclinical and clinical studies to support the notion that cancer vaccines can induce antitumor immune responses in humans with cancer. New technologies provide more information on the identification of potentially immunogenic tumor antigens that can be utilized to stimulate the patient's immune system to specifically recognize and destroy the tumor cells. Although some therapeutic approaches in use today are nonspecific, most protocols are designed to be antigen specific.

The vast majority of vaccine studies today employ measures designed to activate specific lymphocyte populations, partially because of the identification of the mechanism in which T cells can recognize antigens. The use of whole tumor cells or crude extracts is one of the oldest methods of cancer vaccination. A common approach is to vaccinate with lethally irradiated tumor cells using an adjuvant such as Bacillus Calmette-Guérin (BCG). Presumably, the adjuvant will create an environment in which the irradiated tumor can optimally present its tumor-associated antigen to generate an antigen-specific immune response. In a recent study of patients with stage II colonic cancer who had undergone curative resection of the primary tumor, vaccination with a tumor-BCG mixture reduced the recurrence risk by 61 % [8]. In another approach, studies in mice have shown that the introduction and expression of either cytokine genes, such as granulocyte macrophage-colony-stimulating factor (GM-CSF) or costimulatory genes such as B7 or foreign major histocompatibility (MHC), may significantly improve the effectiveness of tumor cells as a vaccine. These elements are all important in creating a local environment optimally able to initiate an immune response. Although these approaches are advantageous in that it is not necessary to characterize tumor antigens, obtaining and culturing tumor cells can be time-consuming and costly. This perception has led to the emergence of alternative approaches for cancer vaccines.

4 DC as a Potential Anticancer Immunotherapy Approach

In order to be effective, vaccine components are often delivered to patients by different vectors such as DC [9]. Characterization of tumor antigens and greater understanding of the biology of immune reactions have made it possible to construct vaccines based on loading DC with specific antigens, in particular, peptides [4]. Given that DC play a central role in the induction of successful active vaccination, DC-based vaccination is a promising approach to generate efficacious antitumor immunity. Indeed, cellular therapy with DC loaded with tumor peptides or killed tumor cells has shown evidence of an immune response to the vaccine and, occasionally, clinical responses [2, 4, 10–12]. In a recent systematic review with a meta-analysis of clinical studies evaluating the objective clinical and immunologic response to active specific immunotherapy in patients with colorectal cancer, pooled analysis showed an overall response rate (complete response + partial response) of 0.9 % for advanced/metastatic colorectal cancer patients who received different vaccine formulations, including autologous tumor cells, peptide vaccine, DC, idiotypic antibody, and virus-based vaccine [13]. Of these cases, humoral and cellular immune responses were present in 59 % and 44 %, respectively, while minor responses and disease stabilization were described in 1.9 % and 8.3 % of colorectal cancer patients, respectively. Pooled results of clinical trials of active specific immunization procedures available for advanced colorectal cancer reveal a very weak clinical response rate of <1 %. Hence, active vaccination against a weakly immunogenic tumor still requires further investigation exploring novel approaches that can generate more frequent clinical responses. In the following sections, we will describe the developmental pathway of DC and their maturation.

5 Development of DC

Antigen-presenting cells can consist of a number of different cell types, including DC, macrophages, or B cells. Of these, DC are believed to be the cell type most adept at activating naive T cells. Unlike most tumor cells, DC express all the molecules required for appropriate costimulation of T cells, including CD40, CD80, CD86, MHC, and Toll-like receptors (TLR). DC, originally identified by Steinman and his colleagues in 1972, represent the pacemakers of the immune response [14]. They are crucial to the presentation of peptides and proteins to T and B lymphocytes and are widely recognized as the key antigen-presenting cells with the unique capacity to initiate primary immune responses. DC are not a single cell type but a heterogeneous collection of cells that have arisen from distinct, bone marrow-derived, hematopoietic lineages [15–17]. The earliest DC progenitors/precursors are released from the bone marrow and circulate through the blood and lymphoid organs ready to receive differentiation signals [18]. Several studies have been carried out suggesting that there are different pathways for the formation of mature DC from $CD34^+$ or other primitive progenitors, in particular, monocytes. Each pathway differs in terms of progenitors and intermediate stages, cytokine requirements, surface marker expression, and, probably most importantly, biological function [15–17]. In protocols based on monocytes, DC are generated from monocytes circulating in the peripheral blood using GM-CSF and interleukin-4 (IL-4). This pathway gives rise to DC with a myeloid phenotype similar to DC generated from the $CD34^+$ hematopoietic progenitors.

There is considerable evidence from culture studies for a close developmental relationship between DC and cells of the monocyte/macrophage lineage [19]. Adherent peripheral blood mononuclear cells (PBMC) are enriched for monocytes, and this fraction may develop a Langerhans cell (LC) phenotype and function if cultured in the presence of fetal bovine serum (FBS) [20].

Further, among the PBMC, only purified monocytes are capable of expressing the LC marker, CD1a, if cultured in GM-CSF, a cytokine required for the in vitro production of DC from the adherent fraction of PBMC [20, 21]. These studies demonstrated that cultures of PBMC in GM-CSF and IL-4 produced cells that were $CD1a^+$ $CD14^-$ and capable of antigen uptake and processing, the typical profile of immature DC. Yields of up to 8×10^6 DC were obtained from 40 mL of blood [22]. Although the resulting cells resembled immature DC, they were atypical because of the presence of lysozyme, myeloperoxidase, and nonspecific esterase and their lack of CD83 expression [23–25]. In some studies, further differentiation into fully mature DC could be induced by exposing these cells to tumor necrosis factor-alpha (TNF-α) or CD40 [26, 27]. This final maturation was characterized by downregulation of the ability to take up and process antigen, while CD54, HLA-DR, CD83, and CD80 expression increased in parallel with the antigen-presenting function [26, 27]. A well-ordered phenotypic evolution of DC precursors has been demonstrated via $CD13^{low}$ progenitors to $CD13^{high}$ $CD1a^-$ and then $CD13^{high}$ $CD1a^+$ intermediates that also expressed variable levels of CD14 [15].

6 Maturation and Function of DC

In most tissues, DC are present in an immature state and are unable to stimulate T cells and instead induce tolerance because they lack the costimulatory signals required for T-cell activation, including CD40, CD54, CD80, and CD86. These immature cells, however, have several features that make them capable of capturing antigen in peripheral sites including (1) phagocytosis, where particles and microbes are taken up; (2) macropinocytosis, where extracellular particulates are sampled in large pinocytic vesicles; and (3) endocytosis, through different receptors, including lectin receptors and DEC-205, Fcγ, and Fcξ receptors [9, 28]. Due to the specialized MHC class II-rich compartments that are abundant in immature DC, the receptor-mediated antigen uptake and macropinocytosis of DC are very efficient, in which only picomolar and nanomolar concentrations of antigen are required, which is much less than the micromolar levels typically required by other antigen-presenting cells [29]. Therefore, immature DC are the most efficient antigen-presenting cells in antigen sampling and processing. Once DC have captured antigens, however, their ability to capture more antigen rapidly declines and they start to migrate to secondary lymphoid compartments, in particular, draining lymph nodes, to present MHC class I/peptide complexes and MHC class II/peptide complexes to $CD8^+$ and $CD4^+$ T cells, respectively. After their recognition of antigen presented by DC in lymph nodes, $CD4^+$ T cells differentiate into memory helper T cells which support the differentiation and expansion of CD8+ cytotoxic T lymphocytes (CTL). To be capable of killing target tumor cells and exert antitumor activity, CTL need help from CD4+ helper T cells. Therefore, maturation of DC during antigen recognition by T cells is a critical step.

7 DC-Based Vaccination

For clinical use, immature DC can be generated in vitro from CD34+ hematopoietic progenitors mobilized into peripheral blood using Flt3L and IL-13 cytokines [30, 31]. As previously mentioned, immature DC can be generated from monocytes circulating in the peripheral blood using GM-CSF and IL-4 [18, 32]. Maturation can be characterized by downregulation of the ability to take up and process antigen and the upregulation of CD54, HLA-DR, CD83, and CD80 expression and as a consequence their antigen-presenting functions. Furthermore, treatment with immature DC in combination with IL-12 and GM-CSF-coexpressing oncolytic adenovirus resulted in a remarkable therapeutic efficacy on advanced tumors, indicating that DC-based vaccination can be feasibly optimized when combined with oncolytic adenovirus coexpressing IL-12 and GM-CSF in combination [33].

8 Vaccination with Peptide-Pulsed DC

Tumor antigen can be introduced in different forms, including (1) whole tumor lysate, (2) tumor-associated protein, (3) deoxyribonucleic acid (DNA)-encoding a tumor antigen, or (4) antigenic peptides. Delivery of peptide via DC has been tested in different settings and has shown promising effects [34]. Loading DC with epitope(s) can result in induction of antigen-specific T cells with multiple specificities against tumor as has been reported in recent studies [35]. In the following section, we will present studies that investigated the possible use of the HLA-A2-restricted peptides in DC-based vaccination in different cancer settings. We will focus on HLA-A2 peptides derived from carcinoembryonic peptide (CEA), mucin (MUC-1), telomerase reverse transcriptase (hTERT), and survivin as a representative model for DC-based vaccination.

9 Vaccination with hTERT-Loaded DC

Most human cells do not express telomerase and lose telomeric DNA with each cell division [36]. Most human cancer cells, however, express high levels of hTERT which protects their telomeric

DNA from shortening during successive rounds of cell division [37]. The inhibition of telomerase activity in hTERT-positive tumor cells can lead to telomere shortening and cell death by apoptosis. The first immunogenic peptide described from hTERT (I540 (ILAKFLHWL)) is restricted to the MHC class I allele HLA-A2.

The clinical trials of DC loaded with hTERT in advanced or metastatic cancer patients have been recently discussed [38]. The first hTERT vaccination trial was conducted on seven HLA-A2 patients with advanced breast or prostate cancer. They were treated with autologous monocyte-derived DC pulsed *ex vivo* with hTERT I540 peptide and keyhole limpet hemocyanin (KLH) [39]. Immune responses and clinical evidence of antitumor activity were observed without toxicity, where hTERT-specific cells killed $hTERT^+$ tumor cells in an MHC-restricted fashion. The immunotherapeutic effects of the full-length hTERT were also evaluated in 20 patients with metastatic prostate cancer [40]. These patients were administered autologous DC transfected with mRNA encoding hTERT. Induction of hTERT-specific $CD8^+$ T cells was observed in most of the patients. These immune responses were associated with an increase in the prostate-specific antigen doubling time and molecular clearance of circulating micrometastases. In a phase 1 vaccination trial, nine gastric cancer patients received four vaccinations by DC pulsed with the immunodominant HER-2/neu (p369) peptide at 2-week intervals intradermally; HER-2/neu peptide-specific recognition could be demonstrated in six of nine patients after immunization, whereas there was no HER-2/neu peptide-specific recognition before immunization [41]. One of the patients underwent a partial clinical response concurrent with a decrease of tumor marker, indicating that tumor vaccination therapy with DC pulsed with HER-2/neu-peptides may be a potential candidate for the novel treatment of gastric cancer patients.

In a recent study, autologous DC were generated from HLA-0201 patients with advanced cancer from blood $CD14^+$ monocytes in the presence of GM-CSF and IL-4 and TNF-α or TNF-α and interferon-alpha (IFN-α). Each DC preparation was pulsed with only hTERT peptide (p540 or p865) with or without class II cognate help (p766 and p672). Class II cognate help significantly augments peptide-specific T-cell responses. The cells were then administered into separate lymph node draining regions every 2–3 weeks. This DC-based vaccination resulted in clinically favorable responses, particularly in patients who showed low levels of circulating T_{reg} [42]. In another recent study, a female patient who underwent radical surgery for a pancreatic adenocarcinoma was treated with autologous DC loaded with hTERT mRNA for 3 years [43]. Based on the immunomonitoring performed at regular intervals following initiation of vaccination, it was obvious that the patient developed an immune response against several hTERT-derived CD4+ helper and CD8+ cytotoxic T-cell epitopes associated with complete remission but with no serious adverse effects.

10 Vaccination with MUC-1-Loaded DC

MUC-1 mucin molecules are highly glycosylated type I glycoproteins expressed by various normal and malignant epithelial cells. The overexpression of MUC-1 during transformation of epithelial cells to cancer cells results in MUC-1 expression over the entire cell surface with many of the MUC-1 molecules showing under-glycosylation of the protein backbone of this molecule, resulting in its recognition by the immune system as a foreign antigen [44]. MUC-1 is anchored within the cell surface by a transmembrane domain, while the extracellular domain consists of a variable number of tandem repeats of 20 amino acids, which are highly immunogenic. Because the MUC-1 molecule is normally expressed on the apical surface of healthy epithelial cells and is highly glycosylated, its protein backbone is unexposed to the immune system. The protein backbone of MUC-1 contains tandem repeats of 20 amino acids, wherein lies the antigenic epitope recognized by cytotoxic T lymphocytes [45].

In an in vitro study in which DC generated from healthy donors were loaded with two different MUC1 peptides to stimulate MUC1 peptide-specific CTL [46], the generated CTL showed toxicity against leukemic cell lines and patient-derived acute myeloid leukemia blasts, indicating that DC loaded with MUC1 may demonstrate efficacy in clinical vaccination studies. MUC-1-reactive T cells have also been detected in the peripheral blood of patients with pancreatic cancer [47]. Therefore, phase I clinical trials based on the use of MUC-1 peptide were conducted on pancreatic cancer patients. Vaccination with DC loaded with MUC-1 peptide has also been applied as adjuvant therapy in patients with resected pancreatic and biliary tumors [48]. These studies showed that the vaccine plus adjuvant can be a safe therapy and can induce immune responses. Unfortunately, however, these detected immune responses were not associated with any significant changes in survival of these patients as compared with historical survival data. This failure in the clinical responses might be corrected if MUC-1 peptide is delivered with an agent that can induce antigen uptake by DC and their subsequent maturation in vivo. Therefore, one approach to augment vaccination with MUC-1-loaded DC is the coadministration of potent adjuvants such as TLR agonists that would induce maturation of the injected DC and their antigen presentation to T cells.

In a phase I/II study, which was conducted on patients with metastatic breast or ovarian cancer expressing MUC-1, vaccination with matured DC pulsed with HLA-A2-binding MUC-1 peptide, peptide-specific CTL were measurable in the peripheral blood of 50 % of the patients as evidenced by the intracellular interferon-gamma (IFN-γ) and cytolytic assays [49]. These responses lasted for more than 6 months. Interestingly, it appears that antigen spreading in vivo occurred in some patients since one patient that received several vaccinations of MUC-1 peptide-pulsed DC developed CEA- and MAGE-3 peptide-specific T-cell responses. This observed antigen spreading has been suggested to be due to the induction of other tumor antigen-specific CTL as a result of the destruction of the malignant cells by the in vivo-induced CTL and uptake and processing of the killed cells by the antigen-presenting cells [50]. These results indicate that vaccination with MUC-1 peptide-pulsed DC could be a potential approach for inducing effective antitumor responses against poorly immunogenic tumors. In another MUC-1-based vaccination trial, 20 patients with metastatic renal cell carcinoma (RCC) were vaccinated every 2 weeks four times with DC pulsed with the MUC-1-derived peptides M1.1 and M1.2 in addition to the PAN-HLA-DR-binding peptide (PADRE), which induces activation of $CD4^+$ T-helper cells. After the completion of the DC vaccination, patients were also treated with three injections/week of low-dose IL-2 [51]. Regression of metastases was induced with three objective responses and two mixed responses in 30 % of the patients that was associated with MUC-1 peptide-specific T-cell responses in the peripheral blood. After in vitro restimulation, the induced T-cell responses developed CTL that were able to recognize MUC-1^+ target tumor cells in HLA-A2-restricted manner.

11 Vaccination with CEA-Loaded DC

Carcinoembryonic antigen (CEA) is an oncofetal antigen expressed in normal epithelial tissues but is frequently overexpressed in adenocarcinomas, particularly those of the gastrointestinal tract, including pancreatic carcinoma [52]. CEA is overexpressed in 80–90 % of pancreatic carcinomas and contains epitopes recognized by $CD4^+$ T cells. A number of potential MHC class I (MHC A2, A3, and A24) epitopes for CEA have been identified and synthesized for use as vaccine.

Several phase I clinical trials assessing various vaccine approaches against CEA have been performed using CAP-1 or CAP1-6D-pulsed DC in HLA-A2-positive patients with metastatic CEA-expressing malignancies, including pancreatic, colorectal, breast, ovarian, pancreatic, and ampulla of Vater cancers [53]. The treatment was well tolerated, and the patients showed appreciated immune responses including delayed-type hypersensitivity (DTH). A correlation between the frequency of T cells that can recognize

CAP1-6D and clinical response was documented. For instance, comparing the anti-CEA and antiviral CD4+ T cells from 23 normal donors and pancreatic cancer patients undergoing surgical resection revealed that anti-CEA CD4+ T-cell response was higher in normal donors (cells produced mainly GM-CSF and IFN-γ) than pancreatic cancer patients (cells produced mainly IL-5) [54], demonstrating a skew toward a Th2 type in pancreatic cancer patients. Therefore, vaccines aimed at correcting tumor-specific responses in these groups of patients would be able to harness them to lyse CEA-expressing tumor cells.

Several studies have also used CEA-derived peptides to load DC for vaccination. For instance, vaccination of patients with CEA-expressing metastatic gastrointestinal or lung adenocarcinomas with DC loaded with the HLA-A24 peptide CEA_{652} induced long-term stable disease and marked decreases in the serum CEA level [55]. Interestingly, this treatment protocol also induced peptide-specific T-cell responses as measured by DTH test that showed positive skin response to CEA_{652}-pulsed DC (skin test) and the in vitro capability of T cells to lyse target cells. Intranodal vaccination of metastatic colorectal carcinoma patients, who had failed standard chemotherapy, with DC loaded with YLSGANLNL or QYSWFVNGTF + TYACFVSNL CEA-derived peptides induced increases in the number of CEA-specific T cells in about 70 % patients, where 20 % patients showed stable disease for at least 12 weeks [56]. Similarly, intravenous vaccination of CEA-positive colorectal cancer patients with DC ($1–5 \times 10^7$) loaded with altered HLA-binding CEA peptide induced expansion of specific CD8+ T cells as measured by IFN-γ secretion and lysis of target cells [57]. Interestingly, the expanded T cells recognized the native CEA peptide, indicating that this peptide-based vaccination protocol may be a promising alternative for cancer immunotherapy. Vaccination of patients with resectable liver metastases of colorectal cancer with DC pulsed with DC loaded with CEA-derived HLA-A2 binding peptide induced T-cell responses in about 75 % of the vaccinated patients [58, 59]. Interestingly, these T-cell responses were higher than those obtained after vaccination with CEA mRNA-electroporated DC. Taken together, it appears that vaccination with CEA-derived peptide or DC loaded with these peptides is a potential approach to induce antitumor immunity and form a foundation to optimize peptide-based vaccination against cancer.

In a recent clinical study, DC transfected with RNA coding for CEA or pulsed with CEA HLA-A2-binding peptide were used to vaccinate patients with resectable liver metastases of colorectal cancer through intravenous or intradermal injection three times weekly prior to surgical resection of the metastases [58, 60]. To augment its antigen presentation capability, all DC were loaded with KLH as a control protein. Evaluation of vaccine-induced immune response revealed CEA reactivity in T-cell cultures of biopsies of posttreatment DTH skin tests where all patients showed T-cell responses against KLH upon vaccination. CEA peptide-specific T cells were detected in 8 out of 11 patients in the peptide group but in none of the five patients in the RNA group, indicating that the use of peptide-loaded DC is a potential anticancer immunotherapy regimen.

12 Vaccination with Survivin-Loaded DC

Survivin is a recently described inhibitor of apoptosis [61]. Survivin is practically undetectable in normal differentiated tissues but is overexpressed in a variety of tumors, particularly those of the gastrointestinal tract [62]. Survivin is among the candidate antigenic molecules that are currently being targeted for therapy by several different approaches, including DC-based vaccination. By using a reverse-immunology approach, it has been shown that the inhibitor survivin elicited $CD8^+$ T-cell-mediated responses in peripheral blood or in tumor-associated lymphocytes from colorectal cancer patients at different disease stage [63].

Several studies have used survivin-derived peptides in vaccination against several cancers including melanoma [64], colon [65], breast [66], lung [67], as well as pancreatic [68] cancers. DC-based vaccination of either full-length survivin protein or survivin peptides has also been implemented with favorable results [69]. For instance, a complete remission of the liver metastases of pancreatic cancer was observed in a patient whose cancer was refractory to chemotherapy with gemcitabine and endured for 8 months following vaccinations with survivin peptide-loaded DC [68].

13 Optimal Administration Route for Peptide-Loaded DC

For induction of effective immunity, it is important for DC to interact with T cells in the peripheral lymphoid organs, in particular lymph nodes and to some extent the spleen. DC vaccine can be injected through different routes, including intravenous, subcutaneous, intradermal, peritumoral, intratumoral, and intranodal. The route of injection of DC during vaccination, however, can significantly impact the quality and the quantity of the induced immune responses since different routes lead to different sites of accumulation of the vaccinated DC. For instance, murine models have shown that after intravenous injection, the majority of the injected DC accumulate in the spleen and to a lesser extent in the lungs, kidneys, and liver, while hardly any DC end up in peripheral lymph nodes [70]. Several preclinical and clinical studies have also shown that intratumoral injection of DC vaccine is effective [71]. Peritumoral injection of DC vaccine was also found to lead to effective migration of the injected DC to the tumor-draining lymph nodes, where the majority of the injected cells remained in the tumor vicinity. This enhanced DC migration was coincided with tumor necrosis and antitumor cytotoxic activity [72]. Of note, this study showed that loading of DC with antigen is an important factor for the migration since antigen-unloaded DC could not effectively reach the tumor-draining lymph nodes. A recent comparative study, however, demonstrated that subcutaneous injection of antigen DC and intratumoral injection of naive DC were similarly effective in mediating tumor regression and long-term survival [73].

Clinical studies in cancer patients have also showed that about 2–4 % of DC migrate to draining lymph nodes after intradermal injection [74]. These and other independent human studies have also indicated that migration of DC after their subcutaneous injection is much lower as compared with their migration after intradermal injection [75] and that intranodal injection results in a much higher amount of DC accumulating in the injected and subsequent draining lymph nodes [74]. Intranodal injection, however, has been found in recent studies to be complicated by inaccurate delivery where DC were misinjected in the perinodal fat in a considerable number of patients [76]. Indeed, a study performed on melanoma patients found slightly higher peptide-specific T-cell responses after intranodal injection than those obtained after an intradermal or intravenous injection [77], while another study in advanced melanoma patients showed no benefit for intranodal vaccination as compared to intradermal vaccination [78]. In a study in prostate cancer patients, vaccination with DC was compared after injection of DC through three different routes, including intradermal, intravenous, and intralymphatic injection via a cannula in a lymphatic channel in the dorsum of the foot [79]. In this study, no significant difference in the antigen-specific T-cell responses was observed after these different routes of DC delivery. Of note, however, the level of *ex vivo* IFN-γ production was obtained only in the peripheral blood cells obtained from patients injected with DC either via the intradermal or intralymphatic routes. These investigators also found that intravenous injection of DC can be of significant benefit to immunity against visceral melanoma metastases, whereas subcutaneous DC vaccination is important for non-visceral metastases [80], suggesting that delivery of DC via different routes during vaccination can induce systemic T-cell responses in different compartments that can control cancer cells in localized and remote sites [81]. Similar conclusions were drawn from another study in patients with metastatic prostate cancer who received two monthly injections of antigen-pulsed DC by intravenous, intradermal, or intralymphatic injection [79]. All patients developed antigen-specific T-cell responses following immunization, regardless of the route of immunization. Taken together with the above observations, it appears that intradermal and subcutaneous delivery of DC vaccine is an effective means to deliver tumor antigens. More studies are required, however, to define the most effective combinatorial delivery routes of DC with regard to the beneficial effects to clinical outcomes.

14 Safety of DC-Based Vaccination

DC vaccination utilized in many of the clinical studies did not also show a significant toxicity. For instance, DC vaccination in glioblastoma patients induced systemic and intracranial T-cell responses modulated by the local central nervous system tumor microenvironment with no toxicity [82]. In this study, 12 patients were enrolled into a multicohort dose-escalation study and treated with one, five, or ten million autologous DC pulsed with constant amounts of acid-eluted autologous tumor peptides. The DC vaccinations were well tolerated, with no major adverse events (grade 3 or 4) and no clinical or radiological signs of autoimmune reactions observed in any subject during the vaccine cycles. Grade 1 toxicities in the form of low-grade fevers and/or flu-like symptoms, e.g., fatigue and myalgia, were observed. Some patients had nausea and vomiting at some point within the first few weeks of the DC-based vaccination. Erythema, pain, and itching were observed at the injection site and lasted 48–72 h after the first DC injection. There were no treatment-related hematologic, hepatic, renal, or neurologic toxicities. In a recent phase II study on patients with hepatocellular carcinoma, intravenous vaccination with DC pulsed with tumor lysate was safe and well tolerated [83]. Toxicity was mild and self-limiting. Some patients experienced grade 1 myalgia, occasionally associated with low-grade fever, nausea, and vomiting, thought to be related to disease rather than DC infusion. No grade 3 or 4 toxicity was observed in any patient with no hepatic toxicity and no autoantibody formation was observed. Vaccination of patients with progressive malignant melanoma with autologous monocyte-derived mature DC pulsed with five high-affinity peptides induced immune responses in six out of ten analyzed HLA-$A2^+$ patients against these peptides in the peripheral blood [84]. Taken together, it appears that DC-based vaccination is a safe approach to deliver the immunogenic antigens in vivo.

15 Blocking the Regulatory Molecules That Negatively Impact DC

Improvement of the adjuvant effects of DC to peptide-based vaccination could involve suppression of the negative intrinsic and extrinsic regulators of DC. Intrinsic regulators include factors such as the programmed death (PD; B7-H) receptor [85], suppressor of cytokine signaling (SOCS) [86], and indoleamine-2,3-dioxygenase (IDO) [87]. Extrinsic regulators are factors such as regulatory cells, in particular regulatory T (T_{reg}) cells [88] and myeloid-derived suppressor cells (MDSC) [89], and their immunosuppressive mediators, in particular transforming growth factor-beta (TGF-β) and reactive oxygen radicals [90]. Indeed, recent studies showed that inhibition of these suppressive factors can enhance DC-based vaccination [91].

TGF-β signaling can be directly blocked by using inhibitory peptides such as P17 and P144 [92]. Treatment with these peptides has been found to augment T-cell responses. Alternatively, application of potent stimulatory adjuvants such as IL-2, IL-7, and IL-15, and TLR agonists may block the regulatory effects of TGF-β [93]. In line with this notion, it has been demonstrated that the adjuvant effects of IL-7 to augment antitumor responses are mediated by upregulating the expression of Nedd4 and smurf2 and by downregulating the expression levels of Cbl-b and smad in T cells, rendering $CD8^+$ T cells refractory to the inhibitor effect of TGF-β [93]. Because IL-7 has been found to be produced and acts directly on DC [94], it is important to investigate how it impacts the TGF-β signaling.

16 The Role of Immunoregulatory Cells

The dysfunction of DC in cancer patients has been attributed to the ability of the cancer cells to inhibit the tumor-reactive T cells indirectly through facilitating the development of suppressive immune cells such as regulatory $CD4^+CD25^+$ T (T_{reg}) cells and MDSC ($CD11b^-CD31^+$HLA-DR) [95]. Recently, it was suggested that MDSC detection in peripheral blood using definitive biomarkers for $CD33^+$ and $CD11b^+$ subsets can distinguish cancer patients from healthy individuals [96].

17 The Regulatory Role of T_{reg} Cells

T_{reg} cells exist naturally in the steady state and constitute about 5–10 % of $CD4^+$ T cells in normal humans and mice [97]. Conventional $CD4^+$ T cells can also convert into T_{reg} cells upon certain antigen recognition [97]. T_{reg} cells are required in the steady state to prevent autoimmune diseases [97] and in pathological conditions to control the infection-induced immunopathology [98]. The presence of T_{reg} cells is also considered as one of the escape mechanisms by cancer and microbes from immune responses [98]. Phenotypically, T_{reg} cells constitutively express the high-affinity α-chain of the IL-2 receptor (CD25), glucocorticoid-induced tumor necrosis factor receptor (GITR), and cytotoxic T lymphocyte-associated antigen (CTLA-4), and Forkhead box P3 (Foxp3), a transcription factor required for T_{reg} cell development and function [99]. They are functionally characterized by their secretion of the suppressive cytokines IL-10 and TGF-β. $CD4^+CD25^+$ T_{reg} effectively suppress the proliferation and activity of $CD4^+CD25^-$ and $CD8^+$ T cells in a contact-dependent manner through inhibition of IL-2 production [100]. Accumulating data have indicated that T_{reg} enriched in tumor mass can potently inhibit the antitumor immunity mediated by $CD4^+$Th1 and $CD8^+$ CTL; however, the mechanism is not fully understood. The proliferation of T_{reg} cells, as well as conversion of nonregulatory T cells into T_{reg} and migration of T_{reg}, was found to be crucial for their enrichment and suppressive capacity in tumor masses [101].

18 The Regulatory Role of MDSC

Recent research, including ours, has established that tumor progression associates with a systemic accumulation of MDSC [102], which results in defective DC function and an inhibition of antigen-specific T-cell responses [95]. Presence of MDSC is considered as one of the escape mechanisms by which cancer cells overcome the effectiveness of the host immune responses [95]. Phenotypically, MDSC can be identified as double negative for the MHC class II molecule (HLA-DR) and any other surface markers of mature lymphoid or myeloid cells (CD3, CD19, CD57, CD14) or Lin^- but positive for both CD33 and CD11b [95]. MDSC might inhibit DC by several mechanisms, including increased production of reactive oxygen species and increased metabolism of the amino acid L-arginine by arginase I and nitric oxide synthase 2 [95]. MDSC have recently been recognized as a subset of innate immune cells that can alter adaptive immunity and produce immunosuppression [103]. MDSC inhibit T-cell effector functions through a range of mechanisms, including arginase 1 (ARG-1)-mediated depletion of L-arginine [104], inducible nitric oxide synthase (iNOS) and nicotinamide adenine dinucleotide phosphate-oxidase (NOX2) production of reactive nitrogen and oxygen species [105], vascular endothelial growth factor (VEGF) overexpression cysteine depletion, and the expansion of T_{reg} cell populations [96]. They create a tolerogenic environment via cytokine production, manipulation of L-arginine metabolism, and dysregulation of both CD4 and CD8 T-cell function [106].

MDSC also produce high levels of indoleamine-2,3-dioxygenase (IDO), which catalyzes the degradation of tryptophan into kynurenine and results in T-cell starvation and apoptosis [107]. Similar to T cells, it is possible that DC are affected by IDO by a similar mechanism. MDSC infiltrate into tumors and accumulate at the invasive front where they promote tumor angiogenesis as well as tumor cell invasion and metastasis via regulation of protease activity [108]. MDSC also confer resistance to cancer therapies. Hence, MDSC are a viable target for therapeutic intervention [109].

19 Blocking the Regulatory Function of T_{reg} Cells and MDSC

MDSC are plastic and depending on specific growth factors and microenvironment can differentiate into DC, macrophages, or endothelial cells [91, 95]. Recent studies suggest the possibility of preventing the suppressor function of MDSC by treatment with certain drugs such as the multitargeted receptor tyrosine kinase inhibitors: sunitinib [110] and ATRA [111] or with the IDO inhibitor 1-methyl-D-tryptophan (D-1mT) [112].

Potential strategies that can block the regulatory cells include low dose of the anticancer drug cyclophosphamide and anti-CD25 (IL-2Rα) antibodies such as anti-Tac (Daclizumab) [113] and RFT5-SMPT-dg [114]. Denileukin diftitox (DD; ONTAK) can also induce T_{reg} cell death [115]. ONTAK is a recombinant fusion protein consisting of peptide sequences for the enzymatically active and membrane translocation domain of diphtheria toxin linked to human IL-2. It specifically binds to IL-2 receptors on the cell membrane, is internalized via receptor-mediated endocytosis, and inhibits protein synthesis by adenosine triphosphate ribosylation of elongation factor 2, resulting in cell death. The multitargeted receptor tyrosine kinase inhibitor sunitinib has also shown to block the regulatory effects of T_{reg} cells [116]. Ultimately, depletion of T_{reg} cells can enhance the development of protective T-cell responses during antitumor immunity [117]. Given the successful application of these approaches in cancer settings, their application to interfere with T_{reg} cell function during DC-based vaccination can accentuate the resultant antitumor immune responses.

20 Induction of Maturation of DC with TLR Agonists

DC maturation, characterized by the increased surface expression of MHC and costimulatory molecules, is crucial for the initiation of antitumor immunity. The full maturation of DC is completed only upon interaction with T cells. This interaction requires expression of several other accessory molecules expressed in DC, including LFA-3/CD58, ICAM-1/CD54, B7-1/CD80, B7-2/CD86, and CD83. Expression of at least one or both of the costimulatory molecules B7-1 and B7-2, which bind the CD28 molecules on T cells, on DC is critical for the generation of effective T cells [118]. Matured DC can produce several inflammatory cytokines, in particular IFN-α, IL-12, and IL-15, and also produce the inflammatory chemokine macrophage inflammatory protein (MIP-1) and macrophage chemotactic protein 1 (MCP-1 or CCL2), which are important in the elicitation of effective primary immune responses [30]. Several strategies have been applied in vivo and in vitro to induce full maturation of DC [10]. Because DC are equipped with receptors that sense different microbial "danger signals" such as TLR agonists [119], triggering of TLR in DC by their specific TLR agonists has been found to be an attractive approach and has showed promising effects in preclinical and clinical studies.

So far, about 13 TLR that can sense different classes of TLR agonists have been characterized. TLR are members of a family of transmembrane proteins with an extracellular leucine-rich domain and a conserved cytoplasmic domain homologous to that of the interleukin-1 receptor (IL-1R), termed the Toll/IL-1R homology (TIR) domain [120]. This structure allows TLR to recognize microbial products (pathogen-associated molecular patterns; PAMPs) and activate, via the TIR domain, a series of downstream pathways that result in immune and inflammatory responses [120]. After binding to their specific ligands on innate immune cells, TLR dimerize and undergo conformational changes which are required for the recruitment of adaptor molecules to the TIR domain [120]. Once the adaptors have been recruited, a complex of IL-1R-associated kinases (IRAks), TRAF6, and IRF-5 is formed and results in the downstream phosphorylation of IκB, which in turn frees NF-κB. Unbound NF-κB translocates into the nucleus where it directly regulates the transcription of proinflammatory genes. When triggered, TLR signaling induces proinflammatory mediators, including cytokines and chemokines, and maturation of DC. These mediators, in combination with mature DC, activate CTL and natural killer (NK) cells, promoting adaptive immunity. In this context, we and others have reported that addition of certain TLR agonists, in particular, TLR3 agonist poly(I:C), TLR7/8 agonist (imiquimod), and TLR9 agonist (CpG), to different immunization regimens, leads to marked adjuvant effects to postvaccination $CD8^+$ T-cell responses, coinciding with antitumor and antiviral immunity [121–128]. In response to TLR agonists, resident immature DC at the site of vaccination undergo a maturation program and migrate to the draining lymph nodes. Therefore, utilizing TLR is a potential approach to induce activation of immature DC and maximize their contribution to memory cell responses.

Furthermore, in vitro treatment of DC with these TLR agonists can induce their full maturation, resulting in substantial increases in antigen-specific T-cell responses [129–133]. These studies led to the application of treatment with TLR agonists in different clinical settings that require the development of strong Th1-type responses [134]. We and others have reported that poly(I:C) is an excellent inducer of DC activation and function due to the rapid release of inflammatory cytokines, including IFN-α [124, 131, 135–139]. Our further analysis showed that poly(I:C) is essential for the effectiveness of antitumor T-cell responses through the rapid induction of a plethora of inflammatory cytokines, including IFN-α and IFN-γ, IL-6, TNF-α, IL-12, and CCL2 [123, 124]. Most importantly, we have found that the adjuvant effects of poly(I:C) to antitumor immune responses were coincided with marked activation of DC in the peripheral blood and liver [123]. Indeed, in vitro treatment of DC, generated from peripheral blood of healthy donors, with Hiltonol® or Ampligen®, two different clinical grade forms of the TLR3 agonist poly(I:C), induced DC activation [135–137, 140–142]. Previous studies have also established the adjuvant effects of several TLR agonists, in particular, TLR3 poly(I:C), TLR7/8 agonist (imiquimod), and TLR9 agonist (CpG) agonists, to the antitumor $CD8^+$ T-cell responses [123–126, 131, 136, 143]. These beneficial effects of TLR agonists to immunotherapy could be because of their induction of maturation of resident immature DC at the site of vaccination and their subsequent migration to the draining lymph nodes [29, 144–148].

Taking the above studies together, it appears that TLR agonists are a potential approach to induce activation of immature DC and maximize their contribution to enhanced T-cell responses. Therefore, it is possible that treatment of a host with cancer with TLR agonists, in particular the TLR3 agonist poly(I:C), the TLR9 agonist CpG-ODN, and the TLR7/8 agonist imiquimod, concomitant with vaccination with DC pulsed with single or multiple peptides, can induce the maturation of the injected DC and their migration to draining lymph nodes where effective antigen presentation can occur, resulting in efficacious antitumor immunity. Meanwhile, administration of a TLR agonist would also elicit the activation of endogenous NK cells and DC and their production of inflammatory cytokines, resulting in a beneficial microenvironment that will further enhance the overall antitumor immunity. These events may lead to significant clinical responses.

The use of TLR agonists as a potent stimulator of DC-based vaccination in cancer as discussed above is likely to be a working hypothesis since treatment of cancer with other TLR agonists has been found to induce significant antitumor effects even in the absence of active vaccination. For instance, intratumoral or systemic administration of the TLR2/6 agonist "macrophage-activating lipopeptide-2" resulted in induction of infiltration of lymphocytes in the pancreatic [149, 150] and melanoma [151] tumor bed with significant tumor suppression. These studies led to a clinical trial based on the intratumoral injection of this TLR2/6 agonist in patients with pancreatic carcinoma. This treatment resulted in the induction of influx of lymphocytes and monocytes in the tumor and abolishment of inhibition of NK activity [149].

Furthermore, treatment with the TLR9 agonist CpG-ODN in an orthotopic murine model of human pancreatic cancer induced an improvement of survival of the tumor-bearing mice [152]. These induced antitumor effects after treatment with these TLR (TLR2/6 and TLR9) agonists were more effective in combination with the chemotherapeutic drug gemcitabine, the drug of choice in pancreatic cancer. In a recent study, vaccination with elutriated monocyte-derived DC matured with TLR2/4-agonist (FMKp, available in clinical grade) in combination with IFN-γ (FIcocktail) induced twofold increases in the induction of cytotoxic T cells against a known tumor antigen when compared with vaccination with DC matured with TNF-alpha/PGE-2, i.e., TP-cocktail, the DC in current clinical trials [153].

Taking the adjuvant antitumor effects of these TLRs with the adjuvant antitumor effects of vaccination with antigen-pulsed DC, it can be suggested that the combination of these two modalities would induce higher antitumor responses than the use of either of them alone. Although activation of DC with TLR agonists in vitro is safe, previous studies have shown that in vitro maturation alone is not sufficient to induce therapeutic antitumor effects against an advanced bulky tumor and that in vivo adjuvants are a prerequisite to the establishment of antitumor responses [113, 154, 155]. The advantage of administration of TLR agonists is to induce the contribution of the endogenous innate immune cells and their cross talk to the exogenous DC. These events can overcome the immunosuppressive effects in the tumor-bearing host and lead to effective antigen-specific immune responses. The application of TLR-based therapy in the clinical setting can open new avenues for cancer immunotherapy; in particular, the agonists for TLR3 (poly(I:C)), TLR7/8 (imiquimod), and TLR9 (CpG) have ranked as potential adjuvants for cancer immunotherapy among the 12 agents listed by the Immunotherapy Agent Workshop held at NIH, July 2007 [156, 157]. Taken together, these studies suggest that coadministration of TLR agonists with DC loaded with multiple epitopes would lead to an effective immunotherapeutic regimen in pancreatic cancer.

21 Conclusion

Vaccination with DC is a potential approach to induce antitumor immunity. However, the recognition of tumor cells by the T-cell responses generated was limited. This could be because vaccination has been mostly based on the use of a single antigen. Therefore, one approach to augment DC-based vaccination is to load DC with multiple epitopes to increase the frequency of the antigen-specific T cells with specificity toward multiple tumor antigens, in particular in the antigen loss setting. DC-based vaccination can also be enhanced by preconditioning the host with inflammatory signals (cytokines or TLR agonists) to increase the maturation and migration of the exogenous peptide-loaded DC from the peripheral tissues to the lymph nodes where effective antigen presentation would occur resulting in a robust tumor-specific immunity. The inflammatory signals would also elicit the activation of the endogenous NK cells and DC and their production of inflammatory cytokines, creating a beneficial microenvironment that would block the intrinsic regulatory elements in DC and allow for a more efficacious antigen presentation. Additionally, blocking the suppressor elements such as T_{reg} cells and MDSC before or during vaccination with peptide-loaded DC would release the brakes regulating the antigen-specific T cells to interact with the antigen-bearing DC, resulting in a robust antitumor immunity.

References

1. Matzinger P (2002) The danger model: a renewed sense of self. Science 296(5566): 301–305
2. Finn OJ (2008) Cancer immunology. N Engl J Med 358(25):2704–2715
3. McCarthy EF (2006) The toxins of William B. Coley and the treatment of bone and soft-tissue sarcomas. Iowa Orthop J 26:154–158
4. Finn OJ (2008) Immunological weapons acquired early in life win battles with cancer late in life. J Immunol 181(3):1589–1592
5. Pejawar-Gaddy S, Finn OJ (2008) Cancer vaccines: accomplishments and challenges. Crit Rev Oncol Hematol 67(2):93–102
6. Salem ML et al (2007) Tumours: immunotherapy. Encyclopedia of life sciences, 2007, John Wiley & Sons, Ltd. www.els.net
7. Yannelli JR, Wroblewski JM (2004) On the road to a tumor cell vaccine: 20 years of cellular immunotherapy. Vaccine 23(1):97–113
8. Vermorken JB et al (1999) Active specific immunotherapy for stage II and stage III human colon cancer: a randomised trial. Lancet 353(9150):345–350
9. Melief CJ (2008) Cancer immunotherapy by dendritic cells. Immunity 29(3):372–383
10. Banchereau J et al (2003) Dendritic cells: controllers of the immune system and a new promise for immunotherapy. Novartis Found Symp 252:226–235, discussion 235–228, 257–267
11. Stift A et al (2003) Dendritic cell-based vaccination in solid cancer. J Clin Oncol 21(1): 135–142
12. Brossart P (2002) Dendritic cells in vaccination therapies of malignant diseases. Transfus Apher Sci 27(2):183–186
13. Nagorsen D, Thiel E (2006) Clinical and immunologic responses to active specific cancer vaccines in human colorectal cancer. Clin Cancer Res 12(10):3064–3069
14. Steinman RM, Cohn ZA (1973) Identification of a novel cell type in peripheral lymphoid organs of mice. I. Morphology, quantitation, tissue distribution. J Exp Med 137(5): 1142–1162
15. Rosenzwajg M et al (1996) Human dendritic cell differentiation pathway from $CD34^+$ hematopoietic precursor cells. Blood 87(2): 535–544
16. Strobl H et al (1996) TGF-beta 1 promotes in vitro development of dendritic cells from $CD34^+$ hemopoietic progenitors. J Immunol 157(4):1499–1507
17. Yao V et al (2002) Dendritic cells. ANZ J Surg 72(7):501–506
18. Reid CD (1997) The dendritic cell lineage in haemopoiesis. Br J Haematol 96(2):217–223
19. Szabolcs P et al (1996) Dendritic cells and macrophages can mature independently from a human bone marrow-derived, post-colony-forming unit intermediate. Blood 87(11): 4520–4530
20. Rossi G et al (1992) Development of a Langerhans cell phenotype from peripheral blood monocytes. Immunol Lett 31(2): 189–197
21. Kasinrerk W et al (1993) CD1 molecule expression on human monocytes induced by granulocyte-macrophage colony-stimulating factor. J Immunol 150(2):579–584
22. Zhou LJ, Tedder TF (1996) $CD14^+$ blood monocytes can differentiate into functionally mature $CD83^+$ dendritic cells. Proc Natl Acad Sci USA 93(6):2588–2592
23. den Brok MH et al (2005) Dendritic cells: tools and targets for antitumor vaccination. Expert Rev Vaccines 4(5):699–710

24. Morisaki T et al (2003) Dendritic cell-based combined immunotherapy with autologous tumor-pulsed dendritic cell vaccine and activated T cells for cancer patients: rationale, current progress, and perspectives. Hum Cell 16(4):175–182
25. Tacken PJ et al (2007) Dendritic-cell immunotherapy: from *ex vivo* loading to *in vivo* targeting. Nat Rev Immunol 7(10):790–802
26. Caux C et al (1992) GM-CSF and TNF-alpha cooperate in the generation of dendritic Langerhans cells. Nature 360(6401): 258–261
27. Cella M et al (1996) Ligation of CD40 on dendritic cells triggers production of high levels of interleukin-12 and enhances T cell stimulatory capacity: T-T help via APC activation. J Exp Med 184(2):747–752
28. Whiteside TL, Odoux C (2004) Dendritic cell biology and cancer therapy. Cancer Immunol Immunother 53(3):240–248
29. Banchereau J, Steinman RM (1998) Dendritic cells and the control of immunity. Nature 392(6673):245–252
30. Aarntzen EH et al (2008) Dendritic cell vaccination and immune monitoring. Cancer Immunol Immunother 57(10):1559–1568
31. Nicola M et al (1999) The influence of interleukin (IL)-4 and IL-13 on human dendritic cell differentiation from $CD34^+$ progenitor cells: the importance of the source of serum. Exp Hematol 27(2):386–387
32. Esche C et al (1999) The use of dendritic cells for cancer vaccination. Curr Opin Mol Ther 1(1):72–81
33. Zhang SN et al (2011) Optimizing DC vaccination by combination with oncolytic adenovirus coexpressing IL-12 and GM-CSF. [Research Support, Non-U.S. Gov't]. Mol Ther 19(8):1558–1568
34. Brinkman JA et al (2004) Peptide-based vaccines for cancer immunotherapy. Expert Opin Biol Ther 4(2):181–198
35. Kavanagh B et al (2007) Vaccination of metastatic colorectal cancer patients with matured dendritic cells loaded with multiple major histocompatibility complex class I peptides. J Immunother 30(7):762–772
36. Harley CB et al (1990) Telomeres shorten during ageing of human fibroblasts. Nature 345(6274):458–460
37. Cong YS et al (2002) Human telomerase and its regulation. Microbiol Mol Biol Rev 66(3):407–425
38. Vonderheide RH (2008) Prospects and challenges of building a cancer vaccine targeting telomerase. Biochimie 90(1):173–180
39. Vonderheide RH et al (2004) Vaccination of cancer patients against telomerase induces functional antitumor $CD8^+$ T lymphocytes. Clin Cancer Res 10(3):828–839
40. Su Z et al (2005) Telomerase mRNA-transfected dendritic cells stimulate antigen-specific $CD8^+$ and $CD4^+$ T cell responses in patients with metastatic prostate cancer. J Immunol 174(6):3798–3807
41. Kono K et al (2002) Dendritic cells pulsed with HER-2/neu-derived peptides can induce specific T-cell responses in patients with gastric cancer. Clin Cancer Res 8(11):3394–3400
42. Aloysius M et al (2009) Generation *in vivo* of peptide-specific cytotoxic T cells and presence of regulatory T cells during vaccination with hTERT (class I and II) peptide-pulsed DCs. [Research Support, Non-U.S. Gov't]. J Transl Med 7:18
43. Suso EM et al (2011) hTERT mRNA dendritic cell vaccination: complete response in a pancreatic cancer patient associated with response against several hTERT epitopes. Cancer Immunol Immunother 60(6):809–818
44. Terada T et al (1996) Expression of MUC apomucins in normal pancreas and pancreatic tumours. J Pathol 180(2):160–165
45. Taylor-Papadimitriou J et al (1999) MUC1 and cancer. Biochim Biophys Acta 1455(2–3): 301–313
46. Brossart P et al (2001) The epithelial tumor antigen MUC1 is expressed in hematological malignancies and is recognized by MUC1-specific cytotoxic T-lymphocytes. Cancer Res 61(18):6846–6850
47. Jerome KR et al (1993) Tumor-specific cytotoxic T cell clones from patients with breast and pancreatic adenocarcinoma recognize EBV-immortalized B cells transfected with polymorphic epithelial mucin complementary DNA. J Immunol 151(3):1654–1662
48. Yamamoto K et al (2005) MUC1 peptide vaccination in patients with advanced pancreas or biliary tract cancer. Anticancer Res 25(5):3575–3579
49. Brossart P et al (2000) Induction of cytotoxic T-lymphocyte responses in vivo after vaccinations with peptide-pulsed dendritic cells. Blood 96(9):3102–3108
50. Brossart P, Bevan MJ (1997) Presentation of exogenous protein antigens on major histocompatibility complex class I molecules by dendritic cells: pathway of presentation and regulation by cytokines. Blood 90(4): 1594–1599
51. Wierecky J et al (2006) Immunologic and clinical responses after vaccinations with peptide-pulsed dendritic cells in metastatic renal cancer patients. Cancer Res 66(11): 5910–5918

52. Kim Y et al (2003) Gastrointestinal tract cancer screening using fecal carcinoembryonic antigen. Ann Clin Lab Sci 33(1):32–38
53. Kaufman HL et al (2007) Poxvirus-based vaccine therapy for patients with advanced pancreatic cancer. J Transl Med 5:60
54. Tassi E et al (2008) Carcinoembryonic antigen-specific but not antiviral $CD4^+$ T cell immunity is impaired in pancreatic carcinoma patients. J Immunol 181(9):6595–6603
55. Ueda Y et al (2004) Dendritic cell-based immunotherapy of cancer with carcinoembryonic antigen-derived, HLA-A24-restricted CTL epitope: clinical outcomes of 18 patients with metastatic gastrointestinal or lung adenocarcinomas. [Clinical trial]. Int J Oncol 24(4):909–917
56. Liu KJ et al (2004) Generation of carcinoembryonic antigen (CEA)-specific T-cell responses in HLA-A*0201 and HLA-A*2402 late-stage colorectal cancer patients after vaccination with dendritic cells loaded with CEA peptides. Clin Cancer Res 10(8):2645–2651
57. Babatz J et al (2006) Induction of cellular immune responses against carcinoembryonic antigen in patients with metastatic tumors after vaccination with altered peptide ligand-loaded dendritic cells. Cancer Immunol Immunother 55(3):268–276
58. Lesterhuis WJ et al (2006) Vaccination of colorectal cancer patients with CEA-loaded dendritic cells: antigen-specific T cell responses in DTH skin tests. Ann Oncol 17(6): 974–980
59. Lesterhuis WJ et al (2008) Dendritic cell vaccines in melanoma: from promise to proof? Crit Rev Oncol Hematol 66(2):118–134
60. Lesterhuis WJ et al (2010) Immunogenicity of dendritic cells pulsed with CEA peptide or transfected with CEA mRNA for vaccination of colorectal cancer patients. Anticancer Res 30(12):5091–5097
61. Ambrosini G et al (1997) A novel anti-apoptosis gene, survivin, expressed in cancer and lymphoma. Nat Med 3(8):917–921
62. Lopes RB et al (2007) Expression of the IAP protein family is dysregulated in pancreatic cancer cells and is important for resistance to chemotherapy. Int J Cancer 120(11):2344–2352
63. Casati C et al (2003) The apoptosis inhibitor protein survivin induces tumor-specific $CD8^+$ and $CD4^+$ T cells in colorectal cancer patients. Cancer Res 63(15):4507–4515
64. Otto K et al (2005) Lack of toxicity of therapy-induced T cell responses against the universal tumour antigen survivin. Vaccine 23(7):884–889
65. Tsuruma T et al (2004) Phase I clinical study of anti-apoptosis protein, survivin-derived peptide vaccine therapy for patients with advanced or recurrent colorectal cancer. J Transl Med 2(1):19
66. Tsuruma T et al (2008) Clinical and immunological evaluation of anti-apoptosis protein, survivin-derived peptide vaccine in phase I clinical study for patients with advanced or recurrent breast cancer. J Transl Med 6:24
67. Karanikas V et al (2008) Baseline levels of $CD8^+$ T cells against survivin and survivin-2B in the blood of lung cancer patients and cancer-free individuals. Clin Immunol 129(2):230–240
68. Wobser M et al (2006) Complete remission of liver metastasis of pancreatic cancer under vaccination with a HLA-A2 restricted peptide derived from the universal tumor antigen survivin. Cancer Immunol Immunother 55(10): 1294–1298
69. Nagaraj S et al (2007) Dendritic cell-based full-length survivin vaccine in treatment of experimental tumors. J Immunother 30(2): 169–179
70. Eggert AA et al (1999) Biodistribution and vaccine efficiency of murine dendritic cells are dependent on the route of administration. Cancer Res 59(14):3340–3345
71. Moyer JS et al (2008) Intratumoral dendritic cells and chemoradiation for the treatment of murine squamous cell carcinoma. J Immunother 31(9):885–895
72. Rossowska J et al (2007) Tissue localization of tumor antigen-loaded mouse dendritic cells applied as an anti-tumor vaccine and their influence on immune response. Folia Histochem Cytobiol 45(4):349–355
73. Cohen S et al (2009) Dendritic cell-based therapeutic vaccination against myeloma: vaccine formulation determines efficacy against light chain myeloma. J Immunol 182(3):1667–1673
74. De Vries IJ et al (2003) Effective migration of antigen-pulsed dendritic cells to lymph nodes in melanoma patients is determined by their maturation state. Cancer Res 63(1):12–17
75. Trakatelli M et al (2006) A new dendritic cell vaccine generated with interleukin-3 and interferon-beta induces $CD8^+$ T cell responses against NA17-A2 tumor peptide in melanoma patients. Cancer Immunol Immunother 55(4):469–474
76. Zitvogel L, Tursz T (2005) *In vivo* veritas. Nat Biotechnol 23(11):1372–1374
77. Bedrosian I et al (2003) Intranodal administration of peptide-pulsed mature dendritic cell vaccines results in superior $CD8^+$ T-cell function in melanoma patients. J Clin Oncol 21(20):3826–3835
78. Kyte JA et al (2006) Phase I/II trial of melanoma therapy with dendritic cells transfected with autologous tumor-mRNA. Cancer Gene Ther 13(10):905–918

79. Fong L et al (2001) Dendritic cells injected via different routes induce immunity in cancer patients. J Immunol 166(6):4254–4259
80. Mullins DW et al (2003) Route of immunization with peptide-pulsed dendritic cells controls the distribution of memory and effector T cells in lymphoid tissues and determines the pattern of regional tumor control. J Exp Med 198(7):1023–1034
81. Adema GJ et al (2005) Migration of dendritic cell based cancer vaccines: in vivo veritas? Curr Opin Immunol 17(2):170–174
82. Liau LM et al (2005) Dendritic cell vaccination in glioblastoma patients induces systemic and intracranial T-cell responses modulated by the local central nervous system tumor microenvironment. Clin Cancer Res 11(15): 5515–5525
83. Palmer DH et al (2009) A phase II study of adoptive immunotherapy using dendritic cells pulsed with tumor lysate in patients with hepatocellular carcinoma. Hepatology 49(1): 124–132
84. Trepiakas R et al (2010) Vaccination with autologous dendritic cells pulsed with multiple tumor antigens for treatment of patients with malignant melanoma: results from a phase I/II trial. Cytotherapy 12(6):721–734
85. Waisman A, Yogev N (2009) B7-H1 and $CD8^+$ Treg: the enigmatic role of B7-H1 in peripheral tolerance. Eur J Immunol 39(6): 1448–1451
86. Yoshimura A (2009) Regulation of cytokine signaling by the SOCS and Spred family proteins. Keio J Med 58(2):73–83
87. Lob S, Konigsrainer A (2008) Is IDO a key enzyme bridging the gap between tumor escape and tolerance induction? Langenbecks Arch Surg 393(6):995–1003
88. Mahnke K et al (2007) Tolerogenic dendritic cells and regulatory T cells: a two-way relationship. J Dermatol Sci 46(3):159–167
89. Marigo I et al (2008) Tumor-induced tolerance and immune suppression by myeloid derived suppressor cells. Immunol Rev 222: 162–179
90. Li H et al (2009) Cancer-expanded myeloid-derived suppressor cells induce anergy of NK cells through membrane-bound TGF-beta 1. J Immunol 182(1):240–249
91. Bronte V, Mocellin S (2009) Suppressive influences in the immune response to cancer. J Immunother 32(1):1–11
92. Llopiz D et al (2009) Peptide inhibitors of transforming growth factor-beta enhance the efficacy of antitumor immunotherapy. Int J Cancer 125(11):2614–2623
93. Pellegrini M et al (2009) Adjuvant IL-7 antagonizes multiple cellular and molecular inhibitory networks to enhance immunotherapies. Nat Med 15(5):528–536
94. Vogt TK et al (2009) Novel function for interleukin-7 in dendritic cell development. Blood 113(17):3961–3968
95. Gabrilovich DI, Nagaraj S (2009) Myeloid-derived suppressor cells as regulators of the immune system. Nat Rev Immunol 9(3):162–174
96. Lechner MG et al (2011) Functional characterization of human $Cd33^+$ and $Cd11b^+$ myeloid-derived suppressor cell subsets induced from peripheral blood mononuclear cells co-cultured with a diverse set of human tumor cell lines. J Transl Med 9:90
97. Chatila TA (2009) Regulatory T cells: key players in tolerance and autoimmunity. Endocrinol Metab Clin North Am 38(2): 265–272
98. Mills KH (2004) Regulatory T cells: friend or foe in immunity to infection? Nat Rev Immunol 4(11):841–855
99. Sakaguchi S (2005) Naturally arising Foxp3-expressing $CD25^+CD4^+$ regulatory T cells in immunological tolerance to self and non-self. Nat Immunol 6(4):345–352
100. Zhou G et al (2006) Amplification of tumor-specific regulatory T cells following therapeutic cancer vaccines. Blood 107(2): 628–636
101. Xu L et al (2011) In situ prior proliferation of $CD4^+$ $CCR6^+$ regulatory T cells facilitated by TGF-beta secreting DC is crucial for their enrichment and suppression in tumor immunity. PLoS One 6(5):1–10
102. Diaz-Montero CM et al (2009) Increased circulating myeloid-derived suppressor cells correlate with clinical cancer stage, metastatic tumor burden, and doxorubicin-cyclophosphamide chemotherapy. Cancer Immunol Immunother 58(1):49–59
103. Stewart TJ, Smyth MJ (2011) Improving cancer immunotherapy by targeting tumor-induced immune suppression. Cancer Metastasis Rev 30(1):125–140
104. Bak SP et al (2008) Murine ovarian cancer vascular leukocytes require arginase-1 activity for T cell suppression. Mol Immunol 46(2): 258–268
105. Corzo CA et al (2009) Mechanism regulating reactive oxygen species in tumor-induced myeloid-derived suppressor cells. J Immunol 182(9):5693–5701
106. Ray P et al (2011) Lung myeloid-derived suppressor cells and regulation of inflammation. Immunol Res 50(2–3):153–158
107. Wang Z et al (2008) Short-term anti-CD25 monoclonal antibody treatment and neogenetic $CD4(^+)CD25(high)$ regulatory T cells

in kidney transplantation. Transpl Immunol 19(1):69–73
108. Yang L et al (2004) Expansion of myeloid immune suppressor $Gr^{+}CD11b^{+}$ cells in tumor-bearing host directly promotes tumor angiogenesis. Cancer Cell 6(4):409–421
109. Finke J et al (2011) MDSC as a mechanism of tumor escape from sunitinib mediated anti-angiogenic therapy. Int Immunopharmacol 11(7):856–861
110. Ko JS et al (2009) Sunitinib mediates reversal of myeloid-derived suppressor cell accumulation in renal cell carcinoma patients. Clin Cancer Res 15(6):2148–2157
111. Kusmartsev S et al (2008) Reversal of myeloid cell-mediated immunosuppression in patients with metastatic renal cell carcinoma. Clin Cancer Res 14(24):8270–8278
112. Qian F et al (2009) Efficacy of levo-1-methyl tryptophan and dextro-1-methyl tryptophan in reversing indoleamine-2,3-dioxygenase-mediated arrest of T-cell proliferation in human epithelial ovarian cancer. Cancer Res 69(13):5498–5504
113. Wang RF et al (2008) Toll-like receptors and immune regulation: implications for cancer therapy. Oncogene 27(2):181–189
114. Platz KP et al (2005) IL-2 antagonists: the European perspective. Transplant Proc 37(4):1783–1784
115. Duvic M, Talpur R (2008) Optimizing denileukin diftitox (Ontak) therapy. Future Oncol 4(4):457–469
116. Ozao-Choy J et al (2009) The novel role of tyrosine kinase inhibitor in the reversal of immune suppression and modulation of tumor microenvironment for immune-based cancer therapies. Cancer Res 69(6): 2514–2522
117. Chen YL et al (2008) Depletion of CD4(+) CD25(+) regulatory T cells can promote local immunity to suppress tumor growth in benzo[a] pyrene-induced forestomach carcinoma. World J Gastroenterol 14(38):5797–5809
118. Vonderheide RH, June CH (2003) A translational bridge to cancer immunotherapy: exploiting costimulation and target antigens for active and passive T cell immunotherapy. Immunol Res 27(2–3):341–356
119. Kowalczyk DW (2002) Tumors and the danger model. Acta Biochim Pol 49(2):295–302
120. Kawai T, Akira S (2007) TLR signaling. Semin Immunol 19(1):24–32
121. Seya T et al (2006) Role of Toll-like receptors in adjuvant-augmented immune therapies. Evid Based Complement Alternat Med 3(1):31–38, discussion 133–137
122. Salem ML et al (2009) Recovery from cyclophosphamide-induced lymphopenia results in expansion of immature dendritic cells which can mediate enhanced prime-boost vaccination antitumor responses in vivo when stimulated with the TLR3 agonist poly(I:C). J Immunol 182(4):2030–2040
123. Salem ML et al (2009) The TLR3 agonist poly(I:C) targets $CD8^{+}$ T cells and augments their antigen-specific responses upon their adoptive transfer into naive recipient mice. Vaccine 27(4):549–557
124. Salem ML et al (2006) The adjuvant effects of the toll-like receptor 3 ligand polyinosinic-cytidylic acid poly(I:C) on antigen-specific $CD8^{+}$ T cell responses are partially dependent on NK cells with the induction of a beneficial cytokine milieu. Vaccine 24(24):5119–5132
125. Salem ML et al (2005) Defining the antigen-specific T-cell response to vaccination and poly(I:C)/TLR3 signaling: evidence of enhanced primary and memory CD8 T-cell responses and antitumor immunity. J Immunother 28(3):220–228
126. Salem ML et al (2007) Defining the ability of cyclophosphamide preconditioning to enhance the antigen-specific $CD8^{+}$ T-cell response to peptide vaccination: creation of a beneficial host microenvironment involving type I IFNs and myeloid cells. J Immunother 30(1):40–53
127. Banchereau J, Palucka AK (2005) Dendritic cells as therapeutic vaccines against cancer. Nat Rev Immunol 5(4):296–306
128. Fajardo-Moser M et al (2008) Mechanisms of dendritic cell-based vaccination against infection. Int J Med Microbiol 298(1–2):11–20
129. Datta SK et al (2003) A subset of Toll-like receptor ligands induces cross-presentation by bone marrow-derived dendritic cells. J Immunol 170(8):4102–4110
130. Edwards AD et al (2003) Toll-like receptor expression in murine DC subsets: lack of TLR7 expression by CD8 $alpha^{+}$ DC correlates with unresponsiveness to imidazoquinolines. Eur J Immunol 33(4):827–833
131. Lore K et al (2003) Toll-like receptor ligands modulate dendritic cells to augment cytomegalovirus- and HIV-1-specific T cell responses. J Immunol 171(8):4320–4328
132. Kadowaki N et al (2001) Subsets of human dendritic cell precursors express different toll-like receptors and respond to different microbial antigens. J Exp Med 194(6):863–869
133. West MA et al (2004) Enhanced dendritic cell antigen capture via toll-like receptor-induced actin remodeling. Science 305(5687): 1153–1157
134. Meyer T, Stockfleth E (2008) Clinical investigations of Toll-like receptor agonists. Expert Opin Investig Drugs 17(7):1051–1065
135. Boullart AC et al (2008) Maturation of monocyte-derived dendritic cells with Toll-like

receptor 3 and 7/8 ligands combined with prostaglandin E2 results in high interleukin-12 production and cell migration. Cancer Immunol Immunother 57(11):1589–1597
136. Jasani B et al (2009) Ampligen: a potential toll-like 3 receptor adjuvant for immunotherapy of cancer. Vaccine 27(25–26):3401–3404
137. Renn CN et al (2006) TLR activation of Langerhans cell-like dendritic cells triggers an antiviral immune response. J Immunol 177(1):298–305
138. Tirapu I et al (2009) PolyI:C-induced reduction in uptake of soluble antigen is independent of dendritic cell activation. Int Immunol 21(7):871–879
139. Walker J, Tough DF (2006) Modification of TLR-induced activation of human dendritic cells by type I IFN: synergistic interaction with TLR4 but not TLR3 agonists. Eur J Immunol 36(7):1827–1836
140. Adams M et al (2003) Dendritic cell (DC) based therapy for cervical cancer: use of DC pulsed with tumour lysate and matured with a novel synthetic clinically non-toxic double stranded RNA analogue poly [I]:poly [C(12)U] (Ampligen R). Vaccine 21(7–8):787–790
141. Mailliard RB et al (2004) Alpha-type-1 polarized dendritic cells: a novel immunization tool with optimized CTL-inducing activity. Cancer Res 64(17):5934–5937
142. Navabi H et al (2009) A clinical grade poly I:C-analogue (Ampligen) promotes optimal DC maturation and Th1-type T cell responses of healthy donors and cancer patients in vitro. Vaccine 27(1):107–115
143. Zhu X et al (2007) Toll like receptor-3 ligand poly-ICLC promotes the efficacy of peripheral vaccinations with tumor antigen-derived peptide epitopes in murine CNS tumor models. J Transl Med 5:10
144. Austyn JM (1998) Dendritic cells. Curr Opin Hematol 5(1):3–15
145. Satthaporn S, Eremin O (2001) Dendritic cells (I): biological functions. J R Coll Surg Edinb 46(1):9–19
146. Satthaporn S, Eremin O (2001) Dendritic cells (II): role and therapeutic implications in cancer. J R Coll Surg Edinb 46(3):159–167
147. Shortman K, Caux C (1997) Dendritic cell development: multiple pathways to nature's adjuvants. Stem Cells 15(6):409–419
148. Shortman K et al (1997) Dendritic cells and T lymphocytes: developmental and functional interactions. Ciba Found Symp 204:130–138, discussion 138–141
149. Schmidt J et al (2007) Intratumoural injection of the toll-like receptor-2/6 agonist 'macrophage-activating lipopeptide-2' in patients with pancreatic carcinoma: a phase I/II trial. Br J Cancer 97(5):598–604
150. Schneider C et al (2004) Tumour suppression induced by the macrophage activating lipopeptide MALP-2 in an ultrasound guided pancreatic carcinoma mouse model. Gut 53(3):355–361
151. Schill T et al (2012) Stimulation of pulmonary immune responses by the TLR2/6 agonist MALP-2 and effect on melanoma metastasis to the lung. Exp Dermatol 21(2):91–98
152. Pratesi G et al (2005) Therapeutic synergism of gemcitabine and CpG-oligodeoxynucleotides in an orthotopic human pancreatic carcinoma xenograft. Cancer Res 65(14):6388–6393
153. Vanderlocht J et al (2010) Increased tumor-specific $CD8^+$ T cell induction by dendritic cells matured with a clinical grade TLR-agonist in combination with IFN-gamma. Int J Immunopathol Pharmacol 23(1):35–50
154. Okamoto M, Sato M (2003) Toll-like receptor signaling in anti-cancer immunity. J Med Invest 50(1–2):9–24
155. Osada T et al (2006) Dendritic cell-based immunotherapy. Int Rev Immunol 25(5–6):377–413
156. Cheever MA (2008) Twelve immunotherapy drugs that could cure cancers. Immunol Rev 222:357–368
157. Cheever MA et al (2008) Translational Research Working Group developmental pathway for immune response modifiers. Clin Cancer Res 14(18):5692–5699

Chapter 38

Advances in Host and Vector Development for the Production of Plasmid DNA Vaccines

Juergen Mairhofer and Alvaro R. Lara

Abstract

Recent developments in DNA vaccine research provide a new momentum for this rather young and potentially disruptive technology. Gene-based vaccines are capable of eliciting protective immunity in humans to persistent intracellular pathogens, such as HIV, malaria, and tuberculosis, for which the conventional vaccine technologies have failed so far. The recent identification and characterization of genes coding for tumor antigens has stimulated the development of DNA-based antigen-specific cancer vaccines. Although most academic researchers consider the production of reasonable amounts of plasmid DNA (pDNA) for immunological studies relatively easy to solve, problems often arise during this first phase of production. In this chapter we review the current state of the art of pDNA production at small (shake flasks) and mid-scales (lab-scale bioreactor fermentations) and address new trends in vector design and strain engineering. We will guide the reader through the different stages of process design starting from choosing the most appropriate plasmid backbone, choosing the right *Escherichia coli* (*E. coli*) strain for production, and cultivation media and scale-up issues. In addition, we will address some points concerning the safety and potency of the produced plasmids, with special focus on producing antibiotic resistance-free plasmids. The main goal of this chapter is to make immunologists aware of the fact that production of the pDNA vaccine has to be performed with as much as attention and care as the rest of their research.

Key words DNA vaccines, Gene therapy, Plasmid DNA, Marker-free plasmids, Metabolic engineering, Vaccine process technology

1 Introduction

DNA-based biopharmaceuticals are gaining relevance, particularly in the field of specialized vaccination and infection treatment. The DNA delivered to the patient can include genes coding for different therapeutic agents, broadening the spectrum of the treatment. There are several vectors that can be used for DNA delivery to cancerous cells like different type of viruses [1, 2], viruslike particles [3, 4], and plasmid DNA (pDNA) [5]. Due to the relative simplicity of production, molecular development, transport, stability, and administration and being noninfectious, pDNA is an attractive option over other vectors for DNA vaccination. pDNA-based

Michael J.P. Lawman and Patricia D. Lawman (eds.), *Cancer Vaccines: Methods and Protocols*, Methods in Molecular Biology, vol. 1139, DOI 10.1007/978-1-4939-0345-0_38,

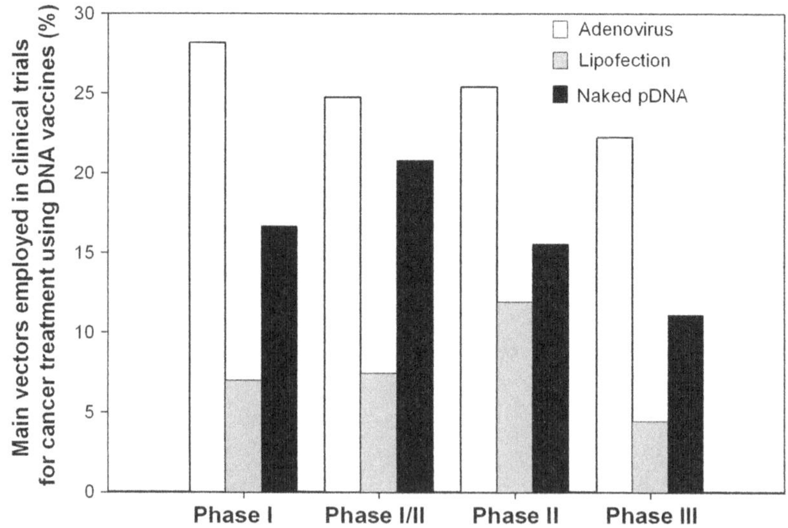

Fig. 1 Main vectors used in current clinical trials for DNA vaccines against cancer. Data represent the percentage of clinical trials using each vector with respect to the total of clinical trials (Data source: *The Journal of Gene Medicine*, 2012)

vaccines are usually produced in bacterial cultivations, which is an additional advantage since cultivation procedures are faster and simpler than those for virus production, and generic industrial facilities can be adapted for the specific purpose of bacterial cultivations for pDNA production.

Figure 1 gives an overview of the vector systems currently used in clinical trials for DNA vaccination against cancer and cancer treatment. Although most of the vectors used in all phases of clinical trials are adenovirus based, an important fraction of the vectors used are naked pDNA. A third important vector class is liposomes, which normally contain pDNA shielded by a lipid bilayer. With the information represented in Fig. 1, the importance of pDNA for vaccine and gene therapy is evident. Current clinical trials involve DNA vaccines against malignant melanoma, pancreatic carcinoma, renal cell carcinoma, head and neck squamous cell carcinoma, metastatic carcinoma, breast cancer, lymphoma, leukemia, prostate carcinomas, lung cancer, multiple myeloma, malignant glioma, colorectal cancer melanoma, and B-cell lymphoma [5]. The amount of pDNA applied per dose varies between 0.1 and 9 mg, and its application can be necessary once or more times per week during several weeks of treatment [6–8]. This represents a challenge for the production of the DNA vaccine, since relatively high amounts of highly purified and supercoiled pDNA should be available from early stages of product development.

In the following sections, the steps involved in pDNA-based vaccines are reviewed with an emphasis on the current advances in strains and vector development, including suggestions for improving pDNA production at laboratory and bench scales.

2 Points to Consider Prior to the Production of Plasmid DNA Vaccines

2.1 Choosing the Right Plasmid

Plasmids have been in biotechnological use for more than four decades [9, 10], and several different replicons have been discovered in the past years. Most commonly used plasmids for gene therapy employ a minimal bacterial backbone containing elements required for maintenance and propagation in the bacterial host—to date exclusively *E. coli*—and for expression of the target gene in the human or animal recipient.

2.1.1 Backbone Sequences

pDNA size is a critical criterion in vector design. Therefore, all nonessential sequences should be removed to yield a plasmid backbone that is reduced to its minimal composition. Besides regulatory and therapeutic challenges, larger pDNAs exert a metabolic burden on the host cell by over-consumption of metabolic precursors [11] and thereby reduce the overall pDNA yield. The backbone sequence typically contains the "plasmid propagation unit," which consists of the *ori* and the selection marker responsible for its replication in the microbial host. During construction of a therapeutic plasmid, a key factor is the choice of the *ori* since it defines technological aspects that become important during the production of the pDNA vaccine. A high plasmid copy number per cell is favorable to meet commercial needs. Because of the importance of this issue, mainly pUC-based plasmids have been used for therapeutic purposes, since they provide high copy number, between 500 and 700 copies/cell, without further modification of the bioprocess. Additionally, these plasmids have a long tradition in biotechnology and therefore have been studied extensively throughout the last several decades. In the course of the development of a DNA vaccine, it is therefore advisable to become aware of the identity of the plasmid backbone. It is necessary to identify the *ori* and all other backbone components to avoid major pitfalls during upstream or downstream processing. In the case of pUC19 and pBR322, the difference between high and low copy is just a single nucleotide mutation (for details *see* Fig. 2) and the absence of the *rom/rop* gene. The *rom/rop* gene (repressor of primer) is a small dimeric protein that participates in the mechanism that controls the copy number of plasmid of the ColE1 family by increasing the affinity between the two regulatory RNAs, RNAI and RNAII, that control the plasmid copy number [12]. To increase the plasmid copy number, *rom/rop* has been deleted in some derivatives of pBR322.

For identification and auto-annotation, the web tool PlasMapper [13] can be recommended. Please bear in mind that

```
pUC19     TTTCCATAGGCTCCGCCCCCCTGACGAGCATCACAAAAATCGACGCTCAAGTCAGAGGTG 60
pBR322    TTTCCATAGGCTCCGCCCCCCTGACGAGCATCACAAAAATCGACGCTCAAGTCAGAGGTG
          ************************************************************

pUC19     GCGAAACCCGACAGGACTATAAAGATACCAGGCGTTTCCCCCTGGAAGCTCCCTCGTGCG 120
pBR322    GCGAAACCCGACAGGACTATAAAGATACCAGGCGTTTCCCCCTGGAAGCTCCCTCGTGCG
          ************************************************************

pUC19     CTCTCCTGTTCCGACCCTGCCGCTTACCGGATACCTGTCCGCCTTTCTCCCTTCGGGAAG 180
pBR322    CTCTCCTGTTCCGACCCTGCCGCTTACCGGATACCTGTCCGCCTTTCTCCCTTCGGGAAG
          ************************************************************

pUC19     CGTGGCGCTTTCTCATAGCTCACGCTGTAGGTATCTCAGTTCGGTGTAGGTCGTTCGCTC 240
pBR322    CGTGGCGCTTTCTCATAGCTCACGCTGTAGGTATCTCAGTTCGGTGTAGGTCGTTCGCTC
          ************************************************************

pUC19     CAAGCTGGGCTGTGTGCACGAACCCCCCGTTCAGCCCGACCGCTGCGCCTTATCCGGTAA 300
pBR322    CAAGCTGGGCTGTGTGCACGAACCCCCCGTTCAGCCCGACCGCTGCGCCTTATCCGGTAA
          ************************************************************

pUC19     CTATCGTCTTGAGTCCAACCCGGTAAGACACGACTTATCGCCACTGGCAGCAGCCACTGG 360
pBR322    CTATCGTCTTGAGTCCAACCCGGTAAGACACGACTTATCGCCACTGGCAGCAGCCACTGG
          ************************************************************

pUC19     TAACAGGATTAGCAGAGCGAGGTATGTAGGCGGTGCTACAGAGTTCTTGAAGTGGTGGCC 420
pBR322    TAACAGGATTAGCAGAGCGAGGTATGTAGGCGGTGCTACAGAGTTCTTGAAGTGGTGGCC
          ************************************************************
                                RNAI
pUC19     TAACTACGGCTACACTAGAAGAACAGTATTTGGTATCTGCGCTCTGCTGAAGCCAGTTAC 480
pBR322    TAACTACGGCTACACTAGAAGGACAGTATTTGGTATCTGCGCTCTGCTGAAGCCAGTTAC
          ********************* **************************************

pUC19     CTTCGGAAAAAGAGTTGGTAGCTCTTGATCCGGCAAACAAACCACCGCTGGTAGCGGTGG 540
pBR322    CTTCGGAAAAAGAGTTGGTAGCTCTTGATCCGGCAAACAAACCACCGCTGGTAGCGGTGG
          ************************************************************

pUC19     TTTTTTTGTTTGCAAGCAGCAGATTACGCGCAGAAAAAAAGGATCTCAA 589
pBR322    TTTTTTTGTTTGCAAGCAGCAGATTACGCGCAGAAAAAAAGGATCTCAA
          *************************************************
                RNAII
```

Fig. 2 ClustalW alignment of the pUC19 ori and the pBR322 ori. The RNAI and RNAII transcripts are indicated by an *arrow*. −10 and −35 *box* of the corresponding promoters driving expression of the two RNA molecules are *boxed*. The difference between pUC19 and pBR322 is indicated in *bold*

PlasMapper is not able to discriminate between pUC-derived and pBR322 (or pMB1)-derived origin of replication (this has to be done by the user; therefore, *see* Fig. 2) but is able to identify the *rom/rop* gene (that lowers the copy number). Additionally, this software tool is able to identify bacterial promoters, e.g., *lac*, *tac*, or T7, often included as artifacts in plasmid backbones, e.g., pVAX1 contains a *lac* promoter upstream of the multiple cloning site (MCS) to allow for blue/white screening. Bacterial promoters that are able to drive expression of the antigen should be avoided at all costs and have to be excluded from the plasmid backbone due to the fact that they can severely hamper cell growth and production yields. It is therefore necessary to thoroughly review all backbone elements. Current state-of-the-art techniques, like restriction-free cloning [14, 15], allow for the easy manipulation of plasmid backbones and therefore should be considered when the redesign of a vector backbone is necessary.

In addition to the sequence necessary for replication, most plasmids contain a selectable marker that ensures selection during the cloning process and stable inheritance of pDNA during bacterial growth. For this purpose, pDNAs carry genes that confer resistance to a drug, mostly antibiotics. Currently, the kanamycin (neomycin) resistance gene (*nptII*) is the most commonly used selection marker, since it is the only one tolerated by regulatory authorities [16]. However, concerns about the spread of antibiotic resistance genes have spurred development of alternative selection mechanisms; *see* Subheading 4.1.1 for details. Please note that, according to the FDA [16] or EMA [17] guidelines, the usage of antibiotics during the manufacturing process should be avoided. Additionally, the EMA clearly states: "…the presence of an antibiotic resistance marker in a plasmid administered in vivo is not recommended. The presence of antibiotic resistance gene should be justified."

Current state-of-the-art production avoids the usage of antibiotics during production due to regulatory compliance. It is therefore advisable to check plasmid yields without the usage of antibiotics and to determine the plasmid retention [18] before scaling up. Additionally, keep in mind that from a regulatory perspective, it is advisable to start the development of a novel DNA vaccine with an antibiotic resistance-free plasmid backbone since it is conceivable that resistance genes on the plasmid backbone will not be tolerated by the regulatory authorities in the future.

2.1.2 Eukaryotic Expression Unit

pDNA vectors to be used as eukaryotic expression vehicles have to contain (1) a constitutive, inducible, or tissue-specific promoter with potent transcriptional activity; (2) a transcription terminator; and (3) elements for optimized mRNA processing and translation, including Kozak sequence, translational termination, mRNA cleavage, polyadenylation, as well as mRNA splicing sites. A schematic overview on a therapeutic pDNA vector can be found in Fig. 3.

Proper vector design is crucial for good and stable DNA yields but also for stable and long-lasting expression in the target tissue. Unfortunately, systematic studies that evaluate how the different structural plasmid components influence each other are rare. Here, we try to highlight the most important points available in the literature.

2.1.3 Eukaryotic Promoters

DNA vaccines typically use viral promoters like the cytomegalovirus (CMV)/immediate-early or the hybrid CMV early enhancer/chicken ß-actin (CAG) promoters to drive high-level expression of the gene of interest. CMV is the most commonly used, but its

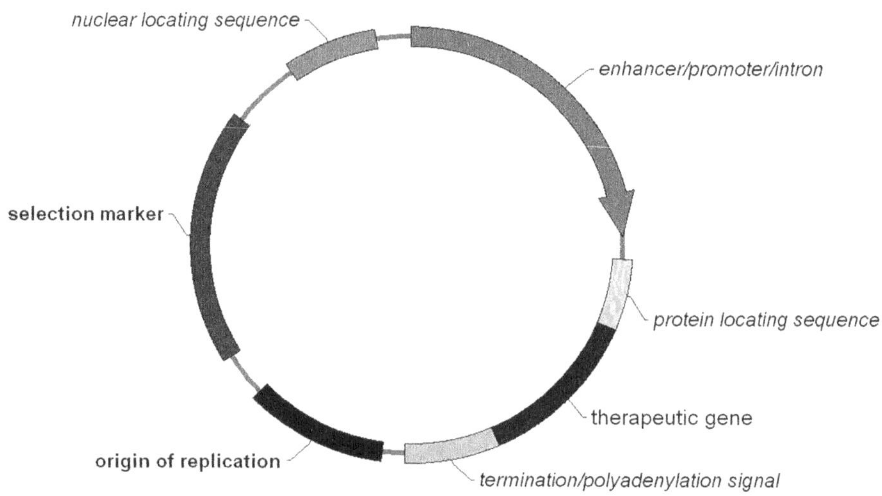

Fig. 3 Schematic drawing of a therapeutic plasmid vector. *Bold* elements are bacterial backbone elements enabling propagation in the microbial host; cursive elements are required for high-level expression of the target protein in mammalian cells and influence plasmid biodistribution, e.g., by increasing nuclear targeting of pDNA

expression has been shown to be downregulated in the presence of INF-γ [19, 20]. Therefore, the development of stronger, orthogonal promoters would be desirable. Work on synthetic promoters that are less tissue and species specific has been conducted [21, 22] and will potentially allow for the design of custom promoters for DNA vaccine approaches. Besides considerations on the strength of the eukaryotic promoter, the position of this element relative to the bacterial backbone elements should be considered as well. For example, Samadashwily et al. [23] reported that termination of plasmid replication at trinucleotide repeats found in eukaryotic transcription and translation control elements, leads to the occurrence of replication intermediates and consequently diminishes the supercoiled content. Due to the fact that those intermediates are smaller than the full-length plasmid, they are considered as an impurity and therefore require additional characterization and purification. Their appearance can be circumvented by inverting the orientation of the *ori* relative to the eukaryotic expression cassette or by increasing the distance between the *ori* and these elements [24]. Additionally, prokaryotic elements have been found to interfere with gene expression in eukaryotic cells [25–28]. For example, the expression from the CMV promoter is affected by the orientation of the antibiotic resistance gene and is dramatically higher when the prokaryotic promoter is distal [24].

These replication intermediates can be visualized in an agarose gel stained with ethidium bromide due to their double-stranded nature. They migrate as an extra-small band below the major supercoiled band and can vary in size between 200 and 700 bp.

2.1.4 Gene of Interest

The gene of interest represents the most essential part of a DNA vaccine, and therefore, care should be taken during the design process of this element. The current state of the art is the synthesis of DNA rather than the cloning of DNA fragments, allowing the optimization and easy removal of detrimental sequence motifs.

2.1.5 Gene Optimization

DNA synthesis allows for codon optimization and for the removal of disadvantageous sequence motifs. There are many companies that offer DNA synthesis using different algorithms for codon optimization. Most approaches either aim at achieving high codon adaption indices (CAI) by using the most frequently used codons in combination with GC content adjustment and the removal of RNA secondary structure [29] or using machine learning algorithms [30]. Codon optimization is a science on its own, and currently there is no absolute consensus on how to design a highly expressed gene. Therefore, it is advisable to use the experience of renowned vendors. To summarize, gene optimization should include adjustment of the Kozak sequence to the consensus sequence (GCC[G/A]CCATG), usage of a dual stop codon to prevent read-through transcription, and the removal of mRNA secondary structure, hairpins, and other inhibitory sequences.

2.1.6 Multiple Antigen Vaccines

In most clinical cases, a pathogen will not be eliminated by the expression of a single antigen. Therefore, strategies that allow for the expression of multiple antigens are of great interest. There are plasmids available that contain a dual promoter construct or an internal ribosomal entry site (IRES) [31, 32] for the expression of two antigens per plasmid. When the IRES element is included in between two ORFs, initiation of translation occurs by the canonical 5′- m^7GpppN cap-dependent mechanism in the first ORF and a cap-independent mechanism in the second ORF downstream of the IRES sequence [31]. Another approach using polyepitopes [33] or multicistronic expression of antigens from a single ORF makes use of altered antigens using such as self-splicing 2A sequences of the foot-and-mouth disease virus (FMDV) [34] or a synthetic consensus immunogen [35, 36].

2.1.7 Poor Immunogenicity of Cancer Antigens

A challenge in the field of cancer vaccines is the poor immunogenicity of cancer antigens [38]. To overcome this limitation, antigens are fused to molecular domains that enhance antigen presentation, thereby creating the so-called DNA fusion vaccines. Promising fusion partners for cancer DNA vaccines are the tetanus toxin fragment C [38–40], the murine antimicrobial β-defensin 2 (mBD2) peptide [41–44], or the human chorionic gonadotropin β-chain (hCGβ) [45–47]. The current state-of-the-art knowledge has been summarized elsewhere [6, 48].

2.1.8 Polyadenylation Signal

It was shown recently that pDNA molecules possessing base sequences that originate from secondary structures with single-stranded regions, mainly homopurine-rich sequences encoded within the polyA signal, are more susceptible to exo-/endonuclease attacks [49]. Two major hot spots were identified by nuclease S1 mapping of a commercial vector designed for the use in the development of DNA vaccines. Results showed that the plasmid was cleaved at spots located within the bovine growth hormone (BGH) polyA signal and within the ColE1 *ori* due to six homopurine-rich sequences within the BGHpolyA and the presence of an 11-base long inverted repeat [50] within the prokaryotic *ori*. Consequently, pDNA variants were created wherein the BGHpolyA was replaced by the SV40polyA or a synthetic polyA signal. When these nuclease hot spots were removed, the half-life of supercoiled isoforms in eukaryotic cell lysates or mice plasma could be extended significantly [50]. The influence of different polyA signals in combination with an antibiotic resistance-free plasmid selection approach was also investigated in human and mouse stem cells [51].

Keep in mind that the polyA signal used does influence the stability of the mRNA. In addition, some vectors used for DNA vaccines contain sequences between the gene of interest (GOI) and the polyA signal. Keep in mind that, according to Luke et al. [52], the 3′-UTR region is translated as well. Expression of cryptic peptides or proteins may cause regulatory issues.

2.2 Influence of the DNA Composition on the Structural Stability of the Plasmid

The conformation of pDNA molecules is a major quality factor for formulated vaccines and is influenced to a large extent by their sequence composition. DNA exists in various possible conformations, and so far, several have been identified: A-DNA, B-DNA [53], C-DNA [54], D-DNA [55], E-DNA [56], H-DNA [57, 58], L-DNA [58], P-DNA [59], T-DNA [60], and Z-DNA [61]. Respectively, the conformation depends on the DNA sequence, the amount and direction of supercoiling, chemical modifications of the bases, and also environmental conditions, e.g., the concentration of metal ions. Under physiological conditions, only the A-, B-, E-, and Z-DNA conformations have been observed. The B-form is the major physiological form. The A-form occurs under nonphysiological conditions in dehydrated samples of DNA or while hybrid pairings of DNA and RNA strands are formed, as well as in enzyme–DNA complexes. The E-form represents a kind of intermediate between the A- and B-forms, and the Z-DNA is a left-handed helix with a structure that repeats every two base pairs.

2.2.1 Supercoiled Plasmid DNA Content

It is generally believed that the supercoiled (SC) form of pDNA is the physiologically active conformation and that this form is optimal for the transfection of mammalian cells [62]. Therefore, care has to be taken to produce this as the main isoform during bacterial cultivation and to enrich the SC isoform during downstream processing. Certain sequences contain elements that promote poor supercoiling due to the formation of intramolecular triplexes (H-DNA), such as segments with predominantly purines in one strand and AT-rich sequences. These segments are overrepresented in eukaryotic DNA [63], and their presence can induce nicking by endogenous nucleases due to the occurrence of single-stranded DNA along the pDNA molecule. It was shown recently that these intramolecular triplexes are able to reduce the relative amount of plasmid in the SC form and that this behavior is enhanced by freeze–thawing [64]. In addition to certain sequence motifs, the choice of the host strain does significantly influence content of SC pDNA [65].

It is therefore advisable to keep the number of freeze–thaw cycles constant in case the performance of two or more different plasmids is compared in order to avoid a bias introduced by degradation.

2.2.2 Instabilities Mediated by Direct/Inverted Repeats or DNA Secondary Structure

Replicating eukaryotic DNA accurately in prokaryotic cells can be difficult due to the fact that eukaryotic DNA may contain inverted repeats or secondary structures, such as Z-DNA, that can be rearranged or deleted by the *E. coli* DNA repair systems. One prominent sequence feature that induces plasmid recombination is the chi sequence (5′-GCTGGTGG-3′), which is able to cause deletions or dimerization [66]. The occurrence of this motif should be avoided whenever possible. Direct repeats can induce the formation of DNA hairpins and loops leading to rearrangements caused by misalignment during replication [67], whereas inverted repeats cause a *recA*-independent formation of circular inverted head-to-head plasmid dimers [68]. In addition, alternating purine–pyrimidine/oligopurine–oligopyrimidine or G-rich sequences do induce the formation of Z-DNA, triplexes, or quadruplexes that are involved in deletions or reduction of the final plasmid DNA yield [64]. A very comprehensive review on the structural instability of plasmid biopharmaceuticals has been performed recently [69]. The relative recombination potential (RRP) was calculated by Oliveira and co-workers for vectors used as backbones for DNA vaccine development [70]. According to their calculation, pCIneo (Promega/U47120) has a rather high RRP, whereas pVAX1 (Invitrogen) has a much lower RRP value. This high value for pCI-neo is in accordance with an observation published previously [71]. It is therefore vital to carefully analyze the nucleotide sequence in order to become sensitive for possible mutational hot spots.

It is advisable to in silico screen the plasmid sequence for possible sequences that may cause pitfalls like direct/inverted repeats, chi-sites, or Z-DNA-forming motifs. Exact repeats in a DNA sequence can be found using REPFIND (http://zlab.bu.edu/repfind/form.html) [72]. In addition, the European Molecular

Biology Open Software Suite (EMBOSS) explorer is a valuable tool for the detection of direct or inverted repeats using the tools available in the "Nucleic repeats" section (http://emboss.bioinformatics.nl). Z-DNA can be tracked down using the Z-hunt web tool (http://gac-web.cgrb.oregonstate.edu/zDNA/) [73]. Repeats which are larger than 14 bp and divided by spacers smaller than 1,000 bp should be considered as possible sources for recombination events [74]. We recommend that researchers be aware of the information provided in the section above and that they redesign plasmid vectors as soon as problems do arise. If inconsistencies in plasmid size are observed, deletion, duplication, or insertion events can be elucidated using sequencing of the plasmid. According to the in silico analysis, it should then be possible to identify the sequence motif responsible for the structural instability and to remove it accordingly.

2.2.3 Structural Instabilities Mediated by Transposable Elements

In prokaryotes, transposable elements provide a significant share of genetic variation through insertional inactivation or enhancing deletions, inversions, or duplications because they provide substrates for homologous recombination [75]. Plasmid-based DNA vaccines often do encode gene products detrimental for growth of the bacterial host. If spurious expression of these genes occurs, inactivation of this gene product might occur by insertion of sequence elements abundant in the genome of *E. coli* [76]. For example, Prather et al. found several IS1 insertions near the gene for neomycin resistance in an HIV DNA vaccine, which affected replication and amplification of the plasmid [77]. Another example, involving an IS2 insertion site, was recently found in the mammalian expression vector, pCIneo [78]. Umenhoffer et al. [79] performed a bioinformatic analysis of raw data from various shotgun sequencing projects, where *E. coli* served as a host for fosmid libraries, and were able to show that the inactivation of ectopic genes inhibiting the growth of the host is not negligible [79]. Structural instabilities due to transposition can be circumvented by using multiple-deletion series (MDS) strains of *E. coli* [80].

2.3 Choosing the Right *E. coli* Host Strain

As in any biotechnological production process, the *E. coli* strain used for pDNA production should be genetically stable, able to maintain fast growth in simple media, and detailed physiological information about the specific strain should be available. In general, *E. coli* strains lacking *recA* and *endA* genes are the preferred hosts for pDNA production. Those genes influence the stability of pDNA and have been deactivated in the most common pDNA producers like *E. coli* DH5α, DH1, JM109, and XL1 Blue [81]. The product of the *endA* gene is the periplasmic enzyme, endonuclease I, that degrades pDNA upon cell lysis [81], whereas the *recA* gene codes for a DNA strand exchange and recombination protein, RecA, with a variety of functions such as ATP-dependent recombination, which it accomplishes by catalyzing DNA strand exchange and insertions. The RecA protein degrades a second protein, RepA, which is necessary for replication of pCO11-derived plasmids [82, 83, 84]. RecA also has a proteolytic activity that activates the Cop protein, a repressor of plasmid replication [84]. Consequently, *recA* mutants generally display higher segregational plasmid stability and higher pDNA production than parental strains [65, 85]. Deletion of the *relA* gene, which is involved in the stringent response to amino acid depletion, is also common in strains used for pDNA production. The relevance of *relA* mutants is explained in Subheading 3.2.1.

The selection of the abovementioned strains for pDNA production has been based on previous experience in lab-scale cultivations. Nevertheless, recent evidence shows that such strains may be not good options for commercial pDNA production. For instance, currently used strains for pDNA production tend to be unstable, i.e., they have a relatively high mutation rate leading to changes of the chromosomal as well as the plasmid DNA [86]. In fact, it has been shown that *E. coli* strain DH10B had a 13.5-fold higher mutation rate than its wild-type MG1655, which is mainly attributed to the higher rates of insertion sequence transposition of DH10B [86]. DH5α has been used in most of the published studies and patents dealing with pDNA production and is consistently reported as one of the most productive strains in small-scale cultivations [65, 87]. There is, however, a lack of detailed physiological information on this highly mutated strain, which is disadvantageous for precise modeling and process development. For instance, DH5α has been generally assumed to lack the *deoR* gene, which codes for a regulator of deoxyribose synthesis [81]. However, it has been recently demonstrated that *deoR* is present in DH5α [88]. Moreover, some of the common pDNA producers like DH5α and DH1 display an elevated overflow metabolism, i.e., aerobic acetate production as detailed in Subheading 3.1 [87], which represents a serious disadvantage for high-cell-density cultivations. Another factor that is dependent on the producer strain is the supercoiled pDNA fraction that can be obtained. This factor is of relevance for the overall quality of the final pDNA product, as will be explained below. Less is known about the influence of the strain on the events of transposition. It has been reported that transposition occurred in the production of clinical grade pDNA by *E. coli* DH5 [89] and that fed-batch conditions promoted the transposition events.

Up to now, there has been no evidence of a “best pDNA producer.” Instead, results point to the fact that factors such as productivity, pDNA supercoiled fraction, growth rates, yields, and by-product formation depend largely on the combination of strain, plasmid [65, 87], and process characteristics [90]. Also, the typical screening conditions, such as batch mode and uncontrolled pH, can mask the potential advantages of different strains. There is also a general lack of information about cell physiology, i.e., metabolic fluxes, gene expression, and protein formation patterns, under the particular conditions of processes for pDNA production.

For initial assessment of a potential pDNA vaccine, the use of commercially available pDNA production strains with *recA*, *endA*, and *relA* mutations is sufficient. Keep in mind that some of these strains can accumulate elevated amounts of acetate, limiting the usable amount of glucose as a carbon source to around 10–15 g/L in batch cultivations. If glycerol is used, it may be possible to provide higher initial concentrations. If further cultivations are to be carried out, or larger amounts of the vaccine candidate are needed for its evaluation, it is advisable to evaluate several strains for the particular application.

2.4 Considerations for the Production of Plasmid DNA in Small Scale: Influence of Cultivation Media

As with any cell cultivation process, the medium should provide all the necessary elements to guarantee efficient growth and product formation. *E. coli* can grow at relatively high rates in a simple medium containing mineral salts like M9. Subsequent enrichment of the medium usually includes trace elements such as enzyme cofactors and growth factors, most commonly thiamine. Further additions to the medium can result in higher growth rates and biomass yield. Depending on the specific application, chemically defined or complex media can be used. For initial studies intended for pDNA evaluation as a therapeutic agent, complex media are frequently the first option. Although there is a variety of media for *E. coli* cultivation, the lysogeny broth, also known as LB and in many cases referred to as Luria-Bertani, is the most widely used formulation for initial screening. This medium is composed of two complex sources, yeast extract and tryptone, and provides vitamins, peptides, trace elements, and minerals which allow reaching cell densities between 0.8 and 1.5 g/L. If tryptone is used in any media formulation, it is advisable to use animal component-free formulations, e.g., tryptone derived from vegetables instead of casein- or meat-derived tryptone, to assure regulatory compliance from the very beginning of the project. For increasing cell densities or yields, the composition can be doubled (with the consequent osmolality increase) or a carbon source can be added. For instance, Zheng et al. [91] evaluated the impact of different carbon sources added to LB medium for the production of a 7 kb plasmid by *E. coli* DH5α. The authors showed that the Y_{px} values of cells grown on D-lactose, mannitose, and sucrose were almost twofold higher than when grown on glucose. Another complex medium that has been reported by several authors for pDNA production is terrific broth (TB), which contains yeast extract and tryptone, although at higher concentrations than LB, plus phosphate buffer and glycerol as a carbon source. As TB medium contains more nutrients than LB, higher cell densities can be obtained with the former. Nevertheless, pDNA production, and particularly pDNA yields on biomass, Y_{px}, has been reported to be higher [92–94] or lower [91, 95] than those achieved using LB medium in shake flask studies. Such results illustrate that pDNA productivity is not only determined by the specific growth conditions but is also strongly dependent on the host/vector combination used. The use of different nitrogen sources like proteose peptone, casein peptone [91], or casamino acids [96] can also increase pDNA yields. One such medium that combined yeast extract, tryptone, glucose, phosphates, ammonium, and magnesium has supported Y_{px} values of 11.17 mg/g [93] in shake flasks, and the same medium in a 20 L bioreactor maintained Y_{px} values of 9.8 mg/g [94].

Duttweiler and Gross [92] proposed a medium formulation for increasing pDNA yields in shake flasks. This medium, named H15, contains typical components like glucose, yeast extract, and casamino acids and is enriched with torula yeast RNA and RNase I to provide nucleotides. Interestingly, H15 medium combines MOPS and TRIS in order to buffer the pH within 6.5–7.5. Several plasmids of sizes ranging from 2.7 to 8.4 kb were produced, and the titers reached using H15 medium were 6–30 times higher than in LB medium and 2–6 times higher than those in LB medium.

Chemically defined media are frequently preferred over complex or semi-defined media for pilot- or large-scale production, since they allow a better physiology control and reproducibility of the batches. Chemically defined media can contain a large number of nutrients in order to support a fast growth of *E. coli* under well-defined conditions. For instance, Zawada and Swartz [97] used a medium containing three mineral salts plus citrate, trace elements, nine vitamins, and ten amino acids in order to achieve cell densities of around 20 g/L while maintaining a growth rate of 0.87–1.10 h^{-1}. For the particular case of pDNA production, several studies on the growth medium composition are available. For such a purpose, the specific demand of intermediaries for nucleotide and DNA synthesis is provided (Fig. 4). For example, Voss et al. [98] reported the use of two ammonia sources and glutamate for a 7 L bioreactor cultivation for pDNA production. A medium design based on a stoichiometric model [99] contained all the 20 proteinogenic amino acids, plus nucleosides, phosphate, and glucose in order to optimize pDNA production. This medium supported a Y_{px} value of nearly 17 mg/g [99]. It has also been shown that the phosphate concentration has an influence on the final pDNA yields [95]. A noteworthy point is that all the mentioned Y_{px} values were obtained in cultivations at constant temperatures. Temperature upshift can significantly increase pDNA yields, as discussed below.

The use of complex sources of nitrogen will, in most cases, improve either growth rate, Y_{px}, or both. However, attention

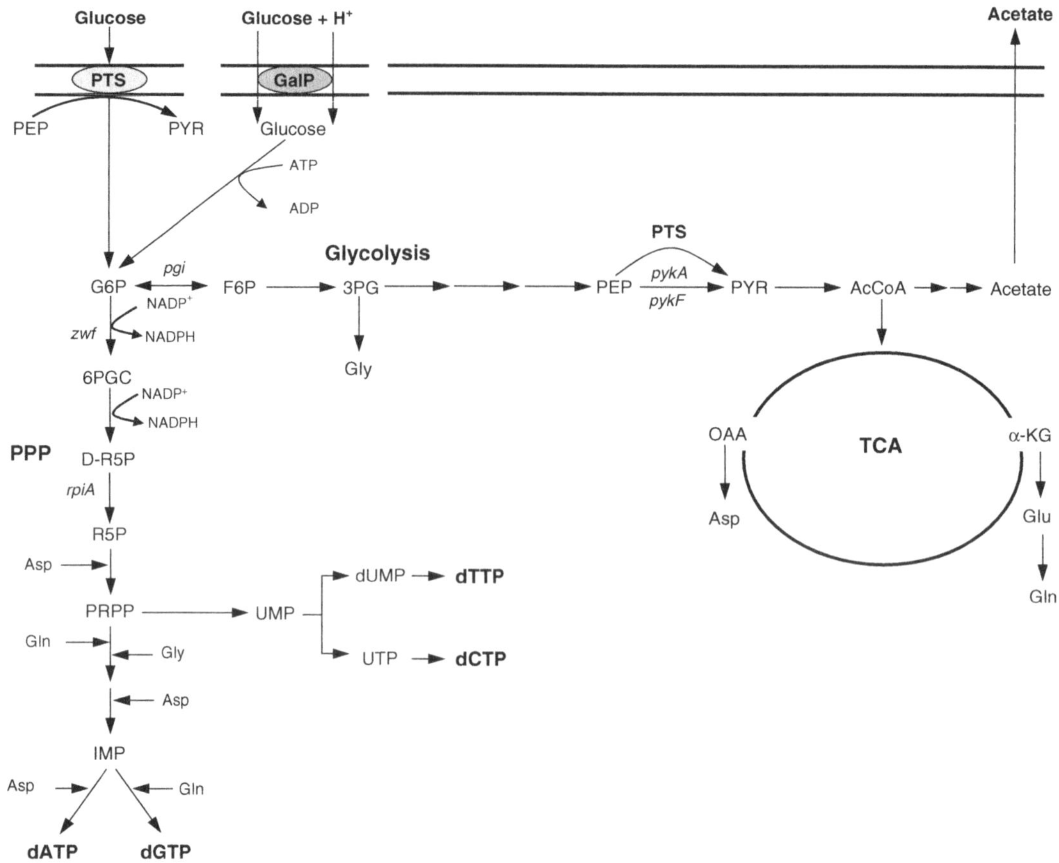

Fig. 4 Simplified metabolic pathways involved in nucleotide biosynthesis and overflow metabolism. *PPP* pentose phosphate pathway, *TCA* tricarboxylic acid cycle, *PTS* phosphotransferase system, *GalP* galactose permease, *PEP* phosphoenol pyruvate, *PYR* pyruvate, *G6P* glucose 6-phosphate, *F6P* fructose 6-phosphate, *3PG* 3-phosphoglycerate, *AcCoA* acetyl coenzyme A, *6PGC* 6-phosphogluconate, *D5RP* D-5-ribulose phosphate, *R5P* ribose 5-phosphate, *PRPP* phosphoribosyl pyrophosphate, *IMP* inosine 5'-phosphate, *UMP* uridine monophosphate, *UTP* uridine triphosphate, *OAA* oxaloacetate, *αKG* alpha-ketoglutarate, *dTTP* deoxythymidine triphosphate, *dCTP* deoxycytidine triphosphate, *dATP* deoxyadenosine triphosphate, *dGTP* deoxyguanosine triphosphate, *Asp* aspartate, *Gln* glutamine, *Gly* glycine, *pgi* gene coding for phosphoglucoisomerase, *pykA*, *pykF* genes coding for pyruvate kinases A and F, respectively, *zwf* gene coding for glucose 6-phosphate-I-dehydrogenase, *rpiA* gene coding for ribose-S-phosphate isomerase A. The genes are shown over the *arrows* to represent the reactions whose coding enzyme catalyzes

should be paid to the physical growth conditions. For instance, a fast growth rate will lead to rapid oxygen consumption and may increase acetate production by overflow metabolism. If microaerobic conditions arise, other organic acids will be produced. Employing baffled shake flasks improves oxygen transfer if the adequate filling volume is used. To avoid a drop in pH, not only due to acid production but also due to basic nutrients consumption, addition (or increase of the amount) of buffers should be considered. Another factor to consider is that highly enriched medium will very probably produce foam, which finally reduces the oxygen transfer rate. If there is no other alternative, antifoam agents can be added to the medium. An option to increase the attainable cell density is the use of slow glucose-release techniques in which glucose or a glucose polymer is entrapped in a gel and glucose is released by diffusion or enzymatic digestion of the glucose polymer [100, 101]. If a slow glucose delivery is maintained, the specific growth rate (and oxygen demand) will be lower, which can be of benefit for pDNA production. Some of these systems are commercially available and their utility for pDNA production should be probed.

3 How to Improve the Production of pDNA Vaccines

Improvement of pDNA production can be achieved by several approaches in addition to medium design, like increasing the Υ_{px} by means of metabolic modifications or manipulation of the process conditions and increasing the number of cells in cultivation. The present section will discuss some of the different advances reported.

3.1 Metabolic Engineering to Increase Plasmid Yields

Although there are a variety of strains available for pDNA production, they are far from being optimal for this purpose. Compared to the relatively abundant information on the metabolic modifications of *E. coli* for the production of recombinant proteins [102], the published work about strain engineering for improving pDNA production is scarce. The alternatives proposed up to now consist of the deregulation of plasmid replication control and the increase of carbon availability for nucleotide biosynthesis. Important advances for reducing the metabolic burden imposed by the expression of the antibiotic resistance marker gene will be discussed in Subheading 4.1.1.

Figure 4 shows a simplified illustration of the metabolic pathways leading to nucleotide production and also illustrates acetate synthesis by overflow metabolism. Since there are several amino acids of relevance for nucleotide biosynthesis, their origin is also shown. As can be seen, glucose is converted to glucose 6-phosphate (G6P) that can follow the glycolytic pathway or the pentose phosphate pathway (PPP). The latter pathway is important not only for the formation of reducing biosynthetic power in the form of NADPH but also for the synthesis of ribose 5-phosphate, which is a precursor of nucleotides. Subsequent steps allow for the biosynthesis of purine and pyrimidine deoxynucleotides (Fig. 4). It is important to note that aspartate is required for the synthesis of phosphoribosyl pyrophosphate (PRPP) and that, additionally, glycine and glutamine are needed for the synthesis of purine deoxynucleotides. If G6P is incorporated in glycolysis, the final product of this pathway, pyruvate (PYR), can be converted either to acetyl-CoA (AcCoA) or to acetate. AcCoA is subsequently integrated in the tricarboxylic acid (TCA) cycle, whereas acetate is excreted. In addition to the important role of the TCA cycle as a provider of NADH + H^+ for aerobic respiration, this pathway also provides precursors for the synthesis of aspartate and glutamine. Acetate is mainly produced if AcCoA cannot efficiently be incorporated in the TCA cycle. Aerobic acetate production, also known as overflow metabolism, is a negative metabolic deviation, since carbon is wasted and pH is affected, whereas growth rate can also be decreased as a consequence of acetate accumulation [103].

The initial efforts to improve pDNA production are related to the mentioned pathways. For instance, increasing carbon flux to the PPP has been explored. In order to recover the growth rate of plasmid-bearing strains intended for the production of recombinant proteins, Flores et al. [104] overexpressed the gene coding for the enzyme glucose 6-phosphate-l-dehydrogenase (*zwf*), which catalyzes the first reaction of the PPP (Fig. 4). This allowed a remarkable growth rate recovery. Unfortunately, the authors did not report pDNA content of the strains. However, when *zwf* was overexpressed in DH5α with the aim of increasing pDNA production, no improvement was observed [105]. A second option to increase carbon flux to the PPP is to reduce the flux to glycolysis. This can be done, for example, by reducing the activity of pyruvate kinase (*pyk*), which catalyzes the last reaction of glycolysis (Fig. 4). By deleting both genes coding for pyruvate kinase subunits (*pykA* and *pykF*), a ninefold increase in plasmid copy number has been reported [106] with the additional advantage of a reduction of acetate accumulation. Mutation of *pykA* or *pykF*, however, had no effect in DH5α, whereas improvement in Y_{px} was observed for strain MG1655 [107]. The glycolytic flux can also be reduced by inactivating the *pgi* gene, which codes for the phosphoglucoisomerase (Fig. 4). Such a modification effectively deviates G6P to the PPP [108]. This mutation successfully increased plasmid production in strain MG1655 cultivated in a complex medium [107]. However, *pgi* mutants display a severely reduced growth rate, and only a modest increase in pDNA production has been observed for PTS mutants grown in mineral medium (Lara et al., unpublished results). Based on DNA microarray and metabolic flux analysis, Wang et al. [109] overexpressed the *rpiA* gene, coding for the enzyme ribulose-5-phosphate isomerase A (Fig. 4), in order to increase the nucleotide biosynthesis. When *rpiA* was overexpressed in the strain BL21, a threefold increase in plasmid copy number was achieved [109]. Overexpression of *rpiA* and *zwf* in strain DH5α has also improved Y_{px} under temperature-induced and uninduced conditions [105].

Other modifications reported to increase pDNA production or quality include the overexpression of *polI* (coding for DNA polymerase I), *ligA* (coding for DNA ligase) [105], and *priA*, *priB*, and *priC* to increase the availability of primosomes [105].

In order to reduce pDNA degradation, inactivation of the *dcm* gene (coding for DNA cytosine methyltransferase) has also been reported [110]. All the mentioned modifications have been made to the strain DH5α. By deleting the fructose repressor gene (*fruR*), a global regulator of central carbon pathways, Y_{px}, and growth rate have also been increased in DH5α [111, 112]. Although the reason for this increase is not totally clear, the authors decided to delete *fruR* based on previous transcriptional analysis aimed to understand the metabolic burden imposed by plasmid presence in *E. coli* [113].

An interesting approach to improve pDNA production is to design a strategy to control the plasmid copy number making use of the replication system of pColE1-like plasmids. In such plasmids, replication initiates with the hybridization of an RNA molecule, RNAII (encoded in the plasmid), to the plasmid itself. The hybrid elongates and forms a hairpin structure that is cleaved by RNaseH, giving access to the DNA polymerase to continue DNA elongation [84]. An antisense RNA sequence, RNAI, is complementary to the 5′ of RNAII and can bind to it before the RNAII–DNA hybrid is formed, therefore inhibiting plasmid replication [84]. Recently, a system to modulate pDNA replication with the aim of reducing the metabolic burden caused by pDNA presence [113, 114] during the first stage of the cultivation has been suggested [115]. Lowering the plasmid copy number and thereby the metabolic burden during the first stage of the cultivation is achieved by the expression of a genome-encoded, inducible version of the RNAI molecule and subsequent deletion of the RNAI promoter from the plasmid backbone. For example, a pUC19 plasmid that has the RNAI promoter deleted tolerated a 1000-fold increased concentration of ampicillin. This system allows rapid accumulation of biomass, and once the desired cell density is achieved, the expression of the RNAI molecule is stopped due to metabolization of the inducer such as lactose [115].

It is interesting to note that many of the mentioned modifications have been applied to the strain DH5α. The reason for this may be that this strain is widely used for pDNA amplification in the laboratory, and it was the natural choice for pDNA production in larger scales. However, due to the fact that DH5α and other commercial strains are highly mutated strains and little is known about their particular physiology and precise genotype, they might not be the best option for process applications. For instance, it has been recently reported that strains XL1-Blue and DH5α are *kdgR* mutants due to an IS5 disruption [89].

Another reason for needing better production strains is the performance of these to reach high cell densities. As explained before, overflow metabolism is a drawback for reaching high cell densities. From the usual strains used for pDNA production, DH5α has been shown to display a relatively high overflow metabolism

[87, 116]. From a process point of view, it is desirable to cultivate a strain with a minimal overflow metabolism and high Y_{px} and stability. Only a couple of examples exist on this issue. Phue and co-workers reported the inactivation of the *recA* and *endA* genes in *E. coli* BL21 [85], a strain well known to have a relatively low acetate accumulation. With these mutations, the modified BL21 strain produced more pDNA than DH5α in fed-batch cultivations. With the objective of providing strains with better growth characteristics for process-like conditions, a strain engineered in the substrate uptake system has also been evaluated. In this strain, named VH33, the natural glucose uptake system, phosphotransferase (PTS), was replaced by galactose permease (GalP) overexpressed from the chromosome [117]. The overexpression of GalP allows efficient glucose uptake but with a lower rate than the PTS [118]. As a result, the imbalance between the TCA cycle and glycolytic fluxes is decreased, and an important reduction in acetate production is achieved. As shown in Fig. 4, the phosphate group used to phosphorylate glucose transported through GalP is donated by ATP instead of PEP. This leaves more PEP available for other biosynthetic activities and can also result in a reduced glycolytic rate. Additionally, PTS-defective mutants have shown an increased carbon flux to the PPP [119], which as explained before is advantageous for pDNA production. Strain VH33 has been cultivated in batch mode using up to 130 g/L of initial glucose concentration, where it is able to reach high cell densities [120] and produces only very little amounts of acetate. This strain has also been tested for recombinant protein production in high-cell-density culture (HCDC) in batch mode with excellent results [118]. When compared to its wild-type strain (W3110), VH33 produced twice as much of a pDNA vaccine candidate against mumps [121]. Additional mutations have been applied to strain VH33. For instance, the *pykA* gene was deleted, and as a result, acetate production was reduced to nearly zero, whereas Y_{px} was almost the double of unmodified VH33 [122]. Other genes like *recA*, *nupG*, and *deoR* have also been deleted in VH33. Such a triple VH33 mutant has been cultivated using 100 g/L of initial glucose in batch mode using a simple mineral medium. Under those conditions, the modified strain VH33 produced 187 mg/L of pDNA and just 2 g/L of acetate. In contrast, when strain DH5α was cultivated under the same scheme, less than 80 mg/L of pDNA were produced and almost 10 g/L of acetate accumulated [116]. These examples show the importance of considering the conditions that may be needed for large-scale production when designing a pDNA microbial factory.

Despite the relative success of the explained cellular modifications, there is still ample room to modify the bacterial physiology in order to maximize pDNA production. For example, regulation of plasmid synthesis factors has to be considered. Although several authors have tried to increase carbon flux to the PPP, the regulation of this pathway by the $NADP^+$/NADPH ratio has also to be taken into account. Whereas several genes related to the PPP have been overexpressed with the goal of increasing nucleotide biosynthesis capacity, the gene dosage has to be optimized. Other factors necessary for pDNA synthesis like amino acid supply have not been considered yet. Although such amino acids can be supplied to the medium, it could also be possible to increase the biosynthesis of Asp, Gly, and Gln in the pDNA producer strains. As glutamine can be unstable in solution, glutamic acid is a good alternative, since it is more stable in solution and easily transported in *E. coli* where it can be converted in glutamine by transamination. If the aim is a pDNA production process with high productivity, it can be advisable to perform medium optimization, e.g., by performing factorial design of experiment, thereby testing the addition of different amino acids since the final biomass yields can be elevated significantly by feeding strain-specific amino acids. Carbon sources other than glucose and glycerol can also be attractive. For instance, xylose can increase Y_{px} since this pentose is directly incorporated to the PPP. Nevertheless, the growth rate can be lower than that achieved using glucose. The selection of carbon source should be balanced in terms of specific production rate and not only in terms of Y_{px} [123].

3.2 Fermentation Engineering Approaches to Improve pDNA Production

Several ways to improve cultivation media and producer strains have been explored in previous sections. HCDC is also a basic approach for increasing productivity. In addition to these approaches, the current practice for pDNA production takes advantage of several strategies to induce, or derepress, plasmid replication in *E. coli*. The different strategies can be applied in small and large scales, whereas others are restricted to small-scale cultivation due to economic constraints. It is important to point out that the stress responses will arise as a result of the induction scheme. Such factors are discussed in the following subsections.

3.2.1 Increase of Y_{px} by Changing the Chemical Environment During Cultivation

It is possible to increase Y_{px} by manipulation of the chemical environment. For instance, *relA* mutants, also called "relaxed" *E. coli* cells as stringent response is reduced in such mutants, bearing pColE1 can increase plasmid synthesis upon exhaustion of amino acids like alanine and arginine [124, 125] leading to an increase of pDNA concentration of up to tenfold after arginine exhaustion. It has been proposed that such an increase in plasmid replication occurs due to an interaction between uncharged tRNA with either RNAI or RNAII, which contributes to deregulated pDNA replication [126, 127]. This hypothesis has been the basis to evaluate the effect of adding AMP to *relA* mutants cultivated in LB medium bearing pColE1. Addition of AMP resulted in an increase of pDNA concentration of more than 300 % [128], which has been attributed to an interference of tRNA aminoacylation by AMP, increasing the abundance of uncharged tRNAs that in turn promote pDNA replication [128].

Silva and co-workers [129] compared induction temperature (discussed in the next subsection), amino acid starvation, and AMP addition to increase pDNA production and concluded that AMP addition resulted in the highest Y_{px} (20.94 mg/g).

Another option to increase Y_{px} is the addition of chloramphenicol to the cultivation medium, inhibiting protein synthesis. Since the formation of new proteins is not necessary for pColE1-like plasmid replication, pDNA synthesis can continue regardless of the eventual growth cessation. This has led to an increase in plasmid copy number of up to 50-fold [84]. This strategy can be easily applied in lab-scale cultivations, but is obviously not appropriate for commercial pDNA vaccine production.

Amino acid exhaustion and/or AMP addition is potentially an efficient way to increase Y_{px} that can be applied to small- and large-scale cultivations. The cost of those molecules should be carefully considered, especially if scale-up is intended. In industrial scales, imperfect mixing could cause unequal distribution of AMP, which may lead to heterogeneous induction. This factor should be evaluated before scaling up. Another issue to be considered is the stress that amino acid starvation can trigger in *E. coli* during pDNA production. Detailed information on this regard is still scarce.

3.2.2 Increase of Y_{px} by Temperature Induction of Replication

A point mutation present in pColE1-derived plasmids immediately upstream of the transcription start site of the RNAI sequence (Fig. 2) prevents the proper folding of RNAII upon a temperature increase that in turn avoids the binding of RNAI to RNAII, resulting in replication upregulation. This effect can be suppressed by lowering the cultivation temperature to 30 °C. Therefore, a straightforward approach to take advantage of such properties is to grow the cells at 30 °C until a desired cell density is achieved and then raise the temperature up to 40–45 °C. This strategy has been extensively used and can lead to increasing Y_{px} up to tenfold [85, 87, 95, 105, 130, 131]. Compared to other strategies, like the addition of chemicals or amino acid limitation, temperature induction can be easier to implement at several scales. Bower and Prather [132] found that the expression of plasmid-encoded *repA* is a limiting factor for plasmid replication. By optimizing the start codon for *repA*, the authors showed that the Y_{px} was doubled using the engineered vector in comparison to the original one, after the temperature upshift.

Despite the positive effect of temperature upshift on Y_{px}, it triggers undesirable cellular changes known as the heat-shock response that results in the fast synthesis of chaperones and a general adaptation of carbon fluxes [133–136] as well as the accumulation of acetate and other organic acids [137]. Temperature increase can also trigger the stringent response and SOS response that drains cellular resources for pDNA synthesis and limit the viability of the cultivation and the achievable biomass. In general, information about the effect of temperature induction on the host physiology of *E. coli*-producing pDNA is very scarce. However, some authors have proposed the use of oscillatory or intermittent temperature induction for improving pDNA production [95]. Despite that the reported experiments were carried out in shake flasks (meaning that pH and dissolved oxygen tension were neither monitored nor controlled), there was a clear increase of Y_{px} when temperature was oscillated between 35 and 45 °C compared to the upshift from 37 to 45 °C. The possible reason for this could be that the transient exposure to elevated temperatures could be less aggressive for the general physiology of *E. coli* than the extended upshift. Another option to diminish the impact of temperature increase on cell physiology could be the use of temperature ramps instead of fast upshifts [110, 137]. It has been demonstrated that slow temperature ramps result in a better growth of cells, reducing the amount of produced acetate and increasing the fraction of viable cells during the cultivation, which results in better productivity of the process compared to fast temperature upshifts [138].

3.2.3 Specific Growth Rate Control

In general, it is assumed that Y_{px} is inversely proportional to the specific growth rate (μ) [90, 123, 139–143] mainly due to the fact that plasmid replications occur, to a certain extent, at a rate that can be independent from other cellular activities. Then, if cells divide less frequently, more plasmid copies are carried by daughter cells. However, some other authors have reported that the correlation between Y_{px} and μ can be positive or that Y_{px} can be approximately constant at a relatively wide range of growth rates (0.05–0.17 h^{-1}) [129, 144]. Also, it has been demonstrated that although some mutations can cause a decrease in growth rate, Y_{px} is not always increased [116].

As explained, the mentioned strategies to increase Y_{px} can be applied to shake flasks and small-scale bioreactors. However, special care has to be taken if temperature induction is to be used in shake flasks since oxygen solubility will be strongly affected when raising the temperatures. If pH drops due to acetate accumulation, pH won't be controlled properly in shake flasks. A recent study shows that amino acid depletion, AMP addition, a combination of both, and temperature induction all have a considerable effect on the physiology of *E. coli* [129], causing, for instance, cell filamentation and a decrease on viability at the end of the cultivation. Up to now, temperature induction has been reported to be successfully applied to commercial cultivations, while other strategies have been less exploited. If growth rate reduction is to be implemented in shake flasks, the already mentioned substrate slow-delivery systems can be useful. Again, little information exists in this regard. Other means for reducing growth rate such as temperature reduction, pH changes, and increasing initial substrate concentrations are not advisable since different cellular stresses can be triggered with undesirable effects on pDNA production.

3.3 Downstream Processes

Plasmid should be extracted from *E. coli* cells and purified to meet the regulatory requisites. Although mechanical rupture of cells (bead mills, ultrasound, and pressure) is well established at lab and process scale, it is not applicable to pDNA purification. It has been shown that pDNA is sensitive to shear damage [145, 146], which may cause partial pDNA degradation or generation of chromosomal DNA fragments of similar size of the pDNA that would be difficult to separate. Other protocols for cell disruption and pDNA extraction have been available at lab scale for years and can be adapted to production scales. *E. coli* cells can be disrupted by alkaline agents that at the same time denaturate chromosomal and plasmid DNA [147, 148]. Supercoiled pDNA can be reannealed and solubilized by neutralization, whereas chromosomal DNA and proteins are complexed by agents like sodium dodecyl sulfate (SDS). The pDNA is then concentrated by ethanol precipitation, and in some cases, further purification by phenol extraction is performed. In most cases, purification yields are improved when *endA*⁻ strains are used. The alkaline lysis procedure is appropriate for isolation of plasmid of different sizes, including pDNA of more than 10 kb [149].

Commercial kits for pDNA purification include a pretreatment with RNases and anion exchange columns in order to yield higher purity. The use of such columns increases the cost of the purification processes [149], which can be an issue when scaling up pDNA production. Other matrices for pDNA bonding, like silica oxide, are cheaper but disadvantageous since bacterial lipopolysaccharides are co-purified [149, 150], but refined protocols have been developed [150]. High-throughput protocols have been developed for pDNA extraction based on alkaline lysis [151–156]. Such protocols are useful in cases like media development, strain evaluation, or process optimization, and there are also commercially available products. Other methods like enzymatic lysis can be efficient at the lab scale, but at industrial scales those methods tend to be expensive and may cause regulatory issues [157]. Alkaline lysis has also been refined from a large-scale process point of view [158–160], and heat-induced lysis has been used for pDNA isolation [161] at laboratory [162] and industrial scales. In combination with enzymatic treatments, heat lysis can be more efficient than alkaline lysis for pDNA recovery.

Cell engineering approaches, like the expression of a protease [163] or RNase [164] by the pDNA production host strain, have been proposed to improve downstream processes in order to facilitate cell rupture and reduce contaminants.

Subsequent pDNA purification involves several steps if regulatory specifications are to be met. Proteins, endotoxins, RNA, and chromosomal DNA should be eliminated. Whereas at lab scale, detergents and organic solvents are used, different protocols such as hydrophobic interaction, anion exchange, and size exclusion chromatography are used at industrial scales [157].

A key issue during alkaline lysis is the noticeable viscosity increase after DNA release. Even at lab scales, inefficient mixing will result in pH gradients that may damage pDNA. In fact, mixing during alkaline lysis is of particular importance during the scale-up of a pDNA purification process.

4 Safety and Regulatory Issues

In the last couple of years, numerous efforts have been made to develop optimized plasmid backbones for DNA vaccine and gene therapeutic applications. In this section we will focus on backbone modifications that aim at improving the following: (1) the *safety*, (2) the *productivity*, and the (3) *potency* of the final plasmid product. Special attention will be paid to the state-of-the-art vector design, including the usage of antibiotic resistance-free plasmid backbones.

4.1 State-of-the-Art Vector Design

4.1.1 Improving the Safety Profile by Using Antibiotic Resistance-Free Plasmids

During the last few years, numerous efforts have been made to develop novel plasmid addiction systems for selection and maintenance of pDNA in order to avoid the presence of antibiotic resistance genes [165–172]. The use of antibiotic resistance genes as a selection marker for the production of plasmid DNA has raised concerns, already addressed by the regulatory authorities; *see* Subheading 2.1.1. As already reported, there is the fear of horizontal gene transfer of these resistance genes to the patient's gut microbiome, for instance, or concern about the integration of those resistance genes into the patient's genome, although no proof for such an integration exists so far. Therefore, a new generation of plasmid backbones, devoid of antibiotic resistance genes, has emerged. All these strategies are based on the same principle; growth of the bacterial cell is artificially linked to the presence of pDNA. The drawback in many of these approaches is that they rely on additional sequences that have to be added onto the vector backbone in order to confer properties that are essential for cellular growth. Although no more toxic drugs are involved and some of these sequences might be advantageous in terms of base composition, most of these approaches provide no reduction in the overall plasmid size. Additionally, the expression of these genes from high copy number plasmids exerts an unwanted metabolic burden on the host cell, shifting selection pressure towards a cellular status with lower plasmid copy number [172]. The metabolic precursors consumed to synthesize the antibiotic resistance gene cannot be devoted to plasmid replication, and thus this metabolic burden has an impact on culture performance and final plasmid yield [11, 114, 173]. A detailed list of all the alternative selection approaches can be found in Table 1. Additionally a comprehensive review on that topic has been published recently [174], including information on preclinical and clinical studies using antibiotic resistance-free plasmids.

Table 1
Different antibiotic resistance-free selection approaches either dependent on poison/antidote systems, essential gene completion, or RNA–RNA interaction, respectively

Antibiotic-free selection approach	Length of additional backbone sequence	References
Poison/antidote selection		
• *Genome-encoded ccdB (poison), plasmid-encoded ccdA (antidote); commercially available from Delphi Genetics (Charleroi, Belgium)*	270 bp (*ccdA*)	[169]
Overexpression of a growth essential gene		
• *Overexpression of fabI reduces susceptibility to triclosan*	860 bp (*fabI*)	[166]
Essential gene complementation		
• *Translation initiation factor infA*	219 bp (*infA*)	[168]
• *Amber suppressor tRNA needed for translation of argE*	200 bp (*sup Phe*)	[167]
• *Amber suppressor tRNA needed for translation of thyA*	200 bp (*sup His*)	[170]
• *dapD and operator-repressor titration (ORT)*	20 bp (*lacO*)	[165]
• *Glycine auxotrophy/serine hydroxymethyltransferase (glyA)*	1,254 bp (*glyA*)	[213]
• *NAD⁺ auxotrophy/quinolinic acid phosphoribosyltransferase*	894 bp (*nadC*)	[214]
RNA–RNA interaction		
• *RNA-IN/RNA-OUT interaction in combination with counter-selectable sacB marker*	144 bp	[171]
• *murA and origin-based RNAI repressor titration*	/	[173, 175]

The highest plasmid titers reported so far for these systems have been achieved using the RNA–RNA interaction-based selection systems [171, 173]. Mairhofer et al. [175] reported the near gram-scale production of an antibiotic resistance-free, minimized plasmid, encoding the monocyte chemoattractant protein-1 (MCP-1), that is devoid of any additional sequence element on the plasmid backbone and merely consists of the target expression cassette and the bacterial *ori*. Plasmid maintenance is achieved by functionally linking the RNAI, encoded on the origin of replication of common ColE1-based plasmids, to a repressor protein, encoded on the host genome, that further controls the expression of an essential gene [175]. Therefore, cell growth is only possible when pDNA is present and by deducing the inhibitor of plasmid replication, RNAI, the plasmid copy number is elevated at the same time, leading to increased plasmid titers. Besides the improved safety profile and size reduction, deletion of the antibiotic resistance gene also has an immunomodulatory effect which is addressed in the next subsection.

4.1.2 Considerations on the Nucleotide Sequence Composition to Improve Immunogenicity

Sequence composition and immunogenicity of the plasmid are interconnected and are therefore relevant for stability and efficacy of the pDNA in the animal or human target cell. Invading DNA is being recognized by the immune system and is subject to interactions with specific cellular components. CpG dinucleotides are known to be statistically underrepresented (~fivefold below expectation) within the eukaryotic genome, assumably because they mutate at high rate (~30-fold) since cytosine is prone to deamination, thereby producing thymidine [176]. Throughout the genome, these CG dinucleotides are commonly methylated with the exception of short unmethylated regions, the so-called CpG islands [177] which can be found within gene regulatory elements. pDNA derived from *E. coli* contains short sequences of unmethylated CpG dinucleotides in a certain base context [178, 179]. The immune system of vertebrates has evolved in a way that it is able to recognize bacterial DNA that is rich in unmethylated CpGs. This recognition is mediated by the Toll-like receptor 9 (TLR9) in cells of the innate immune system [180] and triggers an inflammatory reaction (activating B cells, monocytes, macrophages, dendritic cells, and natural killer cells) that in turn drives the adaptive immune response towards the vector-encoded GOI. This response is highly appreciated in the case of DNA vaccines and undesirable in the case of gene therapeutic applications where sustained transgene expression is necessary. Therefore, numerous approaches that either lower the immunogenic profile of pDNA vectors by reducing the CpG content [181–184] or that increase the immunogenicity by the design of potent immunostimulatory CpG-rich sequences [185, 186] have been developed during the last few years. CpG-depleted vectors can be generated by sequence analysis, in silico sequence optimization and DNA synthesis. A series of four CpG-dinucleotide-free plasmids is available from InvivoGen. However, the benefit of complete depletion of CpG motifs, even in the coding sequence of the transgene, is controversial. Recent studies have shown that CpG depletion clearly diminished the de novo transcription of the gene of interest [187, 188]. The molecular mechanism underlying CpG-mediated transcriptional regulation remains elusive but has been reproducible. Another recent study has shown that CpG-free plasmids are taken up more extensively and, in contrast, are cleared faster from mouse lungs than CpG-rich plasmids [189]. For cancer DNA vaccines, the immunostimulatory effect of CpG motifs has been increased by using CpG oligodeoxynucleotides (ODN) as an adjuvant [190–192].

4.1.3 Episomal Transgene Silencing and Considerations on the Overall Plasmid Size

It was reported previously that episomal pDNA is prone to gene silencing, e.g., in liver cells, due to the presence of bacterial DNA [193]. The proposed explanation is that within the plasmid backbone, repressive heterochromatin is formed which then spreads and inactivates the gene of interest leading to a decline in transgene expression. One common feature of bacterial backbone sequences is that they are transcriptionally inactive in mammalian cells. It is proposed that these transcriptionally inert sequences are similar to the heterochromatin found in eukaryotic cells and are therefore responsible for triggering a nucleosome condensation process, finally leading to the silencing of the transgene in the vicinity [193]. There exist several reports that provide evidence that unmethylated CpG motifs in episomal plasmid DNA may play a role in transcriptional silencing of a transgene [181–183, 194, 195]. Due to deletion of the antibiotic resistance gene, the CpG content of antibiotic resistance-free plasmids is significantly reduced as compared to the parental plasmids. In a recent publication, Ribeiro et al. suggested that the effect of gene silencing seems to be dependent on the length of the bacterial backbone sequence and possibly on the CpG content of that sequence [51]. Here, we have to address that the effect of the CpG content of plasmid vectors on episomal gene silencing is discussed controversially [196]. However, there are indications that the transgene silencing effect is more pronounced with larger plasmids than with smaller ones [51, 196, 197]. Therefore, using state-of-the-art strategies to minimize the bacterial plasmid backbone should be encouraged during the development of new vaccines.

Besides the described effect of the composition of the plasmid backbone on transgene silencing, several reports exist on the effect of plasmid size on the transformation efficiency. Kreiss et al. observed that pDNA size modulates the gene transfer efficiency, whereas the transfection activity of lipoplexes containing smaller plasmids was found to be greater than that of lipoplexes containing the same molarity of larger plasmids [198]. Additionally, it was reported that the diffusion of DNA in the cytoplasm of cells is strongly size dependent, with little or no diffusion of DNAs >2,000 bp. Inside the nucleus, DNA fragments of all sizes seem to be immobile [199]. It is believed that binding effects to cytoskeletal elements, acting as molecular sieve, are not primarily responsible for the slowed diffusion of DNA molecules. The major problem seems to be molecular crowding and collisional interactions exerting a strong dependence on intracellular diffusion. Nuclear translocation is more frequently achieved during cell division due to subsequent nuclear envelope disruption [200]. Entry via the nuclear pores seems to be size dependent as well. Kreiss et al. showed that the transfection of nondividing smooth muscle cells by a minicircle, 2.9 kbp in size, was 77 times more efficient than a plasmid 52.5 kbp in length [198], supporting this hypothesis. Yin et al. did a systematic study on the effect of plasmid size on promoter/enhancer activity in transient transfection assays and concluded that expression declined as a function of vector size and that the sharpest decrease in reporter gene activity occurred when a 5.1 kbp plasmid was increased by 0.65 kbp [201]. Walker et al. showed that this lower efficiency of larger plasmids is not due to the lower copy number since equal mass was used instead of equal molarities [202]. However, Carpentier et al. stated that there are more bottlenecks than the cellular uptake of pDNA. They were able to show that after polyethyleneimine-mediated transfection, positive and negative HEK293-EBNA1 cells contained equal amounts of pDNA and that in positive cells, the nuclear plasmid content was threefold higher than in negative cells [203]. It was shown that transformation-negative cells contained significant nuclear amounts of pDNA. However, transcriptional competency of pDNA was impaired and seems to be dependent on the physiological state of the targeted cell as well. However, it seems that any reduction in size enhances the transformation efficiencies and is therefore beneficial for pDNA delivery.

4.2 How to Meet the Regulatory Guidelines

DNA vaccines are considered to be hybrids between gene therapeutic medicinal products and classical vaccines. The regulatory authorities in Europe and the USA do differentiate between DNA vaccines against infectious diseases (FDA/CBER/OVRR) and DNA vaccines for noninfectious therapeutic indications (FDA/CBER/OCTGT; EMA/GTMP). The development of a medicinal product is a well-defined process consisting of the following steps:

- Proof of concept (animal model)
- Design and development of a manufacturing process
- Demonstration of quality and nonclinical safety
- Clinical trial approval
- Demonstration of clinical safety and efficiency
- Marketing authorization application

The regulatory process for Europe and the USA was recently reviewed elsewhere [204, 205]. To support product development, specific guidelines are available from the different regulatory authorities [206–210]. Here we will briefly comment on the relevant points issued for the manufacturing of plasmid DNA.

4.2.1 General Requirements

As for all biotechnological-derived medicinal products, the general manufacturing requirements must be met. This involves a manufacturing process which is highly defined, carefully controlled, and operated under reproducible conditions, i.e., the manufacturing procedure has to be in compliance with the Good Manufacturing Practice (GMP) guidelines. This includes hazardous critical step analysis and implementation of adequate in-process controls as well as application of appropriate tests to characterize intermediate and final products. A few interesting articles on the GMP production of plasmid DNA are available [157, 211, 212].

Critical tests should at least include the following:

- Visual inspection of the in-process control (IPC) samples and the final product on an agarose gel; an open circular (using, e.g., the enzyme N.BstNBI) and linear standard of the plasmid of choice can be prepared easily to confirm the identity of the bands. The gel should also show the absence of *E. coli* host RNA and DNA.

- Plasmid purity should be also determined using anion exchange chromatography (AEX-HPLC). The method should be able to resolve open circular, linear, and supercoiled plasmid. The goal should be to determine the % of supercoiled pDNA since this corresponds to the purity of the product due to the fact that all other conformations are regarded as contaminants.
- UV analysis can be used to determine the concentration and purity of the plasmid solution. Absorbance should be measured at 230, 260, 280, and 320 nm. The ratio 260/280 should be ~1.8 and the 260/230 should be ~2.0–2.2.
- Residual protein content should be determined using an assay such as the bicinchoninic acid (BCA) assay or others.
- Sequencing of the whole plasmid is advisable.
- The bioburden of the final formulation should be determined using viable aerobic count (Ph. 2.6.12).
- Sterility and removal of bacterial endotoxins should be proofed using the filtration method (Ph. 2.6.1) and the amoebocyte lysate (LAL) test (Ph. 2.6.14).
- Stability upon storage should be tested.

4.2.2 Specific Requirements

The development of the plasmid should be documented with care. Information on the origin of the encoded gene should be provided in detail. A description of the molecular cloning steps that have been performed in the course of the construction of the plasmid should be provided together with the sequence data of the gene, a restriction map, and a source list of the distinct regions within the plasmid. It is not advisable to use any other antibiotic resistance gene than the neomycin phosphotransferase gene II (*nptII*). To avoid problems with regulatory authorities, animal-product-free LB broth and plates should be used for cloning of the plasmid. The origin of the host microorganism that will be used for expansion of the plasmid, most likely *E. coli* K-12 or B, should be provided including its species, subtype, and passage history. It is therefore advisable to use a strain from a secured source such as ATCC which is able to provide this necessary information. In the course of the generation of Master Cell Bank and Working Cell Bank, the identity of the plasmid after transformation should be confirmed, and data on the plasmid retention during fermentation should be generated.

Since data on the plasmid retention is necessary, it is advisable to start monitoring the plasmid stability from the very beginning when developing a production process. Keep in mind that usage of antibiotics should be avoided during manufacturing at all costs.

Low plasmid retention without selection pressure is a critical issue and should be solved prior to initiating preclinical immunological trials. Various approaches to improve plasmid retention exist; *see* Subheading 2.3.

In addition to these relevant manufacturing issues, the following points require consideration as well: (1) biodistribution/persistence of the plasmid; (2) integration into the patient's genome; (3) tolerance induction; (4) autoimmunity, an issue that should be especially addressed when developing cancer vaccines; (5) genotoxicity; and (6) reproductive toxicity. Information on how to address these points can be found elsewhere [203].

5 Conclusion

As clinical trials involving pDNA-based biopharmaceuticals progress, the demand for more efficient pDNA production processes is expected to increase. There have been important advances in the design of vectors, strains, and process strategies for pDNA vaccines over the last few years. In this chapter, we have presented an overview of such advances and current trends and emphasized the need for detailed information and knowledge in several different aspects of pDNA production. We expect that the information summarized here will be of use for better vector design and for selecting more productive cultivation schemes at a small scale in order to accelerate product development.

Acknowledgement

This work was supported by CONACyT grant 183911 and PROMEP grant 10828.

References

1. Rein DT et al (2006) Current developments in adenovirus-based cancer gene therapy. Future Oncol 2:137–143
2. Erbs P et al (2008) Modified vaccinia virus Ankara as a vector for suicide gene therapy. Cancer Gene Ther 15:18–28
3. Cubas R et al (2011) Chimeric Trop2 virus-like particles: a potential immunotherapeutic approach against pancreatic cancer. J Immunother 34:251–263
4. Kaczmarczyk SJ et al (2011) Protein delivery using engineered virus-like particles. Proc Natl Acad Sci USA 108:16998–17003
5. Fioretti D et al (2010) DNA vaccines: developing new strategies against cancer. J Biomed Biotechnol 2010:174378
6. Rice J et al (2008) DNA vaccines: precision tools for activating effective immunity against cancer. Nat Rev Cancer 8:108–120
7. Weide B et al (2008) Plasmid DNA- and messenger RNA-based anti-cancer vaccination. Immunol Lett 115:33–42
8. Staff C et al (2011) A Phase I safety study of plasmid DNA immunization targeting carcinoembryonic antigen in colorectal cancer patients. Vaccine 29:6817–6822

9. Cohen S et al (1973) Construction of biologically functional bacterial plasmids in vitro. Proc Natl Acad Sci USA 70:3240–3244
10. Hershfield V et al (1974) Plasmid ColEl as a molecular vehicle for cloning and amplification of DNA. Proc Natl Acad Sci USA 71:3455–3459
11. Cunningham D et al (2009) Factors affecting plasmid production in *Escherichia coli* from a resource allocation standpoint. Microb Cell Fact 8:27
12. Castagnoli L et al (1989) Genetic and structural analysis of the ColE1 Rop (Rom) protein. EMBO J 8:621–629
13. Dong X et al (2004) PlasMapper: a web server for drawing and auto-annotating plasmid maps. Nucleic Acids Res 32:W660–W664
14. Bond SR, Naus CC (2012) RF-Cloning.org: an online tool for the design of restriction-free cloning projects. Nucleic Acids Res 40(W1):W209–W213
15. Bryksin AV, Matsumura I (2010) Overlap extension PCR cloning: a simple and reliable way to create recombinant plasmids. Biotechniques 48:463–465
16. FDA (1996) Points to consider on plasmid DNA vaccines for preventive infectious disease indications. Center for Biologics Evaluation and Research, Docket No. 96N-0400
17. EMEA (2008) Questions and answers on gene therapy. Doc. Ref: EMA/CHMP/GTWP/212377/2008 ed., European Medicines Agency
18. Belt A (1996) Characterization of cultures used for biotechnology and industry. In: Hunter-Cevera JC (ed) Maintaining cultures for biotechnology and industry. Academic Press, London
19. Harms JS, Splitter GA (1995) Interferon-gamma inhibits transgene expression driven by SV40 or CMV promoters but augments expression driven by the mammalian MHC I promoter. Hum Gene Ther 6:1291–1297
20. Gribaudo G et al (1993) Interferons inhibit onset of murine cytomegalovirus immediate-early gene transcription. Virology 197: 303–311
21. Grabherr MG et al (2011) Exploiting nucleotide composition to engineer promoters. PLoS One 6:e20136
22. Baumann M et al (2012) Artificially designed promoters: understanding the role of spatial features and canonical binding sites in transcription. Bioeng Bugs 3(2):120–123
23. Samadashwily G et al (1997) Trinucleotide repeats affect DNA replication in vivo. Nat Genet 17:298–304
24. Williams J et al (2006) pDNAVACCultra vector family: high throughput intracellular targeting DNA vaccine plasmids. Vaccine 24:4671–4676
25. Kushner P et al (1994) Eukaryotic regulatory elements lurking in plasmid DNA: the activator protein-1 site in pUC. Mol Endocrinol 8:405–407
26. Ghersa P et al (1994) Commonly used cat reporter vectors contain a cAMP-inducible, cryptic enhancer that co-operates with NF-kappa B-sites. Gene 151:331–332
27. Tully D, Cidlowski J (1987) pBR322 contains glucocorticoid regulatory element DNA consensus sequences. Biochem Biophys Res Commun 144:1–110
28. Peterson D et al (1987) Context-dependent gene expression: cis-acting negative effects of specific procaryotic plasmid sequences on eucaryotic genes. Mol Cell Biol 7:1563–1567
29. Fath S et al (2011) Multiparameter RNA and codon optimization: a standardized tool to assess and enhance autologous mammalian gene expression. PLoS One 6:e17596
30. Welch M et al (2009) Design parameters to control synthetic gene expression in *Escherichia coli*. PLoS One 4:e7002
31. Hellen CU, Sarnow P (2001) Internal ribosome entry sites in eukaryotic mRNA molecules. Genes Dev 15:1593–1612
32. Jang SK et al (1988) A segment of the 5' non-translated region of encephalomyocarditis virus RNA directs internal entry of ribosomes during in vitro translation. J Virol 62: 2636–2643
33. Bei R, Scardino A (2010) TAA polyepitope DNA-based vaccines: a potential tool for cancer therapy. J Biomed Biotechnol 2010:102758
34. Mir FA et al (2009) A multicistronic DNA vaccine induces significant protection against tuberculosis in mice and offers flexibility in the expressed antigen repertoire. Clin Vaccine Immunol 16:1467–1475
35. Yan J et al (2006) Enhanced cellular immune responses elicited by an engineered HIV-1 Subtype B consensus-based envelope DNA vaccine. Mol Ther 15:411–421
36. Laddy DJ et al (2007) Immunogenicity of novel consensus-based DNA vaccines against avian influenza. Vaccine 25:2984–2989
37. van der Bruggen P, Van den Eynde BJ (2006) Processing and presentation of tumor antigens and vaccination strategies. Curr Opin Immunol 18:98–104
38. Rice J et al (2002) Critical components of a DNA fusion vaccine able to induce protective

cytotoxic T cells against a single epitope of a tumor antigen. J Immunol 169:3908–3913
39. Radcliffe JN et al (2006) Prime-boost with alternating DNA vaccines designed to engage different antigen presentation pathways generates high frequencies of peptide-specific $CD8^+$ T cells. J Immunol 177:6626–6633
40. Oosterhuis K et al (2011) Preclinical development of highly effective and safe DNA vaccines directed against HPV 16 E6 and E7. Int J Cancer 129:397–406
41. Biragyn A et al (2002) Toll-like receptor 4-dependent activation of dendritic cells by β-defensin 2. Science 298:1025–1029
42. Biragyn A et al (2001) Mediators of innate immunity that target immature, but not mature, dendritic cells induce antitumor immunity when genetically fused with nonimmunogenic tumor antigens. J Immunol 167: 6644–6653
43. Wang YS et al (2007) Immunity against tumor angiogenesis induced by a fusion vaccine with murine β-defensin 2 and mFlk-1. Clin Cancer Res 13:6779–6787
44. Mei HF et al (2012) Beta-defensin 2 as an adjuvant promotes anti-melanoma immune responses and inhibits the growth of implanted murine melanoma in vivo. PLoS One 7: e31328
45. Wei Y et al (2012) Enhancement of DNA vaccine efficacy by targeting the xenogeneic human chorionic gonadotropin, survivin and vascular endothelial growth factor receptor 2 combined tumor antigen to the major histocompatibility complex class II pathway. J Gene Med 14:353–362
46. Guan QD et al (2007) The distinct effects of three tandem repeats of C3d in the immune responses against tumor-associated antigen hCGbeta by DNA immunization. Cancer Immunol Immunother 56:875–884
47. Shi SQ et al (2005) The mouse chorionic gonadotropin beta-subunit-like (muCG beta l) molecule produced by tumor cells elicits the switch of T-cell immunity response from TH2 to TH1 in mice immunized with DNA vaccine based on rhesus monkey homologous CG beta (rmCG beta). J Gene Med 7:87–96
48. Holst PJ et al (2010) DNA fusion gene vaccines. Curr Opin Mol Ther 12:47–54
49. Azzoni A et al (2007) The impact of polyadenylation signals on plasmid nuclease-resistance and transgene expression. J Gene Med 9:392–402
50. Ribeiro S et al (2004) The role of polyadenylation signal secondary structures on the resistance of plasmid vectors to nucleases. J Gene Med 6:565–573
51. Ribeiro S et al (2012) Plasmid DNA size does affect nonviral gene delivery efficiency in stem cells. Cell Reprogram 14:130–137
52. Luke JM et al (2011) Improved antibiotic-free plasmid vector design by incorporation of transient expression enhancers. Gene Ther 18:334–343
53. Arnott S (2006) Historical article: DNA polymorphism and the early history of the double helix. Trends Biochem Sci 31:349–354
54. Marvin D et al (1961) The molecular configuration of deoxyribonucleic acid. III. X-ray diffraction study of the C form of the lithium salt. J Mol Biol 3:547–565
55. Arnott S et al (1974) Structural details of double-helix observed for DNAs containing alternating purine and pyrimidine sequences. J Mol Biol 88:523–533
56. Vargason J et al (2000) The extended and eccentric E-DNA structure induced by cytosine methylation or bromination. Nat Struct Biol 7:758–761
57. Mirkin S et al (1987) DNA H form requires a homopurine-homopyrimidine mirror repeat. Nature 330:495–497
58. Hayashi G et al (2005) Application of L-DNA as a molecular tag. Nucleic Acids Symp Ser (Oxf) 49:261–262
59. Allemand J et al (1998) Stretched and overwound DNA forms a Pauling-like structure with exposed bases. Proc Natl Acad Sci USA 95:14152–14157
60. Paddock G, Abelson J (1975) Nucleotide sequence determination of bacteriophage T2 and T6 species I ribonucleic acids. J Biol Chem 250:4207–4219
61. Wang A et al (1979) Molecular structure of a left-handed double helical DNA fragment at atomic resolution. Nature 282:680–686
62. Cherng J et al (1999) Effect of DNA topology on the transfection efficiency of poly((2-dimethylamino)ethyl methacrylate)-plasmid complexes. J Control Release 60:343–353
63. Ussery D et al (2002) Bias of purine stretches in sequenced chromosomes. Comput Chem 26:531–541
64. Cooke J et al (2004) Impact of intrinsic DNA structure on processing of plasmids for gene therapy and DNA vaccines. J Biotechnol 114:239–254
65. Yau S et al (2008) Host strain influences on supercoiled plasmid DNA production in *Escherichia coli*: implications for efficient design of large-scale processes. Biotechnol Bioeng 101:529–544
66. Zaman MM, Boles TC (1996) Plasmid recombination by the RecBCD pathway of *Escherichia coli*. J Bacteriol 178:3840–3845

67. Lovett ST (2004) Encoded errors: mutations and rearrangements mediated by misalignment at repetitive DNA sequences. Mol Microbiol 52:1243–1253
68. Bi X, Liu LF (1996) DNA rearrangement mediated by inverted repeats. Proc Natl Acad Sci USA 93:819–823
69. Oliveira PH et al (2009) Structural instability of plasmid biopharmaceuticals: challenges and implications. Trends Biotechnol 27:503–511
70. Oliveira PH et al (2010) Analysis of DNA repeats in bacterial plasmids reveals the potential for recurrent instability events. Appl Microbiol Biotechnol 87:2157–2167
71. Ribeiro S et al (2008) High frequency plasmid recombination mediated by 28 bp direct repeats. Mol Biotechnol 40:252–260
72. Betley JN et al (2002) A ubiquitous and conserved signal for RNA localization in chordates. Curr Biol 12:1756–1761
73. Ho PS et al (1986) A computer aided thermodynamic approach for predicting the formation of Z-DNA in naturally occurring sequences. EMBO J 5:2737–2744
74. Oliveira PH et al (2008) Recombination frequency in plasmid DNA containing direct repeats–predictive correlation with repeat and intervening sequence length. Plasmid 60:159–165
75. Mahillon J, Chandler M (1998) Insertion sequences. Microbiol Mol Biol Rev 62:725–774
76. Varani AM et al (2011) ISsaga is an ensemble of web-based methods for high throughput identification and semi-automatic annotation of insertion sequences in prokaryotic genomes. Genome Biol 12(3):R30
77. Prather K et al (2006) Identification and characterization of IS1 transposition in plasmid amplification mutants of *E. coli* clones producing DNA vaccines. Appl Microbiol Biotechnol 73:815–826
78. Oliveira PH et al (2009) Deletion formation mutations in plasmid expression vectors are unfavored by runaway amplification conditions and differentially selected under kanamycin stress. J Biotechnol 143:231–238
79. Umenhoffer K et al (2010) Reduced evolvability of *Escherichia coli* MDS42, an IS-less cellular chassis for molecular and synthetic biology applications. Microb Cell Fact 9:38
80. Pósfai G et al (2006) Emergent properties of reduced-genome *Escherichia coli*. Science 312:1044–1046
81. Casali N (2003) *Escherichia coli* host strains. In: Casali N, Preston A (ed) Methods in Molecular Biol 235:27–48
82. Schnarr M et al (1985) Large-scale purification, oligomerization equilibria, and specific interaction of the LexA repressor of *Escherichia coli*. Biochemistry 24:2812–2818
83. Schnarr M et al (1985) The LexA repressor of *Escherichia coli*. Biol Chem Hoppe Seyler 366:847–848
84. Summers D (1996) The biology of plasmids. Blackwell Science Ltd., Oxford, England
85. Phue J et al (2008) Modified *Escherichia coli* B (BL21), a superior producer of plasmid DNA compared with *Escherichia coli* K (DH5 alpha). Biotechnol Bioeng 101:831–836
86. Bower D, Prather K (2009) Engineering of bacterial strains and vectors for the production of plasmid DNA. Appl Microbiol Biotechnol 82:805–813
87. Singer A et al (2009) DNA plasmid production in different host strains of *Escherichia coli*. J Ind Microbiol Biotechnol 36:521–530
88. Xia X et al (2011) Comparative proteomic and genetic analyses reveal unidentified mutations in *Escherichia coli* XL1-Blue and DH5 alpha. Fems Microbiol Lett 314:119–124
89. van der Heijden I et al (2013) Transposon leads to contamination of clinical pDNA vaccine. Vaccine 31:3274–3280
90. O'Kennedy R et al (2003) Effects of fermentation strategy on the characteristics of plasmid DNA production. Biotechnol Appl Biochem 37:83–90
91. Zheng S et al (2007) Optimization of medium components for plasmid production by recombinant *E-coli* DH5 alpha pUK21CMV beta 1.2. Biotechnol Bioprocess Eng 12:213–221
92. Duttweiler H, Gross D (1998) Growth medium that significantly increases the yield of recombinant plasmid (vol 24, pg 438, 1998). Biotechniques 24:992
93. Danquah M, Forde G (2007) Growth medium selection and its economic impact on plasmid DNA production. J Biosci Bioeng 104:490–497
94. Danquah M, Forde G (2008) Development of a pilot-scale bacterial fermentation for plasmid-based biopharmaceutical production using a stoichiometric medium. Biotechnol Bioprocess Eng 13:158–167
95. Ongkudon C et al (2011) Cultivation of *E. coli* carrying a plasmid-based measles vaccine construct (4.2 kbp pcDNA3F) employing medium optimisation and pH-temperature induction techniques. Microb Cell Fact 10:16
96. O'Kennedy R et al (2000) Effects of growth medium selection on plasmid DNA production and initial processing steps. J Biotechnol 76:175–183
97. Zawada J, Swartz J (2005) Maintaining rapid growth in moderate-density *Escherichia coli*

fermentations. Biotechnol Bioeng 89: 407–415

98. Voss C et al (2004) Effect of ammonium chloride on plasmid DNA production in high cell density batch culture for biopharmaceutical use. J Chem Technol Biotechnol 79:57–62
99. Wang Z et al (2001) Medium design for plasmid DNA production based on stoichiometric model. Process Biochem 36:1085–1093
100. Ukkonen K et al (2011) High-yield production of biologically active recombinant protein in shake flask culture by combination of enzyme-based glucose delivery and increased oxygen transfer. Microb Cell Fact 10:107
101. Scheidle M et al (2011) Controlling pH in shake flasks using polymer-based controlled-release discs with pre-determined release kinetics. BMC Biotechnol 11:25
102. Papagianni M (2012) Recent advances in engineering the central carbon metabolism of industrially important bacteria. Microb Cell Fact 11:50
103. Lara AR (2011) Recombinant protein production in *Escherichia coli*. Revista Mexicana De Ingenieria Quimica 10:209–223
104. Flores S et al (2004) Growth-rate recovery of *Escherichia coli* cultures carrying a multicopy plasmid, by engineering of the pentose-phosphate pathway. Biotechnol Bioeng 87:485–494
105. Williams J et al (2009) Generic plasmid DNA production platform incorporating low metabolic burden seed-stock and fed-batch fermentation processes. Biotechnol Bioeng 103:1129–1143
106. Cunningham D et al (2009) Pyruvate kinase-deficient *Escherichia coli* exhibits increased plasmid copy number and cyclic AMP levels. J Bacteriol 191:3041–3049
107. Goncalvez GAL et al. J. De novo creation of MG1655-derived *E. coli* strains specifically designed for plasmid DNA production. Appl Microbiol Biotechnol 97(2):611–620
108. Hua Q et al (2003) Responses of the central metabolism in *Escherichia coli* to phosphoglucose isomerase and glucose-6-phosphate dehydrogenase knockouts. J Bacteriol 185: 7053–7067
109. Wang Z et al (2006) Effect of the presence of ColE1 plasmid DNA in *Escherichia coli* on the host cell metabolism. Microb Cell Fact 5:34
110. Carnes A et al (2011) Plasmid DNA fermentation strain and process-specific effects on vector yield, quality, and transgene expression. Biotechnol Bioeng 108:354–363
111. Ow D et al (2009) Enhancement of plasmid DNA yields during fed-batch culture of a fruR-knockout *Escherichia coli* strain. Biotechnol Appl Biochem 52:53–59
112. Ow D et al (2007) Inactivating FruR global regulator in plasmid-bearing *Escherichia coli* alters metabolic gene expression and improves growth rate. J Biotechnol 131:261–269
113. Ow D et al (2006) Global transcriptional analysis of metabolic burden due to plasmid maintenance in *Escherichia coli* DH5 alpha during batch fermentation. Enzyme Microb Technol 39:391–398
114. Rozkov A et al (2004) Characterization of the metabolic burden on *Escherichia coli* DH1 cells imposed by the presence of a plasmid containing a gene therapy sequence. Biotechnol Bioeng 88:909–915
115. Grabherr R et al (2011) Method for controlling plasmid copy number in *E. coli*. (Organization, W. I. P., Ed.).
116. Borja GM et al (2012) Engineering *Escherichia coli* to increase plasmid DNA production in high cell-density cultivations in batch mode. Microb Cell Fact 11:132
117. De Anda R et al (2006) Replacement of the glucose phosphotransferase transport system by galactose permease reduces acetate accumulation and improves process performance of *Escherichia coli* for recombinant protein production without impairment of growth rate. Metab Eng 8:281–290
118. Lara AR et al (2008) Utility of an *Escherichia coli* strain engineered in the substrate uptake system for improved culture performance at high glucose and cell concentrations: an fed-batch cultures. Biotechnol Bioeng 99:893–901
119. Flores S et al (2002) Analysis of carbon metabolism in *Escherichia coli* strains with an inactive phosphotransferase system by C-13 labeling and NMR spectroscopy. Metab Eng 4:124–137
120. Knabben I et al (2010) High cell-density processes in batch mode of a genetically engineered *Escherichia coli* strain with minimized overflow metabolism using a pressurized bioreactor. J Biotechnol 150:73–79
121. Soto R et al (2011) High cell-density cultivation in batch mode for plasmid DNA production by a metabolically engineered *E-coli* strain with minimized overflow metabolism. Biochem Eng J 56:165–171
122. Pablos T et al (2012) Enhanced production of plasmid DNA by engineered *Escherichia coli* strains. J Biotechnol 158:211–214
123. Bohle K, Ross A (2011) Plasmid DNA Production for pharmaceutical use: role of specific growth rate and impact on process design. Biotechnol Bioeng 108:2099–2106

124. Hecker M et al (1983) Replication of pBR322 DNA in stringent and relaxed strains of *Escherichia coli*. Mol Gen Genet 190:355–357
125. Hofmann K et al (1990) Amplification of pBR322 plasmid DNA in *Escherichia coli* relA strains during batch and fed-batch fermentation. J Basic Microbiol 30:37–41
126. Wang Z et al (2002) A model for regulation of colE1-like plasmid replication by uncharged tRNAs in amino acid-starved *Escherichia coli* cells. Plasmid 47:69–78
127. Wegrzyn G (1999) Replication of plasmids during bacterial response to amino acid starvation. Plasmid 41:1–16
128. Wang Z et al (2007) Adenosine monophosphate-induced amplification of ColE1 plasmid DNA in *Escherichia coli*. Plasmid 57:265–274
129. Silva F et al (2011) Impact of plasmid induction strategy on overall plasmid DNA yield and *E. coli* physiology using flow cytometry and real-time PCR. Process Biochem 46:174–181
130. Carnes A et al (2006) Inducible *Escherichia coli* fermentation for increased plasmid DNA production. Biotechnol Appl Biochem 45:155–166
131. Bower D et al (2012) Fed-batch microbioreactor platform for scale down and analysis of a plasmid DNA production process. Biotechnol Bioeng 109(8):1976–1986
132. Bower DM, Prather KLJ (2012) Development of new plasmid DNA vaccine vectors with R1-based replicons. Microb Cell Fact 11:107
133. Valdez-Cruz N et al (2010) Production of recombinant proteins in *E. coli* by the heat inducible expression system based on the phage lambda pL and/or pR promoters. Microb Cell Fact 9:18
134. Hoffmann F et al (2002) Metabolic adaptation of *Escherichia coli* during temperature-induced recombinant protein production: 1. Readjustment of metabolic enzyme synthesis. Biotechnol Bioeng 80:313–319
135. Weber J et al (2002) Metabolic adaptation of *Escherichia coli* during temperature-induced recombinant protein production: 2. Redirection of metabolic fluxes. Biotechnol Bioeng 80:320–330
136. Wittmann C et al (2007) Response of fluxome and metabolome to temperature-induced recombinant protein synthesis in *Escherichia coli*. J Biotechnol 132:375–384
137. Caspeta L et al (2009) The effect of heating rate on *Escherichia coli* metabolism, physiological stress, transcriptional response, and production of temperature-induced recombinant protein: a scale-down study. Biotechnol Bioeng 102:468–482
138. Jaén KE et al (2013) Effect of heating rate on pDNA production by *E. coli*. Biochem Eng J 79:230–238
139. Bentley W et al (1990) Plasmid-encoded protein – the principal factor in the metabolic burden associated with recombinant bacteria. Biotechnol Bioeng 35:668–681
140. Chen W et al (1997) Automated fed-batch fermentation with feed-back controls based on dissolved oxygen (DO) and pH for production of DNA vaccines. J Ind Microbiol Biotechnol 18:43–48
141. Kim J, Ryu D (1991) The effects of plasmid content, transcription efficiency, and translation efficiency on the productivity of a cloned gene protein in *Escherichia coli*. Biotechnol Bioeng 38:1271–1279
142. Rozkov A et al (2006) Fed batch culture with declining specific growth rate for high-yielding production of a plasmid containing a gene therapy sequence in *Escherichia coli* DH1. Enzyme Microb Technol 39:47–50
143. Ryan W, Parulekar S (1991) Recombinant protein synthesis and plasmid instability in continuous cultures of *Escherichia coli* JM103 harboring a high copy number plasmid. Biotechnol Bioeng 37:415–429
144. Wunderlich M (2010) Kinetic characterization of engineered *Escherichia coli* strains during plasmid DNA vaccine production in chemostats. In: Department of Food and Bioprocess Engineering, Technical University of Dresden, Germany
145. Levy M et al (1999) Effect of shear on plasmid DNA in solution. Bioprocess Eng 20:7–13
146. Levy M et al (2000) Removal of contaminant nucleic acids by nitrocellulose filtration during pharmaceutical-grade plasmid DNA processing. J Biotechnol 76:197–205
147. Birnboim HC, Doly J (1979) A rapid alkaline extraction procedure for screening recombinant plasmid DNA. Nucleic Acids Res 7:1513–1523
148. Birnboim HC (1983) A rapid alkaline extraction method for the rapid isolation of plasmid DNA. Methods Enzymol 100:243–255
149. Grimm S, Voss-Neudecker F (2003) High-purity plasmid isolation using silica oxide. In: Casali N (ed) Methods in Molecular Biol. Humana Press 235:83–87
150. Neudecker F, Grimm S (2000) High-throughput method for isolating plasmid DNA with reduced lipopolysaccharide content. Biotechniques 28:107–109

151. Bankier T (1993) M13 phage growth and DNA purification using 96-well microtiter plates. Methods Mol Biol 23:41–45
152. Gibson T, Sulston J (1987) Preparation of large numbers of plasmid DNA samples in microtiter plates by the alkaline lysis method. Gene Anal Tech 4:41–44
153. Itoh M et al (1997) Simple and rapid preparation of plasmid template by a filtration method using microtiter filter plates. Nucleic Acids Res 25:1315–1316
154. Itoh M et al (1999) Automated filtration-based high-throughput plasmid preparation system. Genome Res 9:463–470
155. Konecki D, Phillips J (1998) TurboPrep II: an inexpensive, high-throughput plasmid template preparation protocol. Biotechniques 24:286–288
156. Marra M et al (1999) High-throughput plasmid DNA purification for 3 cents per sample. Nucleic Acids Res 27(24):e37
157. Urthaler J et al (2012) Industrial Manufacturing of plasmid-DNA products for gene vaccination and therapy. In: Thalhamer J (ed) Gene vaccines. Springer, Vienna, pp 311–330
158. Clemson M, Kelly W (2003) Optimizing alkaline lysis for DNA plasmid recovery. Biotechnol Appl Biochem 37:235–244
159. Chamsart S et al (2001) The impact of fluid-dynamic-generated stresses on chDNA and pDNA stability during alkaline cell lysis for gene therapy products. Biotechnol Bioeng 75:387–392
160. Varley D et al (1998) Production of plasmid DNA for human gene therapy using modified alkaline cell lysis and expanded bed anion exchange chromatography. Bioseparation 8:209–217
161. Holmes D, Quigley M (1981) A rapid boiling method for the preparation of bacterial plasmids. Anal Biochem 114:193–197
162. O'Mahony K et al (2005) Proposal for a better integration of bacterial lysis into the production of plasmid DNA at large scale. J Biotechnol 119:118–132
163. Carnes A et al (2009) Plasmid DNA production combining antibiotic-free selection, inducible high yield fermentation, and novel autolytic purification. Biotechnol Bioeng 104:505–515
164. Cooke G et al (2001) Purification of essentially RNA free plasmid DNA using a modified *Escherichia coli* host strain expressing ribonuclease A. J Biotechnol 85:297–304
165. Cranenburgh R et al (2001) *Escherichia coli* strains that allow antibiotic-free plasmid selection and maintenance by repressor titration. Nucleic Acids Res 29:E26
166. Goh S, Good L (2008) Plasmid selection in *Escherichia coli* using an endogenous essential gene marker. BMC Biotechnol 8:61
167. Soubrier F et al (1999) pCOR: a new design of plasmid vectors for nonviral gene therapy. Gene Ther 6:1482–1488
168. Hägg P et al (2004) A host/plasmid system that is not dependent on antibiotics and antibiotic resistance genes for stable plasmid maintenance in *Escherichia coli*. J Biotechnol 111:17–30
169. Szpirer C, Milinkovitch M (2005) Separate-component-stabilization system for protein and DNA production without the use of antibiotics. Biotechniques 38:775–781
170. Marie C et al (2010) pFARs, plasmids free of antibiotic resistance markers, display high-level transgene expression in muscle, skin and tumour cells. J Gene Med 12:323–332
171. Luke J et al (2009) Improved antibiotic-free DNA vaccine vectors utilizing a novel RNA based plasmid selection system. Vaccine 27:6454–6459
172. Panayotatos N (1988) Recombinant protein production with minimal-antibiotic-resistance vectors. Gene 74:357–363
173. Mairhofer J et al (2010) Marker-free plasmids for gene therapeutic applications-lack of antibiotic resistance gene substantially improves the manufacturing process. J Biotechnol 143(30):130–137
174. Vandermeulen G, Marie C, Scherman D, Preat V (2011) New generation of plasmid backbones devoid of antibiotic resistance marker for gene therapy trials. Mol Ther 19:1942–1949
175. Mairhofer J et al (2008) A novel antibiotic free plasmid selection system: advances in safe and efficient DNA therapy. Biotechnol J 3:83–89
176. Fryxell KJ, Moon WJ (2005) CpG mutation rates in the human genome are highly dependent on local GC content. Mol Biol Evol 22:650–658
177. Suzuki MM, Bird A (2008) DNA methylation landscapes: provocative insights from epigenomics. Nat Rev Genet 9:465–476
178. Yamamoto S et al (1992) Unique palindromic sequences in synthetic oligonucleotides are required to induce IFN [correction of INF] and augment IFN-mediated [correction of INF] natural killer activity. J Immunol 148:4072–4076
179. Krieg AM et al (1995) CpG motifs in bacterial DNA trigger direct B-cell activation. Nature 374:546–549

180. Hemmi H et al (2000) A toll-like receptor recognizes bacterial DNA. Nature 408:740–745
181. Yew N et al (2000) Reduced inflammatory response to plasmid DNA vectors by elimination and inhibition of immunostimulatory CpG motifs. Mol Ther 1:255–262
182. Yew N et al (2002) CpG-depleted plasmid DNA vectors with enhanced safety and long-term gene expression in vivo. Mol Ther 5:731–738
183. Hyde SC et al (2008) CpG-free plasmids confer reduced inflammation and sustained pulmonary gene expression. Nat Biotechnol 26:549–551
184. Navarro G et al (2010) Low generation PAMAM dendrimer and CpG free plasmids allow targeted and extended transgene expression in tumors after systemic delivery. J Control Release 146:99–105
185. Coban C et al (2005) Effect of plasmid backbone modification by different human CpG motifs on the immunogenicity of DNA vaccine vectors. J Leukoc Biol 78:647–655
186. Higgins D et al (2007) Immunostimulatory DNA as a vaccine adjuvant. Expert Rev Vaccines 6:747–759
187. Kosovac D et al (2010) Minimal doses of a sequence-optimized transgene mediate high-level and long-term EPO expression in vivo: challenging CpG-free gene design. Gene Ther 18(2):189–198
188. Bauer AP et al (2010) The impact of intragenic CpG content on gene expression. Nucleic Acids Res 38:3891–3908
189. Lesina E et al (2010) CpG-free plasmid DNA prevents deterioration of pulmonary function in mice. Eur J Pharm Biopharm 74:427–434
190. Šmahel M et al (2011) Systemic administration of CpG oligodeoxynucleotide and levamisole as adjuvants for gene-gun-delivered antitumor DNA vaccines. Clin Dev Immunol 2011:176759
191. Shirota Y et al (2012) Intratumoral injection of cpg oligonucleotides induces the differentiation and reduces the immunosuppressive activity of myeloid-derived suppressor cells. J Immunol 188(4):1592–1599
192. Bolhassani A et al (2011) Improvement of different vaccine delivery systems for cancer therapy. Mol Cancer 10:3
193. Chen Z et al (2004) Silencing of episomal transgene expression by plasmid bacterial DNA elements in vivo. Gene Ther 11:856–864
194. Yew N et al (1999) Contribution of plasmid DNA to inflammation in the lung after administration of cationic lipid:pDNA complexes. Hum Gene Ther 10:223–234
195. Hodges BL et al (2004) Long-term transgene expression from plasmid DNA gene therapy vectors is negatively affected by CpG dinucleotides. Mol Ther 10:269–278
196. Chen ZY et al (2008) Silencing of episomal transgene expression in liver by plasmid bacterial backbone DNA is independent of CpG methylation. Mol Ther 16:548–556
197. Chabot S et al (2012) Minicircle DNA electrotransfer for efficient tissue-targeted gene delivery. Gene Ther 20(1):62–68
198. Kreiss P et al (1999) Plasmid DNA size does not affect the physicochemical properties of lipoplexes but modulates gene transfer efficiency. Nucleic Acids Res 27:3792–3798
199. Lukacs G et al (2000) Size-dependent DNA mobility in cytoplasm and nucleus. J Biol Chem 275:1625–1629
200. Pollard H et al (1998) Polyethylenimine but not cationic lipids promotes transgene delivery to the nucleus in mammalian cells. J Biol Chem 273:7507–7511
201. Yin W et al (2005) Investigations of the effect of DNA size in transient transfection assay using dual luciferase system. Anal Biochem 346:289–294
202. Walker W et al (2004) The effects of plasmid copy number and sequence context upon transfection efficiency. J Control Release 94: 245–252
203. Carpentier E et al (2007) Limiting factors governing protein expression following polyethylenimine-mediated gene transfer in HEK293-EBNA1 cells. J Biotechnol 128: 268–280
204. Klug B et al (2012) Current status of regulations for DNA vaccines. In: Thalhamer J (ed) Gene vaccines. Springer Verlag, Vienna, pp 285–295
205. Klinman DM et al (2010) FDA guidance on prophylactic DNA vaccines: analysis and recommendations. Vaccine 28:2801–2805
206. CPMP/SWP/465/95 (1997) Note for guidance on preclinical pharmacological and toxicological testing of vaccines
207. EMEA/CHMP/VWP/164653/2005 (2006) Guideline on clinical evaluation of new vaccines. The European Medicine Agency
208. Documents FVG (2007) Guidance for industry: considerations for plasmid DNA vaccines for infectious disease indications
209. 941/20, W. T. R. S. N. (2005) Guidelines for assuring the quality and nonclinical safety evaluation of DNA vaccines
210. CPMP/BWP/3088/99 (2001) Note for guidance on the quality, preclinical and

clinical aspects of gene transfer medicinal products. The European Medicines Agency
211. Yang YP et al (2009) Good manufacturing practices production and analysis of a DNA vaccine against dental caries. Acta Pharmacol Sin 30:1513–1521
212. Quaak SG et al (2008) GMP production of pDERMATT for vaccination against melanoma in a phase I clinical trial. Eur J Pharm Biopharm 70:429–438
213. Vidal L et al (2008) Development of an antibiotic-free plasmid selection system based on glycine auxotrophy for recombinant protein overproduction in *Escherichia coli*. J Biotechnol 134:127–136
214. Dong WR et al (2010) Novel antibiotic-free plasmid selection system based on complementation of host auxotrophy in the NAD de novo synthesis pathway. Appl Environ Microbiol 76:2295–2303

Chapter 39

Challenges Facing the Development of Cancer Vaccines

Mayer Fishman

Abstract

Just like any other effective immunization in medicine, cancer vaccines need to have antigens with particular specificity and immunostimulatory features, the immune responses to be elicited in the body, and therapeutic effect—regression or prevention of the cancer—must be meaningful and clinically observable. There are many choices for cancer antigens, such as tissue-specific proteins, cancer-specific proteins, class I- or class II-restricted peptides derived from those, or in situ and whole-cell-derived products are some examples. Another translational issue is that cancer patients are heterogeneous with respect to the extent to which the immune system is already activated with potential to impact the tumor growth or, conversely, the extent to which the immune system has been impaired through a prior and ongoing interaction with the tumor. Conventional or immunologic tests have potential to define a subset of patients with better chance or response, so that particular vaccines can be tested. Treatment of cancer patients is expensive, and trials are slow. To meet these challenges in practical terms will require not only careful scientific technical work for product development, coordination with clinicians to define patient subsets with diseases that can show responses, but also a comprehensive, practical implementation so that we can unlock the full potential of anticancer vaccines.

Key words Cancer vaccines, Tumor antigens, Antigen presentation

1 Introduction

The relationship of the immune system to tumor is complex. On the immune system side of the interaction, the details of the physiological processes of antigen presentation and lymphocyte activation are known in increasing detail. In the other direction, the variety of ways that tumors can interfere with and influence immune functions are similarly being elucidated in model systems, in clinical specimens, and in patients with cancer [1, 2]. The need to realize the potential for immunologic anticancer effects is great. The challenge of modulating or amplifying the immune system into what could be the most potent anticancer approach ever invented is a central goal of oncologic therapeutics, and cancer vaccines have the potential to be a big part of this.

Michael J.P. Lawman and Patricia D. Lawman (eds.), *Cancer Vaccines: Methods and Protocols*, Methods in Molecular Biology, vol. 1139, DOI 10.1007/978-1-4939-0345-0_39, © Springer Science+Business Media New York 2014

As discussed among the chapters of this volume, there are many technically separate approaches to get the immune cells focused on killing and controlling tumor, each with well-founded rationale and laboratory testing. In practical terms, we can consider some details about many translational challenges related to dendritic cell function and maneuvers, to T-cell and NK-cell *ex vivo* modifications, to macrophage polarization, and to introduction of vaccines directly into the patient, in clinical trials.

Other key decisions within the practical process of therapeutics' development are many and not very different from conventional drug development. These include defining target diseases, populations within those diseases, attainable clinical endpoints, and the economic logistics of introducing a new treatment into the practice of medical oncology. The long path for successful translation must move beyond the discovery phase and choose among these elegant and potent models to find those that are not only most relevant, scientifically, but also most amenable for practical application. These processes of practical application involve many choices that are not immediately or scientifically logical outcomes of the extensive preclinical work, and these issues together define the many hurdles to realizing the huge potential of cancer vaccines.

2 Picking the Antigens

Tumor cells populations are different: different from each other and different from the host [3]. Some of the antigenic changes are similar across the population of patients and could be exploited therapeutically. There are antigens that in some cases are reflections of tissue-specific protein expression, such as tyrosinase in melanoma [4, 5], interleukin-13 receptor $\alpha2$ chain in glioma [6, 7], or prostate-specific membrane antigen (PSMA) in prostate cancer [8]. Their uses in pathologic characterization of tumors and relevance for anticancer effect are many. Some antigens have been very successfully targeted with passive antibody-based treatments, a separate consideration from the vaccine approaches described in this book, such as Her2/neu in breast cancer (trastuzumab), CD20 in B-cell non-Hodgkin's lymphoma (rituximab, ofatumumab), and CD30 in Hodgkin's lymphoma (brentuximab vedotin). Those successes in focusing on those molecularly distinctive tumor features are part of the base of enthusiasm for immunologic susceptibility of cancer.

Most of the cancer patients' specimens from these defined disease groups will have these antigens, which is an advantage because the same vaccine preparation can be used in all the patients; also, monitoring for pharmacologic evidence of a response of the body to the vaccination, for example, by titers of T cells stimulated to produce interferon gamma by ex vivo introduction of the antigen (enzyme-linked immunosorbent spot, ELISpot) [9] or titers of antibodies, is relatively straightforward. On the other hand, the interaction of tumor and immune system is a dynamic, continuous relationship. Evolution of the malignant clone that has dispensed with or mutated the target antigen could become a resistance pathway of major clinical concern [10, 11]. Another example target, the muc-1 protein, is translated comparably in malignant cells of adenocarcinoma or in the corresponding benign parenchyma, but differentially (less) glycosylated, exposing epitopes that are only immunologically evident on the tumor cells [12]. Another example is aberrant patterns of PSA glycosylation that may be specific to prostate cancer [13]. The unlikely reacquisition of normal glycosylation patterns could define an immune approach that is less sensitive to escape through clonal evolution.

In other diagnoses there are easily identifiable proteins unique to the clone of cells in the malignant lineage, such as idiotypes of immunoglobulins of B-cell non-Hodgkin lymphoma [14]. In this case, there is a readily accessible and specific protein in the malignant cells, for which unique epitopes can be targeted. The practical disadvantage is that the flexibility and economy of using the same preparation for all the patients are exchanged for an individualized manufacturing process. Obviously, economic estimates based on early development costs could overstate the cost disadvantage of individualized vaccines. To date, individually manufactured vaccines have changed from a far-fetched logistic impossibility to a practical reality, with many examples such as kidney cancer trials (AGS-003 trial, NCT01582672), the completed trial of the vitespen [15] (licensed in Russia), the Reniale product [16], and autologous tumor cells transduced with B7.1-expressing virus [17], among many other examples, as well as sipuleucel-T, a licensed modified autologous cell product indicated for therapy of minimally symptomatic castrate-refractory prostate cancer which is produced at centralized facilities using PSMA/granulocyte-macrophage colony-stimulating factor (GM-CSF) (PA2024) to load and stimulate the leukocytes ex vivo [18]. While society-wide concerns about ballooning expenditures for new medical technologies certainly apply to these individually manufactured immunologically derived anticancer vaccines these concerns are not unique to them.

Some antigens are distinctive for their function in maintaining the malignant phenotype, survivin mitigation of apoptosis [19], telomerase that attenuates senescence of the clone [20], or overexpression of p53 related to aberrant progression through the cell cycle [21]. Vaccines directed at these epitopes of these proteins could mediate a synergistic regression of the tumor, also incorporating drugs or treatments of other modalities.

While those attributes are dependent on pathologic features of the tumors being treated, another dimension of the discussion of antigen selection, particularly for peptide-based vaccinations, is within the alleles of major histocompatibility complex (MHC). The class I MHC alleles HLA-A, HLA-B, and HLA-C display peptides typically with a length of eight to ten amino acids and are recognized by specific T-cell receptor (TCR) clones, each unique to a particular peptide/HLA class I combination. The $CD8^+$ effector T cells each bear a single TCR type, and this identifies a cell for a potential cytotoxic killing interaction. The MHC class II alleles, HLA-DP, HLA-DQ, and HLA-DR, display longer peptides, typically in the 20–24 amino acid range. In contrast to the class I peptide interactions, the particular instance of a single peptide interacting with multiple alleles of class II peptides from the human population is seen frequently. Class II-dependent helper T-cell and B-cell interactions result in amplification of the expansion of T cells. The extent to which helper T cells interact with antigen-presenting cells, principally dendritic cells, is of key interest to more potent vaccine development.

Nonetheless, vaccination with just class I-restricted peptides is of interest in contemporary therapeutic development. Most often, these trials are restricted to a limited number of HLA alleles, most often HLA-A2*0201, which is about 40–50 % of the population (in the UK [22], in the USA of European ancestry [23], and in very many further reports in other ethnic and regional world populations). Counting the populations with either heterozygotic or homozygotic expression, the peptides would theoretically only be of therapeutic value for that part of the population, although substitution of other corresponding peptides from other subsequences of the (named or theoretical open reading frame derived) proteins that associate with other HLA class I alleles should be a way to provide a similar therapy to the rest of the population. The relative difficulty of then determining, testing, and manufacturing the other peptides would represent a project in its own right, presumably the motivation and capital to realize that would be driven by the "proof of principle" success in the HLA-A2*0201 population.

In summary, specific target antigen, whether peptides, proteins, modified proteins, or whole-cell-derived preparation, must be selected for a particular immune treatment plan to be implemented. Many approaches can be taken to meet this challenge. However, there may be many combinations that ultimately could work, in different situations.

3 Selecting an Immune Maneuver

There are many immune maneuvers; naturally, in the course of preclinical development, each approach will have its advocates among the scientists invested in its development, working in somewhat (or completely) disconnected model systems.

However, some general considerations can be made. Many of the methods discussed above are centered on specific or synthetic antigenic material. On the other hand, whole-cell-based vaccinations have a "holistic" appeal, seeming to sidestep the antigen picking process.

Everything that is distinctive (and bad) in the tumor can be prepared and presented to the immune system to be processed and amplified [24, 25]. The whole tumor cell can be represented by lysates of surgical specimens, short-term cultures of tumor cells in special conditions, irradiation (with its associated induced expression of potential neoantigens), or nucleic acid-derived extracts—either DNA or mRNA. As a group, the advantages to consider are several. The features that are unique to a particular patient's tumor are not overlooked, whether these are "public" mutations of the patient's disease process or "private" mutations that are particular to a metastatic site of disease. Cancer clones that have acquired point mutations of various proteins would seem to be likely to have potential for immune attack, since to the perspective of the repertoire of T cells available in the patient, there would be no prior exposure. On the other hand, disadvantages can be considered too—the relative proportion of the different proteins in the cell is related to the cellular physiology, not to their individual potentials for immunogenic response. The better, or more important, rejection antigens could be swamped out by irrelevant, nonimmunogenic proteins. At a further extreme, some tolerogenic features of the tumor could be surreptitiously introduced into the vaccine product. Some features of the tumor cell that attenuate or dilute the immune response may be unwanted "fellow travelers," or variable in different patients or clinical situations. Different adjuvants, haptens, and viral transfections of costimulatory molecules have some promise to make the whole-cell-based product immunogenic in a more potent way.

Another angle of attack on the problem is represented by lymphocyte maneuvers. Some of these are very antigen specific, modification of T helpers to express tumor antigen, or chimeric antigen receptors, which would indirectly amplify the expansion and activity of effector $CD8^+$ lymphocytes. Others, such as suppression of regulatory T cells (identified as $CD4^+$, $CD25^+$ for $Foxp3^+$ lymphocytes) [26] or toll-like receptor (TLR-9) agonists [27], are general immune modulators, which could be paired with almost any antigen supply strategy. Indeed, one main difference among the various ways to load dendritic cells, whether in situ or ex vivo, is to influence their phenotype and the propensity to activate the relevant lymphocytes after administration. There appear to be many ways to influence lymphocyte and dendritic cells behavior during the process of antigen introduction [28]. These can be considered whether a whole-cell or specific antigen approach is being applied.

On the one hand, it is encouraging that there are many antigens to choose from, many ways to process cellular material that could be used to load dendritic cells and reorient or expand antigen-specific T cells, and increasing understanding of how to influence the conventional interaction of antigen presentation process with the lymphocytes. On the other hand, this leads to a natural conundrum: What preclinical data should drive the process for moving to clinical testing? Some drivers can include issues that are not overtly (or remotely) biologic, such as disease prevalence or intellectual property considerations. The challenge of selecting the optimal way of getting the immune system focused on a particular antigen is the fundamental issue in defining the best immune maneuver.

4 Development of a Translational Strategy

In a clinical trial setting, a direct comparison of two different strategies would entail separate early-phase clinical trials encompassing pharmacodynamic endpoints. One could ask, for example, for which peptides in a multi-peptide vaccine are the highest titers of cytotoxic T lymphocytes or for which are epitope-spreading observable. Alternatively, one could evaluate the patients (immunologic hosts) to define a threshold number or phenotype of antigen-presenting cells below which an immunologic response cannot be induced or a therapeutic context where patients would be relatively more uniform than the disease group defined by simple stage-specific clinical parameters, for example, after debulking surgery or a couple months off of steroids and chemotherapy.

This approach could define a vaccine/host combination for which at the least there can be an expectation of a uniform immunologic behavior. In the setting of a murine model system, these are tightly controlled parameters; it is a high bar, however, to get a level of uniformity of host features for the development of a clinical trial. For example, the same antigen could be subjected to several different dendritic cell loading strategies; conversely, autologous dendritic cells could be loaded in similar ways with a variety of different proteins or peptides, with concurrent application of modulators of the dendritic cell phenotype. And then, the selection of a specific disease population for testing the issue of clinical efficacy (specifically distinguishing that from immune pharmacodynamics) could begin. This is a usual consideration, for example, in conventional drug development where a few candidate drugs from the same class have been developed, such as novel taxanes.

Similarly, this is a difficult standard for a process of selection among dendritic cell loading strategies. The practical reality is that in contemporary therapeutics, the standard of care for any given cancer patient subset is described without any reference to immune-based treatment. Thus, the usual comparator for introducing an immune treatment is to compare that isolated immune treatment to no immune treatment. On the one hand, this is a straightforward trial design. On the other hand, the immunologic question of what is the best way, among a dozen different routes, to introduce antigen to dendritic cells is not addressed. The logistics behind the scale of such a trial or series of clinical trials is daunting—the single marketed ex vivo antigen-loading product, sipuleucel-T autologous cell infusions [18], had a development timeline over a decade long. There are no peptide anticancer vaccines in commercial use. Thus, a major challenge is to select strategically from among what may be similarly promising but technically divergent dendritic cell loading processes, for example, as enumerated among the chapters in the dendritic cell loading section of this volume. The current pattern, where circumstances of grant funding or commercial development interests push forward along various patterns are a practical reality. However, one must recognize that it is somewhat disconnected from an idealized scientific method.

Thus, another key challenge of selecting among the many seemingly effective strategies for dendritic cell loading is that they are not compared directly in clinical testing. Those with good features in preclinical models and pharmacodynamic endpoints (eliciting measurable specific immune response) can advance with appropriate financial backing to clinical testing. If those data are promising, a large-scale, registrational randomized trial can be undertaken.

5 Which Patients Can Benefit?

Another key challenge is unmasked at the point of defining inclusion criteria for the trial. This is a consequence of how contemporary medical treatment of cancer is fragmented into hundreds of pathways, individual to particular histologic diagnoses, at particular stages of spread. When a vaccine is translated from a model system to the clinic, the carefully defined, syngeneic hosts with uniform age and tumor burden are left at the lab, for the most part. These are swapped out for a subset of the incident population for some specific histologically defined diagnosis that has been rendered to some level of uniformity by some clinical features, such as PSA level, age, absence of chronic viral infection, and absence of use of exogenous corticosteroid [18]. Many such inclusion and exclusion strategies have been implemented in various studies.

While in a murine system, it is very straightforward to specify that immunotherapy is for the immune competent or conversely that there are defined defects of immune function that prevent acquisition of useful antitumor immunity. Actually, some of those defined defects usually are apparent as "control group" mice characteristics. However, in the clinical context the criteria for definition of competency are defined in very limited comparably rudimentary criteria, such as circulating vascular endothelial growth factor (VEGF) level, ratio of dendritic cells to myeloid-derived suppressor cells (MDSC), or regulatory T cell ($Cd25^+$, $FoxP3^+$ lymphocytes). In terms of disease burden and immunologic competency, the controlled environment of the laboratory is exchanged for a "come as you are" party.

Similarly, goals of treatment of different diagnoses are heterogeneous. Immune anticancer responses of interest can include changes of lymphocytes, antibodies, or tumor markers (such as PSA or CA 19-9), radiologically identified progression-free survival (PFS), objective tumor regression (overall response rate, ORR), increments of overall survival (OS), or durable complete remissions (CR). Obviously, the last is the goal of the most interest, but the earlier steps are recognized as tangible steps for validation of clinical development, or for PFS, ORR, or OS, concrete endpoints that could be a basis for regulatory approval for marketed application. By working with clinicians with specializations and experiences centered around these diagnoses, a strategic plan can be developed. That plan can be coordinated with expertise in implementation of the cancer vaccine approach and a realistic understanding of competition from nonimmunotherapy technologies and regulatory and marketing requirements. In this way, one could hope for progress toward implementation of translational trials with defined goals to impact on clinical practice. Ultimately, a marketable product will require a large-scale investment in a pivotal trial to take a vaccine approach from a scientific, controlled system into an applied, clinically relevant product. Capital markets will analyze these implementation and markets from a critical, independent approach, grounded in the quality of the responses seen in preclinical development, but responsive to many other forces and perspectives.

The process of going from a working murine model system or a proof of principle early-phase trial with a core of patients that have done unexpectedly well to a licensed drug preparation with a particularly targeted clinical base is expensive and resource consuming. Economic risks are big and biotechnology evolves in real time during a clinical trial development. Intellectual property considerations may drive some technologies ahead of others which may seem scientifically better.

Figure 1 illustrates four abstracted variables (antigen selection, loading method, target disease, and types of hosts) as wheels of a slot machine, where many combinations would seem to have a potential payoff for some patients, in some circumstances. Many combinations seem dependent on antigens that are specific to a particular diagnosis. Some payoffs are better than others. While murine systems typically demonstrate objective improvement of survival, in clinical trial development, progress is not limited to a

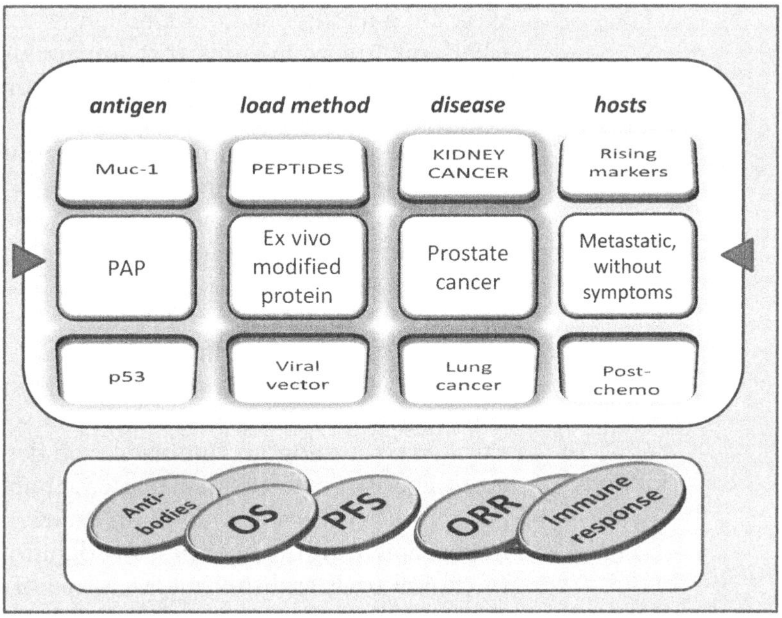

Fig. 1 An illustration of four abstracted variables (antigen selection, loading method, target disease, and types of hosts) as wheels of a slot machine, where many combinations would seem to have a potential payoff for some patients

single jackpot payoff. But every combination will not work; while some development choices seem random and interchangeable, most have not led to clinical progress. The financial challenge is that these selections must not be made like a slot machine gambler, investing a coin in many random combinations. These anticancer vaccine development choices are not random and interchangeable. So many vaccine strategies seem valid, and there are many levels of payoff (illustrated as labels on the coins in the payoff slot). Some contribute to the scientific development of other vaccine strategies without obvious success in the clinically defined subset of patients who were treated. The illustrated combination corresponds to sipuleucel-T.

6 Conclusions

A pure scientific method would depend on many direct randomized comparisons among the methods of immune manipulations, in relatively uniform hosts, and comparison in terms of a clinical outcome. This is not going to happen for economic logistic and intellectual property reasons. Abstraction of the separation of process of antigen and dendritic cell loading strategies is one concept that accommodates a potential for anticancer vaccine development to start in one small subset of patients and to then spread to others.

Basic host features such as circulating dendritic cell/MDSC ratio [29] and tumor features that impact the immune system [30], polarization of tumor associated macrophages (TAM) [31] and regulatory T cells [28] can be quantified. This could have far-reaching consequences in the optimization and successful development of anticancer vaccine, as competency for anticancer response is reconstructed in patients with clinically homogeneous features.

In conclusion, anticancer vaccine development is advancing on many fronts. Isolated immune treatments of today—CTLA-4 blockade in melanoma (ipilimumab), cytokines (interleukin-2 in melanoma and kidney cancer), sipuleucel-T (prostate cancer)—will be augmented at some point by others in advanced development, e.g., anti-PD1/PDL1 axis drugs, and some of the many peptide vaccines or autologous tumor-derived dendritic cell loading strategies. The carefully defined implementation of translational trials contributes in a stepwise, if irregular, way toward meaningful improvement of therapeutics. Recognition that the long timelines of clinical trials and shifting landscape of other anticancer innovations means that a degree of flexibility and openness in the design of trials and goals of immunotherapy will help to meet the challenge of attaining rapid, applied progress for development of concrete, meaningful clinical applications of anticancer vaccines.

References

1. Palucka K et al (2001) Dendritic cells and immunity against cancer. J Intern Med 269(1):64–73
2. Janikashvili N et al (2011) The dendritic cell-regulatory T lymphocyte crosstalk contributes to tumor-induced tolerance. Clin Dev Immunol 430394. Epub 2011 Nov 3
3. Gerlinger M et al (2012) Intratumor heterogeneity and branched evolution revealed by multiregion sequencing. N Engl J Med 366(10): 883–892
4. Frankel TL et al (2010) Both CD4 and CD8 T cells mediate equally effective in vivo tumor treatment when engineered with a highly avid TCR targeting tyrosinase. J Immunol 184(11): 5988–5998
5. Dalerba P et al (1998) High homogeneity of MAGE, BAGE, GAGE, tyrosinase and Melan-A/MART-1 gene expression in clusters of multiple simultaneous metastases of human melanoma: implications for protocol design of therapeutic antigen-specific vaccination strategies. Int J Cancer 77(2):200–204
6. Iwami K et al (2012) Peptide-pulsed dendritic cell vaccination targeting interleukin-13 receptor α2 chain in recurrent malignant glioma patients with HLA-A*24/A*02 allele. Cytotherapy 14(6):733–742
7. Shimato S et al (2008) Identification of a human leukocyte antigen-A24-restricted T-cell epitope derived from interleukin-13 receptor alpha2 chain, a glioma-associated antigen. J Neurosurg 109(1):117–122
8. Fishman M (2009) A changing world for DCvax: a PSMA loaded autologous dendritic cell vaccine for prostate cancer. Expert Opin Biol Ther 9(12):1565–1575
9. Slota M et al (2011) ELISpot for measuring human immune responses to vaccines. Expert Rev Vaccines 10(3):299–306
10. Reiman JM et al (2007) Tumor immunoediting and immunosculpting pathways to cancer progression. Semin Cancer Biol 17(4):275–287
11. Kim R et al (2007) Cancer immunoediting from immune surveillance to immune escape. Immunology 121(1):1–14
12. Tarp MA, Clausen H (2008) Mucin-type O-glycosylation and its potential use in drug and vaccine development. Biochim Biophys Acta 1780(3):546–563
13. Saldova R et al (2011) Core fucosylation and alpha2-3 sialylation in serum N-glycome is significantly increased in prostate cancer comparing to benign prostate hyperplasia. Glycobiology 21(2):195–205

14. Schuster SJ et al (2011) Vaccination with patient-specific tumor-derived antigen in first remission improves disease-free survival in follicular lymphoma. J Clin Oncol 29(20):2787–2794
15. Wood C, C-100-12 RCC Study Group et al (2008) An adjuvant autologous therapeutic vaccine (HSPPC-96; vitespen) versus observation alone for patients at high risk of recurrence after nephrectomy for renal cell carcinoma: a multicentre, open-label, randomised phase III trial. Lancet 372(9633):145–154
16. Jocham D et al (2004) Adjuvant autologous renal tumour cell vaccine and risk of tumour progression in patients with renal-cell carcinoma after radical nephrectomy: phase III, randomised controlled trial. Lancet 363(9409): 594–599
17. Fishman M et al (2008) Phase II trial of B7-1 (CD-86) transduced, cultured autologous tumor cell vaccine plus subcutaneous interleukin-2 for treatment of stage IV renal cell carcinoma. J Immunother 1:72–80
18. Kantoff PW et al (2010) Sipuleucel-T immunotherapy for castration-resistant prostate cancer. N Engl J Med 363(5):411–422
19. Nagaraj S et al (2007) Dendritic cell-based full-length survivin vaccine in treatment of experimental tumors. J Immunother 30(2):169–179
20. Pendino F et al (2006) Telomeres and telomerase: pharmacological targets for new anticancer strategies? Curr Cancer Drug Targets 6(2):147–180
21. Lane DP et al (2010) p53-based cancer therapy. Cold Spring Harb Perspect Biol 2(9):a001222, Epub May 12
22. Burt C et al (2013) HLA-A, -B, -DR allele group frequencies in 7007 kidney transplant list patients in 27 UK centres. Int J Immunogenet 2013 Jun;40(3):209–215
23. Mack SJ et al (2009) HLA-A, -B, -C, and -DRB1 allele and haplotype frequencies distinguish Eastern European Americans from the general European American population. Tissue Antigens 73(1):17–32
24. de Gruijl TD et al (2008) Whole-cell cancer vaccination: from autologous to allogeneic tumor- and dendritic cell-based vaccines. Cancer Immunol Immunother 57(10):1569–1577
25. Le DT et al (2010) Cellular vaccine approaches. Cancer J 16(4):304–310
26. Facciabene A et al (2012) T-regulatory cells: key players in tumor immune escape and angiogenesis. Cancer Res 72(9):2162–2171
27. So EY, Ouchi T (2010) The application of Toll like receptors for cancer therapy. Int J Biol Sci 6(7):675–681
28. Chiang CL et al (2011) Adjuvants for enhancing the immunogenicity of whole tumor cell vaccines. Int Rev Immunol 30(2–3):150–182
29. Kusmartsev S, Gabrilovich DI (2002) Immature myeloid cells and cancer-associated immune suppression. Cancer Immunol Immunother 51(6):293–298
30. Gabrilovich DI et al (2012) Coordinated regulation of myeloid cells by tumours. Nat Rev Immunol 12(4):253–268
31. Ruffell B et al (2012) Differential macrophage programming in the tumor microenvironment. Trends Immunol 33(3):119–126, Epub 2012 Jan 23

Chapter 40

Future of Cancer Vaccines

Hauke Winter, Bernard A. Fox, and Dominik Rüttinger

Abstract

Extensive research in the area of active-specific immunotherapy has led to the approval of the first therapeutic cancer vaccine sipuleucel-T (Provenge™) in 2010. Even though a major milestone for the field of cancer immunotherapy, many obstacles towards successful integration of vaccination strategies into the oncologists' armamentarium remain. This chapter discusses possible future perspectives for cancer vaccines as a treatment modality in oncology with special focus on biomarkers (response prediction and patient selection), requirements for clinical trial design, and combination therapies (standard of care and new molecular entities).

Key words Cancer vaccines, Future perspective, Biomarkers, Immunotherapy, Clinical trial

1 Introduction

On April 29, 2010, the United States' Federal Drug Administration (FDA) approved sipuleucel-T (Provenge™) as the first therapeutic cellular immunotherapy for the treatment of minimal or non-symptomatic metastatic castrate-resistant prostate cancer (mCRPC). Without doubt a major milestone for the field of (active-specific) immunotherapy, most importantly it was approved based on statistically relevant and clinically meaningful improvement in median overall survival (OS) of 4.1 months within the Phase III IMPACT trial [1]. Unlike sipuleucel-T, other novel agents now approved for the treatment of prostate cancer, e.g., abiraterone acetate (Zytiga™), have demonstrated objective clinical responses according to established response criteria and have been able to alter the time to disease progression in a majority of patients on top of improving OS. Thus, the hurdles for the future development of therapeutic prostate cancer vaccines to successfully meet the threshold for regulatory approval will likely further increase in the post-sipuleucel-T era and not be lowered as suggested in verve about approval of the first therapeutic cancer vaccine. These challenges may currently be specific for clinical development strategies in prostate cancer; however,

Michael J.P. Lawman and Patricia D. Lawman (eds.), *Cancer Vaccines: Methods and Protocols*, Methods in Molecular Biology, vol. 1139, DOI 10.1007/978-1-4939-0345-0_40, © Springer Science+Business Media New York 2014

very likely the pressure in particular on early-phase clinical vaccine trials to inform on patient selection markers, indicators for response predication, but also to identify and validate clinical, biologic, and molecular surrogates for survival will further increase, irrespective of the tumor histology.

The future development of cancer vaccines will involve more clinical combination trials (both combinations with standard treatment modalities and immunotherapeutic approaches), and it will depend on identifying those patient populations most likely to respond to a cancer vaccine. Likely, these will be patients with more indolent metastatic disease and settings involving adjuvant, neoadjuvant, and additive treatment. There will also be less reliance on objective tumor response criteria established for the clinical assessment of small molecules but increased use of OS or newly created immune-related response criteria. There may also be an increased focus on patients with a high risk to develop cancer, e.g., genetic predisposition, and strategies to identify cancer vaccine targets for these patients. The absence of adequate tools to study immunotherapeutic approaches in cancer may, indeed, have been the main reason for the only marginal success thus far. However, the still incomplete knowledge of human immunology and the lack of critical assessment of ineffective or marginally effective agents may have also contributed to the failure of many clinical cancer vaccine trials. The abovementioned aspects of the future development of cancer vaccine will be discussed in this chapter.

2 Future Clinical Trial Design for Cancer Vaccines

Clinical trial endpoints chosen to gain regulatory approval of oncology drug products and biologics are designed to demonstrate that the active agent provides clinical benefit as evidenced by an improved OS (and ideally also improved quality of life) or an equally favorable effect on an established surrogate for an improved OS. Thus, an improvement in median OS is generally regarded as the gold standard to demonstrate superiority versus an active comparator or placebo, preferably tested in a blinded and randomized fashion. However, assessment of OS usually requires testing large patient cohorts resulting in long follow-up timelines. Therefore, clinical endpoints such as progression-free survival (PFS), time to progression (TTP), objective response rates (according to RECIST or WHO criteria), and at some occasions some novel endpoints have been used as surrogate markers for OS. These endpoints can be determined earlier and are less influenced by other causes of death, and results are less likely to be diluted by subsequent lines of therapy. On the other hand, OS is the only endpoint measured on a continuous basis and is, obviously, not affected by measurement errors (for both timing and technique).

Data from several clinical cancer vaccine trials now suggest that PFS or TTP may not be the appropriate endpoints. More importantly, the IMPACT Phase III trial has demonstrated that an improved OS can be achieved without significant changes in, e.g., PFS [1]. At the same time, this is a critical issue as it is the early signs of clinical activity, measured by objective response rate or PFS/TTP in Phase I and II trials that are needed to generate enough excitement around a novel compound to warrant further investment in expensive larger Phase III trials. Therefore, there has been an intense search for immunologic endpoints that clearly correlate with clinical outcome measures. Unlike prophylactic vaccines against infectious disease, cancer vaccines have mainly failed to show that correlation. This may be attributable to several reasons, such as (1) the failure of the vaccine to induce a robust immune response; (2) the lack of immune-monitoring techniques to capture and quantify an immune response; (3) the relevant tumor rejection antigens are not available for monitoring, e.g., antigen spreading; or (4) tumors continue to grow despite an immune response induced by vaccination, e.g., escape variants, inhibitory ligands, or suppressive elements.

Clearly, future clinical trials for cancer vaccines will require novel paradigms. In this context the following approaches seem particularly attractive and important to consider:

- Assessment of individual tumor growth kinetics and regression rate constants, which have been shown to correlate with survival and may serve as an early marker for therapeutic efficacy [3]
- Implementation of immune response-related criteria instead of or on top of established response criteria to allow enough time for potentially delayed detection of clinical activity [4, 5]
- Exclusion of early patient withdrawal criteria (such as determination of "progressive disease" by radiologic criteria) and early study termination criteria (sequential adaptive trial design) routinely included in early phase clinical trials

Regulatory bodies have started initiatives to meet the new challenges, and both the FDA (guidance issued in 2009) [6] and the European Medicines Agency (EMA) (concept paper released in 2010 to request public feedback) are addressing these issues.

3 Clinical Phase III Cancer Vaccine Trials

Next to sipuleucel-T for mCRPC, more recently two additional vaccine approaches have successfully passed the confirmatory Phase III of clinical development.

In June 2012, a formal notification was submitted to the EMA with the intent to file a Marketing Authorization Application

(MAA) seeking approval in the European Union (EU) for BiovaxID®, a vaccine for the treatment of follicular non-Hodgkin's lymphoma, consisting of hybridoma-derived autologous tumor immunoglobulin idiotype (Id) conjugated to keyhole limpet hemocyanin (KLH) and administered with granulocyte-monocyte colony-stimulating factor (GM-CSF). If approved, this would be the first therapeutic cancer vaccine available in Europe for non-Hodgkin's lymphoma, with regulatory approval for sipuleucel-T in the EU being expected for 2013. The MAA will be based on results of a Phase III clinical trial that randomly assigned 177 patients having achieved a complete response after cisplatin, doxorubicin, cyclophosphamide, and etoposide (PACE) chemotherapy to treatment with the Id vaccine or KLH + GM-CSF alone. After a median follow-up of 56.6 months, the median time to relapse for the vaccine arm was 44.2 months vs. 30.6 months for the control arm receiving KLH + GM-CSF [7]. The key difference of this Phase III clinical test compared to previous Phase III clinical vaccine trials for lymphoma patients was the low tumor burden, i.e., complete response following standard chemotherapy.

Schwartzentruber et al. recently reported on another vaccine approach in patients with stage IV or locally advanced stage III cutaneous melanoma expressing HLA*A0201 [8]. Patients ($n = 185$) were randomly assigned to receive interleukin-2 (IL-2) alone or gp100:209-217(210 M) peptide plus incomplete Freund's adjuvant (Montanide ISA-51) followed by IL-2. The patients treated with the peptide vaccine plus IL-2 demonstrated a significant improvement in objective response rate compared to patients receiving high-dose IL-2 alone (16 % vs. 6 %) and also had a slightly longer PFS, 2.2 months vs. 1.6 months. The median OS was also longer, with 17.8 months vs. 11.1 months. These results were in contrast to previously reported Phase II results for gp100 peptide vaccines in melanoma [9]. However, these Phase II studies did not include an IL-2 alone control arm, thus, making it difficult to draw conclusions about the vaccine itself. Additionally, the 6 % response to IL-2 alone was lower than previously reported, further complicating the interpretation [10].

There are several other Phase III trials ongoing employing different vaccine platforms in a range of human cancers. A bit surprisingly, non-small cell lung cancer (NSCLC), which for a long time was not considered an immune-sensitive disease, now has experienced a resurgence with at least four Phase III clinical studies ongoing evaluating active-specific immunotherapeutic approaches. Final results of the first Phase III trials are expected for later in 2013.

Table 1 summarizes recent positive clinical Phase III cancer vaccine trials and currently ongoing randomized Phase III trials for patients suffering from NSCLC.

Table 1

Recent positive clinical Phase III cancer vaccine trials (*upper panel*) and currently ongoing randomized Phase III vaccine trials in non-small cell lung cancer (*lower panel*)

Vaccine	Target/approach	Patients/treatment	Results (vs. control)	Trial/references
Provenge® (sipuleucel-T)	Dendritic cells + prostatic acid phosphatase (PAP)	• Metastatic, androgen-independent prostatic adenocarcinoma ($n = 512$) • Coadministration with GM-CSF	• Median survival 25.8 months vs. 21.7 months • 31.7 % 3-year survival rate vs. 23.0 %	IMPACT/[1]
BiovaxID®	Autologous tumor cells fused with murine/human heterohybridoma to produce idiotype (conjugated to KLH)	• Follicular lymphoma in complete remission for at least 6 months following PACE CTX • Coadministration with GM-CSF	• Of 177 randomized patients, 117 maintained CR ≥ 6 months after PACE CTX • Median time to relapse: 44.2 months vs. 30.6 months	BV 301/[7]
Gp100 antigen + Montanide ISA	Modified gp100:209–217 (210 M) peptide	• HLA-A0201 positive, locally advanced stage III or IV cutaneous melanoma • Vaccine followed by high-dose IL-2 vs. IL-2 alone	• Objective response rate 16 % vs. 6 % • Median OS 17.8 months vs. 11.1 months	CCCGHS-NCI-T98-0085/[8]
Stimuvax® (L-BLP 25)	MUC1	• Unresectable stage III NSCLC • SD or better after first-line RCT • Estimated enrollment: 1514 • Primary endpoint: survival	Pending	START/ NCT00409188
recMAGE-A3 + AS15	MAGE-A3	• Resectable stages IB-IIIA NSCLC • MAGE-A3 expression on tumor • Estimated enrollment: 2270 • Primary endpoint: DFS		MAGRIT/ NCT00480025/ [11]
EGF-rP64K + Montanide ISA51	EGF	• +Low-dose cyclophosphamide • NSCLC stage IIIB/IV • Primary endpoint: OS		NCT01444118
Lucanix® (belagenpumatucel-L)	Allogeneic cell lines + TGFβ antisense	• NSCLC stages III/IV • SD or better following frontline platinum-based CTX • Estimated enrollment: 506 • Primary endpoint: OS		STOP/ NCT00676507

GM-CSF granulocyte-macrophage colony-stimulating factor; *KLH* keyhole limpet hemocyanin; *PACE* prednisone, doxorubicin, cyclophosphamide, etoposide; *CTX* chemotherapy, *HLA* human leukocyte antigen; *IL-2* interleukin-2; *DFS* disease-free survival; *OS* overall survival

4 Combination Therapy

It is now commonly acknowledged that cancer vaccines may show improved antitumor activity, both in preclinical models and clinical studies, when combined with other treatment modalities such as radiation, chemotherapy, targeted agents, and other immunotherapies. These combinations have demonstrated to broaden the response and potentially also to treat resistance. For future approaches, it will be of upmost importance to assess the anticipated interactions of the combination(s) both for clinical activity and overlapping toxicities. If the selected combination partner(s) acts on those immune cells necessary to prime and entertain an antitumor immune response, e.g., chemotherapy blocking dendritic cell and/or T cell function, or modifies the tumor microenvironment in a way that will antagonize the development of immunity, it will be critical to understand the exact mechanism, and it may still be possible to combine. For example, chemotherapy was generally believed to have a negative effect on vaccine-induced immune responses and antitumor activity; however, it may very well also be immunostimulatory dependent on the dose and regimen selected [12]. Other combination partners may reveal properties that had not been anticipated based on their conventional use, such as the mechanistic target of rapamycin or mTOR inhibitor, which is usually used as an immunosuppressive drug, but has recently be shown to exert—under certain circumstances—immunostimulatory effects [13]. Therefore, special attention needs to be given to better understand potentially synergistic effects, but also to the design of clinical studies with regard to sequencing and dosing of combinations.

The most frequently applied combination approaches for cancer vaccines have been those with standard (or modified) chemotherapy. Here, the proposed synergistic mechanisms have now been studied extensively. Some of the suggested effects are based on (1) cross-priming of tumor associated antigens (TAA) and subsequent T cell activation following chemotherapy-induced tumor cell death, e.g., oxaliplatin and anthracyclines; (2) depletion of regulatory T cells or myeloid-derived suppressor cells, e.g., cyclophosphamide, gemcitabine, and taxanes; (3) induction of homeostatic proliferation of immune cells, e.g., cisplatin and vinorelbine; (4) agonist effect on toll-like receptors, e.g., docetaxel; and (5) direct stimulation of T cell proliferation, e.g., lenalidomide.

Combining vaccines with cyclophosphamide is a common strategy and has resulted in increased survival in two Phase II studies [14, 15]. Both studies included GM-CSF, underscoring the possible importance of adjuvant selection in vaccine studies.

For the future, multimodality approaches for therapeutic cancer vaccines should be based on well-designed preclinical studies that elucidate the precise scientific rationale for combinations and document the mechanistic synergy. The subsequent clinical studies need to consider these findings and include sufficient flexibility for changes in dosing, schedule, and administration of both the vaccine and the combination partner(s).

5 Biomarkers for Cancer Vaccines

For sipuleucel-T, improved median OS was associated with cumulative CD54 upregulation (the analysis demonstrated a strong correlation, which persisted after adjustment for baseline prognostic factors, such as weight, prostate-specific antigen, lactate dehydrogenase, number of bone lesions, and localization of disease) [2] and also with antibody titers of more than 400 against PA2024 or prostatic acid phosphatase at any time after baseline [1]. For the vast majority of cancer vaccine clinical trials, however, the common biomarker has been the immune response of patients to TAA assessing pre- and postvaccination samples for antibody responses and/or $CD8^+$ and $CD4^+$ T cell responses using various techniques including enzyme-linked immunosorbent assay, enzyme-linked immunosorbent spot assay, and fluorescent antibody cell sorting analysis. Despite the fact that more recent studies have been able to identify associations between clinical outcome and the induction of an immune response [16], these results are far from having identified a true surrogate biomarker for clinical activity of a vaccine. In addition, the limitations in availability of patient samples need to be overcome. The focus will need to shift towards collection of potentially more relevant specimens, i.e., tumor tissue to obtain TAA-specific T cells as opposed to collection of peripheral blood mononuclear cells alone. The inter-patient variability of immune responses may also not allow for identification of 1 surrogate biomarker (or a combination of different markers). Furthermore, the phenomenon of "antigen spreading," i.e., the antigen to monitor for is not a TAA contained in the vaccine but is generated by cross-priming after, e.g., destruction of tumor cells, needs to be taken into consideration.

Identifying the patient population most likely to respond to treatment may be of particular importance for cancer vaccine trials. The ideal candidate may be the 1 with slow-growing and/or low-volume disease combined with minimal prior exposure to chemotherapy. For future trials, instead of trying to define "slow growing" and globally defining an arbitrary maximum number of previous treatment lines, patient selection biomarkers could be defined and potentially combined in a scoring system, allowing for selection of those patients most likely to benefit from treatment. Such markers could consist of the number of regulatory T cells which has been shown to increase with greater tumor burden or the levels of indoleamine-2,3-dioxygenase and other immunosuppressive cytokines such as transforming growth factor-ß or interleukin-10, all of which may inhibit T cell function and proliferation. Alternatively, evidence of a preexisting T cell response may predict for response to therapy. Recently, it was reported that patients who respond to therapy have a gene "signature" at their tumor sites pretreatment [17]. This gene signature, while not fully defined, appears to assess both immune and tumor markers. Further, patients who are gene signature positive have increased disease-free survival following vaccination, while those without a positive signature fail to elicit T cell responses and have outcomes similar to the placebo group. These findings are consistent with the observations of Mlecnik and colleagues who identified the presence of CD8 memory T cells at the invading margin and center of primary colon cancers as being prognostic for disease-free survival [18]. These studies utilized digital imaging and software to objectively quantitate T cell numbers and identify an "immunoscore." This immunoscore provided a significantly better prognostic factor than TNM staging and a recent report reviewed literature suggesting a similar pattern may exist for 20 other malignancies [19].

To assess these patient selection and potential response prediction, biomarkers will require strict assay standardization and sample handling guidelines. This is reflected in recommendations published recently by a large group of academic, pharmaceutical, and regulatory stakeholders [20]. A retrospective study aimed at validating immunoscore as a prognostic biomarker is underway, and additional studies will assess whether it is also a predictive biomarker [21].

6 Perspectives for the Future

Future studies using therapeutic cancer vaccines will include assessment in combination with a wide range of partners early in development after characterizing the single-agent features of the vaccine. The targeted patient population will shift towards more indolent metastatic disease or adjuvant or additive treatment settings. Patient selection and response prediction biomarkers will help to identify those patients most likely to benefit from vaccine treatment and to spare others from unnecessary treatment-related procedures and toxicities. By far, the greatest challenge for the future of cancer vaccines will be to demonstrate evidence of clinical activity early in the development. Employing new immune-related response criteria and establishing long-term survival as a clinical trial endpoint will facilitate clinical assessment of cancer vaccines, but only accepted surrogate endpoints/biomarkers for survival, used for population enrichment and stratification, will be able to provide the critical momentum in cancer vaccine development when competing with other anticancer agents that show both PFS/TTP or objective responses and OS benefit, for regulatory approval.

One of the strongest arguments in favor of active-specific immunotherapy is the largely very benign safety profile in the clinic. This observation may direct future efforts towards using cancer vaccines in patients that are at high risk of developing cancer. Potential target populations would be familial adenomatous polyposis patients (high risk for colorectal cancer), high-grade intraepithelial prostatic neoplasia (high risk for prostate cancer), or other hereditary forms of breast, ovarian, or thyroid carcinomas.

The post-sipuleucel-T era of cancer vaccines holds many promises but also significant hurdles. If all stakeholders adopt that the mechanism of action proposed for cancer vaccines is so distinct from cytotoxic drugs for which clinical development standards had been established a generation ago, the recently emerging preclinical and clinical data will eventually result in inclusion of cancer vaccines into standard oncology treatment.

Acknowledgments

This work was supported in part by a grant from the Chiles Foundation, Portland, Oregon, NIH RO1 CA080964, and the Walter-Schulz-Foundation, Munich, Germany.

References

1. Kantoff PW et al (2010) Sipuleucel-T immunotherapy for castration-resistant prostate cancer. N Engl J Med 363:411–422
2. Higano CS et al (2009) Integrated data from 2 randomized, double-blind, placebo-controlled phase 3 trials of active cellular immunotherapy with sipuleucel-T in advanced prostate cancer. Cancer 115:3670–3679
3. Stein WD et al (2011) Tumor regression and growth rates determined in five intramural NCI prostate cancer trials: the growth rate constant as an indicator of therapeutic efficacy. Clin Cancer Res 17:907–917
4. Wolchok JD et al (2009) Guidelines for the evaluation of immune therapy activity in solid tumors: immune-related response criteria. Clin Cancer Res 15:7412–7420
5. Hoos A et al (2010) Improved endpoints for cancer immunotherapy trials. J Natl Cancer Inst 102:1388–1397
6. Guidance for industry: Clinical considerations for therapeutic cancer vaccines (2011) US Department of Health and Human Services, Food and Drug Administration, Center for Biologics Evaluation and Research. http://www.fda.gov/biologicsbloodvaccines/guidancecomplianceregulatoryinformation
7. Schuster SJ et al (2011) Vaccination with patient-specific tumor-derived antigen in first remission improves disease-free survival in follicular lymphoma. J Clin Oncol 29:2787–2794
8. Schwartzentruber DJ et al (2011) Gp100 peptide vaccine and interleukin-2 in patients with advanced melanoma. N Engl J Med 364:2119–2127
9. Sosman JA et al (2008) Three phase II cytokine working group trials of gp100 (210 M) peptide plus high-dose interleukin-2 in patients with HLA-A2-positive advanced melanoma. J Clin Oncol 26:2292–2298
10. Rosenberg SA et al (1998) Durability of complete responses in patients with metastatic cancer treated with high-dose interleukin-2:

identification of the antigens mediating response. Ann Surg 228:307–319
11. Tyagi P, Mirakhur B (2009) MAGRIT: the largest-ever phase III lung cancer trial aims to establish a novel tumor-specific approach to therapy. Clin Lung Cancer 10:371–374
12. Hodge JW et al (2012) The tipping point for combination therapy: cancer vaccines with radiation, chemotherapy, or targeted small molecule inhibitors. Semin Oncol 39: 323–339
13. Ferrer IR et al (2011) Paradoxical aspects of rapamycin immunobiology in transplantation. Am J Transplant 11:654–659
14. Laheru D et al (2008) Allogeneic granulocyte macrophage colony-stimulating factor-secreting tumor immunotherapy alone or in sequence with cyclophosphamide for metastatic pancreatic cancer: a pilot study of safety, feasibility, and immune activation. Clin Cancer Res 14:1455–1463
15. Walter S et al (2012) Multipeptide immune response to cancer vaccine IMA901 after single-dose cyclophosphamide associates with longer patient survival. Nat Med 18(8): 1254–1261
16. Disis ML (2011) Immunologic biomarkers as correlates of clinical response to cancer immunotherapy. Cancer Immunol Immunother 60:433–442
17. Gajewski TF et al (2010) Gene signature in melanoma associated with clinical activity: a potential clue to unlock cancer immunotherapy. Cancer J 16:399–403
18. Mlecnik B et al (2011) Histopathologic-based prognostic factors of colorectal cancers are associated with the state of the local immune reaction. J Clin Oncol 29:610–618
19. Fridman WH et al (2012) The immune contexture in human tumours: impact on clinical outcome. Nat Rev Cancer 12:298–306
20. Butterfield LH et al (2011) Recommendations from the iSBTc-SITC/FDA/NCI workshop on immunotherapy biomarkers. Clin Cancer Res 17:3064–3076
21. Galon J et al (2012) The immune score as a new possible approach for the classification of cancer. J Transl Med 10:1

INDEX

Michael J.P. Lawman and Patricia D. Lawman (eds.), *Cancer Vaccines: Methods and Protocols*, Methods in Molecular Biology, vol. 1139, DOI 10.1007/978-1-4939-0345-0,

Lightning Source UK Ltd.
Milton Keynes UK
UKOW07n1518140515

251441UK00004B/34/P

9 781493 903443